The Journal of Infectious Diseases

Published by the John McCormick Institute for Infectious Diseases

EDITED BY

LUDVIG HEKTOEN AND EDWIN O. JORDAN

IN CONJUNCTION WITH

FRANK BILLINGS F. G. NOVY

H. GIDEON WELLS KARL F. MEYER

Volume 30

1922

Chicago, 1922

Composed and Printed by
American Medical Association Press
Chicago, Illinois, U. S. A.

THE STUDY OF COLONY FORMATION IN DEEP AGAR *

STUDIES ON PATHOGENIC ANAEROBES VI

Hilda Hempl Heller

From the George Williams Hooper Foundatiin for Medical Research, University of California Medical School, San Francisco

Under uniform conditions living creatures of the same species vary in shape only within comparatively narrow limits. Morphology is, in the case of the majority of living things, the character that is the most easily observable, and for this reason it has been used as a basis for the classification of all forms of life. Among the bacteria such use of morphologic criteria for systematic purposes is frequently avoided because the form of these organisms is exceedingly simple and because the bacteria are highly specialized, not as to shape but as to the enzymes with which they split the substances surrounding them. Higher plants are classified not according to the shape of their stems and leaves, but according to that of their reproductive organs. For purposes of bacterial classification, we may well let chemical characters take the place of those morphologic ones that the bacteria do not possess. A chemical classification will then serve to build a skeleton structure which will group and divide the bacteria into genera [1] that are comparable with those of the higher plants. The trend followed in dividing the bacteria has usually been to employ morphologic characters for the making of major divisions and chemical ones for the finer differentiations. For many reasons pointed out in a former paper [2] morphologic criteria fail to furnish a means for logically subdividing the major group of anaerobic rods. Chief among these are the facts that most morphologic characters appear in various groups, that there is a general overlapping of such characters and that there is a lack of correspondence between chemical and morphologic differ-

Received for publication, July 5, 1921.

* The present paper is intended as an introduction to others in which the colony formation of anaerobic strains will be discussed.

1 Heller, H. H.: J. Bacteriol., 1922, 7 (Jan.).

2 Ibid., 1921, 6, p. 521.

ences. It is the purpose now to indicate the exploitation of a so-called morphologic character for purposes of finer differentiation.

Anaerobic bacilli form within a solid nutrient agar mass colonies of very different shapes, but many types are constant in their behavior if the conditions surrounding the organisms are uniform. This constancy is such that if a strain of anaerobic bacilli be inoculated, on various occasions, from a culture of the same age grown on a similar medium, always onto the same variety of deep agar, and if it be incubated for the same period at an identical temperature, it will produce colonies that are enough alike to furnish the systematist with an excellent means for the comparison and identification of cultures. This constancy is such that the slight variations in conditions that occur when technic is faithfully imitated by conscientious workers in different laboratories are not sufficient seriously to impair the use of deep colonies for systematic purposes in certain of the anaerobic groups when simple mediums are employed. The colonies are similar enough to warrant their comparison to the leaves and stems of higher plants. The same overlapping of characters of vegetative portions appears among higher plants as among bacterial colonies. Thus some senecios look more like cacti than they do like other senecios; the foliage of a hakea resembles that of some accacias more than that of other hakeas; remarkable resemblances of foliage occur among members of the genera Juniperus, Cupressus and Chamycyparis. But sort out the senecios and the hakeas on the basis of the morphology of their reproductive organs, then their leaves and stems differentiate their species from each other; sort out the bifermentans from the Welch bacilli and the vibrion septique from the sporogenes on the basis of their chemical reactions, and the morphology of their colonies will serve to group strains that have thus been sorted into genera into smaller groups which may or may not be considered as species, depending on the constancy of colony formation in those genera. The only great difference in such a comparison between the higher plants and the bacteria is that the latter, immersed in gels containing liquids of widely different composition, are far more subject to such variation as is determined by external conditions than are the former.

Surface colonies of aerobic organisms have been used for systematic purposes and for the study of mutations for many years. Such colonies are frequently characteristic in shape, but colony characters other than form, such as pigment formation and opacity, have been frequently used for these types of investigation. The aerobe surface colony is much more characteristic and uniform in contour than the anaerobe surface colony. The former is automatically limited in size because grown in the dry air of the incubator, while the latter is subject to such different moisture and gas conditions that though specifically fairly characteristic, it is not very uniform in behavior. Anaerobic surface colonies have been described in most detail by McIntosh,[3] Henry,[4] Adamson [5] and Zeissler.[6] The latter has used colonies on glucose blood agar as a basis for the subdivision of the vibrion septique group; [7] his method has the advantage of showing hemolysis. In the depths of an agar medium gas and moisture conditions are so controlled that their disturbing effects are eliminated, and colonies growing therein are more uniform in behavior, and their study permits much more accurate determination than does that of surface growths.[8] Deep colonies have been figured most extensively by von Hibler [9] and by Weinberg and Seguin.[10]

Illustration of the way in which certain of the anaerobic genera may be subdivided by colony determination will be given in subsequent papers. A collection of colony photographs of organisms that do not belong in the groups to be later discussed is included in the present paper (plates 1-5).

The shape of a bacterial colony is not to be thought of as a matter of chance nor, on the other hand, is it in any degree so dependent on the inherent germ plasm as are the shape and histologic arrangement of the tissues of the higher plants. It is dependent, first, on the moisture content of the medium, secondly, on the texture of the colloid mass as determined by the rapidity of cooling, thirdly on the ability of the organism to multiply in the medium, and fourthly on the motility of the organism in the medium. Intrinsically characteristic generic or specific colony form, if it exists, is subordinate to these four factors. All the chemical phenomena that are observable in bacterial growth in liquid medium must be thought of as contributing to shape the colony in a solid medium. Pabulum—split proteins, sugars and vitamins;

[3] Med. Research Committee, Special Report 12, 1917.
[4] J. Path. & Bacteriol., 1917, 21, p. 344.
[5] Ibid., 1919, 22, p. 345.
[6] Ztschr. f. Infektionskr. d. Haustiere, 1920, 21, p. 1.
[7] Heller, H. H.: J. Infect. Dis., 1921, 27, p. 385. Reprints, Hooper Foundation, 1921, 6.
[8] Heller, H. H.: J. Bacteriol., 1921, 6, p. 521.
[9] Ueber die pathog. Anaeroben, 1908.
[10] La gangrène gazeuse, 1918.

lag; initial reaction, buffers, acid inhibition, neutralization by alkaline end-products. Temperature, acid, and autointoxication have their effect on motility as well as on growth.

Therefore the acquisition by an individual bacillus of the ability to split and assimilate a nutritive element present in a substratum will make itself known by an increase in the size of the colony formed by the mutating bacillus. Likewise the loss of a power involved in the assimilation of nutriment from a medium will cause the formation of smaller colonies in that medium. Other mutations involving the formation of autointoxication products, the motility, or even the rate of disintegration of bacillary bodies, will also affect the size or transparency of the colonies.

Colony shape may then be used in the case of anaerobic bacilli as a technical means of spotting mutations. Mutating forms may then be isolated, studied on the medium in which they appeared, and suitable experiments may then be arranged to demonstrate, if possible, what was the metabolic cause of the change in colony form.

As emphasized before,[2] the mutations of anaerobes, though little studied, cannot be essentially different from those of other living things. Careful work makes it seem highly improbable that such mutations ever involve many characteristics at once. The anaerobic bacilli are relatively stable types. A Welch bacillus cannot be changed into an amylobacter, nor a blackleg bacillus into a Welch bacillus or sporogenes bacillus or aerobic bacillus. On the other hand, to claim that mutations do not occur among these organisms would be to state that they lack one of the best recognized attributes of living matter. So far as we know, they have originated by descent and not by spontaneous generation—if not by mutation, then how? Apparently mutation, such as may be recognized by a change in colony form, occurs far more frequently in some groups of anaerobic organisms than in others. In such groups colony form is not available for systematic purposes.

A colony differing from its neighbors, when fished onto a new series of agar tubes, may or may not give new colonies like itself. For the observation of such colonies a control series of the normal type present should always be inoculated, and the appearance of the colonies should be noted at several different time intervals. Occasionally two colonies will be found in a culture derived from a single colony, whose descendants pass through the same morphologic history, but do so at consistently different speeds. There is, then, a difference between these strains, and the new form may be accepted as a mutant of the other. On the other hand, one may often fish two colonies of different appearance from a tube containing a considerable number of colonies, and their offspring may be all alike or show similar variations that are clearly not mutations. One more set of dilution tubes will usually be sufficient to settle the question whether a mixture of two types is present or whether the differences noted lie within the limits of variation for the species. Some anaerobic strains occasionally show in thickly seeded tubes one or a few colonies several times larger than the others. These are usually constellations of small colonies derived from minute chunks of infected inoculum. When planted on a new series of tubes, the same forms may appear in about the same proportion as before, and repeated selection from such colonies does not increase their number. These large colonies do not breed true and are thus not mutations.

Technical Considerations Involved in the Study of Anaerobic Colonies

Inoculation of material for photographic representation of the colonies hereafter pictured was as follows: Liquid from meat cultures was used for inoculum. In the case of rapidly growing anaerobes one or two day cultures only were employed. In the case of proteolytic organisms a somewhat older culture was occasionally used, but old run out cultures were avoided. Tubes of agar were melted in the water bath and were then tapped and shaken sharply and replaced in the water bath for a few minutes and then shaken again. This method removes the air without soaking the plugs with steam. The tubes were then cooled to 42 C., and the first was inoculated with a small loopful of culture and shaken; the second was usually inoculated from the first with the amount of agar that would fill the capillary of a large bore Pasteur pipet; the pipet was then well flamed, and the third or third and fourth tubes were inoculated with somewhere between 0.25 and 0.75 c c of material from the second tube. Colonies were well distributed by rolling and tipping. The tubes were allowed to cool in air at room temperature.

Twenty-four hours was chosen as the standard time for incubation unless there was a reason for choosing another period. Thus blackleg colonies are invisible at 24 hours, as are those of some strains of tetanus. For some organisms a comparatively early stage is characteristic and for others a later stage is more so.

Preparation of colonies for photographing is carried out as follows: The tube containing colonies to be photographed is held with the mouth slanting toward an open Petri dish, and an open large bore Pasteur pipet bent at a right angle is inserted along one side to the bottom. This pipet is then removed and the agar bdown out of it, and it is then reinserted and through it the column of agar in the culture tube is blown out into the Petri dish. A safety razor blade may be used to section the medium, usually at right angles, and slices about 2 mm. thick are placed on a slide with a drop of water and covered with a small coverslip. These are examined directly on the ground glass of the camera.

Photographic Technic: The microscope and camera are arranged on the plan designed by Dr. L. B. Wilson,[11] the lens of the camera being removed. The source of illumination for most of the pictures was a Spencer light placed under the stage of the instrument. Mirror and condenser were removed. A ground glass disk such as accompanies Leitz microscopes was placed on the stage under the slide. For later work a nitrogen light[12] and a mirror without condenser have been employed. The ocular used in all cases has been a Zeiss projection ocular No. 4, and two objectives have been employed, Zeiss No. A_2 arranged to give on the ground glass of the camera a magnification of 15 diameters, and a Leitz No. 3 which gives an enlargement of 50 diameters. For work in which a wide range of lighting conditions must be recorded, such as one finds in general colony work, Seed's "Non-halation-L-Ortho" plate has been found superior, and Seed's "26" plate is also excellent. These two are fairly rapid and give, apparently, a maximum of detail in contour and in the minute fuzzy halos surrounding many colonies. For representation of the interior structure of smooth-contoured colonies, Dr. K. F. Meyer tells me that he finds "Process" plates excellent. Their range is not sufficient for general work. Seed's "23" plate also gives too much contrast for most purposes. Orthonon plates were found to be too thin. All the exposed plates were developed in a tank according to the directions accompanying them. It is well to choose a type of emulsion that may always be had and to use that type constantly for comparative work. Regular glossy Velox paper was used for the prints.

All conditions regarding age of colonies and age of inoculum, medium, incubation temperature and photography, are made as uniform as possible and are carefully recorded.

Contamination.—For ordinary laboratory purposes it is sufficient for the investigator of anaerobes to inoculate his cultures in a small quiet room where no other people are moving about. For a worker with considerable practice and skill contaminations occur rarely under such conditions, at least in an atmosphere that contains little dust. It is hopeless to try to do accurate work in a busy room.

Crowding.—The number of colonies present in a tube has a striking effect not only on the size but also on the shape of the colonies in the tube. Many types of colonies originate as lenticular masses and then send out protuberances or downy strands. If colonies with such a habit are abundant, they pass through the various morphologic phases in a shorter period of time than if they are few, and different colonies in the tube pass through their development at different speeds, so that from a single tube with many colonies the entire history of colony

[11] Spencer photomicrographic outfit 4336B.

[12] Bausch and Lomb adjustable microscope lamp No. 1784.

formation may be traced. This point is illustrated by the series of photographs showing the process of colony formation of a *Rivoltillus*[1] (vibrion septique) strain (Plate 6). Where colonies are numerous they are, of course, smaller than where they are few. For these two reasons therefore, types should always be chosen from tubes with so few colonies that they do not interfere with each other. A striking case of difference not only in form of the colony but in its texture is shown by the series of photographs of colonies of an unidentified anaerobic organism (Plate 7). To designate the number of colonies present in a tube, I have usually employed the following rough scale:

Sole colony	1
Colonies few	1— 20
Colonies not numerous	20— 60
Colonies moderately abundant	60—400
Photographed for history of development	
Colonies, abundant	over 400
Rarely photographed	

Permeating Growth.—The more rapidly proliferating species of anaerobes, motile and nonmotile, frequently leave their colonies and multiply in the agar gel as though it were a broth.[8] When this happens the colonies abruptly stop growing. Tubes containing this permeating growth may be readily identified by holding them to the light with a control. When there is more than a suspicion of this phenomenon the colonies should not be used for systematic measurements unless the permeation of the medium is a constant character of the strain. Plate 8 shows the effect of permeating growth on the size of the colonies. Colonies in agar cooled rapidly in water or ice water are more sharply delimited than those in agar that is cooled at room temperature. Uniform procedure should be adopted with regard to cooling the agar, or if the procedure be varied to diminish permeating growth note should be made of the fact.

Uniform Conditions.—An instance may be given of the difficulties encountered by the student desirous of identifying an anaerobic strain. No worker has time to duplicate the mediums and technic of von Hibler,[9] who gives excellent photographs of colonies in his book. Plate 2 of his book may be taken as an example. Among the mediums used for the growth of the colonies represented on this page are glucose cat-meat agar, spleen-broth agar, sodium formate spleen-broth agar, rabbit-meat agar, guinea-pig-meat agar, and for illustrations on other plates fish-meat agar and various other queer concoctions have been employed. Far better be it to give the conditions of growth as von Hibler does than not to give them at all. One appreciates his effort to study the organisms under different conditions, but he made his work hopeless to follow. He gives us a single page with 4 pictures of the morphology of 3 species of bacteria in the animal body. Then come 12 photographs of deep colonies and two of surface colonies of 8 species of organisms. These are photographed at 10 different ages ranging from 10 hours to 3 days, the organisms have grown on 9 different mediums from 4 or more different kinds of animals (it is to be hoped that he never confused his mediums) represented in 7 different enlargements. The anaerobist working on bibliography is surely a creature to be pitied, and is not to be blamed for failing to follow the work of others conscientiously and thoroughly. Von Hibler is also to be criticized for terming colonies formed on one kind of medium "typical" and on another kind "atypical."

Photographs of colonies should always be accompanied by the name of the strain that gave rise to them. The beautiful lithographs of oedematiens colonies shown by Weinberg and Seguin [10] represent colonies very different in aspect, but there is no indication which forms are characteristic for the various strains that another worker might consider to belong to distinct species.

One photograph is usually insufficient to give a fair idea of the possible variations of a strain. Several colonies should be depicted, the number depending on the limits of variation in the strain.

The medium chosen should be one on which as many species as possible will grow, but a universally suitable one is probably not to be hoped for. Liver agar has been found eminently satisfactory for most types of anaerobes but affords too fertile a substratum for some. It was excellent for producing a suitable colony formation with blackleg, oedematiens, tetanus and botulinus organisms. Vibrion septique strains grew too rapidly in it so that at 24 hours colonies descended from spores were smaller than those descended from vegetative rods; at 48 hours, they were uniform in size but permeating growth was so frequent that many tubes had to be discarded, and the growth was so luxuriant that the colonies of different strains could not be so nicely grouped as in the case of other genera. A search should be made in such cases for a less nutrient substratum or for a firmer medium. But there are indications that liver agar is so complex a medium that it furnishes too much chance for mutations to affect the shape of the colonies, and simpler mediums may have to be adopted. Agar more than a month old should not be used for colony photographs as it is too dry. For most types of anaerobes sufficiently uniform colonies may be secured on medium from 1 to 30 days old. Blackleg strains will not grow after the medium is from 6 to 10 days old. Agar that is too fresh or that contains too much moisture will also give misleading results (Plate 7). Such agar may be incubated to dry it out before using.

Liver Agar.—This is made up of beef liver 1 part, distilled water 4 parts. Infuse over night in the refrigerator, bring to a boil, strain through cheesecloth, add 1½% Difco peptone, 0.5% salt and 2% agar. Melt the agar, titrate and adjust to P_H 7.2, cool to 60 degrees, add white of egg and serum; autoclave for one hour, titrate again and adjust to P_H 7.2; filter through cotton, tube, and sterilize in the autoclave.

CONCLUSIONS

Under constant conditions members of a pure strain (biotype) of anaerobic bacteria make deep colonies that differ from each other scarcely more than do the vegetative portions of individuals of a species of higher plants.

It is found that a collection of anaerobic bacilli that correspond in all ordinary cultural characteristics may be broken up into groups of strains on the basis of colony formation in deep agar. These groups are, in some genera, when the medium employed is simple, to be termed "species," in others not. The observation of colonies may thus be of great value to the systematist.

The shape of a colony in an agar medium depends primarily on the reproductive power of the organism and its motility in that medium. The reproductive power depends on its enzymes and metabolic activities. Therefore, any mutation involving the metabolic activities of the organism on a given medium may demonstrate its occurrence by causing a change in the colony morphology of the mutating organisms in the strain. Colony formation in deep agar is, then, a phenomenon whose study will be most closely observed by the student of mutation.

The colony shape must thus be thought of as a chemical character as well as a morphologic one, and the possibilities of its exploitation on specially prepared mediums to test the nature of mutations are infinite.

Technical considerations and various pitfalls are discussed: preparation of colonies and their photography, contamination, crowding, permeating growth, uniform conditions and choice of medium.

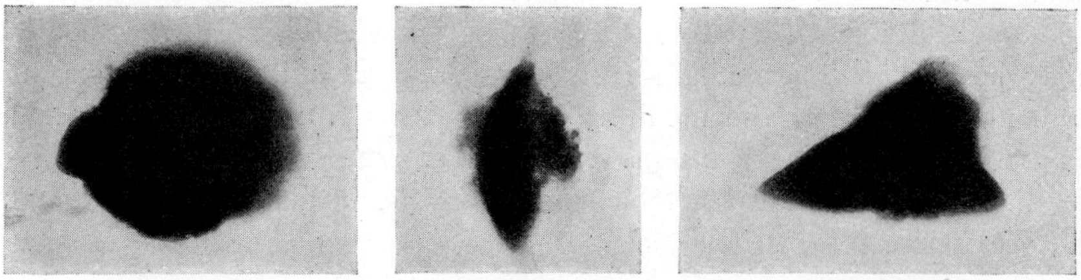

Bacillus 12 of McIntosh, type strain. Colonies not numerous; × 50.

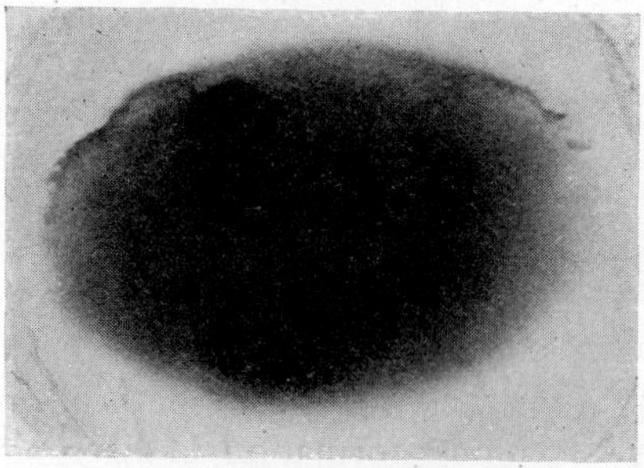

An unidentified mildly proteolytic organism isolated from stools of infants by Miss J. Easton. Colonies few; × 50.

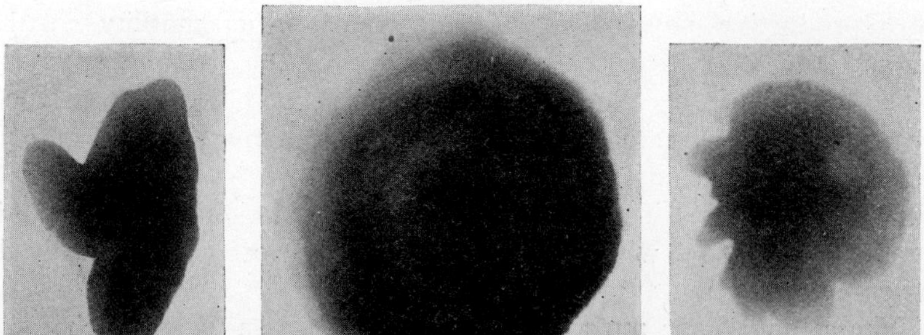

Fig. 1.—Lenticular and modified lenticular types. Except where otherwise noted, the colonies photographed in this series were grown on beef liver peptone agar for 24 hours at 37 degrees. The nomenclature employed is explained in another paper.[1]

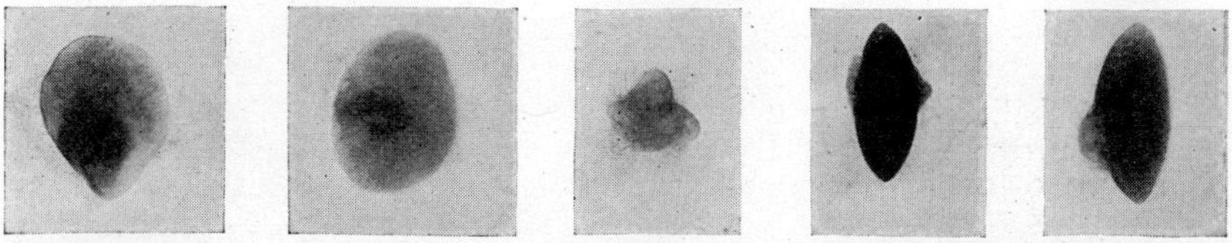

Putrificus sp.; strain IOR from septic wound. This corresponds more nearly to Bienstock's description of B. putrificus than any other strain in the collection. Colonies moderately abundant; × 50.

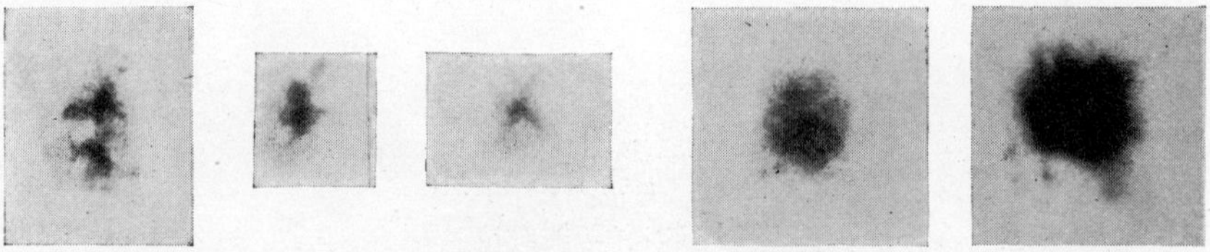

Many colonies present, 18 hours. Few colonies present, 24 hours.
Weinbergillus histolyticus, type strain, HW; × 50.

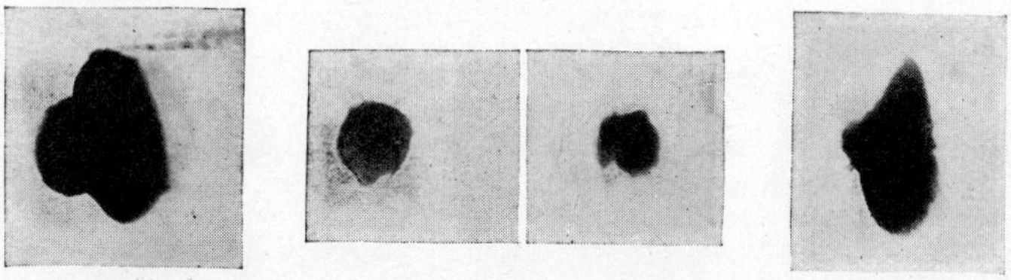

Seguinillus aerofoetidus, type strain, AW. Colonies few; × 15.

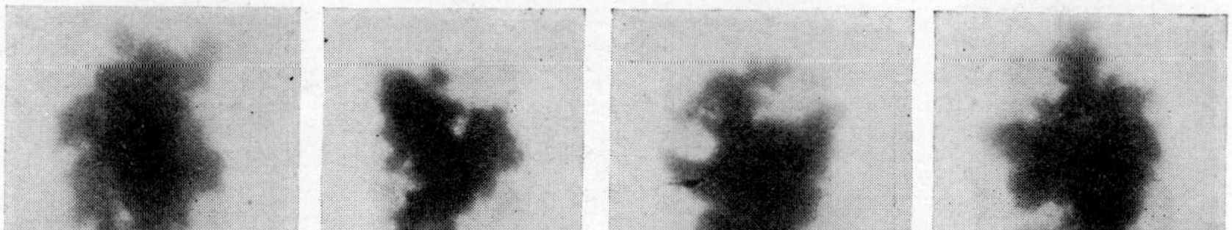

Vallorillus fallax, type strain, FW. Colonies few, 4 days old. Note diffuseness of outline due to permeating growth; × 50.

Fig. 2.—Colony forms.

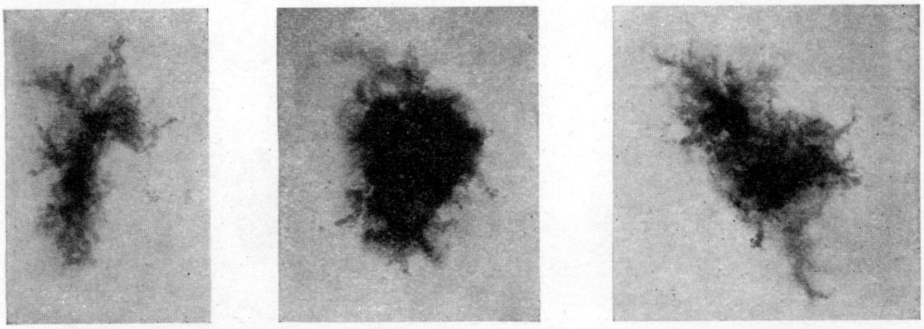

Martellillus proteolyticus; type strain, F, from septic wound, man. Colonies few; × 50.

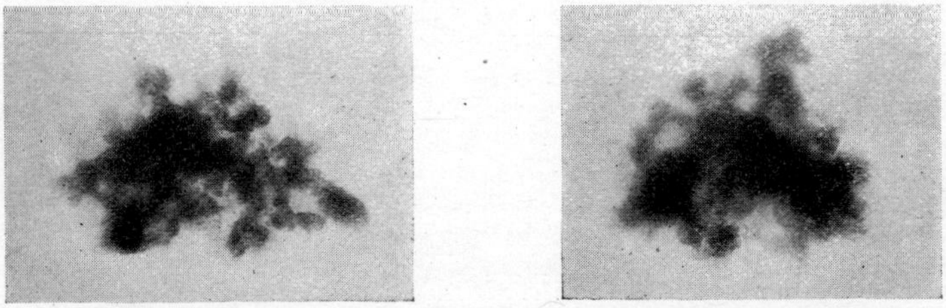

Martellillus sp. Strain JC, from Bradsot material. Conditions as above.

THE BIFERMENTANS TYPE

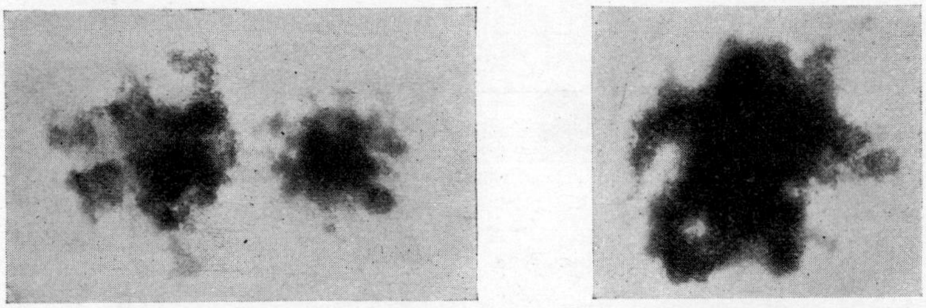

Eighteen hours, colonies few.

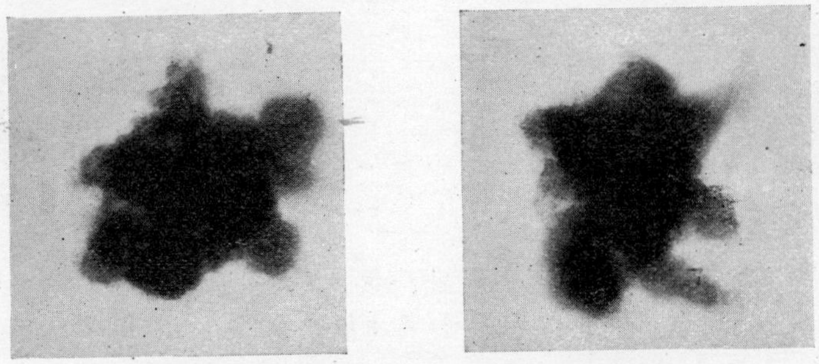

Twenty-four hours, colonies moderately abundant.
Robertsonillus primus. Type strain, L, from septic wound, man; × 50.

Fig. 3.—Colony forms.

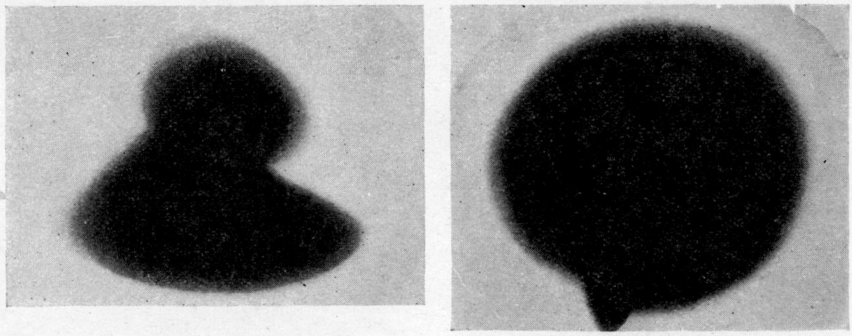

Strain WM; few colonies.

Strain WAT; few colonies.

Welchillus (B. Welchii) colonies; × 50. Note dulness of outline due to permeating growth.

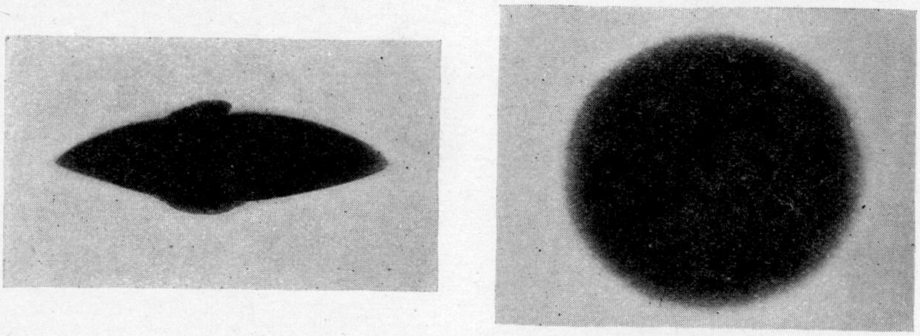

Strain P 11; isolation of Robertson; few colonies.

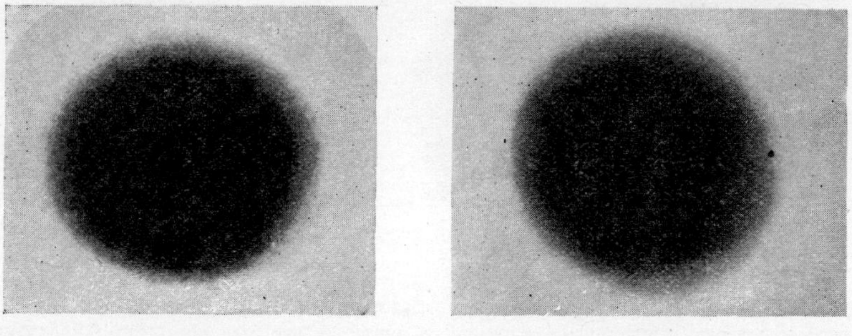

Strain P 7; isolation of Robertson; few colonies. Henrillus (B. tertius) colonies; × 50.

Fig. 4.—Nonmotile organisms.

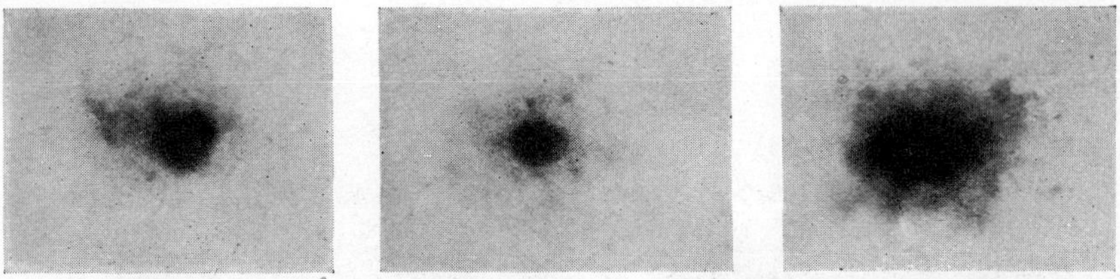

Eighteen hours old, colonies not numerous; × 50.

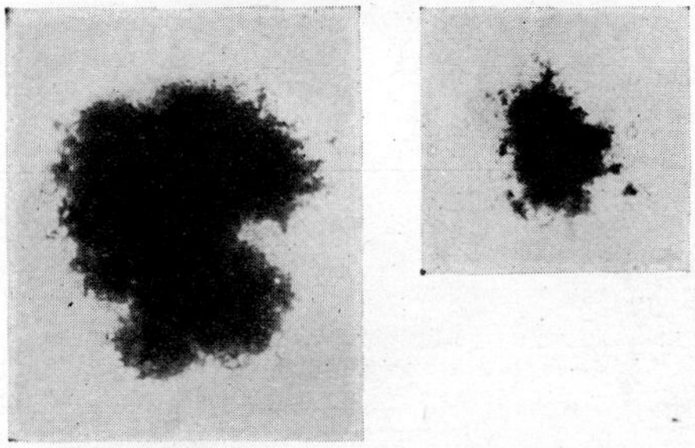

Two days old, not numerous; × 15. Note difference in size of colonies.

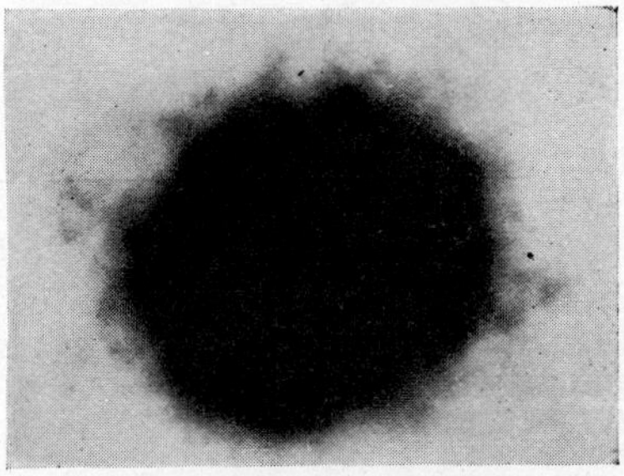

Veal infusion agar; eighteen hours; × 50.

Metchnikovillus sporogenes; Strain MR; isolation of Robertson.

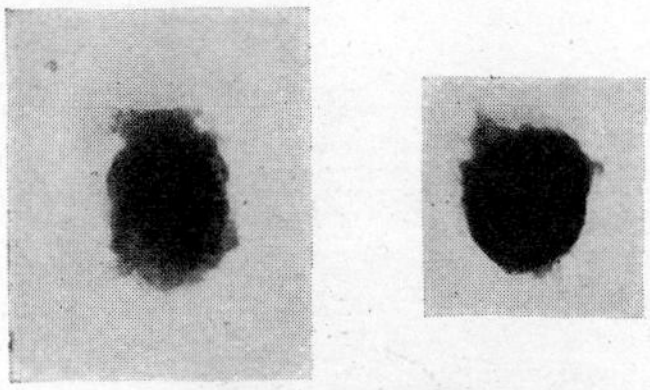

Eighteen hours; × 50.

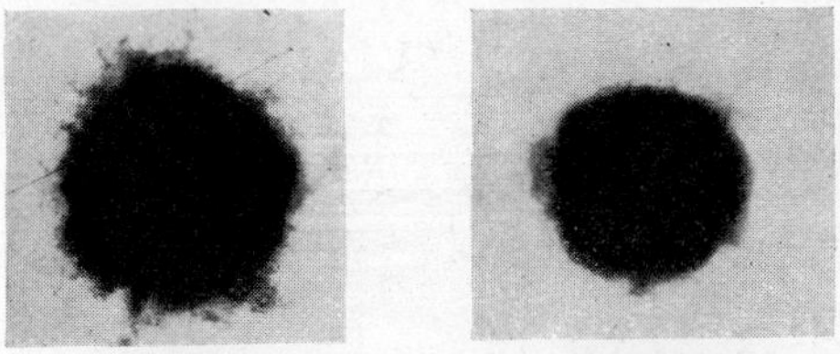

Eighteen hours, veal infusion agar.

Metchnikovillus parasporogenes McIntosh; strain R 60.

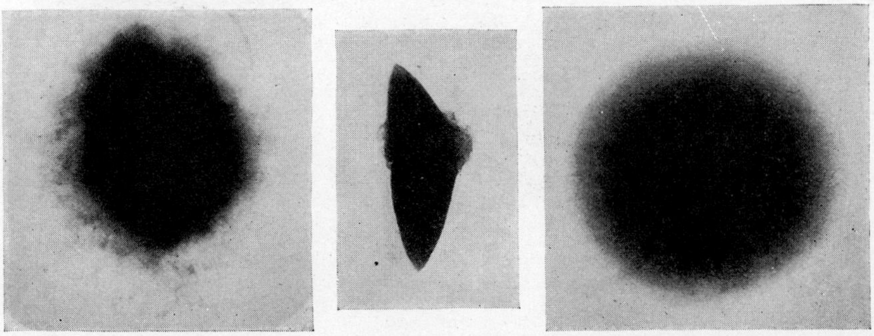

A culture of "Malignant oedema bacillus" from Germany resolved itself into two species, a typical sporogenes strain (at the left) and a nonmotile less strongly proteolytic organism (at the right).

Fig. 5.—Highly motile organisms.

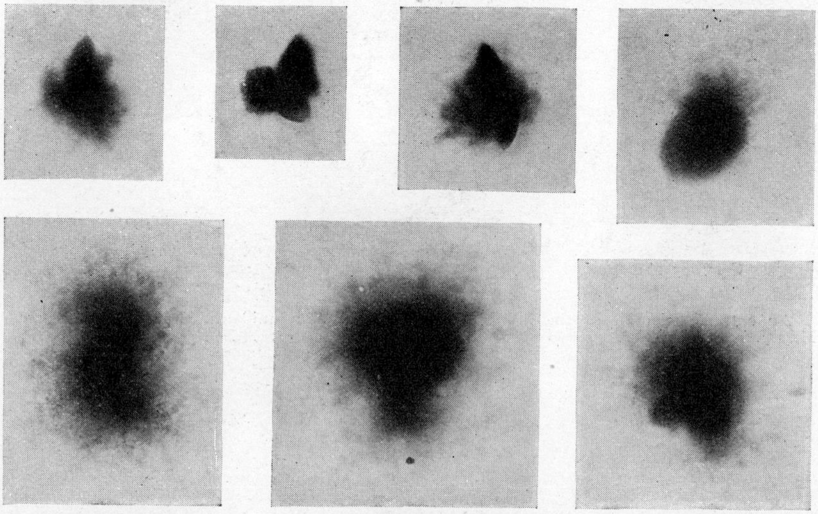

Colonies moderately abundant.

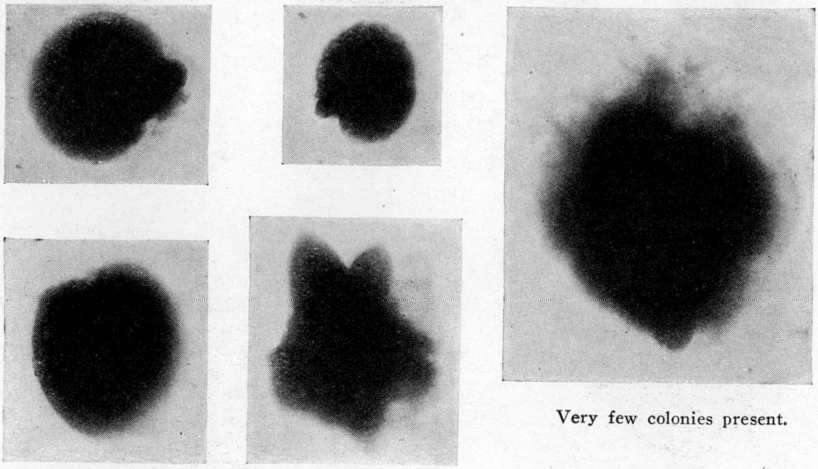

Very few colonies present.

Fig. 6.—The development of a vibrion septique colony. Vibrion septique strain VS that retains its lenticular form unusually long (24 hours); × 50. The influence of crowding is well shown. The second group of colonies developed in a tube inoculated from the first. A greater dilution of inoculum was the only difference in the conditions in the two tubes.

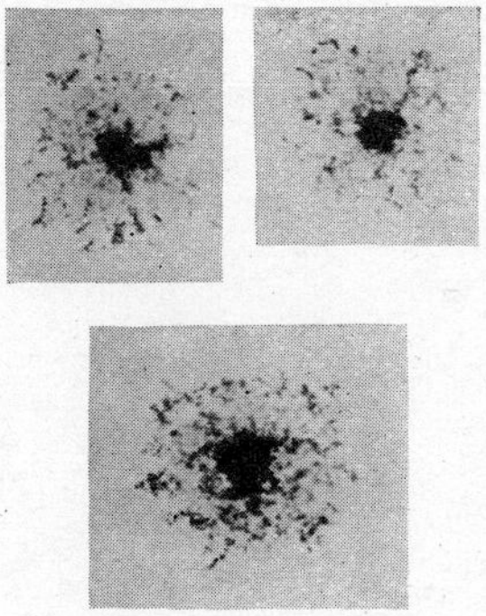

Colonies abundant.

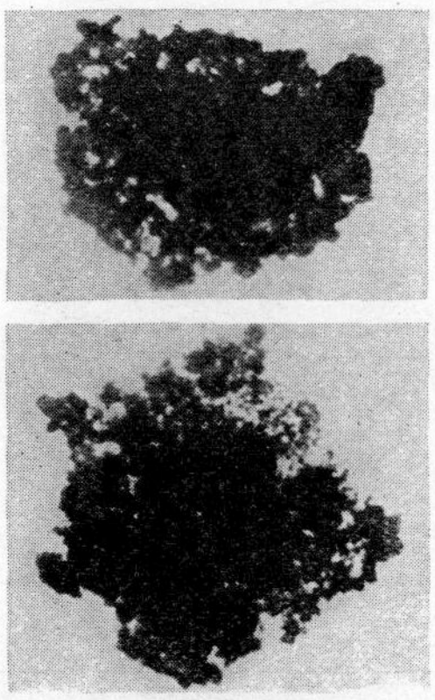

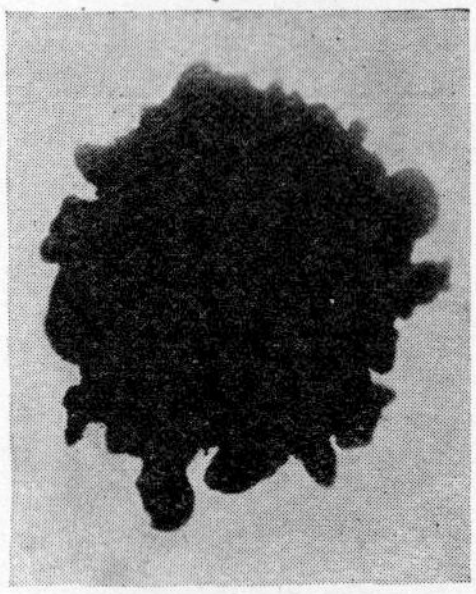

Above, colonies few. Left, colonies not so numerous.

An extreme example of the influence of crowding. An unidentified organism isolated by Miss J. Easton. Three successive dilutions of a pure culture; × 50.

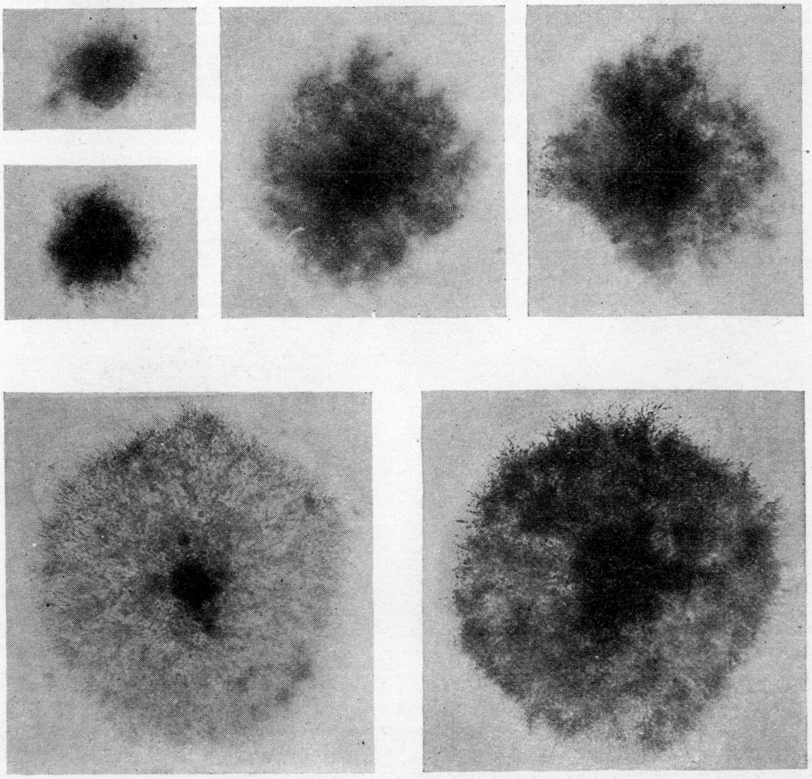

An instance of the influence of moisture in the agar on colony formation. Tetanus strain T 087, grown under otherwise identical conditions in "2%" agar that was (above left) old and dry (above right), fresh, and (below) unusually soft.

Fig. 7.—Influence of crowding and of moisture.

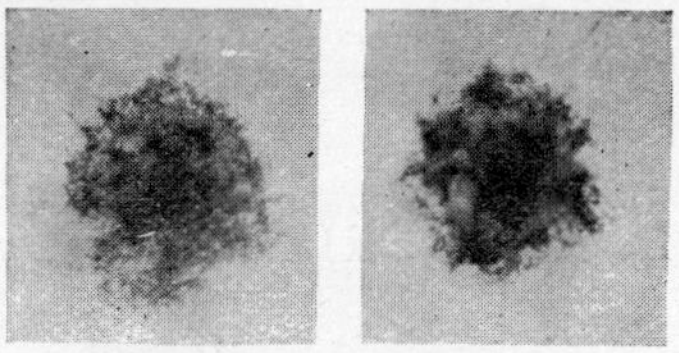

Strain HV; 7 colonies; permeating growth +.

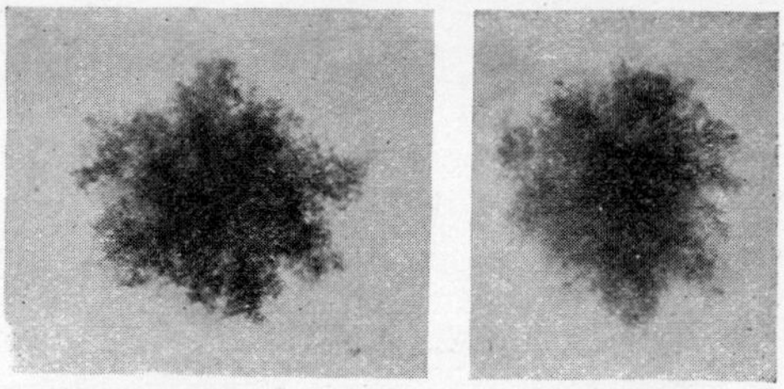

Eight colonies; permeating growth —.

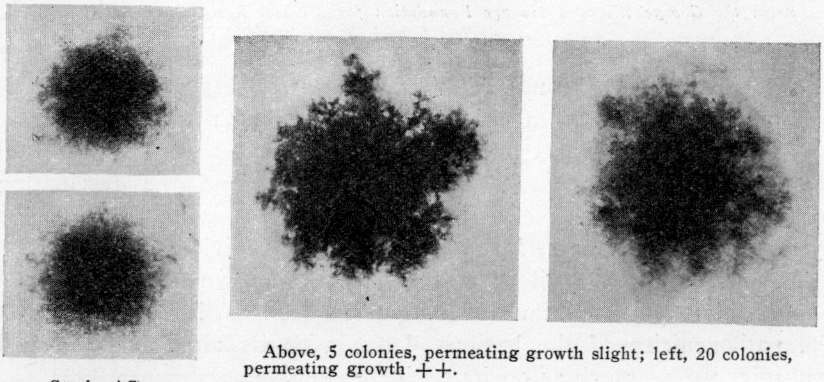

Above, 5 colonies, permeating growth slight; left, 20 colonies, permeating growth ++.

Strain AS

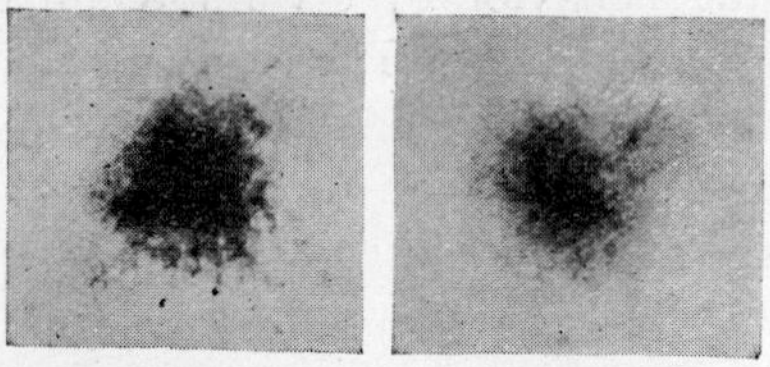

Strain BN; 3 colonies; permeating growth slight.

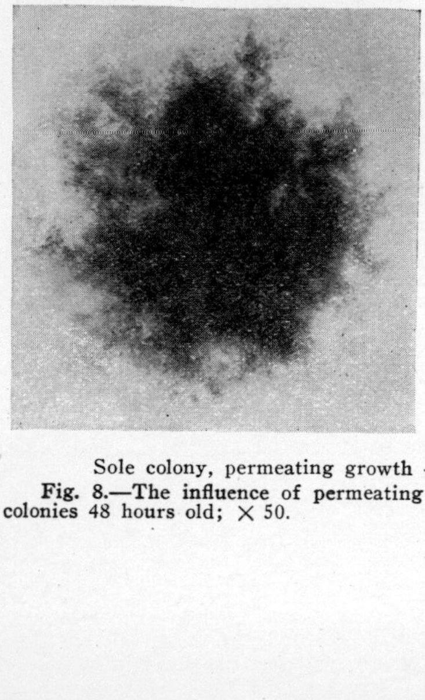

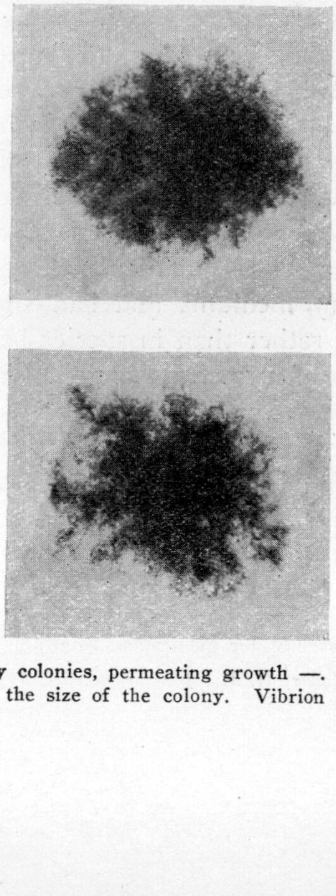

Sole colony, permeating growth —. Twenty colonies, permeating growth —.

Fig. 8.—The influence of permeating growth on the size of the colony. Vibrion septique colonies 48 hours old; × 50.

NOTES ON THE GENUS NICOLAIERILLUS (B. TETANI)

STUDIES ON PATHOGENIC ANAEROBES VII

HILDA HEMPL HELLER

From the George Williams Hooper Foundation for Medical Research, University of California Medical School, San Francisco

As one searches through the literature on the tetanus bacillus he is forcibly struck by its meagerness. The biology of the organism itself has been largely neglected because of the interest centering around the powerful toxin that it produces, and around the fascinating mechanism governing the distribution of the toxin in the nervous system. In the history of few diseases have individual case reports been so frequently detailed; in few diseases known to be infectious has the biology of the causative organism been so little studied. Yet the pathogenicity of the bacillus depends on its ability to live and multiply just as much as on its toxin production.

This paper gives a few notes on the behavior of certain tetanus strains that have found their way to this laboratory. The study of the tetanus organisms was not undertaken as other than a side line during the investigation of tissue invading pathogens. These notes make no pretense of being in any way exhaustive, and are intended simply to serve as an introduction to several papers by myself and other workers who have studied the same strains.

The anaerobic bacilli that cause tetanus have long been referred to one species under the name Bacillus tetani. In a recent classification [1] it was pointed out that such anaerobic bacilli as behaved similarly on ordinary mediums and had similar morphology should be placed in genera rather than in species because in such groups it is usually possible to demonstrate common types that differ consistently in minor characters and correspond to the general taxonomist's idea of species. Systematic bacteriology is so little developed that it is at present very difficult to find characters that are acceptable for the differentiation of strains. Especially is this true in the groups of anaerobic rods. One finds that a type of character that is apparently consistent in one genus is subject to variation in another and for each group various

Received for publication, Aug. 18, 1921.

[1] Heller, H. H.: Jour. Bacteriol., 1921, 6, p. 521.

characters must be studied before a logical classification can be formulated. Such study cannot be attempted for many genera by any one investigator. Certain points of interest bearing on the classification of the tetanus bacilli are deserving of publication.

The genus Nicolaierillus was defined [2] as follows:

"Putrificoideae that in meat medium produce gas and various color changes: yellowish, pink, grey or mauve, dependent on the medium; the particles of meat are gradually suffused with a black pigment, and bleach at the top. The meat is softened but the particles do not greatly diminish in size. Do not attack sugars. Gram-negative (weak methyl violet) rods that form terminal spherical spores. Colonies in deep agar diverse. Common in soil, found in horse feces, may multiply in wounds, but do not normally invade tissue. Produce a characteristic neuro-toxin."

The known strains referable to this genus are probably all toxigenic because it is the toxigenic phenomenon that usually leads to their isolation. Other anaerobes of similar morphology have been isolated; they are nontoxigenic and are culturally referable to other genera. The organisms producing the neurotoxin that causes clinical tetanus are apparently all referable to the genus Nicolaierillus. Nevertheless, it is probably unwise to restrict the generic definition to such strains as are toxigenic; many times difficulty is experienced in obtaining toxin from known toxigenic strains, and the nature of toxin and the process of toxin formation are too little understood for us to use the production of a poison as a critical generic character.

The Tetanus Committee, under the chairmanship of Sir David Bruce, determined, in 1916, to investigate the cause of the occurrence of cases of tetanus that proved refractory to tetanus antitoxin. Tulloch undertook a serologic investigation of the strains of B. tetani obtainable from laboratories and isolable from septic wounds. In three reports [3] he published his results. He succeeded in demonstrating that the agglutination reaction separated the group into four distinct types. The toxins produced by these types were apparently identical. Agressins were produced that were relatively specific to each type and were apparently unfiltrable or highly labile.

COLONY FORMATION OF NICOLAIERILLUS STRAINS—MUTATION

A search for descriptions of tetanus colonies in deep agar is not very illuminating. Kitasato [4] pictures a deep colony, apparently in

[2] Heller, H. H.: Ibid., 1922, 7, Jan.

[3] J. Roy. Army Med. Corps, 1917, 29, p. 631; Proc. Roy. Soc., B, 1919, 90, p. 145 and p. 529.

[4] Ztschr. f. Hyg. u. Infectionskrankh., 1889, 7, p. 225.

gelatine, that is a very dense symmetrical sphere with encircling fine short radiations. He states that old colonies consist of thread-like masses. Kitasato is credited with being the first to isolate the tetanus bacillus in pure culture. This he probably did, but his critique of the purity of a tetanus culture was not reliable, for the cut accompanying the description of a pure culture shows two typical sporulating rods of undeniable sporogenes type. I have never found any such subterminal oval sporulating organism in a pure tetanus culture.

Apparently the work of Sanchez-Toledo and Veillon [5] was careful. They describe agar colonies, as well as gelatine colonies, finding the agar colonies the less characteristic. The "clouds" are less transparent, and the "needles" less fine. Their pictures of deep gelatine colonies may have been of pure cultures and may not. The cuts (lithographs) leave some room for doubt as to whether a slender oval endsporulating organism may not have been present, but the sporogenes type is apparently absent.

Fränkel and Pfeiffer,[6] in 1892, depicted a dilution shake of tetanus colonies in deep gelatine, and this has been extensively copied in textbooks. Apparently two forms were present. Were the culture one of another anaerobe than the tetanus bacillus, one would be justified in concluding that a mixed culture had been studied. But colonies of a mutated tetanus strain may well have been the subject of the photograph.

Sanfelice [7] (p. 356) states that gelatine colonies are not characteristic, but that the deep agar ones may be distinguished from those of other anaerobes by the fineness of their filaments; he pictures two sorts of deep agar colonies (Figs. 41 and 42).

Righi [8] found a fluffy colony with a dense nucleus characteristic for tetanus organisms, in spite of the serious contamination of his cultures. Grixoni [9] recognized the same type.

Von Hibler's [10] critique of the purity of tetanus cultures was exceedingly at fault. Strain 14 (pl. II, fig. 15) shows only clostridial forms with oval spores, and strain 15 (fig. 16) shows two thirds of the bacilli of sporogenes type and one third of tetanus type. Von Hibler tells us of the behavior of strain 11, that was long grown on glycogen-

[5] Arch. de méd. expér., 1890, 2, p. 709.
[6] Mikrogr. Atlas d. Bakterienkunde, 1890, plates 27-41.
[7] Ztschr. f. Hyg. u. Infektionskrankh., 1893, 14, p. 339.
[8] Riforma med., 1894, 3, p. 651.
[9] Ibid., p. 698.
[10] Ueber di path. Anaeroben, 1908.

containing serum medium. Many bacilli thereafter "lost" the power of liquefying gelatine, but regained it after growing six days in the muscles of a living guinea-pig. Von Hibler makes many interesting statements on atypical colonies, on injuring of the bacterial protoplasm by growing the organisms on unfavorable mediums, etc. Some of his observations may refer to real mutations, but in view of his astounding ignorance of the morphology of tetanus bacilli his notes cannot be considered of value. It is of interest that von Hibler's critique of the purity of non-proteolytic anaerobic cultures was, in the main, fair, while the distinctions between one proteolytic type and another were not duly appreciated. Von Hibler states that deep tetanus colonies in gelatine are spherical with radiations, and a concentric space of liquefaction develops within them. In agar deep colonies are "zerschlissen" or of rough contour. A cut (pl. 3, fig. 6) shows an irregular woolly colony. Atypical ones pictured (pl. 4, figs. 2, 3 and 4) are lenticular with woolly projections.

McIntosh [11] states that "Shake colonies are best obtained in glucose agar; in the medium the colonies in twenty-four hours are relatively large, and at the end of forty-eight hours may measure 2-3 mm. in diameter. The growth is delicate and forms a light, cloudy mass consisting of very delicate intermingled filaments, spreading out from a small central nucleus." McIntosh pictures two colonies that do not look alike. The Medical Research Committee [12] give a similar account of tetanus colonies in deep agar.

Textbooks quote Kitasato's original description almost verbatim. These descriptions of deep and surface gelatine colonies are not readily applicable to our present day technic that employs agar almost exclusively. Yet one modern textbook after another gives us solely observations dating back to 1889. Von Lingelsheim,[13] in an elaborate compilation, apparently wonders whether a deep agar tetanus colony may be distinctive in morphology, but leaves the matter for the future to decide.

While anaerobes of most groups or genera make colonies of somewhat similar structure, the strains of this genus form colonies of exceedingly diverse types. A series of these is illustrated by the photographs accompanying this article. Of interest is the extreme variation noticed in the size of the colonies produced by the different strains. The

[11] Med. Research Committee, Special Report Series 12, 1917.
[12] Ibid., 39, 1919.
[13] Kolle u. Wassermann: Handbuch d. path. Mikroorg., 1912, 4, p. 737.

range in size of colonies of 24 hours is from invisible spots 0.02 mm. in diameter to huge fluffs 3 mm. in diameter. Form also is diverse. The slow-growing types are apparently nonmotile and form colonies of fundamentally lenticular contour. These lenticular colonies are complex and often form peculiar lengthened structures (plate 1). Such shapes are unusual in other groups of anaerobes. The large colonies owe their size to higher motility and to greater powers of utilization of their substratum as food.

The colony forms illustrated may be loosely divided into several types. These types should probably not be termed species. A relationship is not necessarily implied between the various strains that form each type of colony. A similar utilization of nutriment and a similar motility are all that connect the strains that form colonies resembling one another. Thus strains that agglutinate differently may make colonies of the same type, although the agglutination reaction is probably much more fundamentally specific than is the shape of the colonies.

Neither do the differences between these colonies represent, in the majority of cases, what is usually termed variation. When the variations for a given strain are once understood, it is found that mutations occur that in turn breed true, and may be sharply distinguished from variations. The colony form becomes the chief expression of any mutation that may take place in the metabolism of the organism. De Vries [14] employed specific and not subspecific names for what he supposed to be the products of single mutations in the genus Oenothera. These later proved to be recombinations representing sums of single mutations that had occurred previously, any one of which would not deserve specific differentiation. In other groups such as the insects, whose mutations have been well studied, a trinomial nomenclature is resorted to, and the specific name of the original wild type has been retained, while a Latin or vernacular name has been applied to the mutant, which is termed a biotype, the name subspecies being reserved for groups that are delimited by their geographic distribution. Biotype, then, is a name that may be used for these elementary species that differ from one another and breed true, but we should not term two similar colony forms of different history the same biotype, as one might do with two strains of similar higher forms developed from two different types of parents, for the reason that the colony character is not so well understood as are the characters of higher plants and animals, is not so significant or so truly an essential part of the organism as are

[14] Mutation Theory, 1909, 1.

the leaves or stems of complex forms, and there is more chance for a colony type to represent various elementary species than in the case of more elaborately detailed characters. But we should expect that different strains and species of our organisms, like those of more complex forms, should frequently mutate independently in the same fashion.

A description of some of the mutations of Nicolaierillus strains will be presented in a future paper. They are frequent enough to explain the wide range of colony form found in the genus. The bearing of this phenomenon on the taxonomy of the genus is probably nil. Other workers in this laboratory that are using the same strains may be able to confirm the results of Tulloch or to assign certain colony types to various other groups of their own; in other words, to attach some chemical significance to the change in colony form. It is premature even to select a "type species" for the genus. Till further study is made, type 1 of Tulloch, identifiable only by an agglutinating serum, may be taken for a so-called "type species" with the name "N. tetani." A chemical or morphologic character rather than a serologic one is of course preferable for the subdivision of a group.

THE ISOLATION OF NICOLAIERILLUS STRAINS

Many complaints have been made of the difficulty encountered in isolating these organisms. This is due to several factors. In mixed cultures the organisms are recognized only when they form spores—a comparatively late period—and their early active multiplication phase in the vegetative form is not taken advantage of. In many mediums they are somewhat overgrown by other proteolytic organisms. It is extremely difficult to get tetanus bacilli to grow on the surface of an agar plate that is free from blood. In deep agar the colonies of different strains are so unlike that no widely representative "type" can be recognized. The strains that form minute colonies are perforce incapable of easy isolation from gross mixtures. Of interest is the fact that Righi accepted as typical of tentaus bacilli colonies with a dense center and loose radiations, while a collection of cultures sent me by Dr. Duval of New Orleans that were probably isolated by one worker, all made large opaque woolly colonies. Tulloch devised a selective medium for B. tetani by means of which Robertson was able to isolate the organism from wound cultures by the Barber technic. McCoy and Bengtson [15] isolated a series of strains which they were

[15] Am. J. Publ. Health, 1919, 9, p. 427.

so kind as to furnish this laboratory. Their isolations were made as follows: Fermentation tubes were filled with freshly boiled veal infusion, inoculated with suspected material, and incubated at 37 C. until spherical spores were observable in the cultures. Such a fermentation tube was then heated at 70 degrees for 30 minutes and material from it was inoculated into deep agar shakes of veal infusion agar, and the colonies were fished after 3 days' incubation. I have not tried this method in its details, but give it here because it is so simple. When tetanus strains have become contaminated in the laboratory I have had little or no difficulty in isolating the types of active growth by deep colony procedure from liver peptone agar. For some time I was baffled by mutating colonies, and I believe that many supposed contaminations by other anaerobes were cases of mutation. Meat medium should be avoided as a substratum on which to propagate contaminated tetanus strains as it encourages too many other forms. When dealing with badly overgrown cultures or with material from wounds, feces or soil, such a medium as Tulloch's is to be recommended, followed by a deep-colony procedure. The only element that will then make the isolation of the bacilli difficult is the worker's ignorance of the colony form of the particular strain that he desires to isolate. He must, in most cases, fish more colonies than he would were he dealing with a genus of uniform colony formation. The illustrations will help somewhat in recognizing various sorts of tetanus colonies. In case a strain is present that forms minute colonies, one may try other agar substrata, or Barber's technic,[16] or one may use many dilution tubes and incubate for 3 or 4 days until the minute colonies in one or other of the tubes are large enough to be fished readily. Tetanus colonies grow with fair speed at room temperature, and in some cases it may be found advantageous to incubate at a low temperature. For fishing crowded colonies the binocular is of great assistance.

Robertson (per. com.) notes that tetanus cultures become more readily contaminated than do those of other anaerobes. I formerly noted the same phenomenon, and believe it to be due to the fact that she and I usually reincubated tetanus cultures in anaerobe jars to observe spore formation. Long incubation in anaerobe jars frequently causes contamination, as does also the exhaustion of meat tubes containing gas, in which the medium is allowed to boil up onto the cotton plugs. I find that incubation of meat medium cultures of tetanus bacilli in air with or without vaseline allows characteristic development of the cultures.

[16] Phil. J. Sc., 1914, 9, p. 307.

THE BEHAVIOR OF NICOLAIERILLUS STRAINS IN MEAT MEDIUM

Statements concerning the proteolytic activity of the tetanus bacilli vary considerably. There is almost entire unanimity that gelatine is liquefied. Von Hibler [10] and Zeissler,[17] on the one hand, ascribe to tetanus organisms an intense proteolytic activity. Von Hibler worked with badly mixed cultures. He states, however, (p. 95) that many strains of tetanus bacilli do not blacken brain deeply. Zeissler goes so far as to state that brain is blackened intensely and that the odor varies between a pungent odor, and a very bad one, and that milk is peptonized in from 4 to 14 days. His photograph apparently shows a culture contaminated by oval-end-sporulating organisms. On the other hand, the Medical Research Committee [12] state: "Meat medium: Pink color or no change in the medium according to the samples of meat; softening of the consistency of the meat. The odor is characteristic but not putrefactive. Milk: Poor growth; no change in medium. Coagulated serum: Little or no liquefaction." Adamson [18] found the organism mildly proteolytic.

My experience would lead me to emphasize the proteolytic action of the organism a little more than do the members of the Committee. Perhaps they worked with a peptone-free meat medium that did not afford so much nutriment for the ogranism as that employed in this laboratory. But such descriptions as that of Zeissler cannot be construed as applying to pure cultures of tetanus bacilli, for these are among the less active proteolytic anaerobes. The Committee is certainly correct in stating that the color change in meat medium varies with the batch of medium. A series of pure tetanus strains inoculated and incubated uniformly on one batch of medium behave with striking similarity—those that form minute colonies on agar cause changes in the medium with less rapidity than do those that form large colonies. Meat medium is made in this laboratory of one part of coarsely ground beef heart with two parts of distilled water. Five hundred c c of Martin's peptic-digest broth is added to 3 liters of meat medium. The reaction is P_H 7.2. For a long time it was thought that the behavior of tetanus bacilli on this medium was exceedingly uniform and characteristic. Later other assistants made the medium and separate batches were found to give very different results. All batches with an initial reaction in the neighborhood of P_H 7.2 gave evidences of moderate proteolysis inside of a few days and showed slight softening

[17] Ztschr. f. Infektionskrankh. d. Haustiere, 1920, 21, p. 1.
[18] J. Path. & Bacteriol., 1920, 23, p. 241.

of the medium, and never, even on long incubation enough softening to cause more than a slight settling of the meat particles. In odor they were much the same, and the morphologic aspect of the bacilli was much the same. But the color changes were different in the various batches of medium.

The most usual type of color change noted was an initial yellowing of the meat, followed shortly by the appearance of a pinkish shade that changes later to a light terra cotta, rarely to a dark terra cotta. A black pigment is usually noted suffusing the particles nearest the surface and a few of the morsels lower down. If the particles be finely ground, the top layer later bleaches in a few days to pale yellow. If the incubation is in hydrogen a diaphanous black ring appears at the surface of the liquid, but disappears on exposure to the air. Some batches of medium show the initial yellowish stage protracted, and the pink color does not become intense. The black pigment is then very tardy in making its appearance, or it may be absent. In other batches neither pink nor yellow appear. The meat becomes gray and apparently allows good growth of the bacilli. Black pigment may be present. Another batch that apparently afforded excellent growth early gave a mauve color suffused with black pigment. A lot of meat medium that titrated P_H 6.6 sometimes failed to give any growth with tetanus bacilli, but when it did the organisms did not change its appearance. A collection of meat medium tetanus cultures that was three months old showed considerable variation in reddening and blackening. This is consistent with the ready mutation observed with some strains on protein medium. Cultures a year old that have been left at room temperature in air are not uncharacteristic in appearance. If the column of meat is high, it will be noted that all sharp edges of the particles of meat have disappeared, but that the particles have not settled greatly in the tubes. Their basic color may still be red, but this color is almost coated by a thin black film. The top layer of meat a quarter of an inch thick is almost white, the boundary between this layer and the blackened meat below being sharp if the meat has been finely ground.

Gas production is abundant early and becomes less after a few days.

Most authors agree that the odor of tetanus cultures is characteristic and not like that of other proteolytic anaerobes. A young meat culture is faintly and not unpleasantly proteolytic and no butyric acid or sourish smell is noticeable. After 10 days the odor at the mouth of the tube is of hydrogen sulphide only, that of meat smeared on a slide is pungent and different from that of most proteolytic anaerobes. Most people would term it unpleasant. At 3 months the odor is rank, pungent and almost overpowering.

Bacilli are moderately abundant in 24-hour meat medium cultures whether incubated in air, under vaseline or in hydrogen. They are most abundant in 48-hour cultures and do not drop off in numbers abruptly after this time as do so many anaerobes. This is the most marked distinction to be noted between the tetanus bacilli and the nonproteolytic Macintoshillus bacilli (Bacillus tetanomorphus [10, 11]) when stained cultures are observed. Vegetative rods are quite characteristic in their morphology. Their thickness is very uniform, rarely far from 0.8: 1.0 micron. The length may vary from 1 micron to very long filamentous rods. The usual length is from 2-8 microns and filaments and long rods and attached bacilli are rare. The rods are nearly always straight and the ends neatly rounded. They are uniformly and consistently gram-negative when treated with a weak solution of methyl violet, and are gram-positive after treatment with a strong violet stain, such as Sterling's. The gram-negative bacilli are remarkably clear in their staining with the carbol-fuchsin counterstain, and there are no pale forms and no bacilli showing irregularities of protoplasm in cultures under 5 days of age. The morphology of the nonsporulating tetanus bacillus, at first insignificant and hard to distinguish from that of other organisms, becomes to the experienced eye characteristic and definite, and contaminations of tetanus cultures are usually readily noticed. The anaerobic tetanomorphous bacillus of McIntosh and doubtless some other organisms are, however, not definitely to be distinguished by their morphology alone.

Spore formation may commence within forty-eight hours but usually begins on the third or fourth day and is active for a long period; occasionally it fails to appear. Spores vary considerably as to the time of their formation and as to their abundance in the different strains. Spores are invariably spherical and orgonts [19] (p. 4 or 389) show an oval end only in the very early stages. Swelling of the rods takes place apparently only in the portion where spore formation occurs. Spores remain in the rod for a long period. Orgonts are not abundant, sporulating rods are frequent, and only after 10 days or so does one note numerous free spores. The majority of spores are, in most strains, strictly terminal, but occasionally a strain is found that repeatedly forms some spores centrally. A tip of protein from the rod is

[19] Heller, H. H.: J. Infect. Dis., 1920, 27, p. 385.

occasionally noted on the distal end of the spore, giving the rod an appearance superficially like that of a sporulating sporogenes or botulinus organism. But the wall of the spherical tetanus spore is thinner than in those species, and the tip of protein more rounded, the sides of the bacillus are more nearly parallel. I have rarely observed two spores in the same rod. The bacterial wall about the spore is thin, and the spore wall is thin; refractility is low. Sometimes the spores themselves retain the methyl violet of the Gram stain to some extent, remaining transparent the while. The spores of Macintoshillus do the same; both types occasionally show young spores thickly covered by the mother cell, and these may stain gram-negatively like the mother cell or they may retain the stain. Macintoshillus bacilli form more spores during the first two days than Nicolaierillus bacilli. Colonies of the former organisms are pictured in this article.

NICOLAIERILLUS STRAINS ON OTHER PROTEIN MEDIUMS

The behavior of tetanus strains on protein mediums other than meat has been so well treated by Adamson [18] that extensive experiments have not been tried. The following notes were made on the behavior of five pure strains that were incubated in hydrogen at 37 C.

Indol broth gave good growth and after five days of incubation a negative test for indol.

The bacilli grew well on brain medium, producing at first a little gas and abundant rods. After four weeks the medium was not blackened, nor did it show any sign of a greenish or grayish tinge. The lower portion was pink as it had been before inoculation. The odor was faint and ester like, in no way repellent and putrefactive.

The organisms apparently refused to grow on alkaline egg.

Deep coagulated beef serum furnished active growth, and at first gas. Spores were formed early and abundantly. The medium soon showed a gray-greenish color, and at the end of a month was suffused with a slightly greenish leaden tinge and was somewhat softened but not liquefied. The odor was faintly proteolytic.

Although there was multiplication on deep Loeffler's serum, the bacilli did not produce a greenish color. The odor was musty.

In deep Dorset's egg gas was formed early and a slight softening of the medium took place. Later lead-colored spots appeared with a general pale suffusion by the lead color. The odor was faintly of hydrogen sulphide.

Brom-cresol milk was clotted by a rennet like enzyme of slow action. The clot appeared during the first week, and at the end of four weeks most of the casein had settled to a somewhat rubber-like clot at the bottom of the tubes. This clot was compact and could be torn in pieces that disintegrated in invisible particles. The mass behaved much like a compactly settled lump of white lead in paint. The supernatant liquid was not clear, but was clearer than normal milk, and alkaline. Peptonization, if present, was certainly not visible to the eye. The odor was musty.

SUMMARY

Certain differences may be found between Nicolaierillus strains on careful search. It is premature to apply these differences to specific differentiation.

Tetanus strains show remarkable powers of mutation on complex protein substrata. These powers are easily observed in colony formation, but do not affect grossly the picture of proteolytic action on meat medium.

The morphologic and staining reactions of the bacilli are very characteristic and permit the accustomed worker to recognize them readily and to spot contaminations with ease. The behavior of pure cultures on meat medium is fairly characteristic and is different from that of most common contaminating anaerobes. Meat medium is probably the best protein medium for the differentiation of tetanus strains from other anaerobic organisms. All strains observed were noticeably proteolytic and none were intensely so.

Such strains as form large colonies are easily isolated by deep colony procedure.

APPENDIX. LIST OF TETANUS STRAINS STUDIED

From the Hygienic Laboratory, Washington, D. C.

Agar stabs. May, 1917.

THL = "Tetanus No. 1 Hyg. Lab."

November, 1918.

TA = "Tetanus Ag. Dept."
TB = "Tetanus 2 NY Dept. June, 1919."
TC = "Tetanus Courtplaster."
TD = "Tetanus P. D. Co."
TE = "Tetanus 089."
TG = "Tetanus from gelatine."
TM = "Tetanus Mulford."
TN = "Tetanus N. Y. Board of Health."
TO = "Tetanus OT 026580."
TP = "Tetanus Smith's from pease."
TR = "Tetanus OTK 02."

TT = "Tetanus Tulloch type I."
TU = "Tetanus U. Chicago."

June, 1919.
TVP = "Tetanus from vaccine virus point."

From Miss Muriel Robertson, Lister Institute, London.
TMcC = "Tetanus of MacConkey" London, Nov., 1916. Meat culture.

November, 1918.
TUSA = "B. tetani USA II" Tulloch's type I. Egg broth.
T220 = "B. tetani R 220 L" Tulloch's type III. Meat culture.
T67 = "B. tetani T 67 V" Tulloch's type II. Egg broth.

From Dr. K. F. Meyer, San Francisco.
VT = "Tetanus from vaccination case." A small boy who had been vaccinated played in a stable and developed tetanus and died. Two types were cultivated from the culture made from the vaccine pustule.

From Parke, Davis and Company, Detroit.
T 087 = "Tetanus 087" Agar stab.

From the Gilliland Laboratories.
TL = "B. tetani" Agar stab.

From Dr. Duval, New Orleans. Agar stabs.
T 2 A = "B. tetani 204A." Isolated from wound.
T 2 B = "B. tetani 204B." Isolated from soil.
T 2 C = "B. tetani 204C." Isolated from wound.
T 2 E = "B. tetani 204E." Isolated at necropsy.
T 2 F = "B. tetani 204F." Isolated from wound.

From the Cutter Laboratory, Berkeley.
T 4 = "B. tetani 4." Agar stab.

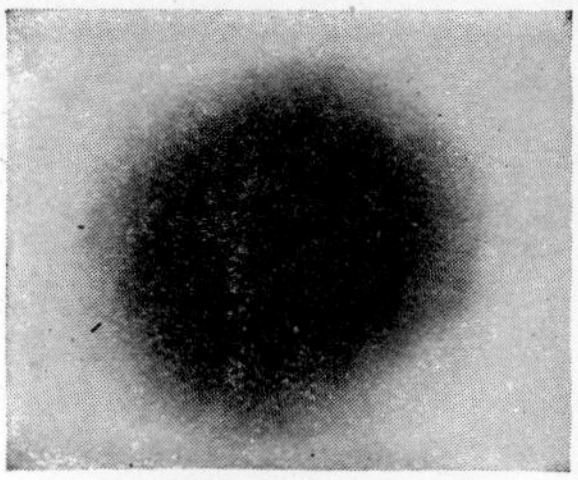

Strain TO;
colonies not numerous.

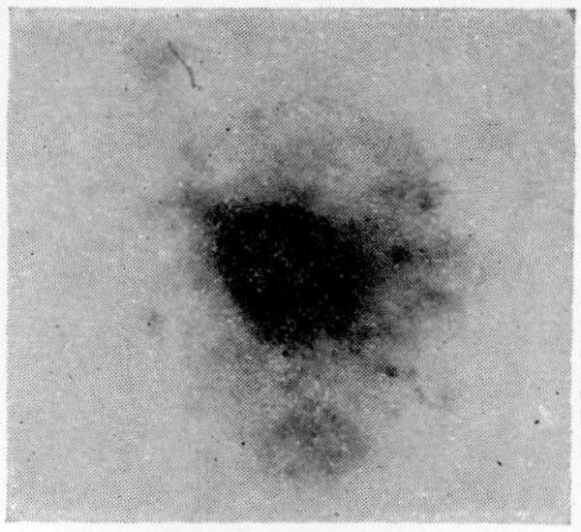

Strain TMcC;
colonies few.

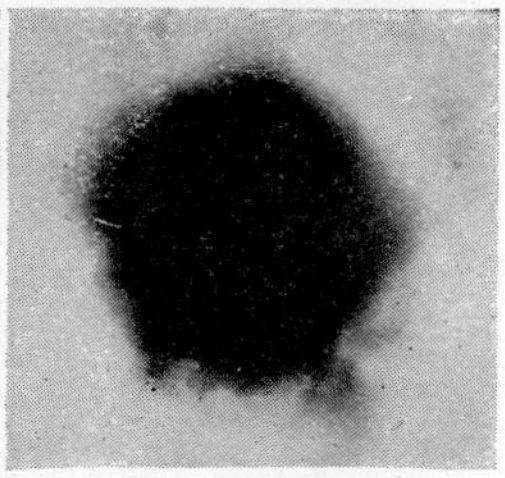

Strain TB;
colonies not numerous.

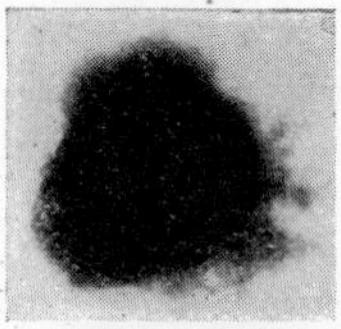

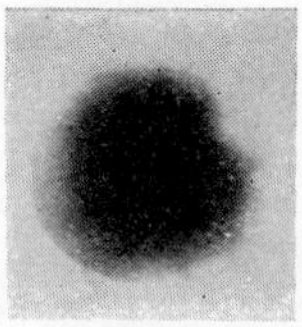

Strain TC;
colonies not numerous.

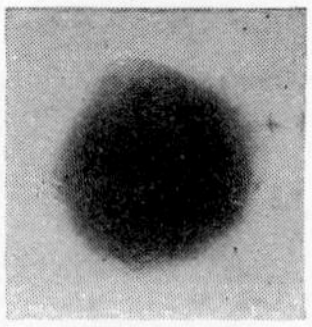

Strain VTS.

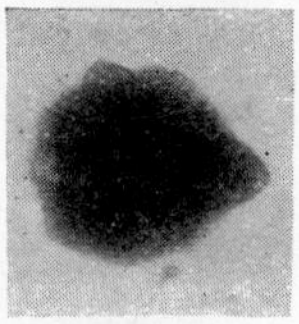

Strain TA.

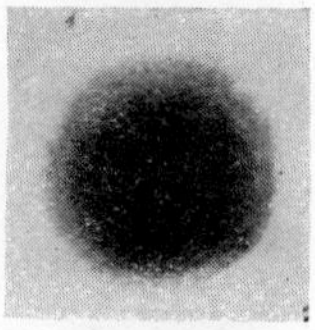

Strain TG.
5 days, × 15.

Colonies few.

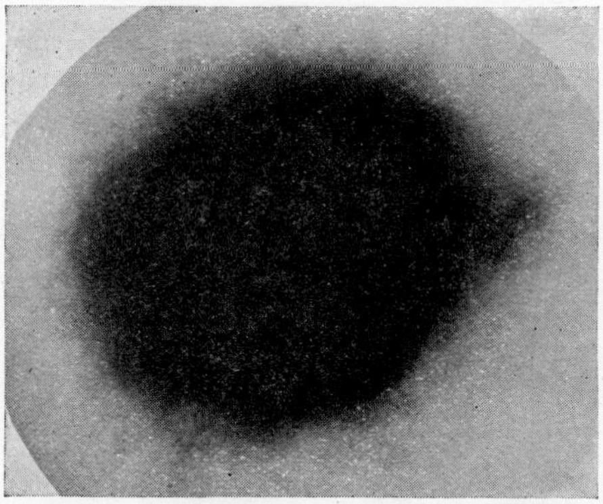

Strain T_2F.

Colonies not numerous.

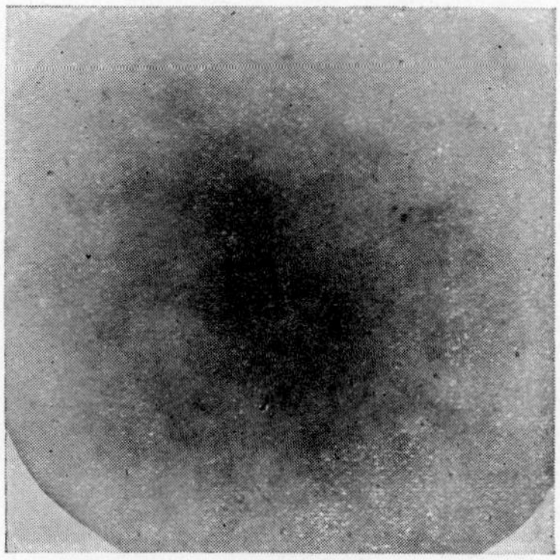

Strain T_4.

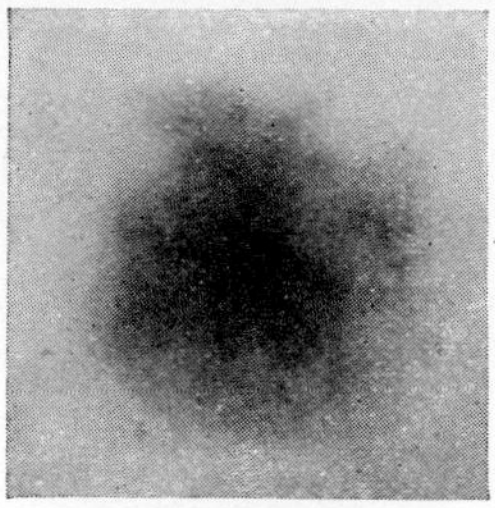

Strain TN;
colonies not numerous.

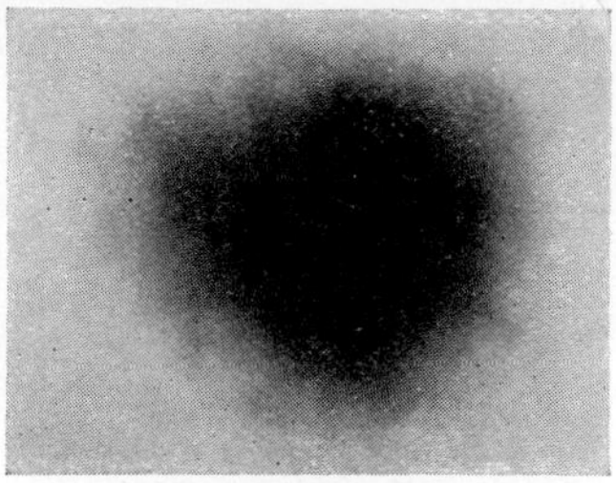

Strain T_2A.

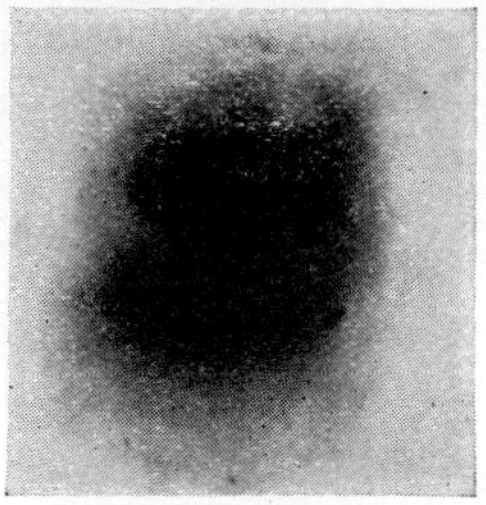

Strain TG; 5 days, × 15.
Colonies few.

Fig. 1.—Various types of Nicolaierillus (Tetanus) colonies. Unless otherwise indicated, these photographs represent colonies that were incubated for 24 hours at 37 C. in deep liver peptone agar and were enlarged 50 diameters.

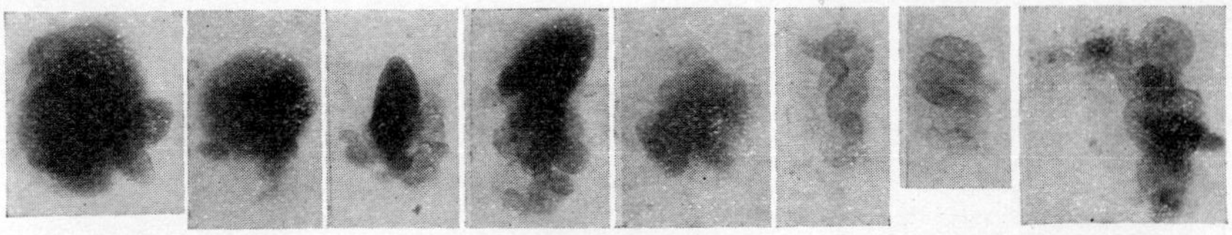

Strain TE; colonies few. Colonies moderately abundant.

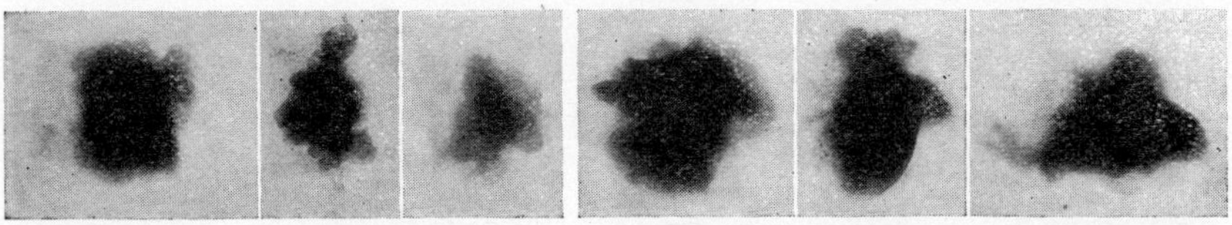

Strain TU; colonies not numerous. Colonies few.

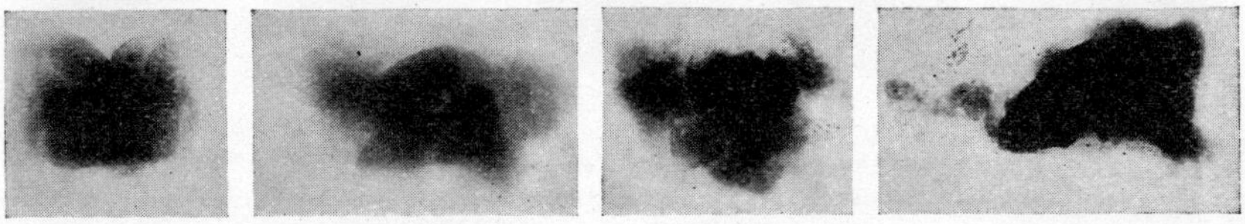

Strain TE; 48 hours' incubation; colonies moderately abundant. Strain TU

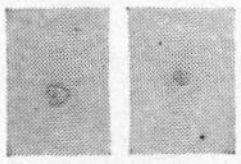

Colonies moderately abundant. Strain TD.

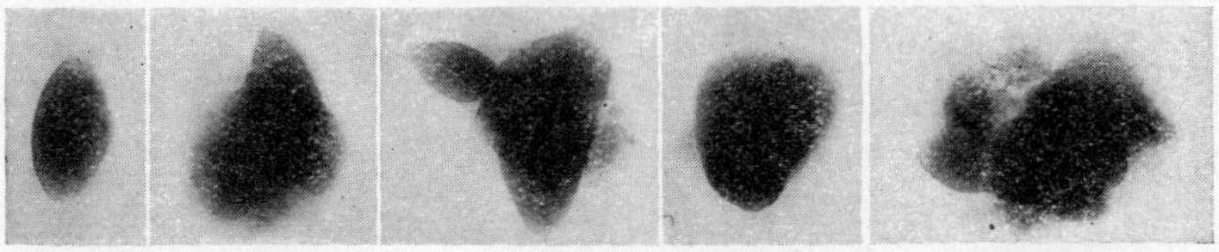

Four days' incubation; colonies few.

NICOLAIERILLUS (TETANUS) COLONIES

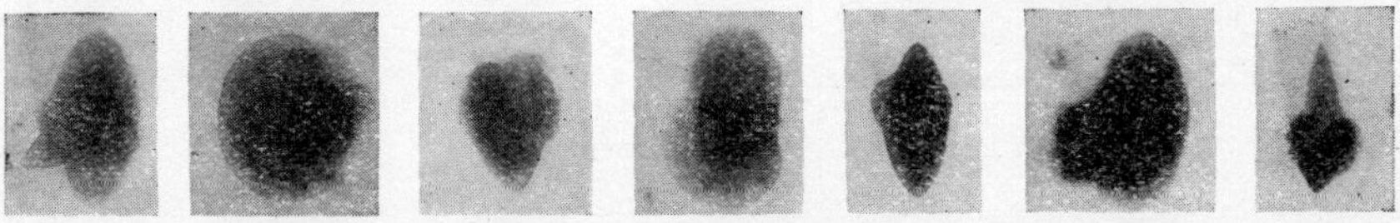

Macintoshillus tetanomorphus, type strain, PT; colonies abundant.

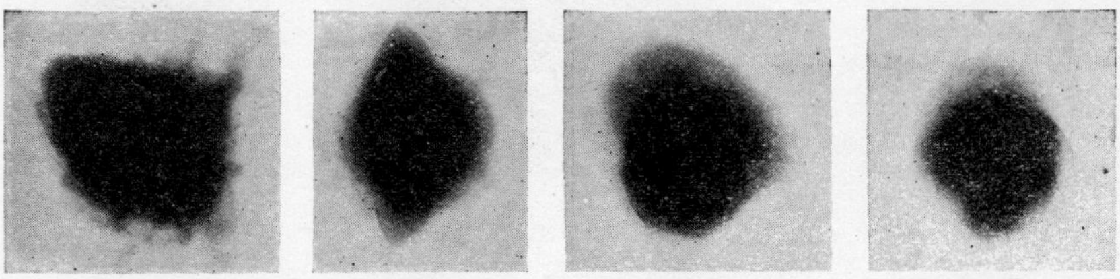

Strain 297. Strain 221.

Colonies moderately abundant.

Fig 2.—Macintoshillus (B. tetanomorphus) colonies.

MUTATIONS IN THE GENUS NICOLAIERILLUS (B. TETANI)

STUDIES ON PATHOGENIC ANAEROBES VIII

From the George Williams Hooper Foundation for Medical Research, University of California Medical School, San Francisco

HILDA HEMPL HELLER

In a former paper,[1] it was suggested that in the study of anaerobic bacilli colony formation in deep agar was available for two purposes: for the differentiation of strains that behaved alike on ordinary mediums, and for the study of mutations. The objection will be made that if anaerobic colonies mutate, they are useless for systematic purposes. This objection holds good for the groups in which mutations occur readily and not for those in which they are rare. No other group studied in this laboratory shows such a wide range of colony types as does the genus Nicolaierillus[2] (B. tetani). The diversity of these colonies has been pictured in a preceding communication.[3] Mutations in deep liver agar are frequent in this proteolytic genus, while among nonproteolytic organisms, although mutations in colony form probably occur, they have not been noted. Moreover, in some genera it has been possible to correlate the different colony types with other characters that may be termed specific, while in the tetanus group it has thus far been impossible to do so. A study of a few mutations in the genus Nicolaierillus is herewith described. Apparently these organisms furnish a most excellent field for the close study of bacterial mutation—here only superficially investigated.

TECHNIC

The technic employed in this study has been described before.[1,4] It is principally the ancient procedure of Liborius.[5] Inoculum was thoroly mixed in the first of three dilution tubes of deep agar. From this tube a suitable amount was removed with a Pasteur pipet to a second tube, this amount depending on the number of organisms in the original inoculum. The second tube was mixed and a larger amount (0.25-0.75) taken from it and placed in a third. Three tubes usually suffice to give a satisfactory picture of the flora

Received for publication Aug. 18, 1921.

[1] J. Infect. Dis., 1922, 30, p. 1.

[2] Heller, H. H.: J. Bacteriol., 1922, 7, Jan.

[3] J. Infect. Dis., 1922, 30, p. 18.

[4] J. Bacteriol., 1921, 6, p. 445.

[5] Ztschr. f. Hyg. u. Infectionskrankh., 1886, 1, p. 115.

of an inoculum. In case more chance for mutation is desired, two or three number 2 tubes may be inoculated. A third dilution tube should always be used to give a chance for obtaining in one tube a pure culture of the predominant biotype.

The shaft of agar from which inoculation is desired is blown from its tube into a Petri dish by means of a large-bore Pasteur pipet. The same pipet, with careful flaming, may be employed many times with no chance of contamination. The location of a desirable colony may be marked by the pipet groove in the agar and by a mark on the glass tube to indicate the distance of the colony from the end of the tube. Small colonies may be fished under the binocular or ordinary microscope but such procedure is seldom necessary for tetanus colonies. Fishing is accomplished with the pipet that is to be used for diluting the agar in the next three tubes. The glass is drawn to a needle point, broken and flamed, and inserted into the agar shaft to the desired colony, which is sucked up and transferred to the first dilution tube of a new series. Agar may be cut with a flamed (not a boiled) razor blade or knife; it is unnecessary to "sear" the agar, which process only melts it anyway.

THE HISTORY OF STRAIN T 087

The culture T 087 was received from Parke, Davis and Co. and is one of their regular toxin-producing strains. When first studied, its colonies in deep liver peptone agar were uniform, small, subspherical, with an irregular outline and no long woolly protuberances (plate I upper left figures). After some months of cultivation on meat medium the strain was thought to be contaminated with an organism forming woolly colonies. The small colony type was isolated but contamination by a woolly colony was again observed, and repeated shakings in agar dilutions showed that the supposed contamination must have been a mutation. The history of the behavior of this strain is here given in detail.

The original agar culture (Nov. 4, 1919) was inoculated onto meat and therefrom onto agar dilution tubes. One colony form was observed, the small type mentioned in the foregoing. A colony of this sort passed through a meat culture and was inoculated onto agar again. Two types of colonies were noted; a small one was fished onto meat, and this culture had had 5 passages on meat when, 9 months later, it was reinoculated onto agar, and showed 2 types of colonies in about equal numbers. The larger of these (TOL, plate 1) was replanted many times on agar of the same batch and no reversion or mutation was noted.

A small colony gave in dilution tubes both types, the small being most abundant. The third tube had 6 colonies of each type. The offspring of 2 large ones from this tube were all fluffy like TOL, with which they were probably identical. One small colony gave, in a series of 4 dilution tubes, only one woolly colony (TO 2), which may have been a contamination by TOL, but by its composition was probably a mutant. Its subsequent history was of interest. This one colony gave two types. In the second tube 58% were large. In the third tube 4, which were carelessly abandoned, were large, one was small, one smooth and larger. The story of the smooth larger colony on reinoculation onto agar tubes follows:

1. Very abundant colonies, 2 types.
2. Large, dense, and smooth, 390; small 96.
3. None. ↓

Large dense smooth type one colony onto agar.

1. ?
2. Eighty-nine large, fluffy; 2 small.
3. Two fluffy (TOM, Plate 1).

The smooth large colony, intermediate type between TOM and TO 2 was, sad to say, not photographed, and it is a question whether it may have been the same as TOM or not.

A small colony from TO 2's first subculture, which represented the original type, gave in dilution tubes uniform small colonies of which a single one was markedly asymmetrical, having a woolly side and a smaller smooth side. Inoculation (fishing was done under the binocular) from the woolly half of this asymmetrical colony gave pure dense woolly colonies (TDW, plate 1). Inoculation from the smooth half gave in the third tube 40 dense woolly colonies and 44 smooth ones.

A smooth colony from a sister tube to that from which TO 2 was derived, a tube in which no woolly colonies existed, gave two types of colonies, 41% of them large. As I was at the time still under the impression that these large mutating colonies were all alike, this mutant was not photographed and was lost. Here is an instance, one of several in this series, in which a colony fished at random, had within it mutants that had caused no change in the shape of that colony. It is better to choose for the demonstration of mutation colonies in tubes that contain no mutant colony, so that the question of contamination by permeating growth is eliminated.

To return to the early tube in which there were 6 small colonies and 6 woolly ones: Another colony showed either contamination with TOL or mutation. Twenty-five % of the colonies were fluffy and the rest smooth. One small colony from this generation gave 0.43% large colonies, another 2.9% large ones. These also probably represent contamination by the other type (TOL). One tube of this series contained 100 smooth colonies and no woolly ones at all. When one such colony was inoculated into agar tubes the second dilution tube showed a mutant, one colony in 250, radiate in structure, which type (TRW) in culture tubes did not resemble TOM so closely as it does in the photograph. The third tube contained only 2 small colonies, no woolly ones. One of these on inoculation into agar showed only one type (small) in the first tube, one type in the second (300 colonies), but in the third dilution tube were 12 small colonies and one woolly mutant (TLW), that was larger than all the others, which was easily isolated in the dilution series on which it was planted.

About as many transplants were made of smooth colonies that gave rise to no mutants as of those that did. Their history is omitted.

The photographs on the plate were made under identical conditions at the end of the experiment.

Three-day meat cultures of these 6 strains (T 087, TDW, TOL, TOM, TRW and TLW) were inoculated subcutaneously into guinea-pigs in 0.75 c c doses. The animals showed no symptoms of tetanus. Ten-day meat cultures gave a like result, and 7-day cultures in glucose-veal toxin broth containing blood inoculated on a third series of guinea-pigs caused no symptoms of tetanus. The behavior of all the T 087 strains was culturally entirely typical of that of tetanus bacilli[3] and strain T 087 had long been known as a standard toxin producing strain. Miss P. Schoenholz was so kind as to investigate the agglutination reactions of the organisms and found that all 6 substrains were agglutinated by serums made from strain TT (Tulloch's type 1) in titers from 1000-6000, strain TE (T 089 of the U. S. Public Health laboratory) in titers from 4000-20000 and strain T 087 (a serum that was made shortly after the arrival of the culture in this laboratory) from 4000-8000. It must be concluded that during the frequent fishing of the small type before the commencement of this experiment a wholly nontoxic mutant had been selected from among the toxin-producing colonies.

We have here a record of 4, or 5 or 6 different mutant types, all but one occurring during the 2 weeks' study of a tetanus strain. Apparently this strain mutates in so many directions that the classic demand that to prove bacterial mutation the mutant must be repeatedly found, cannot be satisfied without long search. Had the colonies not been photographed they would have been thought to be alike, and the requirement would have been technically, apparently, fulfilled. No contamination, either by other anaerobes than tetanus, or by aerobes, was noted during the whole study—and such contamination was feared and rather expected, for the laboratory is full of many kinds of anaerobes. Practically every unusual colony was fished and its behavior studied.

It was noted that if the colonies were fished when 24 hours old, mutants were hard to find, but if they were 48 hours old, in a large series of tubes they were usually to be found. Therefore, old material was investigated in order to find whether many mutant forms existed therein.

THE BEHAVIOR OF STRAIN T USA

This strain was furnished by Miss Muriel Robertson who, I believe, isolated it from a stock American strain by means of the Barber technic[6] during the tetanus investigation. She states that with it Tulloch made the serum with which his type 1 strains were identified.[7] It was received in the form of an egg broth culture in the fall of 1919 and bore the designation T USA II and the date September 6. Previously another culture of what was probably the identical strain had been received from Dr. McCoy of the United States Public Health Laboratory. This (TT) was labeled "Tulloch, Type I" and made large fluffy colonies without an opaque center and, more rarely, large opaque woolly colonies (Fig. 2, top row).

In March, 1920, the egg broth culture "T USA II" was inoculated onto meat and therefrom onto agar. Two types of colonies were observed. One

[6] Phil. J. Sc., B., 1914, 9, p. 307.

[7] J. Roy. Army Med. Corps, 1917, 29, p. 631; Proc. Roy. Soc., B., 1919, 90, p. 145.

was large and fluffy without an opaque center. The other was slightly smaller and was opaque. After isolation, these were photographed (Plate 2, second row), but already after only two successive transplants the original type of clear fluffy colony had been partly replaced by a colony with a small opaque center—T USA W. Both these types were typical tetanus bacilli and later formed high titer toxins that produced typical tetanus symptoms in mice during an immunity experiment.

In October, 1920, a meat culture was again made from the original egg broth tube. On agar its colonies were of only one type, large and fluffy. A sister meat culture was sent to Dr. Ivan C. Hall, who complained that it contained two kinds of tetanus colonies, an opaque one that behaved normally and a fluffy one that could not be purified, the opaque type continually reappearing therein.

In April, 1921, the meat culture made in October, 1920, was planted directly into new agar dilution tubes. Instead of one single fluffy type, such as was found in such a transplant in October, a galaxy of divergent types appeared. From the second dilution tube a number of these were fished into a new series of agar tubes and were isolated in pure culture (Plate 2, large group, all but T USA LC). Some of these were alike but between others of the strains were marked differences. The original fluffy type was, apparently, lost. Certain of the colonies were similar when observed with a hand lens, but differences could be observed between them when they were photographed. Such were T USA M and P. Others can be correlated by photographic procedure (USA X and P). T USA F is a larger form than the original type. T USA LC, the only strain pictured that was not isolated from the second dilution tube from which the others originated, is an independent derivative from the original stock, which was a fluffy clear centered strain, and it resembles F in contour but not in size. T USA O was consistently larger than T USA X and P, which are probably the same sort of mutant as the original T USA S. T USA B is distinctly smaller and more smoothly contoured than any T USA S-like colony observed. And, finally, because the parent tube had lain for some days before it was fished, a successful subculture was obtained of a very minute form, T USA T, which is hardly to be discerned with a hand lens after 24 hours' growth, but forms small spherical colonies when 48 hours old.

Thus we see that a tetanus strain, left long on a medium, like egg, that furnishes little nutriment, retains its type, probably through failure to multiply. But, if it be sown on a well-buffered highly nutrient medium, like meat, it will continue to multiply, in so doing it may mutate, and the mutant forms complete, some dying out, some sporulating and waiting for a better day, others increasing, till after a few months, if mutation be active, the culture tube may contain a multitude of biotypes, some better able to multiply on another substratum like agar, and some less able to multiply on it, and some multiplying as abundantly as the parent type but taking, in colonies, different forms.

These strains—T USA-F, M, LC, O, X, P, and T—were all typical tetanus bacilli; 3-day old meat cultures of them when inoculated subcutaneously into guinea-pigs in doses of 0.75 c c killed the animals with symptoms of tetanus inside of 48 hours.

THE HISTORY OF THE STRAIN TG

This strain was isolated from gelatine at the United States Public Health Laboratory from which I received it in an agar stab in November, 1918. It was planted onto meat on November 6, therefrom onto meat June 25, 1919. July 2, agar shakes from this meat culture gave colonies that were invisible in 24 hours, and are shown at that age magnified 50 diameters in the photographs (Plate 3, top left). Colonies incubated longer than 24 hours grew apace and when 5 days old were as in the series below. A smooth colony was fished from this tube and after passage on meat gave colonies in agar that were denominated "irregular, smooth and minute." On July 14, the meat culture that was planted June 25 was again inoculated onto agar tubes and the result was small irregular colonies, at 24 hours indistinguishable, at 48 hours definitely of two sorts—lenticular and woolly. Subsequent transplants were made from the stock termed "irregular, smooth and minute" in September, and the first agar shake showed small irregular compound lenticular colonies (Plate 3, upper right) that, when 3 days old, were not to be distinguished from one another, but when 5 days old were of 2 types, some loose and woolly, some smooth and lenticular, and 2 with bushy protuberances. Both types were fished, but, sad to say, the smooth type was lost and has never been recovered. The strain now is a woolly one (the 4 colonies below) with an enormous range in colony size that is exceedingly baffling to work with. Three quarters c c of 3-day old meat culture inoculated subcutaneously into a guinea-pig caused the death of the animal in a few hours.

It must be borne in mind that this work was done before the significance of these mutations was comprehended, in order to be sure the strain was pure, and in order to take photographs. Whether the differences seen between the two top groups of figures on plate 3 represents a mutation it is now impossible to say. It is probable that it does. But that the woolly type, now the only one preserved, is a mutation from the smaller type cannot be doubted. Of interest is the fact that when crowded the colonies resemble closely their ancestral form. In crowded tubes these compound lenticular colonies are permanent and do not turn woolly except when the agar has not been thoroughly mixed and there is abundant nutriment for the colonies at the edge of the culture. But no pure lenticular form can be isolated from them, for as soon as they are planted in sufficient dilution lenticular forms are almost impossible to find, practically all the colonies being woolly. These woolly colonies vary greatly in size, but whatever sized colony may be chosen for inoculation into dilution tubes the result is always the same—the colonies vary from minute ones to large fluffs with a clear zone about the center.

STRAIN TL

This was received from Dr. S. H. Gilliland and was apparently a pure biotype that made a transparent colony with a tendency to form a thickened cortical layer (Plate 5, top left). Two years later a meat culture of the strain showed heavy opaque colonies of about the same size as the older ones (TLC, second row, left). Search revealed a few transparent colonies among them. After 2 transplants, the transparent type (TL B, top row, right) was recovered and it was impossible to demonstrate whether or not it was identical with the original type. Both of these strains (TLC and TLB) were highly pathogenic for guinea-pigs, causing marked asymmetry and rigidity of the body followed by the death of the animals inside of 48 hours.

It is of interest that these colonies showed a very small range of variation in size. The strain TG in its woolly form shows similar colonies that are a little more irregular in contour than those of TL, but they have a very wide range of variation in size. Strain TP ("Smith, from Pease" sent me by Dr. G. W. McCoy) forms more opaque colonies with a great range in size, utterly unsuited to the study of mutations.

STRAIN TVP

Strain TVP was isolated from an ivory vaccine point by Miss Bengtson and sent to me by Dr. G. W. McCoy. It forms the largest colonies in the whole collection, which is of interest from an epidemiologic point of view when one considers its origin. On first transplantation 2 kinds of colonies were noted. A loose fluffy type was isolated, and gave rise to colonies somewhat inconsistent in behavior, shown in Fig. 4, top and center. Two years later, 2 types, TVPF and TVPD which is derived from TVPF, were discovered in the original tube. What relationships these bear to the colonies pictured earlier is not clear. Three-day meat cultures of TVPF and TVPD killed guinea-pigs in doses of 0.75 c c with symptoms of tetanus in 24 and 48 hours, respectively.

STRAIN T McC

T McC was a culture given by Dr. A. T. MacConkey to Miss Robertson who gave it to me in 1916. The agar colonies depicted in the first photographs (plate 5, second row, center) were derived from a single colony in agar. The second photographs (second row, right) were later derived from the original culture without intermediate fishing, the batch of medium was a different one, but the conditions were the same. These photographs represent, in all probability, different biotypes, and the opaque form may have been derived from the other.

STRAIN T 220

This was received in meat culture, in 1918, from Miss Robertson who isolated it from a wound. With it Tulloch[7] made the agglutinating serum that enabled him to establish his type 3. It apparently existed in 2 forms in the meat culture as it was received, for transplants shortly from that culture have twice shown 2 forms (plate 5, third row). These have been worked with quite extensively and no other type has been noted in the cultures. It is not known which form gives rise to the other. Strong toxins that produced typical tetanus in mice were produced by both strains.

STRAIN VT

This was given me by Dr. K. F. Meyer, who secured it from a vaccine process in a fatal case of tetanus in a little boy who probably became infected through playing in a stable. When first studied, 2 very different types of colonies were noted that, when isolated, were photographed (plate 6, first and second rows). Strong toxins that produced typical tetanus in mice were formed by both strains.

THEORETICAL CONSIDERATIONS

Tetanus strains mutate readily in protein mediums in which they are able to multiply actively. This mutation is apparently much more frequent than in the case of nonproteolytic anaerobes. The phenomenon is in accordance with the hypothesis,[2] that proteolytic anaerobes are the products of a more far-reaching evolution than nonproteolytic ones. That is, the proteolytic anaerobes always have mutated more frequently on protein mediums than the others, and that is why they have attained their specialization.

Some strains of tetanus bacilli apparently mutate more readily than others.

The mutations of these organisms, frequent and striking as they are, never, so far as I have been able to observe, result in anything but the formation of typical tetanus bacilli. The derivation of forms differing from their ancestors in several important characters should be considered as possible only after the passing of a far longer period than that noted by certain workers with anaerobes (Grassberger and Schattenfroh;[8] Kolle, Ritz and Schlossberger[9]). A worker claiming to change a blackleg bacillus into a Welch bacillus would, in my opinion, in order to substantiate his claims, have to show pure cultures of several intermediate biotypes, for apparently mutation of several important characters does not occur, either at once, or in rapid succession. It is improbable that radical changes involving many characters of an anaerobe occur in short spaces of geologic time; otherwise we would not find universal common types all over the world.

As in the case of higher organisms, mutation may be either favorable or unfavorable to the existence of the organism. Probably numerous mutations affect the metabolism neither favorably nor unfavorably. The chances of detecting a favorable mutation are far greater than are those of detecting an unfavorable one. This does not correspond with the findings that Beijerinck[10] and others have made with aerobes;

[8] Arch. f. Hyg., 1901, 48, p. 50; p. 1312; 1905, 53, p. 58.

[9] Med. Klin., 1918, 14, p. 281; München. med. Wchnschr., 1919, 66, p. 348.

[10] Folia mikrobiologia, 1912, 1.

Beijerinck believes that acquisition of characters by mutation has not been demonstrated for aerobic organisms. This is doubtless a matter of interpretation, but it is far easier to demonstrate the acquisition of a power by an anaerobe than the loss of one, when deep colony methods are used. The process of identifying mutations in the study of strain TO87 depended frequently on the detection of the mutation in the very colony in which it occurred—one among perhaps 100 or 500 others. This was easy because such colonies are bigger or fluffier than their neighbors, or they are asymmetrical. The chances of deliberately fishing a mixed colony in which a less capable mutant exists are remote—unless, indeed, there should appear an inhibitive or autolytic action like that noted for the colon bacillus by Bordet and Ciuca.[11] But in old cultures such less capable forms may exist and may be discovered by careful search. In the process of this investigation many minute colonies were fished before any were found that bred true. Colonies descended from spores and colonies near the wall of the tube may be smaller than their neighbors, but are usually of the same biotype.

No case of reversion has, in this brief study, been discovered. Beijerinck terms the reappearance of pigment forming prodigiosus colonies in nonpigment-producing strains "reversion." Pigment is a substance that may be analyzed and such reversions may thus be definitely proved. But when a mere matter of colony form is under consideration, it will not be wise to call the reappearance of an ancestral form in a pure mutant culture a reversion, unless we know something of the chemical nature of the processes involved.

According to Dr. Thomas Morgan (pers. com.), there are two kinds of possibilities that may determine reversion in bacteria, a recombination of two genes to produce a remote ancestral type being probably restricted to forms in which amphimixis occurs. The reversions which we should consider may depend on the tautomeric action of a gene that is always present and that may balance one way or another, or they may depend on an entirely new mutation that produces the same character as was possessed by an ancestral type. In the first case, the reversion will occur repeatedly in a certain percentage of cases; in the second case it will be exceedingly rare.

The study of mutating colonies will enable the systematist to deduce which metabolic characters are least constant by making special mediums containing substances that are to be investigated, and studying the colony formation in deep agar shakes made of such medium. This

[11] Compt. rend. Soc. de biol., 1920, 83, p. 1293.

method is analogous to the well-known one of putting indicator in special sugar mediums for use with aerobes. If an indicator could be found that would not be reduced in the presence of anaerobic growth, it would be of great value in determining anaerobic mutations on carbohydrates. Such substances as furnish material on which the bacteria readily mutate, may be rigorously excluded from a standard medium on which the habits of various strains may be compared. An easy way is thus offered of avoiding expensive and time consuming tests of the behavior of certain organisms when such tests should never be used for systematic purposes on account of the mutation of the organisms under the conditions afforded by those tests.

The significance of these mutations to the biochemist is great. His road is a difficult one to plan. He must make quantitative determinations and yet know that they may be impossible to confirm. Specific chemical action exists, surely, but it will be difficult to determine what is specific and what is not. The chemical behavior of anaerobes should be studied for several strains of the same group that differ in every known way.

Mutations are also of importance to the therapeutist. DeKruif [12] has recently found two types of the bacillus of rabbit septicemia living side by side, both virulent for rabbits, one far more so than the other. For organisms whose pathogenicity is dependent on their invasive power, such mutations are of great significance for purposes of immunization. Virulence depends very much on the ability of the organism to multiply in its environment. It has been customary of late for surgeons to depend, in certain types of tetanus cases, on antitoxin to help the body to fight off an infection that would otherwise remain somewhere near equilibrium, instead of operating to sterilize the seat of the infection. Theoretical considerations are radically against such procedure. Any day a new form of tetanus bacillus may arise that is four or five times as well able to multiply as were its ancestors, and this type may upset the equilibrium. Such a phenomenon may explain many cases of latent tetanus.

No effect of these observed colony mutations on toxin production has been noted, although it is reasonable to presume that by multiplying more extensively a strain will produce a stronger toxin. Filtered toxins prepared from some of the mutant strains had similar titers. All strains tested produced strong toxins in 3-day meat cultures except T 087 and its derivatives which behaved consistently with one another.

[12] Jour. Am. Med. Assn., 1921, 76, p. 651.

Miss McRoberts of this laboratory is investigating the agglutination reactions of these strains and will report on them separately. One is forced to presume that these nutritional mutations are more frequent and superficial than such as would be discovered by immune reactions where a large protein fraction of the bacterium or a secreted toxin is the substance estimated.

TECHNICAL DEDUCTIONS

In choosing anaerobic material for the study of mutations one may seek in the literature or in his own notes for evidences of irregularity in the behavior of certain types of organisms. The worker should first investigate whether the irregularities are due to contamination, for the literature is permeated with reports based on the behavior of contaminated cultures. If pure cultures have been found that behave peculiarly, a medium may be chosen that will emphasize the peculiarity. Deep colonies in this medium should be craefully observed, and, if the work is undertaken seriously, the colonies should be occasionally photographed. A species of organism should be chosen that does not form much gas or grow readily through agar mediums as though they were broth. Strains selected for particular observation should make symmetrical colonies that show little variation. A strain that normally is lenticular but occasionally sends out woolly processes, such a character being quite within the limits of variation for the biotype, is not well adapted for the study of mutation.

One should use the same batch of medium throughout a given experiment whenever possible (plate 5, lower series).

A type of photographic plate should be used that covers a wide range of lighting conditions and can always be procured. Detail, in the photography of colonies, is more important than contrast.

One should refuse to undertake to study mutations in a dusty room where there are draughts or people pass frequently—otherwise other types of anaerobes will probably make their appearance in the culture.

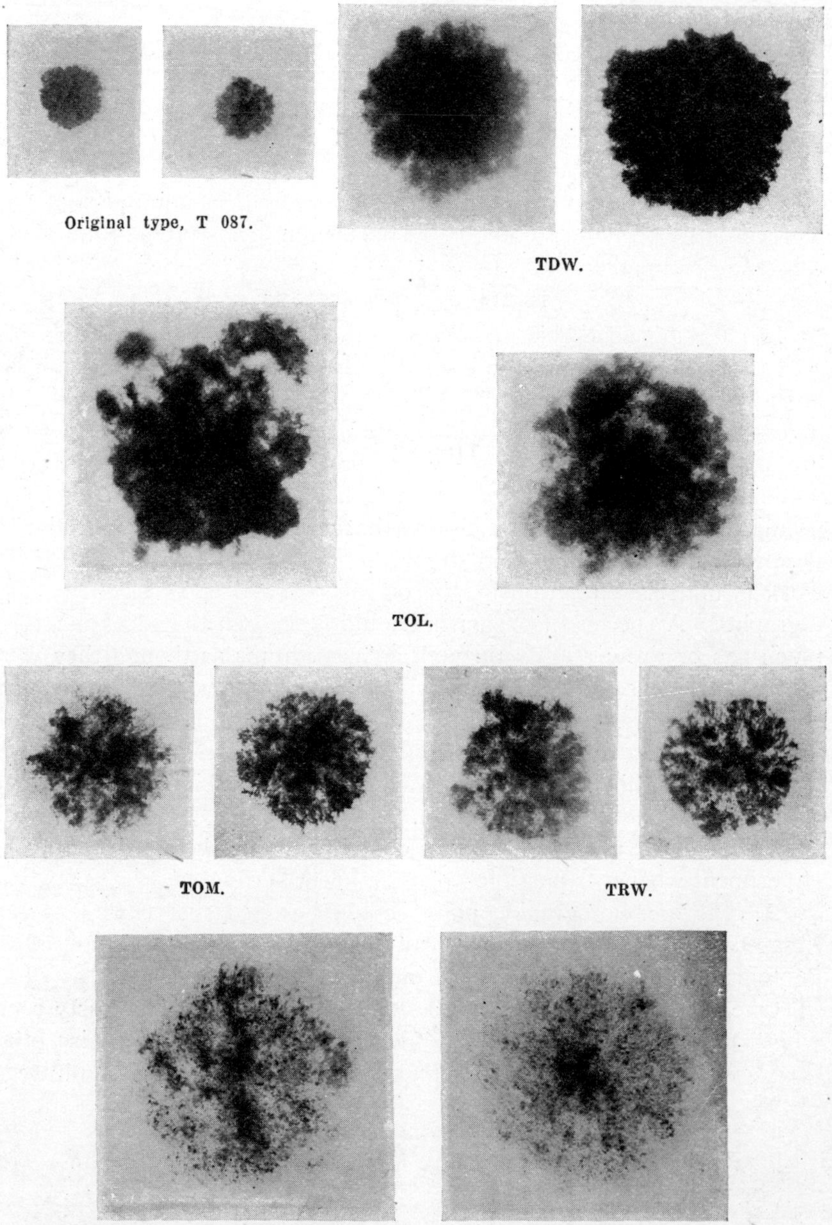

Fig. 1.—The mutations of strain T 087. Five pairs of photographs show what are probably 4 types of mutants derived from the minute type in the upper left hand corner. They arose during two weeks' study of the behavior of this strain on deep liver peptone agar. All were grown simultaneously for 24 hours on the same batch of medium under identical conditions; colonies few; × 50.

Unless otherwise indicated this and the following illustrations represent colonies that were incubated for 24 hours at 37 C. in deep liver peptone agar and were enlarged 50 diameters.

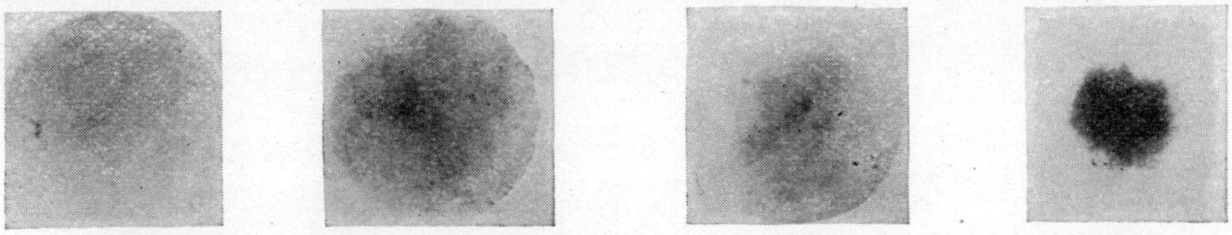

Strain TT, probably identical with strain T USA; colonies not numerous, 1919.

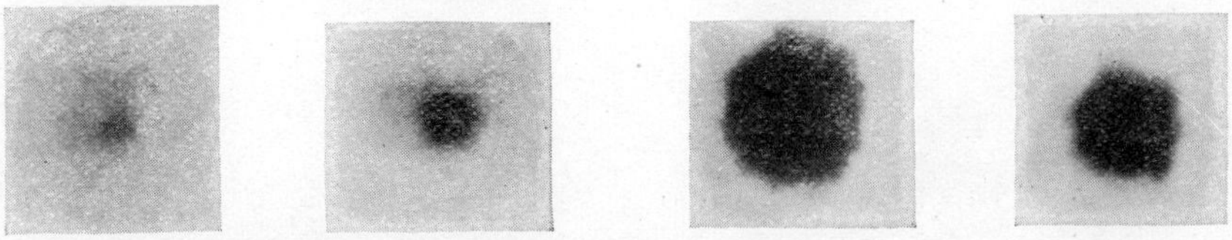

Strain T USA W. Colonies not numerous, 1919. Strain T USA S.

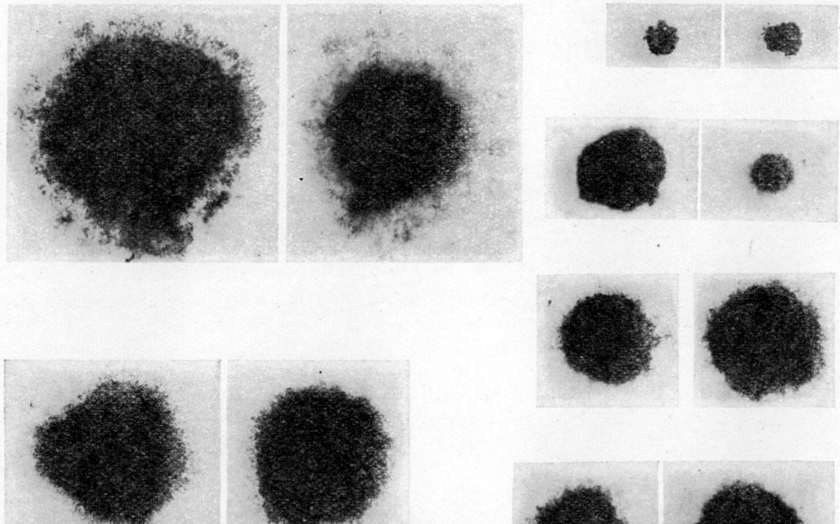

Fig. 2.—Mutations of strain T USA. In October, 1920, a meat culture of T USA (W) showed the fluffy type only. In March, 1921, the same meat medium tube that had long stood at room temperature showed a number of biotypes. The original form was apparently lost; some new types were larger than the original; all were denser and two smaller. The conditions of growth for the members of each of the three series were identical. The lower series were all taken on a Seed No. 23 plate; colonies few; × 15. The upper series were taken on softer plates at 50 diameters and were reduced to 15 diameters.

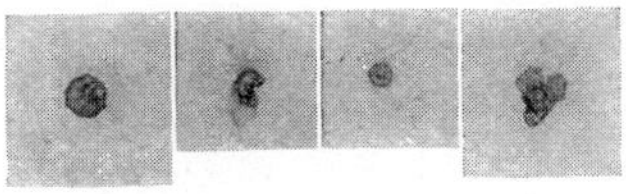

July 3, 1919; colonies moderately abundant; × 50

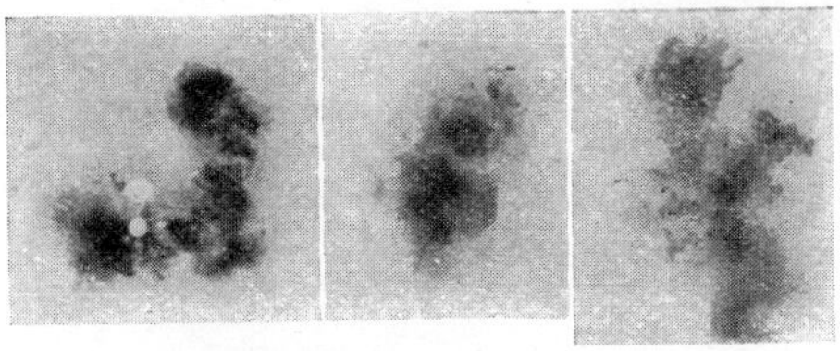

Oct. 2, 1919; colonies few.

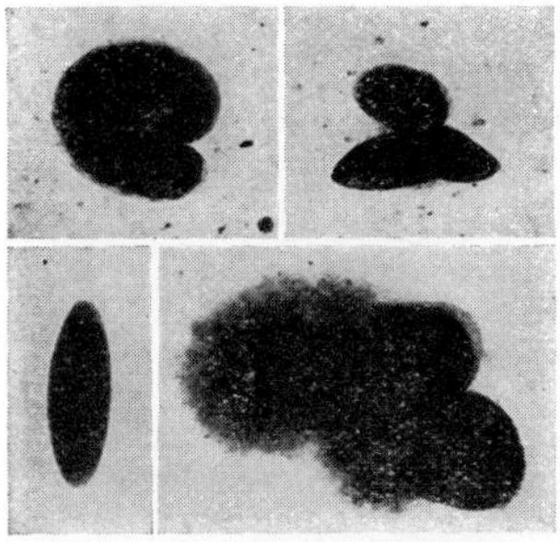

The above type, 5 days at 37 C.; colonies few; × 15.

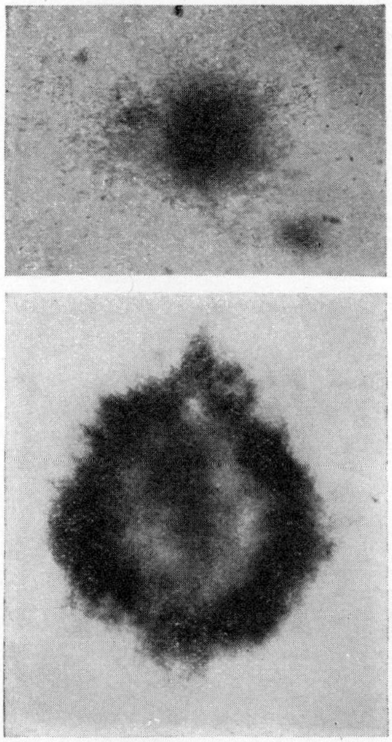

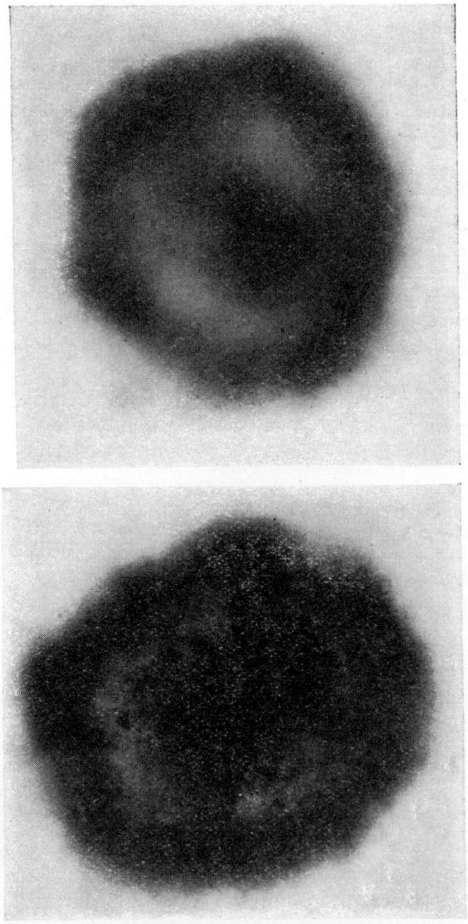

March, 1921, colonies not numerous.

Fig. 3.—Changes in the behavior of strain TG. The origin of the woolly form from that of Oct. 2, 1919, was observed. This is a type with great range in size of colony.

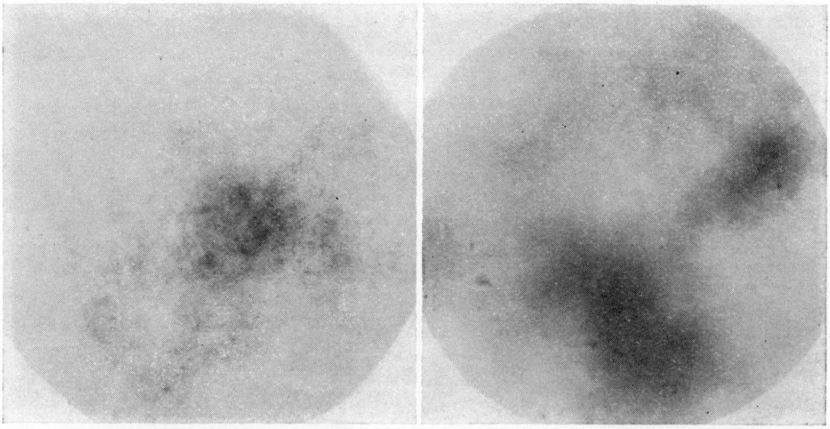

Oct. 28, 1919. Colonies few. December, 1919.

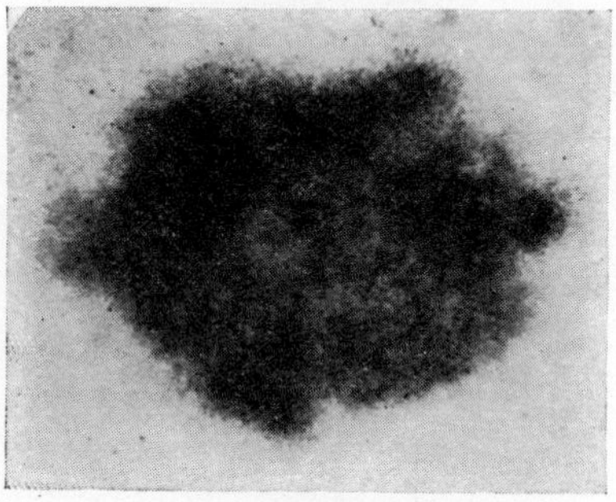

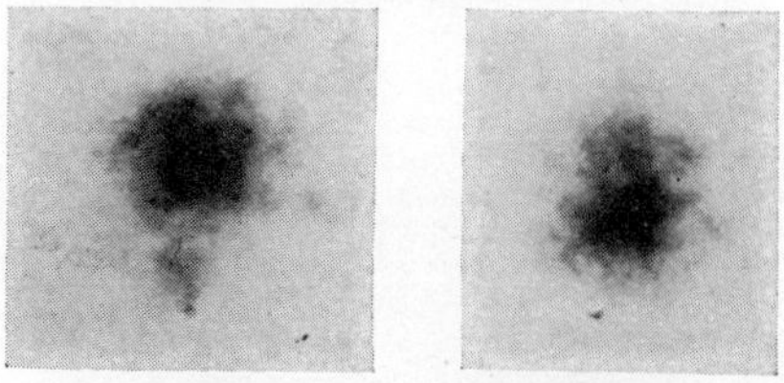

Oct. 28, 1919; colonies few; × 15.

Oct. 22; colonies few; × 15.

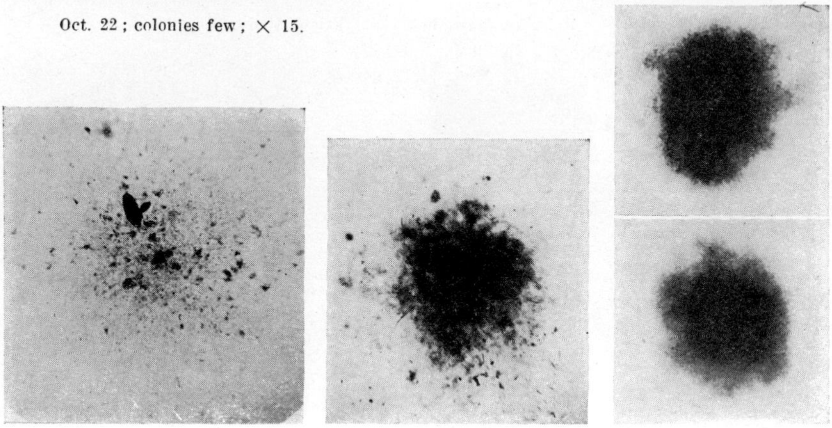

Strain TVP F. Strain TVP D.

Colonies few; × 15.

Fig. 4—The behavior of strain TVP. The upper 5 photographs show the inconsistent behavior of the strain. The lower ones, taken under identical conditions, show 2 types isolated from the original material in April, 1921.

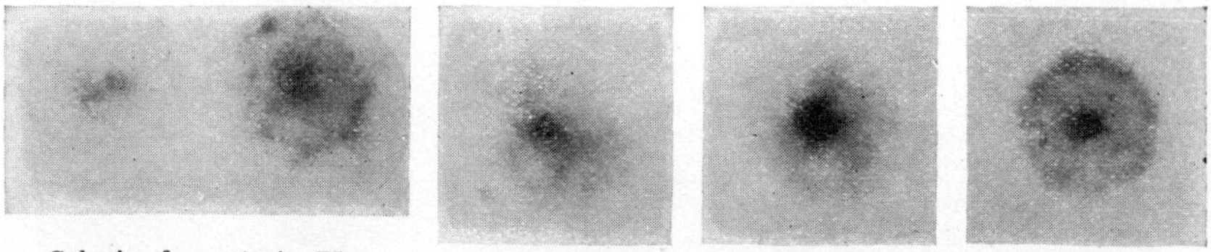

Colonies few; strain TL, December, 1919.

Colonies not numerous. Sole colony.
Strain TLB, April, 1921.

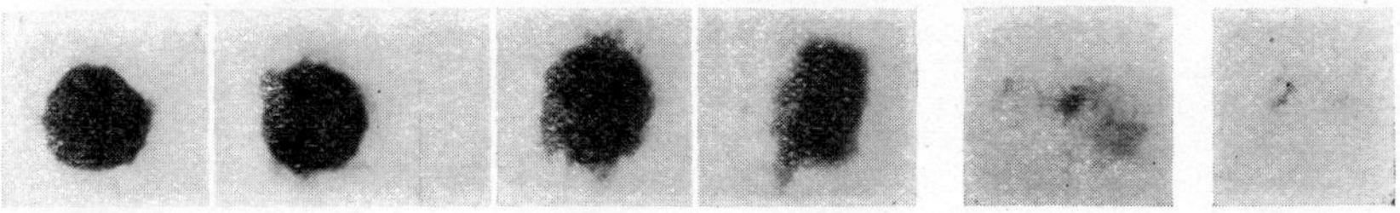

Strain TLC, April, 1921; colonies few.

July 7, 1919. Sept. 30, 1919.
Strain TMcC.

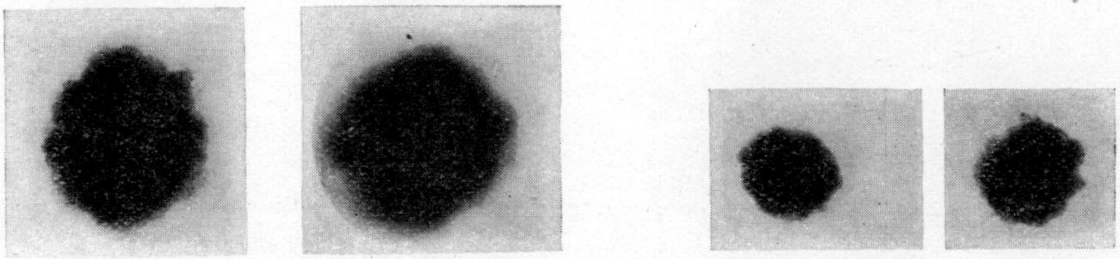

Strain T 220 W. Strain T 220 S.

Colonies not numerous.

Pairs of types noted at various times.

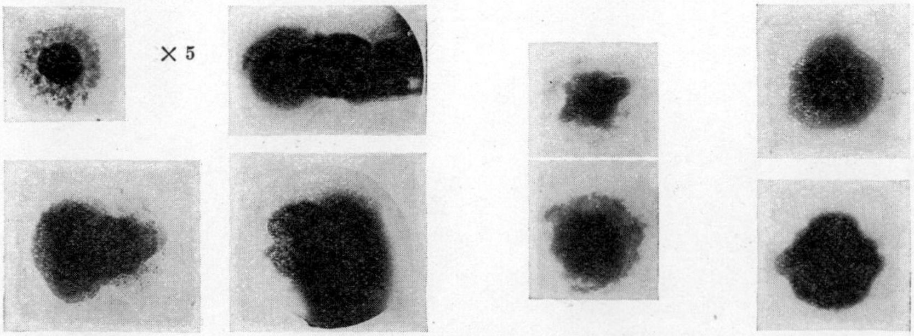

Fig. 5.—Simulated mutation strain T 220 S. This strain forms in 5 days colonies like the first (× 5) of this series. Cultures from the center gave dense woolly colonies (on the right) on stiff agar; cultures from the edge gave compound lenticular ones (the 3 flat colonies on the left) on soft agar. Subsequent transplants on the same batch of medium showed that the strains were identical. The two middle forms are from an intermediate medium. Colonies few; 48 hours old; × 15.

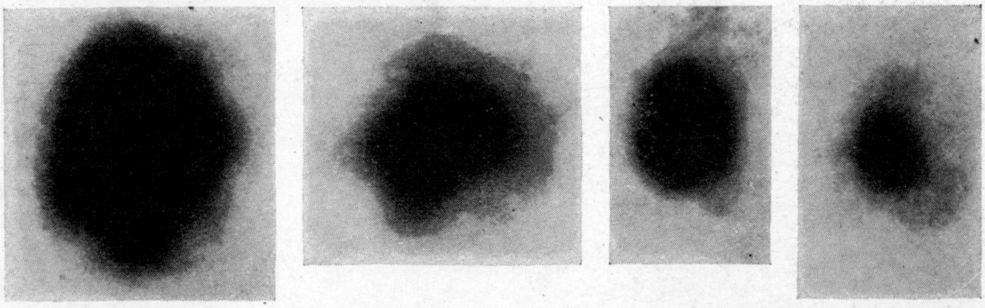

Strain VTW; colonies few. Colonies moderately abundant.

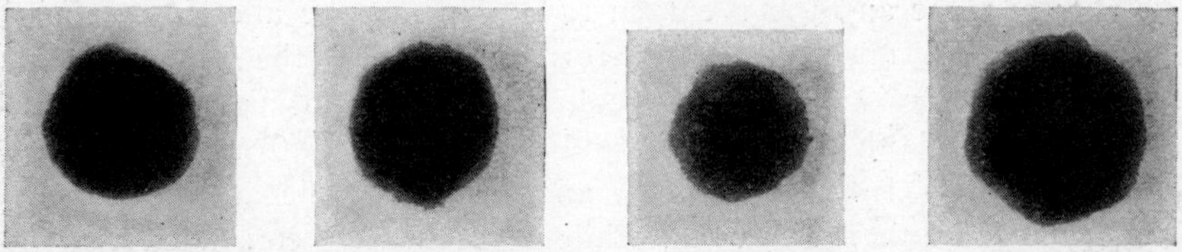

Strain VTS; colonies few.

Strain VT gave the two types when first observed in meat culture.

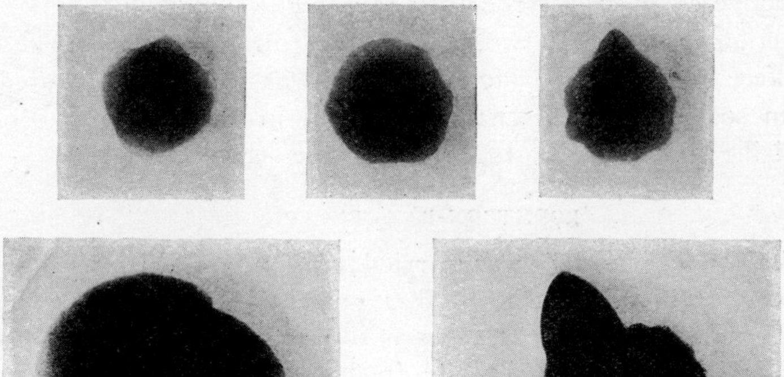

Fig. 6.—Strain TA: the upper colonies were taken in June, 1919, the lower ones in April, 1921, under approximately identical conditions; colonies few; × 50. It is obviously impossible to determine from these data whether mutation occurred or not.

THE EFFECT OF THE ROENTGEN RAY AND MUSTARD GAS (DICHLORETHYLSULPHID) ON ACTIVE ANAPHYLAXIS IN THE GUINEA-PIG

H. J. Corper; Louisa T. Black and Mary Moore

From the Research Department, National Jewish Hospital for Consumptives, Denver, Colo.

The importance attributed to allergy in the resistance to tuberculosis makes it advisable to study this state in as many ways as possible. In view of the report that certain leukotoxic agents, notably benzene and the roentgen ray, influence the allergic condition, a way seemed open to gain information as to the importance of allergy in the resistance to tuberculosis, especially as the guinea-pig is susceptible to both tuberculosis and sensitization. Corper [1] failed to note any effect from thorium x, another leukotoxic agent, on active anaphylaxis in the guinea-pig, while v. Heinrich [2] concluded that the formation of "sensibilisin" was reduced markedly by the roentgen ray, and was most marked when guinea-pigs were treated with the roentgen ray immediately after the sensitizing injection, the reinjection of foreign protein being given 3 weeks later, coincident with the maximum destructive effect of the roentgen ray on the lymphoid tissues. If the reinjection was given 6 weeks after treatment with the roentgen ray, the effect on the anaphylactic reaction was much less marked. The protein solution, horse serum, was used in amounts of 0.01 c c for sensitizing and from 0.05 to 0.5 c c for the second injection.

ROENTGEN-RAY EXPERIMENTS

The study reported was carried out on young male guinea-pigs weighing from about 250 to 300 gm. each, and the roentgen ray was given in three different doses as shown in the tables. Two separate protein mixtures, egg white and fresh normal horse serum were used to produce active anaphylaxis; in both cases the first injection consisted of 0.1 c c of sterile protein mixture mixed with 0.1 c c of sterile 0.9% sodium chloride solution, while the second injection was 1.0 c c of the sterile protein mixture and 1.0 c c of salt solution. These two proteins were chosen because in the doses used the egg white

Received for publication, Aug. 13, 1921.

[1] Jour. Infect. Dis., 1919, 25, p. 248.

[2] Centralbl. f. Bakteriol, O., 1, 1913, 70, p. 421.

produces a severe and frequently fatal anaphylaxis while the normal horse serum usually produces a definite but not fatal anaphylaxis, hence the effect of treatment with the roentgen ray on the anaphylactic reaction in the guinea-pigs could be noted easily. Leukocyte counts were made every second day to note the effect of the roentgen ray on the circulating leukocytes during the experiments. The results of these experiments with egg white are given in table 1. It is to be

TABLE 1
THE EFFECT OF ROENTGEN RAYS ON ANAPHYLAXIS IN THE GUINEA-PIG PRODUCED BY EGG WHITE *

Experiments	Roentgen-Ray Treatment		Maximum Reaction	Time of Maximum Reaction After Injection, Minutes	Lowest Leukocyte Count Attained	Time in Days of Lowest Leukocyte Count After Sensitization	Leukocyte Count on Day of Second Protein Injection
	Exposure	When Given					
Single large exposure	22 cm. spark gap; 5 milliamperes; target 30 cm. away, 15 minutes†	7 days before the first protein injection	+++	30	3,200	4	9,400
			Died	9	3,000	0	10,600
			++	45	4,800	4	8,400
		On same day as first injection	+++	40	4,000	10	10,200
			Died	35	5,600	6	11,400
			+	60	4,800	10	8,600
Repeated medium exposures	17 cm. spark gap; 5 milliamperes; target 30 cm., 15 minutes	Began 7 days before sensitization and repeated every 3 days to keep circulating leukocytes at a low level	Died	75	2,000	17	2,200
			+++	45	2,200	15	2,800
			Died	30	1,400	9	1,800
Repeated small exposures	8 cm. spark gap; 1 milliampere; target 30 cm., 3 minutes	Began 2 days before sensitization and repeated every 3 days throughout experiment	++	35	7,600	12	8,200
			+++	45 (died in 3 hours)	10,600	16	10,600
			+++	40	8,200	12	8,800
			++	60	8,000	18	9,200
Single large exposure	22 cm. spark gap; 5 milliamperes; target 30 cm., 15 minutes	7 days before the second protein injection	+++	35	5,600	19	5,600
			Died	20	6,200	18	6,400
			Died	60	6,000	18	6,200
		On same day as second protein injection	+++	45	.....	....	8,000
			+++	35	.....	....	11,000
			+++	45	.....	....	12,400
			++	20	.....	....	12,400
Controls...	....	....	+++	40			
			+++	25			
			+	45			

* The anaphylactic reaction obtained after the second protein injection is graded from — no reaction, mild +, moderate ++, and +++ a severe reaction with subsequent recovery of the animal. When the guinea-pig died during the acute reaction it is designated by "died." The interval between the first and second injection of egg white was 19 days. The first injection of protein, given intraperitoneally was 0.1 c c of egg white with 0.1 c c of salt solution and the second injection, given intraperitoneally, was 1 c c of egg white with 1 c c of salt solution.

† In the experiments in which the 22 cm. spark gap, 5 milliampere current for 15 minutes, or the 17 cm. spark gap, 5 milliampere current for 15 minutes, was used the exposure was made at 3 minute intervals with a 10 minute rest to cool the Coolidge tube.

noted that the maximum nonlethal dose of roentgen ray given before (7 days) or coincident with the first injection of egg white, or before (7 days) or with the second injection, had no ameliorating influence on the anaphylactic reaction after the second injection. Likewise,

TABLE 2

THE EFFECT OF ROENTGEN RAYS ON ANAPHYLAXIS IN THE GUINEA-PIG PRODUCED BY NORMAL HORSE SERUM *

Experiments	Roentgen-Ray Treatment		Maximum Reaction	Time of Maximum Reaction After Injection, Minutes	Lowest Leukocyte Count Attained	Time in Days of Lowest Leukocyte Count After Sensitization	Leukocyte Count on Day of Second Protein Injection
	Exposure	When Given					
Single large exposure	22 cm. spark gap; 5 milliamperes; target 30 cm. away, 15 minutes	7 days before the first protein injection	+++	45	5,200	8	9,200
			Died	50	2,800	1	8,000
			++	45	3,400	3	8,600
		On same day as first injection	++	50	6,000	6	12,000
			++	35	5,600	9	8,800
			+	50	4,400	8	10,400
Repeated medium exposures	17 cm. spark gap; 5 milliamperes; target 30 cm., 15 minutes	Began 7 days before sensitization and repeated every 3 days to keep circulating leukocytes at a low level	++	50 (died in 2.5 hours)	2,200	17	2,400
			+	50	1,200	2	2,000
			++	30	1,000	8	1,600
Repeated small exposures	8 cm. spark gap; 1 milliampere; target 30 cm., 3 minutes	Began 2 days before sensitization and repeated every 3 days throughout experiment	++	25	10,000	7	10 200
			++	40	8,200	17	8,200
			+	45	8,400	7	8,800
			+++	25	9,600	12	10,000
Single large exposure	22 cm. spark gap; 5 milliamperes; target 30 cm., 15 minutes	7 days before the second protein injection	++	45	7,200	19	7,200
			+++	35	5.800	17	6,000
			++	30	6,000	19	6,000
			+++	45	7,200	17	7,400
		On same day as second protein injection	++	50	.....	....	10,200
			+++	35	.....	....	10.200
			++	25	.....	....	12,400
			++	40	.....	....	9,800
Controls...	....	....	+++	30			
			+++	25			
			+	45			
			+	30			

* The anaphylactic reaction is graded as in table 1, from — to +++. The interval between the first and second injection of normal horse serum was 19 days. The first injection of protein given intraperitoneally was 0.1 c c of normal horse serum with 0.1 c c salt solution and the second injection of protein given intraperitoneally was 1 c c of normal horse serum with 1 c c of salt solution.

repeated moderate roentgen-ray treatments, sufficient to maintain the circulating leukocytes at about 2000 per c. mm. of peripheral blood, throughout the incubation period, or very small repeated treatments not noticeably affecting the peripheral leukocytes, had no appreciable ameliorating effect on the anaphylactic reaction. On the contrary, a slight increase in the severity of the reaction was noted, especially in those animals given the second injection when the roentgen ray had exerted a more profound effect as indicated by the level of the peripheral circulating leukocytes.

The results obtained with normal horse serum and roentgen-ray treatments were similar to those obtained with egg white and are given in table 2. The anaphylactic reaction following the second intraperitoneal injection of normal horse serum did not seem to be inhibited or reduced in the guinea-pigs that had been treated with the roentgen ray regardless of whether the treatment was a single large dose 7 days before or coincident with the first injection of horse serum, or before (7 days) or coincident with the second dose of serum. Repeated exposures to the roentgen ray sufficient to maintain a decided leukopenia throughout the incubation period or exposures insufficient to appreciably affect the peripheral leukocytes had no determinable effect on the anaphylactic reaction. When, however, the roentgen ray had exerted a profound effect on the hematopoietic system, as indicated by the reduction in the number of peripherally circulating leukocytes, the severity of the anaphylactic reaction seemed to be slightly increased.

MUSTARD GAS EXPERIMENTS

Mustard gas came into prominence as a result of its use in warfare and although its specific toxic action on the skin, conjunctiva and respiratory tract were recognized early, its action on the hematopoietic system remained undisclosed for some time. Krumbhaar and Krumbhaar [3] noted a direct toxic action on the bone marrow in gassed men, resulting in a depletion of the circulating leukocytes preceded by a preliminary leukocytosis. Pappenheimer and Vance [4] obtained similar results in rabbits; these findings were corroborated by Hektoen and Corper,[5] who found that mustard gas also has an inhibitory action on the development of specific antibodies in both rabbits and dogs, placing it in a class with leukotoxic agents like benzene, the roentgen ray and thorium x.

The study with mustard gas was carried out on young male guinea-pigs. The mustard gas was administered in solution, in 50%

[3] Jour. Amer. Med. Assn., 1919, 72, p. 39, and Jour. Med. Res., 1919, 40, p. 497.
[4] Jour. Exper. Med., 1920, 31, p. 72.
[5] Jour. Infect. Dis., 1921, 28, p. 279.

glycerol in 0.9% Na Cl solution, subcutaneously in 3 different doses as shown in the tables. The proteins used to produce anaphylaxis were egg white and normal horse serum, the mode of adminstration and dosage being the same as in the roentgen-ray experiments. Leukocyte

TABLE 3

THE EFFECT OF MUSTARD GAS ON ANAPHYLAXIS IN THE GUINEA-PIG PRODUCED BY EGG WHITE *

Experiments	Mustard Gas Injections		Maximum Reaction	Time of Maximum Reaction After Injection, Minutes	Lowest Leukocyte Count Attained	Time in Days of Lowest Leukocyte Count After Sensitization	Leukocyte Count on Day of Second Protein Injection
	Dose	When Given					
Single large dose	0.5 c c 0.2%	7 days before the first protein injection	Died	40	5,200	8	9,200
			+++	50	8,200	4	10.400
		On same day as first injection	+++	30	8,000	15	12,800
			+++	55	9,800	4	11,200
			+++	50	7,800	9	10,400
			+++	40	9,600	6	12,000
Repeated medium doses	0.5 c c 0.02%	Began 5 days before sensitization and repeated every 3 or 4 days throughout experiment	Died	80	9,600	4	12,400
			+++	45	6,000	8	10,400
			+++	40 (died in 3 hours)	4,000	12	7,800
			+++	55	6,600	15	7,200
Repeated small doses	0.5 c c 0.002%	Began 3 days before sensitization and repeated every 3 days throughout experiment	+++	40	6,200	20	6,200
			Died	55	8,400	12	9,200
			+++	45	9,400	4	14,800
			Died	105	6,000	12	8,000
Single large dose	0.5 c c 0.2%	7 days before the second protein injection	+++	35	10,000	17	10,000
			+++	45	7,200	17	8,000
			Died	2 hours	10,000	20	10,0C0
			+++	50	6,200	17	8,400
		On same day as second protein injection	+++	75	.....	....	11,800
			Died	25	.....	....	10,000
			+++	45 (died in 3 hours)	.....	....	13,600
			+++	55	.....	....	13,800
Controls...	....	....	+++	40	.....	....	13,200
			Died	35	.....	....	8,800
			+++	55	.....	....	10,800
			Died	75	.....	....	12,400

* The anaphylactic reaction in this table and table 4 is graded as in table 1, from — to +++. The interval between the first and second injection of egg white was 20 days. The first injection of protein given intraperitoneally was 0.1 c c of egg white with 0.1 c c salt solution and the second injection of protein given intraperitoneally was 1 c c of egg white with 1 c c of salt solution.

counts were made every second day during the experiments, the last count on the day of and preceding the second protein injection. The results of these experiments are given in tables 3 and 4.

Mustard gas does not produce as profound effects on the leukocytes in the guinea-pig as the roentgen ray or thorium x, especially in doses consistent with the life of the animal, and it may produce a leukocytosis. The results seem to indicate, however, that like the roentgen ray and thorium x, mustard gas has no appreciable influence on the allergic or anaphylactic reaction whether given subcutaneously 7 days before

TABLE 4
THE EFFECT OF MUSTARD GAS ON ANAPHYLAXIS IN THE GUINEA-PIG PRODUCED BY NORMAL HORSE SERUM

Experiments	Mustard Gas Injections		Maximum Reaction	Time of Maximum Reaction After Injection, Minutes	Lowest Leukocyte Count Attained	Time in Days of Lowest Leukocyte Count After Sensitization	Leukocyte Count on Day of Second Protein Injection
	Dose	When Given					
Single large dose	0.5 c c 0.2%	7 days before the first protein injection	+++	40 (died in 3 hours)	5,000	8	12,000
			+++	60	6,800	2	11,200
		On same day as first injection	+++	35	6,200	9	9,600
			+++	60	8,200	6	10.000
			+++	60	9,400	9	14,800
			++	40	6,600	6	9,200
Repeated medium doses	0.5 c c 0.02%	Began 5 days before sensitization and repeated every 3 or 4 days throughout experiment	+++	45	8,000	8	11,000
			+++	50	6,000	15	6,200
			Died	110	6,000	12	10,600
			+++	60	8,400	8	9,000
Repeated small doses	0.5 c c 0.002%	Began 3 days before sensitization and repeated every 3 days throughout experiment	++	45	9,800	15	11,600
			+++	35	8,400	15	12,800
			+++	55	7,000	4	9,800
			+++	45	5,200	4	10.200
Single large dose	0.5 c c 0.2%	7 days before the second protein injection	++	60	7,400	20	7,400
			Died	90	7,200	20	7,200
			++	45	9,600	15	11,200
			+++	50	9,000	17	9,400
		On same day as second protein injection	++	35	.....	....	10,000
			++	55	.....	....	8,200
			+++	60	.....	....	14,200
			+++	50	.....	....	7,600
Controls...	....	....	+++	40	.....	....	9,600
			++	50	.....	....	11,400
			+++	60 (died in 3 hours)	.....	....	12,000
			+++	45	.....	....	10,000

or coincident with the first protein injection or 7 days before or with the second injection, in maximum nonlethal doses. Likewise, repeated small or medium doses throughout the entire incubation period and initiated a few days before the primary injection are without appreciable effect.

DISCUSSION

Von Heinrich[2] was inclined to view his results as indicating that the roentgen ray restrained the formation of the "sensibilisin" by its action on the lymphoid tissues and interference with antibody formation. If we were certain that anaphylaxis is of antigen-antibody nature, we might be able to draw more definite conclusions regarding the effect of the roentgen ray on the antibodies concerned. Hektoen and his colleagues[6] found that not all antibodies were affected equally by leukotoxic agents; thorium x may interfere with the production of precipitin but not of lysin. Thus we are confronted with the possibility that the antibodies, if such they are, involved in the complicated reaction of anaphylaxis may belong to the class of those not appreciably influenced in vivo by the roentgen ray, or it may be that the crudeness of the quantitative estimation in the anaphylactic reaction makes it impossible to detect slight differences as is possible in the estimations of lysins, precipitins and agglutinins. There is another consideration to which Corper[1] called attention in his work on thorium x and anaphylaxis, namely, that we are dealing with a chronic poisoning by the roentgen ray, whose action, combined with that of the anaphylaxis may slightly increase the severity of the latter, especially when the reaction is precipitated at the height of the action of the roentgen ray.

SUMMARY

In guinea-pigs a maximum nonlethal dose of roentgen ray given 7 days before or coincident with the sensitizing injection of egg white or normal horse serum, or 7 days before or with the second injection, causes no appreciable ameliorating influence on the reaction resulting from the second injection of these proteins. Likewise, repeated moderate roentgen ray treatments, sufficient to maintain a low level of the peripheral circulating leukocytes, about 2,000 leukocytes per c mm, throughout the incubation period, or very small repeated treatments not noticeably affecting the number of peripheral circulating leukocytes, has no appreciable ameliorating effect on the severity of the anaphylactic reaction. A slight increase in the severity of the reaction was noted, however, especially in guinea-pigs given the second or exciting injection of protein when the roentgen ray had exerted a profound influence on the hematoipoetic system as indicated by the

[6] Jour. Infect. Dis., 1916, 19, p. 69; 1915, 17, p. 415; 1918, 22, p. 28; 1920, 26, p. 330.

level of the leukocytes. As pointed out by Corper in the case of thorium x and anaphylaxis, this result may be due to the intoxication with the roentgen ray coincidently with the anaphylactic reaction.

Subcutaneous injections of mustard gas in maximum nonlethal doses given 7 days before or coincident with the sensitizing injection of egg white or normal horse serum, or 7 days before, or with the second injection, are without appreciable influence on the reaction resulting from the second injection of these proteins. Likewise, repeated small or medium doses administered throughout the incubation period, being initiated a few days before the first protein injection, are without appreciable effect.

CULTIVATION OF TUBERCLE BACILLI

E. Louis Goodman and Mary Moore

Research Department, National Jewish Hospital for Consumptives, Denver

The factors, respiratory and nutritional, which influence the growth of the tubercle bacillus in the test tube are numerous and complicated. The literature is burdened with reports on methods to hasten the development of this bacillus both in the culture tube and in the animal body. The true tubercle bacillus, however, persists in growing slowly and a careful analysis of the available studies reveals that there are many sources of misinterpretation, especially when it is reported that it can be grown luxuriantly within a few days. In such cases the organisms are usually not pathogenic and frequently prove to be some other acid-fast organism, the mere property of acid-fastness being used to classify them erroneously as tubercle bacilli. Thus, we have heard that certain animal tissues and other substances incorporated into mediums have an especially hastening influence on the growth of these organisms. In spite of these reports, reliable laboratories continue to grow tubercle bacilli on certain simple standard mediums, i.e., glycerol agar, Dorset's egg medium or modifications thereof, inspissated serums and glycerol broth.[1] When Nocard and Roux [2] found that the addition of glycerol to the medium markedly enhanced the growth of human tubercle bacilli, a decided progress was made, while Dorset's [3] introduction of the egg medium gave the laboratory a universally obtainable and easily preserved material for suitable medium for this bacillus.

In 1915 Petroff [4] described his method for the primary cultivation of human tubercle bacilli from contaminated material, such as sputum and feces, in which the material is given a preliminary treatment with an equal volume of 3% sodium hydroxide solution for 20 to 30 minutes at incubator temperature and, after removal of the alkali the residue seeded on Dorset's egg medium containing a 1:10,000 dilution of gentian violet to inhibit the development of organisms not killed by the sodium hydroxide. He isolated the tubercle bacillus from 129 of

Received for publication, August 13, 1921.

[1] Corper, H. J.: Amer. Rev. Tuberc., 1919, 3, p. 461.
[2] Ann. de l'inst. Pasteur, 1887, 1, p. 19.
[3] Amer. Med., 1902, 3, p. 555.
[4] Jour. Exper. Med., 1915, 21, p. 38.

135 sputum specimens.[5] Stewart[6] obtained cultures by Petroff's method from 24 of 37 sputums positive microscopically. Corper, Fiala and Kallen[7] in cultivating 526 microscopically positive sputums obtained macroscopic cultures in only 27.3% (144). At that time no discrepancies could be found in the procedure used by them, and Petroff's high percentage could not be accounted for since the mediums and details of technic used were well controlled.[8] In recent observations by Corper, Gauss and Rensch[9] it was found that carbon dioxide in concentrations as low as 3% can inhibit the growth of tubercle bacilli and that bacilli seeded on glycerol agar contained in fairly large culture tubes (6x1 inches) and subsequently glass sealed and incubated would not grow sufficiently to be visible macroscopically, while the contained gases would reach about 5% carbon dioxide concentration. These observations made it seem highly desirable to study the effect of tin-foil capping on the growth of tubercle bacilli in tubes, it being thought that the tin-foil capping may possibly prevent ready access of air to the cultures and thus the amount of carbon dioxide developed by the bacilli and retained in the tube rise sufficiently to account for some of the negative cultures in the observations cited. In order to study the effect of this part of the manipulation 100 culture tubes (5/8 by 6 inches) similar to those used in the routine cultivation of tubercle bacilli from the sputum, were prepared with a sterile 5% glycerol agar slant, neutral to litmus, sterilized by autoclaving, and 100 tubes of the same size containing a sterile slant of egg medium with 1 : 10,000 dilution of gentian violet (Petroff), sterilized by inspissation. After inoculation these tubes were divided into groups of 20 of each medium, half of which were stoppered with paraffined cotton and then covered with paraffined cloth to prevent the medium from drying out and to allow easy access of atmospheric air, and the other half stoppered with paraffin cotton stoppers and then carefully covered with tin-foil using every precaution to avoid tears or breaks in the tin-foil and to seal as tightly as possible by using 3 small rubber bands tightly drawn around the top of the culture tube and tin-foil cover. Each set of 20 of one kind of medium was inoculated with a separate culture of tubercle bacilli. The cultures used were 3 human cultures, one old laboratory avirulent strain "human," and two recently isolated virulent human

[5] Bull. Johns Hopkins Hosp., 1915, 26, p. 276.
[6] Jour. Exper. Med., 1917, 26, p. 755.
[7] J. Infect. Dis., 1918, 23, p. 267.
[8] Personal communication.
[9] J. Amer. Med. Assn., 1921, 76, p. 1216, and Amer. Rev. Tuberc., 1921, 5, p. 562.

strains "Gluckson" and "Weisbrod," and 2 bovine strains, an old laboratory culture "Bov. D" and a recently isolated culture "Bov. V." The tubes were read after one and two months' incubation at 37.5 C. (table 1).

TABLE 1

THE GROWTH OF TUBERCLE BACILLI ON GLYCEROL AGAR AND PETROFF'S MEDIUM IN CULTURE TUBES WITH PARAFFINED AND TIN-FOIL CAPS

Culture	Medium	Tube Sealed with	Number of Culture Tube: Growth One Month After Inoculation										Growth Two Months After Inoculation									
			1	2	3	4	5	6	7	8	9	10	1	2	3	4	5	6	7	8	9	10
"Human"	Glycerol agar	P	3	3	3	2	2	2	1	1	0	C	4	4	4	4	4	4	4	4	4	C
		T	3	2	2	2	2	2	1	1	1	0	4	4	4	4	4	4	4	4	4	3
	Petroff's	P	3	3	2	2	2	2	2	1	1	1	4	4	4	4	4	4	4	3d	3d	2d
		T	3	2	2	2	1	1	1	1	0	C	4	4	4	4	4	4	4	4	3	C
"Gluckson"	Glycerol agar	P	3	3	3	3	3	3	3	3	3	2	4	4	4	4	4	4	4	4	4	4
		T	3	3	3	3	3	3	2	2	2	2	4	4	4	4	4	4	4	4	4	4
	Petroff's	P	3	3	3	3	2	2	2	1	0	0	4	4	4	4	4	4	2	2	1d	0d
		T	3	3	3	3	3	2	2	2	2	0	4	4	4	4	4	3	3	3	2	2
"Weisbrod"	Glycerol agar	P	3	2	2	2	1	1	1	1	0	0	4	4	4	4	4	4	4	3d	3	3
		T	3	2	2	2	2	1	1	1	1	1	4	4	4	4	4	4	4	3	3	2d
	Petroff's	P	0	0	0	0	0	0	0	0	0	0	4	4	4	3	2	1	1	0	0	0
		T	1	0	0	0	0	0	0	0	0	0	4	4	4	4	4	3	1	1C	C	0
"Bov. D."	Glycerol agar	P	2	2	2	1	1	1	1	1	1	1	4	4	4	4	4	4	4	4	4	4
		T	2	2	1	1	1	1	1	1	1	C	4	4	4	4	4	4	4	4	4	C
	Petroff's	P	3	3	2	2	2	2	2	2	2	1	4	4	4	4	4	4	4	4	2d	2C
		T	3	3	3	3	2	2	2	2	2	2	4	4	4	4	4	4	4	4	4	4
"Bov. V."	Glycerol agar	P	2	2	2	2	2	1	1	1	1	0	4	4	4	4	4	4	4	4	3	3
		T	2	2	2	2	1	1	1	1	1	0	4	4	4	4	4	4	4	4	4	3
	Petroff's	P	3	3	3	3	3	3	3	2	2	1	4	4	4	4	4	4	4	4	4	3d
		T	3	3	3	3	3	3	3	3	2	2	4	4	4	4	4	4	4	4	4	4

The tubes in line P were stoppered with sterile cotton plugs dipped in sterile melted paraffine and covered with paraffine cloth held in place by a rubber band.

The tubes in line T were stoppered with sterile cotton plugs dipped in sterile melted paraffin and covered carefully with tin-foil snugly bound with three small rubber bands.

The figures indicate the amount of growth in the culture tube and are graded from "0" indicating no growth to "4" indicating a luxuriant and maximum growth. "C" indicates the culture was contaminated and "d" after a numeral indicates the medium dried up and growth indicated by the numeral is still visible.

Table 1 reveals that tin-foil capping held in place by rubber bands drawn as tightly as possible around the neck of the culture tube planted with tubercle bacilli does not seal these tubes well enough to permit an accumulation of sufficient of the respiratory gases (carbon dioxide) to in any way inhibit or prevent the growth of these bacilli. The tin-foil capping can, therefore, not account for the negative cultures (72.7% of positive microscopic sputums) obtained by Corper, Fiala and Kallen.

The tubercle bacillus was originally grown by Koch on inspissated blood serum mediums. Being a surface grower, an aerobe, it does not do so well in liquid mediums, so that unless special purposes are in view, such as the preparation of "old tuberculin," it is usual to grow the bacillus on either an inspissated serum or egg medium or glycerol agar. On glycerol broth prepared in the same way as glycerol agar with the exception that the agar is omitted, the cultures usually require a longer time to become luxuriant and frequent cultural failures are obtained. The factors involved in these differences in the results obtained on the two mediums may be due to the difficulty in obtaining satisfactory surface seeding in the glycerol broth, the tendency of the glycerol broth to form a liquid film about the bacilli preventing satisfactory respiratory exchange, the differences in physical composition of the two mediums and probably other equally important factors. In order to obviate the difficulty of surface seeding in broth cultures a number of suggestions have been made, i. e., to rub the culture on the glass at the liquid level, to use a small amount of serum which has been coagulated at the liquid level on the glass, to put cotton into the medium, etc. Comparative studies on these points are, however, lacking. It is also to be noted that small lumps of tubercle bacilli are more apt to give cultures than fine emulsions. Recently Masucci[10] found that the addition of amino-acids in the form of "aminoids" (Arlington Chemical Co.) to the ordinary glycerol broth markedly increased and hastened the growth of tubercle bacilli on this medium. The glycerol broth he used was prepared from fresh meat juice to which were added 1.7% "Difco" peptone and 0.3% "aminoids." From the standpoint of technic a test of the value of the addition of "aminoids" to broth for growing tubercle bacilli seemed worth while. Two types of "aminoids," beef aminoids with 75% amino-nitrogen, biuret free, and milk (casein) aminoids with 65% amino-nitrogen were used in these experiments. In the first experiment ordinary glycerol broth, prepared from meat juice, peptone and glycerol, neutral to litmus was made and put into 250 c c sterile cotton stoppered nursing bottles in amounts of about 90 c c. To test the value of the beef blood "aminoids" this was added to the broth in 0.3% amounts, after which the reaction was again adjusted to neutrality to litmus. The broth was then put into bottles in 90 c c amounts, the mediums were sterilized by autoclaving and were then planted with

[10] Jour. Lab. & Clin. Med., 1920, 6, p. 96.

an avirulent laboratory "human" strain, and "Gluckson," a virulent recently isolated culture. In the same way 0.3% milk "aminoids" were added to the broth, and the bottles were planted with the tubercle bacilli. The bottles were kept at 37.5 C. for two months with the results recorded in table 2.

TABLE 2

THE EFFECT OF THE ADDITION OF "AMINOIDS" TO GLYCEROL BOUILLON ON THE GROWTH OF HUMAN TUBERCLE BACILLI

Tubercle Bacilli	"Aminoids"	Series	Glycerol Bouillon Culture Flasks		
			1	2	3
"Human"	Beef	Controls	+++*	+++	+
		Test	—	—	—
	Casein	Controls	++	++	+
		Test	+++	++	—
"Gluckson"	Beef	Controls	+++	+++	++
		Test	—	—	—
	Casein	Controls	+++	++	++
		Test	++	+	

* The culture flasks after inoculation were incubated at 37.5 C. for two months after which the readings were made and recorded. — Indicates no growth and +++ a luxuriant maximum growth covering the entire surface of the broth. The flasks were observed at weekly intervals throughout the period of incubation.

These results do not indicate that the addition of "aminoids" in 0.3% amount to the ordinary glycerol broth in any way hastened the growth of human tubercle bacilli. There would seem to be rather a retarding (as noted with the beef "aminoids") effect on the growth, indicating that there are probably other factors instrumental in determining the rate or luxuriance of growth rather than the mere presence or absence of amino acids in the form of "aminoids." Complete studies of the metabolism and chemistry of the tubercle bacillus, such as are being carried on by Long,[11] and comparative culture rate experiments carefully controlled as suggested by our study will throw more light on the exact conditions necessary for the maximum growth of the tubercle bacillus in different mediums.

SUMMARY

The human tubercle bacillus grows equally well on culture tubes containing slants of glycerol agar or egg medium (Petroff's) regardless of whether the tubes have been capped with waxed cloth or with tin-foil, securely held in place with rubber bands, thus indicating a

[11] Am. Rev. Tuberc., 1920, 4, p. 842.

ready access of atmospheric air in the folds of the tin-foil in spite of precautions to prevent this means of the escape of the carbon dioxide produced by the respiration of the bacilli. Tin-foil capping does not account for the low percentage (27.3%) positive cultures obtained by Corper, Fiala and Kallen in cultivating microscopically positive sputums. The addition of "aminoids" beef or casein to the ordinary laboratory glycerol broth has no appreciable effect on the growth of human tubercle bacilli on this medium; such an addition may even markedly retard the growth of the bacilli as was found to be the case with beef "aminoids."

SPIROCHETAL ORGANISMS IN THE TISSUES IN ACUTE YELLOW ATROPHY OF THE LIVER

N. Hayashi and T. Kibata

From the Department of Pathology of the College of Physicians and Surgeons, Columbia University, and the Pathological Laboratory of the Presbyterian Hospital, New York

In the course of our study of a typical case of acute yellow atrophy of the liver in the Presbyterian Hospital, New York, we have been able to demonstrate histologically the occurrence of a species of spirochete in the tissues. In view of the possible etiologic interest of the finding, its brief description will be given in the present paper.

MATERIAL AND METHODS

Material for the present study came from a man, 27 years old, admitted Oct. 13, who died Oct. 16, 1919. Clinically, the case was one of acute yellow atrophy of the liver with typical symptoms. The total duration of the illness was one week. Necropsy two hours after death, and microscopic examinations further demonstrated typical acute yellow atrophy of the liver. In addition, general jaundice, multiple capillary hemorrhages of the peritoneum, lung, liver, kidney, pelvis, stomach and duodenum, bronchopneumonia of the left lobule, and pleuritic adhesions, edema of the lungs, acute tubular nephritis, fatty liver, heart and kidney were noted.

Inoculation and cultures of postmortem material, made by Dr. Hideyo Noguchi, failed to demonstrate Leptospira ictero-hemorrhagica in this case.

Various tissues were stained by Giemsa as well as with the Levaditi methods, and were carefully examined microscopically.

Intestines.—Widely scattered in the necrotic tissue of the intestine were found groups of long threadlike organisms, measuring 10-12 microns, staining reddish violet with Giemsa stain. These elongated organisms were clearly brought out also by Levaditi stain.

Liver.—A number of rod or thread-like organisms, measuring 2-4 microns, similar to those that were seen in the intestine, were found in the necrotic tissue of the liver. In addition, numerous minute bodies of diplococcoid or diphtheroid type, were found intra- as well as inter-cellularly. These minute bodies show polar staining with

Received for publication Aug. 18, 1921.

Giemsa stain, resembling the Prowaschek's body in typhus. Morphologically, there is a series of forms which may be transitional between the long thread-like and coccoid forms. The coccoid body was not demonstrated by the Levaditi method.

Kidney.—The necrotic epithelium of the tubules showed typical examples of a spiral organism, in addition to the two types of bodies as seen in the liver. The spiral form is well stained by the Levaditi method and is seen to consist of 10-15 curves. It measures 8-25 microns (Fig. 4).

Pancreas.—Coccoid bodies were found in abundance, especially in association with blood vessels. Some of these bodies were slightly elongated, approaching the thread-like form seen in the liver (Fig. 3).

Through the kindness of Dr. Symmers, cases of epidemic acute hemorrhagic jaundice in the Bellevue Hospital, New York, have been studied for comparison. These cases in which Leptospira icterohemorrhagica could not be demonstrated directly or by inoculation have been reported by Dr. Symmers.[1] In 3 of 6 of these cases, we found three types of bodies similar to those that were just described. These bodies occurred in the pancreas, liver and intestine, but were particularly abundant in the kidney.

Control examinations have been made of normal human intestines (5 cases), normal guinea-pigs (10 cases), and the intestine of a man with an undetermined type of spirochetal infection. It has not been possible to demonstrate in any of this material the types of bodies that we found in the acute yellow atrophy of the liver.

DISCUSSION

That the coccoid body is not a bacterium may be judged from the occurrence of two or more chromatic spots and from the positive Levaditi reaction. It is more like the Prowaschek's body in typhus. Morphologic intergradation among the three types of bodies described suggests that they may represent stages in the life cycle of a single species of organism, namely, that of a spirochete. In connection with this assumption, it may be mentioned that Fry and Balfour[2] in the spirochetal infection of the fowl, and Kitogawa and Mukoyama,[3] in the rat-bite fever, have described the development of typical spiral organisms out of the granular forms.

[1] Jour. Am. Med. Assn., 1920, 74, p. 1153.
[2] Parasitology, 1912.
[3] Arch. Int. Med., 1917, 20, p. 318.

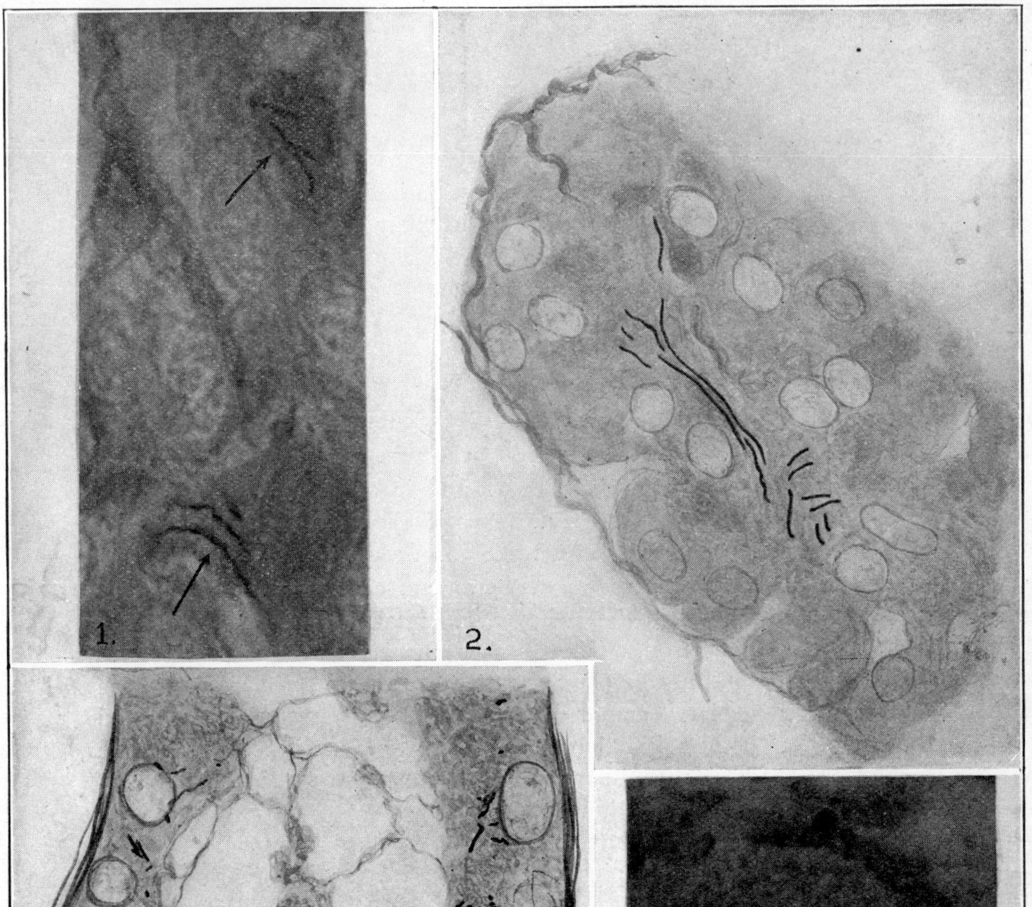

Fig. 1.—Pancreas, showing about a dozen thread-like forms, and one typical spiral form. This illustration and fig. 2 were drawn from Levaditi material.

Fig. 2.—Kidney, showing several thread-like forms, in addition to coccoid ones, in the epithelium of the tubule. Some of the thread-like forms show curves.

Fig. 3.—Pancreas; several thread-like and spiral forms on the left. Three spirals on the right. This illustration and fig. 4 were photographed from Levaditi material.

Fig. 4.—Kidney; a typical spiral form with several curves.

It is not possible on the basis of the present findings alone to determine the etiologic significance of the spirochete in acute yellow atrophy of the liver. However, in view of the fact that the organism was most abundant in the liver, where the lesion was most prominent, and less abundant in the intestines, kidneys, and pancreas, which showed only slight lesions, it is at least conceivable that the organism may be etiologically related to the disease. It may be said as a general rule, that the relative abundance of an etiologic agent is parallel with the degree of severity of the lesion.

SUMMARY

What appears to be the stages in the life cycle of a species of spirochete have been demonstrated in the liver and certain other affected organs from a typical case of acute yellow atrophy of the liver. While the definite etiologic relation of the organism to the disease cannot at once be determined, the parallelism existing between the abundance of the organism and severity of the lesion suggests the probability of such a relation.

JOHNE'S DISEASE AND ITS DETECTION

B. A. Beach and E. G. Hastings

From the College of Agriculture, University of Wisconsin, Madison

The condition to which the name Johne's disease is commonly applied has been called by some chronic dysentery. It has also been called paratuberculosis. The first of these names owes it origin to the German veterinarian who, together with Frothingham of this country, discovered the causal organism in 1895. The second name reflects one of the most striking symptoms of the disease, while the third term expresses the group relationship of the organism which is one of the acidfast bacilli. It would seem that the name Johne's disease is preferable to the others, since it is the term that has been used most widely. A multiplicity of names leads to confusion.

The disease has been studied by Meyer who gives a complete bibliography.[1] The papers to which reference is made in this article have been published mostly since 1913. The most extended study of the various aspects of the disease have been made by M'Fadyean,[2] and his associates. The work of M'Fadyean relates to the experimental transmission of the disease, to its histology and to its detection by means of a product, johnin, prepared from the specific organism. In the isolation and cultivation of this organism, and in the preparation of johnin, M'Fadyean followed the path originally marked by Twort and Ingram.[3]

Johnin has been used by the investigators referred to on animals showing evident symptoms of the disease and on animals artificially infected. The present paper deals primarily with the tests of entire herds with this product. The purpose was to determine whether an infected herd could be freed from the disease by its use, as a herd can be freed from tuberculosis by the use of tuberculin. The results obtained will not permit us to give a definite answer to this question. They are presented with the hope of attracting attention to a disease which is apparently becoming more widespread in our country each year.

Distribution.—Comparatively little is known concerning the extent of the disease in the great cattle-producing countries. Attention has

Received for publication Aug. 20, 1921.

[1] Jour. Med. Research, 1913, 29, p. 147.

[2] Jour. Comp. Path. and Therap., 25, 1912, p. 217; 29, 1916, pp. 62, 134 and 201; 31, 1918, p. 73.

[3] Johne's disease, 1913.

been directed to it chiefly by the work of investigators rather than by the losses it occasions. The work concerning the disease has been done chiefly in Switzerland by Meyer, in Denmark by Bang, and in England by M'Faydean and others. The extent to which the disease is present in these countries has scarcely been mentioned by the writers. The importance of the disease in Denmark is reflected in this statement credited to Bang: "The future of a certain breed of dairy cattle in Denmark depends on the ability to eliminate Johne's disease."

The disease was first reported in this country in 1908 by Leonard Pearson of Philadelphia who found acid-fast bacilli in a piece of thickened intestine from an animal which had shown clinical manifestations of Johne's disease. Since that time it has been reported from several parts of the country. Meyer, following his work in Switzerland, studied the disease in this country. He made no observations on the frequency of occurrence. Our experience has led us to believe that the disease is more prevalent than has been supposed, especially in the pure bred herds. Our present information indicates that the disease is spreading quite rapidly through the transfer of animals from herd to herd and that the disease is one that the breeder will be forced to consider because of the economic loss it will occasion.

TABLE 1

LOSSES OCCASIONED BY JOHNE'S DISEASE

Herd	Number in Herd	Duration of Infection	Animals Removed from Herd on Account of Disease	Percentage of Yearly Loss
1	50	17 years	41	4.7
2	40	15 years	20	2.2
3	35	10 years	22	6.2
4	18	10 years	22	12.0

The history of losses occasioned by this disease in a number of herds with which we have worked is presented in summary form in table 1. A yearly loss of from 2 to 12% extending over a period of years is a serious matter.

It seems probable that animals are being removed from many herds because of this disease without its nature being recognized. The slow development, the inconstancy of the most marked symptom, diarrhea, and the gradual loss of flesh by the animal are not likely to cause the owner to suspect that he has a transmissible disease in his herd. The animal is sold for slaughter, and the cause of its decline passes unrecognized. The slow spread of the disease in the herd again militates against the recognition of its transmissible nature and makes difficult any estimation of the losses caused by it.

The disease is one unknown to many veterinarians and therefore passes unrecognized by them, a fact that interferes with gaining knowledge of its occurrence.

Isolation of Johne's Bacillus.—The cultivation of the organism by Twort, and the preparation by Twort, and Ingram of johnin, an agent similar in many respects to tuberculin, led us to attempt the isolation of the organism.

In the summer of 1915 tissues were received from an animal that supposedly had died of Johne's disease. The infection had been known to be present in the herd for a number of years. Cultures were made from the wall of the intestine and from the mesenteric lymph nodes on nutrient agar which contained human tubercle bacilli and to which sterile blood serum had been added, following the method of Twort and Ingram. Out of a large number of tubes, 2 showed no development of rapidly growing saprophytic organisms. After several months' incubation both of these tubes showed in stained preparations such numbers of acid-fast organisms corresponding to the description given by Twort and Ingram that it seemed probable that actual growth of the Johne's bacillus had taken place in the tubes. The growth was so slight that from the macroscopic appearance of the agar cultures, one could not be certain that reproduction had occurred. Transfers were made to slopes of the same medium. After several months' incubation, it seemed certain that growth had taken place in the subcultures. The organism has been maintained on agar of similar composition for approximately 6 years. With prolonged cultivation the growth has become more free until at present the organism may be said to give a fair growth.

The growth of the organism is very erratic. At one time and on one batch of medium the growth may be excellent, as measured by the growth of such an organism as the tubercle bacillus. At another time and on another batch of medium of composition similar to the other, the growth will be most meager. This inconsistency of growth has been noted by others.

From our most recent results it seems probable that the medium is a more important factor in determining the profuseness of growth than is the period during which the culture has been grown on artificial medium. Apparently some slight variation in the medium exerts a marked influence on the growth of the organism. It is hoped that further work may make the cultivation of the organism an easier task. Under present conditions the preparation of any considerable amounts of johnin is very difficult. A medium which would insure a certain and good growth of the organism would be of great assistance in overcoming this difficulty.

With the hope of securing some of the diagnostic agent, johnin, transfers were made to a liquid medium the base of which consisted of the broth in which certain nonpathogenic acid-fast organisms had grown. After nine months' incubation it was apparent that growth had occurred. In the liquid medium the organism occurred in small masses at the bottom of the flasks. There was no clouding of the medium, even on shaking. The organism has also been maintained in the liquid medium. After many trials a surface growth in liquid medium was secured. It was thought that a surface growth might be more profuse than that beneath the surface and thus a johnin of greater potency be secured. It has not been possible up to the present to maintain the growth on the surface of the medium as is so easily done with tubercle cultures, when the surface growth is once obtained.

As the culture became somewhat more free growing, efforts were made to cultivate it in mediums to which no blood serum had been added or which contained serum heated to 55 C. Very little, if any, growth was obtained in such mediums. The raw serum seems to be an essential ingredient of the medium. Horse serum has been used exclusively in this work.

In June, 1917, an opportunity was presented to test a herd known to be infected with this disease. The results of this test led to a continuation of the work. The detailed description of the methods now used for the preparation of the johnin follows. As far as we are aware, this was the first time johnin had been used in this country, and, so far as we are aware, was the first test of an entire herd.

Avian tuberculin has been used by a number of investigators both in this country and abroad following the suggestion of Bang. There is no indication in the nature of the disease to relate its cause to the avian tubercle bacillus, and there would seem to be equally as few reasons for believing that a tuberculin made with the avian tubercle bacillus would prove a valuable diagnostic agent. The results of a number of investigators have shown that avian tuberculin will give positive reactions in a portion of the animals manifesting clinical symptoms. There is, however, no positive indication that avian tuberculin will reveal the disease in the less advanced cases.

The identity of the culture which we have isolated and used rests largely on its cultural characters, on its morphology and staining reactions, and on what is more important, the preparation of an agent which seems to be specific for the diagnosis of Johne's disease. The isolation of an acidfast bacillus from what are apparently lesions of Johne's disease is inadequate proof that the true Johne's bacillus has been obtained. A number of investigators speak of having isolated Johne's bacillus and say that the culture grew rapidly and profusely. It would seem from our experience and from that of others that such cultures must have been other types of acidfast bacilli, for certainly exceedingly slow and meager growth is one of the most striking characteristics of the Johne's baccilus.

Preparation of Johnin.—The basal portion of the medium is a broth in which certain nonpathogenic acidfast organisms have grown. A medium is prepared as follows: Four hundred fifty gm. of chopped lean beef is extracted with 1,000 c c of water for 3 hours. The temperature of the water is brought to 45 C. After about one hour the temperature is raised to 50 C., and during the third hour, to 55 C. The mixture is stirred frequently. The major portion of the liquid is removed from the meat, which is then heated to 100 C. in the remaining liquid. This causes the meat particles to shrink and serves the purpose of securing the maximum amount of liquid.

To the liquid is now added 1% of peptone (Difco product has been used), 0.5% K_2HPO_4, 0.2 % Liebig's beef extract and 5% of glycerol by volume. The reaction is adjusted to a pH of 7.5-8. The medium is placed in 500 Erlenmeyer flasks, 100 c c in each flask and sterilized in the autoclave. One-half the flasks are seeded with the grass bacillus of Karlensky, the remainder with the grass bacillus of Moeller. They are incubated at 37.5 C. for two weeks. They are then heated to 100 C. The cultures are filtered and the filtrate made up to the original volume of the medium before incubation. The following ingredients are then added: Five-tenths per cent. peptone, 0.25% K_2HPO_4, 0.2% Liebig's beef extract, 0.5% by volume of glycerol, and 0.5% of aminoid peptone from beef (Arlco). The reaction is left unchanged. The medium is filtered, 50 c c portions are placed in 500 c c Erlenmeyer flasks, and sterilized in the autoclave. Before the flasks are inoculated 5 c c of sterile blood serum is added to each flask.

The flasks receive a heavy inoculation from previous liquid cultures or from a suspension of growth removed from an agar culture. They are incubated at 37.5 C. from 10 to 16 weeks. The tops of the flasks are covered with lead foil to prevent evaporation during the long period of incubation.

On removal from the incubator the flasks are heated to 60 C. for from 1-2 hours, filtered and the volume restored to the original amount. One-half of 1% of phenol is added. The johnin is stored for use. No data have been collected as to the persistency of its potency, nor in regard to the relation of the latter to profuseness of growth in a particular batch of medium.

Application of the Test.—The johnin is injected into the jugular vein, 10 c c being the dose for an average sized animal. The reaction in the case of the affected animal follows quickly in the majority of cases, as is shown in table 2. Ordinarily only one temperature reading has been made previous to injection, and the post-injection temperature readings have been begun one hour or less after the injection. The temperature readings are continued for at least 10 hours. Table 2 shows the hour at which the maximum post-injection temperatures were reached in the case of animals injected intravenously.

The thermal reaction is comparable to that noted in the subcutaneous tuberculin test as is shown in table 3.

TABLE 2

THE HOUR AT WHICH THE MAXIMUM TEMPERATURE WAS REACHED IN CASE OF ANIMALS REACTING TO JOHNIN

Hour After Injection	Number Reacted	Percentage	Hour After Injection	Number Reacted	Percentage
1	None	None	7	15	29.50
2	None	None	8	3	5.88
3	5	9.85	9	1	1.90
4	3	5.88	10	3	5.88
5	17	33.33	11	1	1.9
6	3	5.88	12	None	None

TABLE 3

THE FREQUENCY DISTRIBUTION OF REACTING ANIMALS WITH REFERENCE TO MAXIMUM TEMPERATURE

Maximum Temperatures	Number	Percentage
103–104	13	25 0
104–105	23	44.2
105–106	7	13 5
106–107	7	13.5
107–108	2	3.8

Constitutional Reactions.—There are manifestations of infection following the administration of johnin other than a rise in temperature. The majority of infected cattle exhibit a roughened hair coat from 30 minutes to 4 hours following the intravenous injection. The condition is more noticeable in some cattle than in others. We have never seen a roughened hair coat that was not accompanied by a thermal reaction, and that did not correspond approximately in time of appearance with the initial rise in temperature.

At any time between 4 and 24 hours following the administration of johnin, approximately 25% of infected cattle exhibit a marked softening of the feces. At times a severe diarrhea is noted, the bowel discharges being thin and watery, and rarely streaked with blood. A foul odor is sometimes to be noted.

Sometimes an uneasiness accompanied by muscular tremors and a more or less marked dyspnea may be seen. These symptoms usually appear 15 to 30 minutes after injection and persist for from 1-2 hours.

In 3 instances, of approximately 1,000 cattle tested severe constitutional reactions were noted. The first to come to our attention was an adult cow that had shown clinical symptoms of Johne's disease for about 2 months. About one minute after the intravenous injection of johnin she fell prostrate and remained in an unconscious condition for several minutes; temperature 99; pulse, fast and weak. In 15 minutes she had sufficiently recovered to be able to regain her feet and in an hour's time was apparently normal. This cow was infected, as shown by the fact that she reacted at this time and postmortem revealed the characteristic lesions and the specific organism.

The second subject was a 3 year old heifer that had been tested 6 months before, but did not react. About 1½ hours after injection this heifer fell prostrate; dyspnea was marked; the temperature was 102.6. The highest preinjection temperature was 101.2. The pulse was not perceptible. In about 1½ hours recovery had apparently taken place. She reacted at this time. Postmortem examination revealed infection with Johne's bacillus.

The third instance was that of a 6 months old heifer. About 15 minutes after injection she was markedly dyspnec with a pronounced flank breathing, the tongue protruded and the temperature had risen from 101.8 to 102.6. In about 30 minutes she was dead. Postmortem examination revealed marked congestion of about 12 inches of the ileum situated about 2 feet from the ileocecal juncture. Acidfasts were demonstrated microscopically.

Twenty-five to 30% of the cattle we have tested exhibited urticaria or serum sickness. This appears a few minutes after injection and is manifested by inflammation of the conjunctiva, excessive lachrymation, swelling around the anus and vulva, and wartlike elevations anywhere on the body. This condition is often seen following the injection of other biologic products. Recovery is usually rapid. So far as we are aware, deaths never occur. This condition has no diagnostic significance, and it may be manifested by both infected and noninfected animals alikelike.

Confirmation of the Test by Retests on Reacting Animals.—In a part of the cattle reacting to the johnin test, we have had opportunity for confirmation of the results by a retest. In one herd, consisting of 18 animals ranging in age from 2 to 12 years, 5 reactors were found.

These reactions were all definite; the lowest post-injection maximum temperature was 104.2. This herd was kept intact and retested one year later with the result that the same animals again gave definite reactions, and in addition a 4 year old cow that had failed to react the year before. In the meantime, no clinical cases had developed. The only irregularity in connection with this herd was the fact that one cow gave a suspicious reaction to the first test and failed to react on retest. Five cows in another herd reacted to the johnin test. On retest 5 months later 2 gave definite reactions and one a suspicious reaction.

Confirmation of the Test by Postmortem Examination of Reacting Animals.—In a portion of the reacting animals, opportunity for postmortem examination has been presented. No lesions outside the digestive tract and adjacent lymph glands which could be attributed to this disease have ever been noted. Our observations are based on 24 postmortem examinations of cattle reacting to the johnin test. Four of this number revealed no macroscopic lesions of disease; 3, a slight enlargement and reddening of the ileocecal valve with no visible intestinal lesions; 4, a marked enlargement and reddening of the ileocecal valve with no visible intestinal involvement; 2, a marked intestinal thickening with no visible changes in the valve; and 7, a marked involvement of both intestine and valve. Four showed a slight involvement of both valve and intestine.

The macroscopic appearance of pieces of infected gut varies widely in different animals. The anatomic changes are always quite insignificant in comparison to the state of emaciation to which the animals are reduced. In cases of long standing there is a thickening of the ileum, frequently 25 to 30 feet in extent. Cases are reported of a thickening of the entire intestinal tract. Involvement extensive as this is rare. Inflammation of the ileocecal valve is frequently observed. At times the valve is greatly swollen, becoming from 15 to 20 times its normal size. On the other hand, macroscopic evidence may be lacking, yet acidfasts may be demonstrated microscopically. A piece of thickened bowel presents on its mucous surface a peculiar wrinkled appearance; the mucosa seems to be thrown into folds and ridges. Normal gut at times presents wrinkling; these wrinkles will, however, disappear on stretching. This thickening is not uniform.

It is not uncommon for a piece of normal bowel to be interposed between two thickened pieces. This patchy tendency is frequently noted in cases in which the cecum is involved. We have noted nothing characteristic as to the color of infected mucosa. Occasionally there may be small petechiae irregular in outline and distribution. Twort and Ingram note a characteristic pinkish yellow color. This yellow color does occur, but it has not been constant with us. At times the intense inflammation in the region of the valve will impart a dark red color. It is entirely possible that these acute inflammatory changes are due to the secondary invasion with other types of bacteria. Part of the reacting cattle slaughtered by us had never shown symptoms of Johne's disease. In several of these animals the ileocecal valve was markedly enlarged and inflamed. On the other hand, in some of the cases of long standing inflammatory changes were slight, or entirely absent. We have never observed ulcers or nodules. The macroscopic changes of the lymphatic glands are meager and confined to a slight enlargement and softening of the substance. In sections a serous fluid frequently exudes. In one case of long standing a marked induration was noted.

Confirmation of the Test by Microscopic Examination.—The appearance of a piece of infected gut in Johne's disease is no indication as to the number of acidfast organisms which can be demonstrated microscopically. They may be numerous in material showing slight lesions and difficult to demonstrate in a markedly thickened gut.

The specific organisms can usually be demonstrated by histologic section and many times also by smears. In specimens in which we have been unable to demonstrate acid-fasts readily by direct examination we have substituted a method of concentration by means of antiformin. The mode of procedure has been as follows:

A small piece, not more than ¼ inch square, of the suspected intestine is placed in full strength formaldehyde for from 1-2 hours, depending on the size of the tissue. It is then removed and placed in the incubator or drying chamber until thoroughly hard and dry. The tissue is then ground to a fine powder in a mortar and this powder treated for 2 hours with a 25% antiformin solution. This is diluted with an equal volume of distilled water and centrifuged. The supernatant liquid is decanted, the tube filled with distilled water and again centrifuged. The sediment is examined for acid-fasts. This method has given good results.

Acid-fast organisms have been found in the tissues of 29 of the 30 reacting animals from which it has been possible for us to obtain material for such examination.

Results Obtained from Herd Tests.—It was stated earlier in this paper that the work was undertaken with the hope of determining the value of the test in eliminating the disease from infected herds. It was recognized that the slow progress of the disease in the individual animal would undoubtedly make the task of freeing a herd from the disease a long one. Practically nothing is known concerning the length of the period of incubation, nor is anything known concerning the stages of the disease in which an animal may not react to the test.

The herd on which the most work has been done has been known to have been infected for 14 years at the time the work was begun. During this period 20 animals had been lost because of the disease. The average number of animals in the herd was 45. Table 4 presents the results obtained in the various tests made on this herd.

The results do not indicate that the elimination of the disease from the herd by the use of the test will be an easy task. We are not at all certain that additional reactors will not be found in this herd in spite of the negative results obtained in the last test.

TABLE 4

RESULTS OF TESTS ON HERD I

Date	Reactors
June, 1917	5
November, 1917	4
February, 1919	6
June, 1919	3
November, 1919	4
June, 1920	4
December, 1920	2
June, 1921	0

The owner of this herd has felt very hopeless in his struggle against this disease because of the fact that there was no way of ascertaining which were the infected animals until clinical symptoms appeared. It is probably true that long before these symptoms are to be noted the organisms are being given off by the affected animal. It was hoped that the test would enable the affected animal to be recognized before she became a source of danger to the other members of the herd. It is this hope that has led the owner to continue the use of the test in his herd.

The specific organism has been found in the tissues of all but one of the 28 animals reacting in this herd. In the test made in June, 1919, one adult animal gave a suspicious reaction. At the following test in Nov., 1919, there was no indication of a reaction to the johnin. The animal did, however, give a clear cut reaction in June, 1920, and was removed from the herd.

Another herd has been tested once yearly for 3 years. One reactor was found in the first test. No animals have reacted during the 2nd and 3rd tests. One clinical case developed in this herd. The infection was demonstrated by postmortem examination in both the clinical case and the animal reacting to the test. The work on the other herds which we have under observation has not been extended enough to warrant its inclusion here.

Spread of the Disease in a Herd.—Some observations have been made on the rapidity with which the disease spreads in a herd. In 1910, three animals were introduced into a herd. Two of these showed clinical symptoms in 1912 and were sold. The other showed symptoms of the disease in 1913. The disease was undoubtedly introduced into this herd by these animals. During the period 1913-21, 15 animals have been removed from the herd because of this disease.

Another herd became infected in 1905 through the introduction of an animal that apparently at that time was showing clinical symptoms. Two years later another animal was disposed of because of marked symptoms of the disease. In 1909, six animals were removed from the herd because they were in the last stages of the disease. No other clinical cases developed until May, 1916, when 2 animals were removed. Between June, 1918, and Jan. 1, 1919, five clinical cases developed, and the animals were disposed of. In Jan., 1920, the herd was first tested. Seven animals reacted and were removed. In Dec., 1920, the test detected 11 reacting animals; 6 of these were removed from the herd and the remaining 5 were retested in May, 1921. Two gave positive reactions and one a suspicious reaction. No rise in temperature was noted in the other two.

It is evident from these observations that the disease is one which at times may spread rapidly in a herd, and at other times it may spread exceedingly slowly.

SUMMARY

The work herein reported is an attempt to eliminate Johne's disease from infected herds by the use of the diagnostic johnin, a product prepared by the use of the specific organism of the disease. It is comparable to tuberculin in its action on the infected animal. The preparation of johnin is described and its method of application.

One herd has been tested eight times in four years. Reactors were obtained in each except the last test.

The results of the test have been confirmed by macroscopic and microscopic examinations of the tissues, and in a few instances by retests on reacting animals. Acidfast bacilli have been found in 29 of the 30 reacting animals.

CONCLUSION

The results obtained indicate the possibility of eliminating Johne's disease from infected herds by the use of johnin, a product comparable to tuberculin.

A STUDY OF STREPTOCOCCI FROM POST-GONORRHEAL PROSTATITIS BY A QUANTITATIVE METHOD OF AGGLUTINATION AND ABSORPTION

Russell D. Herrold

From the John McCormick Institute for Infectious Diseases, Chicago

This study includes 28 strains of streptococci from a series of chronic postgonorrheal infections of the prostate, 4 strains of streptococci from the normal urethra and 16 from various sources outside the genito-urinary tract (feces, nasopharynx, sputum of chronic bronchitis, empyema, tonsillitis, pleural fluid, scarlet fever throat, puerperal sepsis, and mastoid infection).

The general grouping of these streptococcal strains according to their action on blood agar is indicated in table 1.

Rabbits were immunized with 6 selected strains (table 1), all of which were found present in 2 successive cultures of prostatic exudate. Three of these were typical streptococci of the viridans type, causing the alpha type of hemolysis of Smith and Brown; one caused a narrow zone of hemolysis corresponding (alpha prime); the other two were typical hemolytic streptococci causing the wide hemolytic zones (beta). The rabbits were injected once a week with a 16-hour growth on ascites phosphate agar. Suspensions were made in salt solution and heated for 30 minutes at 53-56 C. The first injection was ¼ of a slant intravenously and with each succeeding injection the dose was increased by that amount until a maximum of one slant was given. The animals were bled and tested on the seventh day after the fourth injection. In the case of those animals whose serums did not contain sufficient agglutinins, the injections were continued at weekly intervals until a satisfactory titer was obtained, serum being taken for tests preceding each later inoculation.

The green streptococci generally seemed to produce agglutinins more readily than the hemolytic.

A standard technic for agglutination was used which gave consistent results on repeated trials.

A solid medium was used because homogenous suspensions then could be obtained regularly. The basis of this medium was nutrient agar in which dibasic sodium phosphate was substituted for sodium

Received for publication Aug. 22, 1921.

TABLE 1

AGGLUTINATION TITERS OF ANTISTREPTOCOCCIC SERUMS BEFORE AND AFTER ABSORPTION

Source of Streptococci	Classification of Streptococci According to Growth on Blood Agar	No. of Strain	Agglutination Titers of Serums for Prostatic Streptococci						Agglutination Titers of Serums for Homologous Prostatic Streptococci After Absorption						Nos. of Strepto-coccus Strains With Which Serums Were Treated
			Serum Against Strain 1	Serum Against Strain 12	Serum Against Strain 13	Serum Against Strain 14	Serum Against Strain 20	Serum Against Strain 22	Serum 1	Serum 12	Serum 13	Serum 14	Serum 20	Serum 22	
Prostate........	Viridans-alpha	1	3200	400	100	10	0	0	0	4000	1200	800	400	600	1
Prostate........	Viridans-alpha	2	3200	400	10	10	0	0							
Prostate........	Viridans-alpha	3	3200	400	100	10	0	10	0	4000	800	800	400	800	3
Prostate........	Viridans-alpha	4	3200	400	100	10	0	0							
Prostate........	Viridans-alpha	5	3200	400	10	10	0	0	0	4000	800	800	400	800	5
Prostate........	Viridans-alpha	6	3200	200	100	10	0	0							
Prostate........	Viridans-alpha	7	3200	200	100	10	0	10							
Prostate........	Viridans-alpha	8	3200	400	100	10	0	0	0	6000	800	800	400	800	8
Prostate........	Viridans-alpha[1]	9	2800	200	10	10	0	10	0	4000	800	600	400	800	9
Prostate........	Viridans-alpha	10	3200	400	100	10	0	0	0	6000	800	800	400	600	10
Prostate........	Viridans-alpha[1]	11	3200	100	100	10	0	0							
Prostate........	Viridans-alpha	12	1600	8000	800	800	0	10	2800	0	0	0	200	800	12
Prostate........	Viridans-alpha	13	1600	8000	1200	800	0	10	2800	0	0	0	400	800	13
Prostate........	Viridans-alpha[1]	14	1200	4000	1200	800	0	10	2400	0	0	0	400	600	14
Prostate........	Viridans-alpha	15	1600	8000	800	800	0	10							
Prostate........	Viridans-alpha	16	1600	8000	1200	800	0	0	2800	0	0	0	200	800	16
Prostate........	Viridans alpha	17	1600	8000	1200	800	0	10							
Prostate........	Viridans-alpha	18	1200	8000	1200	800	0	10							
Prostate........	Viridans-alpha[1]	19	1600	8000	1200	800	0	10							
Prostate........	Hemolytic-beta	20	10	10	10	10	400	10	2400	4000	1200	800	0	800	20
Prostate........	Hemolytic-beta	21	0	0	0	10	400	0	2800	4000	800	800	0	600	21
Prostate........	Hemolytic-beta	22	0	0	0	0	0	800	2800	6000	800	800	400	0	22
Prostate........	Hemolytic-beta	23	0	0	0	0	0	800	2800	4000	800	800	400	0	23
Prostate........	Viridans-alpha[1]	24	0	0	100	10	0	0	2400	6000	800	600	200	800	24
Prostate........	Viridans-alpha	25	0	0	0	10	0	10	2800	4000	800	800	400	800	25
Prostate........	Hemolytic-beta	26	10	10	10	10	0	0							
Prostate........	Hemolytic-beta	27	10	0	0	10	0	0							
Prostate........	Viridans-alpha	28	0	0	0	10	0	0							
Normal urethra..	Hemolytic-beta	29	0	0	0	0	0	0	2800	6000	800	800	400	800	29
Normal urethra..	Hemolytic-beta	30	0	0	0	10	0	0	2800	4000	800	600	400	800	30
Normal urethra..	Viridans-alpha	31	0	0	0	0	0	0	2800	4000	800	800	400	600	31
Normal urethra..	Viridans-alpha	32	0	0	0	0	0	0							
Feces...........	Viridans-alpha	33	2800	400	100	10	0	0	0	4000	800	800	400	800	33
Feces...........	Hemolytic-beta	34	0	0	0	0	0	0							
Nasopharynx....	Hemolytic-beta	35	10	10	10	10	10	10							
Nasopharynx....	Hemolytic-beta	36	10	10	10	10	0	100	2800	4000	800	800	400	600	36
Nasopharynx....	Hemolytic-beta	37	10	10	10	100	0	10							
Nasopharynx....	Viridans-alpha	38	100	10	0	10	0	10							
Sputum.........	Viridans alpha	39	10	100	0	10	0	0	2800	4000	800	600	400	800	39
Sputum.........	Viridans-alpha[1]	40	0	0	0	0	0	10							
Sputum.........	Hemolytic-beta	41	0	0	0	10	0	0							
Empyema.......	Hemolytic-beta	42	0	0	10	10	0	0							
Tonsil...........	Hemolytic-beta	43	0	0	0	10	0	10	2800	6000	800	800	400	800	43
Tonsil...........	Viridans-alpha	44	0	10	0	0	0	0	2400	4000	800	800	400	600	44
Pleural fluid.....	Hemolytic-beta	45	10	10	0	10	0	10							
Scarlet fever throat.........	Hemolytic-beta	46	10	10	0	0	0	0	2800	6000	1200	800	400	600	46
Puerperal sepsis.	Hemolytic-beta	47	10	10	10	10	10	10							
Mastoid.........	Hemolytic-beta	48	10	10	10	10	0	10	2800	4000	800	800	400	800	48

chloride. The buffer effect of the phosphate is well known. Ascites fluid was added to the melted agar in the proportion of 1 part of fluid to 3 parts of agar. The ascites fluid was previously heated to 56 C. for one hour. Plates were used because the surface available is several times that of a slant with an equal quantity of medium. Approximately the 12-hour growth on one plate of a stock strain was suspended in 1 c c of sterile distilled water. The resulting heavy suspension was taken up with a capillary pipet and 2 or 3 drops placed on the surface of each 10 plates. The pipet was then sealed at the end in the flame and bent at an angle of 90 degrees 4 or 5 cm. from the end; now the drops could be quickly and uniformly spread with the bent pipet in a similar manner to that used in making blood smears, and without tearing a less solid medium than could be inoculated with wire loops. The plates were incubated 12-18 hours, and suspensions of the growth in normal salt solution made in amounts of 1 c c per plate. The surface growth was scraped off with a bent capillary pipet and the suspension transferred to graduated tubes which were centrifugated for 20 minutes at high speed. A 50% suspension was made of the bacterial sediment and placed in the icebox as a stock emulsion for later agglutination and absorption tests. It was found that such concentrated suspensions in salt solution would keep several weeks in the refrigerator without deterioration so far as agglutination and absorption are concerned.

The streptococci and especially the hemolytic, which tend to clump spontaneously when grown in broth or on ordinary blood agar, lost this property after a few successive transfers of young cultures on ascites phosphate agar.

Agglutination tests were made with equal mixtures of serum dilutions and a 0.5% streptococcus suspension which were incubated at 52-56 C. for 2 hours when preliminary readings were made. The tubes were then reincubated over night and final readings made the next morning. However, there were only few variations in the two readings in a large number of tests.

A serum which agglutinated in a maximum dilution of 1 : 1,200 gave the same titers macroscopically with suspensions of 0.25, 0.5 and 1% of streptococci.

The tabulated agglutination results show that antistreptococcus serum 1 contains major agglutinations for 11 prostatic streptococci and minor agglutinins for 8 of similar origin. Only one strain of those tested from other sources gave a like reaction. This strain was isolated from the feces of a patient with pyelonephritis. Three other anti-streptococcus serums—12, 13 and 14—contained specific agglutinins for 8 prostatic streptococci and group agglutinins for 11 other strains. The group agglutinins of serum 1 were present in rather higher dilution than usual but later absorption tests established the specificity. It may be recalled here that Barnes,[1] found group precipitins for streptococcus extracts in relatively high dilutions. Antistreptococcus (hemolytic) serums 20 and 22 each agglutinated its homologous strain and one other. The remaining strains, including 2 hemolytic, 2 viridans, and 1 alpha prime viridans could not be classified with any of the serums. Four streptococcal strains from the normal urethra were not agglutinated, and with the exception of one feces strain, the other 15 strains from sources outside the genito-urinary tract were not agglutinated except in low dilution. There was no cross agglutination between the hemolytic and viridans streptococci except in very low dilutions. Since two thirds of the streptococci or prostatic origin fall into two related groups and as streptococcus viridans is regarded as a heterologous group, the results seem to indicate some degree of specificity in the types which occur in chronic postgonorrheal prostatitis.

Absorption tests were made with selected strains of each group and also with several other strains which did not agglutinate or only in very low dilutions.

It was found that in order to obtain complete absorption in low dilution, it is necessary to use concentrated suspensions, the serums of higher titer requiring proportionately heavier suspensions.

The following method was used: Titration was first made to determine the amount of streptococci necessary to completely exhaust the homologous serum. Varying dilutions of the stock 50% suspensions were made (25, 12.5, 6.25, and 3.125%) in amounts of 0.1 cc each in small precipitin tubes 4-5 mm. in diameter and to these were added 0.1 cc of serum diluted 1:5. The mixtures were incubated for 2 hours at 53-56 C. with occasional agitation. Control serum tubes without bacterial suspension were also incubated. After incubation 0.1 c c of the fluid was withdrawn from each tube and placed in another set of precipitin tubes and an equal amount of 0.5% streptococcus suspension added to each treated serum, the untreated serum, normal serum, and normal salt solution. If the supernatant fluid was not sufficiently clear it was centrifugated; when a large number of strans were being tested about 20 tubes were centrifugated at a time by plugging the tips of the centrifuge tube containers with cotton and placing 4 or 5 small tubes in each container. One and one-fourth times the smallest percentage of streptococcus suspension necessary to remove the agglutinins were used for absorption by heterologous strains in cross absorption tests. Complete absorption could be obtained in 2 hours by this method.

[1] Jour. Infect. Dis., 1918, 22, p. 230.

No advantage was noted by heating the emulsion to 65 C. before use, because these mixtures were incubated at higher temperature than usually the case.

The results of the absorption tests indicate clearly that the two main groups are distinctly specific even though the antiserum for one of them was rather strong in common agglutinins.

DISCUSSION

There is a great deal of interest at the present time in the immunologic classification of streptococci and the relation of streptococci to various diseases. Havens [2] classified 93% of 292 strains of hemolytic streptococci from various sources into 3 groups by agglutination; Tunnicliff,[3] Bliss,[4] and Gordon [5] have established a definite immunologic group of certain hemolytic streptococci, isolated from scarlet fever. Any definite grouping of nonhemolytic streptococci so far has not been established. Krumweide and Valentine,[6] made agglutination tests with antistreptococcus serums, produced with endocarditis and tonsil strains, and noted cross agglutination with 3 endocarditis strains while several other strains of the same origin were not agglutinated. One prostatic streptococcus, which they included was not agglutinated by any of their serums.

Holman,[7] and Kinsella and Swift [8] believe that streptococcus viridans constitute a heterogeneous group members of which cause disease only in states of lowered resistance from preexisting infection or other causes. Howell [9] states that a classification of streptococcus could not be made from the results of complement-fixation tests. Barnes,[1] however, found the precipitins relatively specific in high dilution. Clawson,[10] concludes that the nonhemolytic group is widely heterogeneous from agglutination and complement-fixation tests. Williams, Unneberg, Goldberg and Hussey [11] state that in a series of influenza cases the "alpha streptococci" which were dominant "consist of multiple strains from the results of carbohydrate reactions and the action on standard blood agar medium." Bumpus and Meisser [12]

[2] Jour. Infect. Dis., 1919, 25, p. 315
[3] Jour. Am. Med. Assn., 1920, 74, p. 1387.
[4] Bull. Johns Hopkins Hosp., 1920, 31, p. 174.
[5] Brit. Med. Jour., 1921, 1, p. 632.
[6] Jour. Infect. Dis., 1916, 19, p. 760.
[7] Jour. Med. Research, 1916, 34, p. 377.
[8] Jour. Exper. Med., 1918, 28, p. 169.
[9] Jour. Infect. Dis., 1919, 25, p. 46.
[10] Jour. Infect. Dis., 1920, 26, p. 93.
[11] Jour. Immunol., 1921, 6, p. 53.
[12] Arch. Int. Med., 1921, 27, p. 326.

find that their results from animal experiments indicate that certain green producing streptococci from focal infection of the mouth produce a specific pyelonephritis. However, they do not state whether their strains were all of the same immunologic type. It seems that the streptococci in postgonorrheal prostatitis possess sufficiently specific features to warrant efforts to trace them back to the sources of infection.

SUMMARY

A homogenous emulsion of streptococci can be obtained uniformly from young growths on ascites phosphate agar plates.

The quantitative method of making suspensions of centrifugated packed bacteria is more satisfactory than other methods of computation such as counting or comparison with standard barium sulphate suspensions.

Two thirds of the streptococci isolated from chronic prostatic infections can be classified by agglutination into two related groups. This specificity seems to be limited to the viridans (alpha and alpha prime) types of streptococci.

SUSCEPTIBILITY OF RABBITS TO THE VIRUS OF MEASLES

INOCULATIONS WITH NASOPHARYNGEAL MATERIAL

From the Research Laboratory, New York City Department of Health

M. Grund

The investigation, the results of which are reported now, was undertaken to determine whether the inoculation of nasal secretions from patients with measles would produce definite and characteristic symptoms in rabbits; it was carried on at the same time, and with material from the same patients as were used by Nevin [1] in her work on blood inoculations.

The nasopharynx of patients in the early eruptive, or pre-eruption stage of measles was irrigated with 30-50 cc normal salt solution. Cultures were made from the material thus obtained, on blood-vitamine-agar to establish the prevalent types of bacteria. From 5-10 cc of the washings were injected into the trachea of rabbits, the animals being lightly anesthetized. In most animals this amount of fluid caused a leakage from the nose, showing that the mucous membrane of the upper air passage was thoroughly flooded with infectious material. Unfiltered washings were used in most cases, as it was believed that the usual flora of the upper respiratory tract would not cause characteristic symptoms in rabbits. Only a small number of rabbits received material passed through a Berkefeld V candle. Aerobic cultures from these filtrates were uniformly negative for the test organism (B. prodigiosus).

The majority of rabbits (table 1) gave a certain reaction, yet apparently there are among them a fairly large number of refractory individuals, for in a number of instances in this series, only one animal out of two inoculated with the same nasal washings developed symptoms, and even when both succumbed, there was often considerable difference in the severity of symptoms. In susceptible animals the incubation period varied between two and seven days.

The least reliable and constant symptom seems to be the enanthem; while present in about 20% of the cases, only 5 animals showed what

---

Received for publication Aug. 29, 1921.

[1] J. Infect. Dis., 1921, 29, p. 429.

TABLE 1

RABBIT INOCULATIONS WITH NASOPHARYNGEAL WASHINGS

Case	Rabbit No.	Exanthem: Erythematous			Exanthem: Maculopapular			Desquamation			Coryza			Conjunctivitis			Enanthem		Temperature Extremes	Leukopenia			Remarks
		Intensity	Day of Onset	Duration	Intensity	Day of Onset	Duration	Intensity	Day of Onset	Duration	Intensity	Day of Onset	Duration	Intensity	Day of Onset	Duration	Intensity	Day of Onset		Intensity	Day of Onset	Duration	
M19	191	+	2	2	..	..	..	..	..	..	+	9	2	..	..	..	..	..	102.2-102.8	..	..	..	
	192	+	2	2	..	..	..	..	..	..	..	..	..	..	..	..	..	..	102 -102	..	..	..	Died after 4 days; dysentery
M20	201	..	..	..	..	..	..	..	..	..	+	12	1	..	..	..	..	..	102.6-102.8	+	10	1	
M21	211	..	..	..	..	..	..	..	..	..	+	3	4	+	3	1	+?	6	101.3-103	+	2	1	
	212	++	2	2	..	..	..	..	..	..	+	2	2	+	2	1	..	..	102 -105	++	3	1	Died after 4 days; bronchopneumonia
M22	221	+	2	4	+	4	2	+	5	2	+	4	2	+	4	1	..	..	100.8-102.4	+	3	1	
	222	..	..	..	..	..	..	+	6	3	..	..	..	..	..	..	..	..	99.8-102.2	+	2	2	Filtered material inoculated
M23	231	+	2	4	..	..	..	+	5	6	+	3	1	..	..	..	..	..	102 -104.8	..	..	..	
	232	++	2	5	++	4	3	++	4	7	+	5	3	..	..	..	..	..	100.8-102	+	3	1	
M24	241	+	3	3	..	..	..	+	6	5	..	..	..	..	..	..	..	..	99.4-100.8	..	..	..	
	242	..	..	..	..	..	..	+	7	5	..	..	..	..	..	..	..	..	99.6-103.1	+	3	1	
M25	251	..	..	..	+	7	2	+	10	3	+	5	6	+	10	1	..	..	101.8-104.7	+	7	1	
M26	261	..	..	..	..	..	..	..	..	..	..	..	..	..	..	..	..	..	101.7-105.4	+	4	1	Phlegmon of abdominal wall
	262	..	..	..	..	..	..	+	10	3	+	7	1	..	..	..	..	..	102 -105.8	+	5	1	Died of rabbit septicemia
	263	+	2	7	..	..	..	+	11	5	..	..	..	..	..	..	..	..	101.8-107	±	2	1	
M27	271	++	2	2	..	..	..	..	..	..	..	..	..	..	..	..	..	..	101.4-101.3	++	2	2	Died after 4 days; bronchopneumonia
M29	291	..	..	..	±	3	2	±	12	4	±	2	6	..	..	..	+	2	....	..	..	..	
	292	±	2	2	..	..	..	+	14	5	++	3	4	..	..	..	..	..	....	..	..	..	Filtered material inoculated
R I	R1	..	..	..	..	..	..	..	..	..	..	..	..	..	..	..	..	..	....	..	..	..	Died within 24 hours
D I	D1	..	..	..	+*	2	..	+*	5	..	+	2	..	+	2	..	..	..	....	..	..	..	
D II	D2	..	..	..	..	..	..	..	..	..	..	..	..	..	..	..	..	..	....	..	..	..	
Sc I	S1	..	..	..	..	..	..	+	1	..	..	..	..	..	..	..	..	..	....	..	..	..	
Sc II	S2	+	4	..	..	..	..	+	7	..	+	3	..	..	..	..	..	..	....	..	..	..	

* Scratches ?

TABLE 2

Passage Experiments and Inoculations with Cultivated Virus

Case	Rabbit No.	Exanthem: Erythematous: Intensity	Exanthem: Erythematous: Day of Onset	Exanthem: Erythematous: Duration	Exanthem: Maculopapular: Intensity	Exanthem: Maculopapular: Day of Onset	Exanthem: Maculopapular: Duration	Desquamation: Intensity	Desquamation: Day of Onset	Desquamation: Duration	Coryza: Intensity	Coryza: Day of Onset	Coryza: Duration	Conjunctivitis: Intensity	Conjunctivitis: Day of Onset	Conjunctivitis: Duration	Enanthem: Intensity	Enanthem: Day of Onset	Temperature Extremes	Leukopenia: Intensity	Leukopenia: Day of Onset	Leukopenia: Duration	Remarks
M21	213	+	2	2	..	..	..	±	4	1	+	2	2	+	2	1	±?	2	102.2-102.4	+	3	1	Inoculated with filtered lung tissue from R 212
	214	±	3	1	..	..	..	..	..	..	+	3	1	..	..	..	..	..	101.6-102.2	..	..	..	Inoculated with filtered blood culture R 212
	215	..	..	..	..	..	..	..	..	..	..	..	..	..	..	..	..	..	101.6-102	..	..	..	Inoculated with nasal discharge from R 212
M27	272	..	..	..	+	5	1	+	6	2	+	5	2	..	..	..	..	..	102.3-103.6	++	7	1	Inoculated with unfiltered lung tissue R 271; died 8th day
M28	281	++	2	5	..	..	..	+	5	4	+	2	2	±	2	2	±	1	103 -103	..	..	..	Both inoculated with 2d transfer of a culture of filtered nasal washings, M 28
	282	+	2	2	+	2	2	+	7	7	±	2	2	..	..	..	+	2	102 -102.4	..	..	..	
	283	+	3	2	+	3	2	+	13	6	+	5	1	..	..	..	+	2	....	..	..	..	Inoculated with blood from R 281-282 (pooled)
	284	..	..	..	..	..	..	..	..	..	+	3	4	..	..	..	+?	3	....	..	..	..	Inoculated with blood from R 283
	285	±	3	1	+	5	5	+	10	6	++	4	6	..	..	..	..	..	....	..	..	..	Both inoculated with blood culture from R 281, second transfer
	286	+	3	4	..	..	..	+	10	5	+	3	4	..	..	..	..	..	....	..	..	..	
M29	293	..	..	..	+	6	3	+	11	3	+	2	6	..	..	..	..	..	....	..	..	..	Inoculated with culture from filtered nasal washings; patient M 29, second transfer
	294	++	2	8	..	..	..	+	9	5	++	2	4	..	..	..	++	2	102	..	..	..	
	295	..	..	..	+	4	2	..	..	..	..	..	..	..	..	..	..	..	....	..	..	..	Inoculated with culture from filtered nasal washings; patient M 29, third transfer
	296	+	2	1	+	3	2	..	..	..	+	7	2	+	2	1	+	2	....	..	..	..	
	297	+	4	2	+	5	4	+	10	3	+	5	2	..	..	..	..	..	....	..	..	..	Inoculated with culture from filtered nasal washings; M 29, fifth transfer

one might describe as good typical Koplik spots. The temperature curve also is not at all characteristic; in very few animals did the temperature go above 103. In some of the cases a certain relationship appeared between the temperature curve, the cutaneous symptoms and the leukocyte count; however, it was far from constant, and the fluctuations noted in daily blood counts made for one week before inoculation do not make a "leukopenia" seem a very dependable diagnostic sign in rabbits. In a number of animals a distinct polychromatophilia was noted.

Conjunctivitis and inflammation of the upper respiratory passages, in varying degrees of severity, occurred in 70% of animals; it is not always possible to eliminate "snuffles," but the appearance of coryza together with the rash, and its brief duration in most cases, point against its being an intercurrent infection. Seventy-five per cent. of the rabbits showed some form of cutaneous eruption, either a diffuse, punctate erythema, which in 3 severe (2 fatal) cases became petechial, or, sometimes following the erythema, sometimes occurring without it, a maculopapular rash, which faded after 2-4 days and left pigmentation persisting until desquamation began.

Desquamation, either branny or flaky, occurred in all but 4 animals after the rash and was noted 3 times in cases in which no rash had been noted (3 animals with marked erythema died before desquamation occurred).

Control animals were inoculated with nasopsaryngeal washings from 1 case of nasal catarrh, 2 cases of diphtheria and 2 of scarlet fever. There was desquamation in the 2 scarlet fever animals, preceded in one case by a rash which was, however, different in character from that shown by the measles rabbits. The other animal, showing 2 macules, presented other evidences of clawing and scratching over some of the unshaved portions of his skin.

Passage experiments from rabbit to rabbit were unsuccessful when nasal discharges were used, owing probably to the scantiness of material. Successful inoculations were made in 7 cases, using, 3 times, 2 cc of blood, and, twice, a suspension of lung tissue from severe and fatal cases. The other passage experiments were conducted with rabbit blood cultures. Attempts have also been made to cultivate a specific organism from the filtered nasal washings from patients, and while the work along these lines is incomplete, the reactions obtained in rabbits inoculated with the fifth transfer of such cultures indicated at least that the virus remains alive and virulent at 37 C. for 24 days. The results obtained by reinoculating convalescent animals have thus far been rather contradictory, and frankly successful in only two cases.

It cannot be claimed that the results obtained in any one animal give a clear and typical picture of measles, yet taking the series as a whole, there has been enough conformity to encourage the belief that rabbits are susceptible to the virus of measles and within rather wide limits give a characteristic syndrome.

Note.—E. Harde, in the Compt. Rend. Soc. de biol., 1921, 84, p. 968, makes a short communication on the transmission of measles from man to rabbit by means of intravenous inoculation with blood. She states that an erythema develops within 48 hours and lasts from 24 to 48 hours. The blood of a scarlet fever patient produced only a slight reddening after the same interval of time, but no real erythema. These injections were made at this laboratory a number of years ago, but the results were not considered conclusive enough to follow up or to publish, until Dr. Harde saw the rabbits described in the present articles.

SPONTANEOUS CHRONIC MENINGO-ENCEPHALITIS OF RABBITS

Jean Oliver

From the Pathological Laboratory, School of Medicine, Stanford University, San Francisco, Calif.

During the course of the last year we have been studying reactions which follow arsphenamin administration to rabbits. After each experiment, tissues were taken from all the organs as a routine measure and examined for any lesions that might be present.

In the first group of experiments, animals were given repeated large doses of arsphenamin extending over a period of 10 days, and, as a rule, such animals died from the effects of this procedure. Lesions of various organs were found and especially a peculiar inflammatory process in the brain. A later group of experiments in which the animals died immediately or in the course of a few hours following the injection of massive doses of arsphenamin, also showed these same lesions of the central nervous system, and as in these cases sufficient time had not elapsed for the development of changes of this type, it seemed fairly certain that the lesions must be due to a disease spontaneously occurring in the rabbits. Supposedly normal animals from our stock-room were therefore killed and their brains examined. Brains were also obtained from the public markets. In both instances about 20% of the animals showed the same lesions as had been encountered in the experimental animals.

No gross lesions of the meninges or in frontal sections of the brain could be made out. Microscopic examination, however, showed a widespread inflammatory process most frequently in the cerebral cortex, but also occurring in the neighborhood of the basal ganglions and the medulla.

The pia in all cases showed a varying degree of infiltration with "round cells." This consisted in most part of lymphocytes, though a few plasma cells were occasionally found. The process was often most marked in the cerebral sulci and in such places extended to the depths of the fissures. An extension into the substance of the cerebral cortex was also seen around the small vessels of the pia, which penetrate it. Here a "jacket" of lymphocytes, often of considerable thickness, was

Received for publication Aug. 29, 1921.

commonly found (fig. 1). Similar perivascular infiltrations were found around small vessels in the centrum ovale, the basal ganglions and the medulla (fig. 2).

Besides these perivascular collections of round cells, in those cases in which the lesions were most marked, an extension of the infiltration into the substance of the brain tissue was found. This consisted of focal round areas of cellular infiltration lying, as a rule, beside a small vessel or between two such vessels. Occasionally there seemed

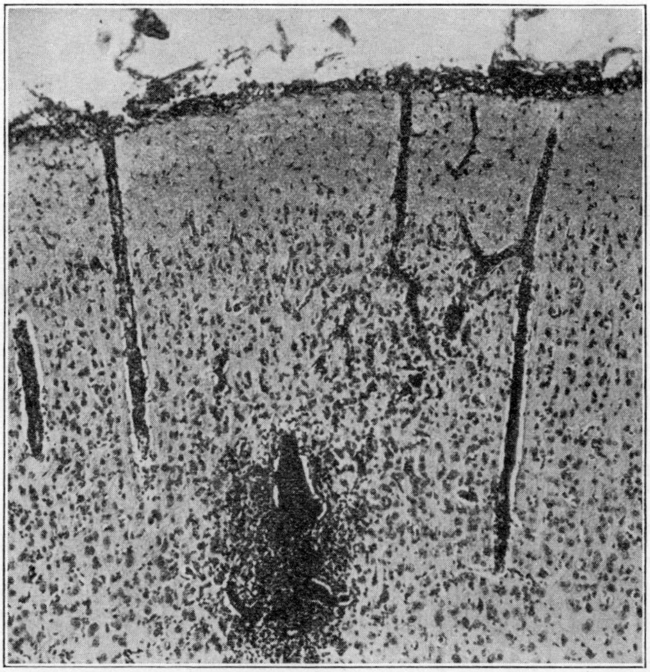

Fig. 1.—Cerebral cortex showing infiltration of pia and small vessels with lymphocytes. In the lower part of the section appears an area of focal infiltration.

to be a proliferation of capillaries into these regions, and in the larger ones the centers were necrotic and filled with nuclear débris. Fat stains of such areas of necrosis showed a large amount of fat, both free in the necrotic material and in the form of fine droplets in the leukocytes surrounding it. Nissl stains of various parts of the brain showed no definite lesions in the ganglion cells, except that those in the immediate neighborhood of the areas of focal infiltration often stained poorly.

The distribution of these inflammatory processes in a single case varied widely depending on the severity of the disease. The least affected showed only a meningeal involvement, others, meningeal and perivascular, while in the most severe cases focal areas of infiltration and necrosis were present. In some ainmals these processes were most marked in the cerebrum, in others the centrum ovale or basal ganglions were more involved. One frequently found combination which anatomically resembles very closely "lethargic encephalitis" of

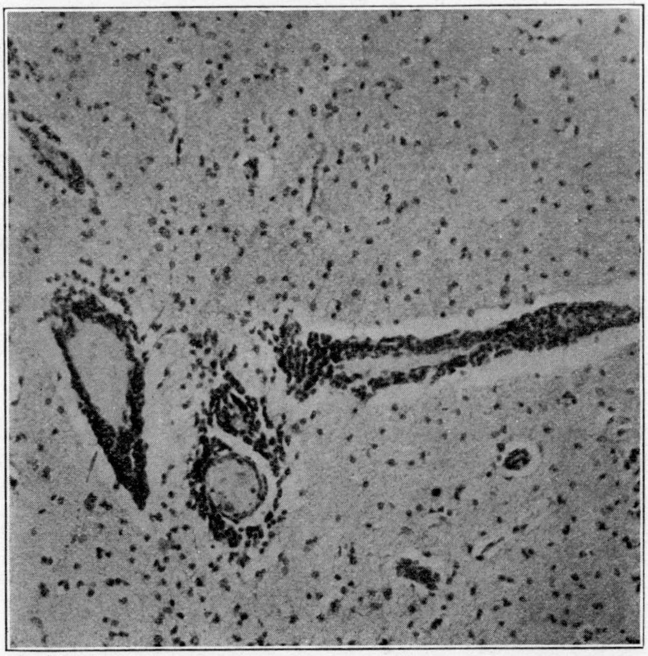

Fig. 2.—Perivascular infiltration with lymphocytes around vessels in neighborhood of basal ganglions.

man, was a slight meningeal and a more marked perivascular infiltration in the region of the basal ganglions, with no areas of focal infiltration and necrosis.

Sections stained for bacteria with the Giemsa, Gram-Weigert and carbol-fuchsin methods showed no organisms in any of the lesions.

The rabbits in our stock-room have been examined for functional disturbances. Their gait is normal, and various reflexes—accommodation of the pupil to light, for instance—are apparently normal. They seem to be as lively as normal rabbits and none have died recently. None of those examined had had "snuffles" recently.

These rabbits are bought in comparatively small numbers from several widely separated sources, and as a rule are used in the course of a week or 10 days. It seems, therefore, on account of the chronicity of the lesions and also from the fact that the same process was found in rabbits from the public markets, that the disease is of widespread distribution in this region. The disease has apparently not been of constant duration, as in 1917 Dr. E. C. Dickson in some experiments on botulism, using rabbits from the same stock-room, examined 60 experimental animals without encountering the condition.

In some experiments on the results of injections of streptococci into rabbits, Bull[1] has described similar lesions to those mentioned. He also examined three control rabbits which had died of a bacillary septicemia associated with snuffles. In one of these animals the same lesions were found.

Our findings show how prevalent such spontaneous lesions may be and also that they may be unassociated with snuffles or with any other demonstrable disturbance in the animals' health. Though the disease seems to be of little importance as far as the general health of the rabbit is concerned, the importance of the lesion as a source of confusion in experimental procedures is obvious. This is especially true as the animals rarely die, and as there is apparently no simple means of determining from a clinical examination whether the rabbit is healthy or not.

[1] Jour. Exper. Med., 1917, 25, p. 557.

A BUFFERED PHYSIOLOGIC SALT SOLUTION

Alice C. Evans

From the Hygienic Laboratory, U. S. Public Health Service, Washington, D. C.

The importance of the relationship between H-ion concentration of the medium and biologic phenomena has received much attention in recent years. But the results of the researches of Sørensen, Michaelis, Henderson, Clark and others have not yet been practically applied to every phase of biologic investigation. In the field of immunology the various tests are generally carried on without the degree of consideration for control of H-ion concentration which it is practically possible to attain. It is the purpose of this paper to present a simple method for the control of the H-ion concentration of physiologic salt solution.

Even when all due care is taken for the cleanliness of receptacles, the range of variation in reaction of unbuffered solutions is considerable. Distilled water standing in hard glass flasks, protected from the atmosphere only by a cotton plug, has been found to absorb enough carbon dioxide to bring the reaction to P_H 5.8. On the other hand, distilled water which had been sterilized and left standing in soft glass cylinders with ground glass stoppers was found with a reaction of P_H 8.8. These figures are merely variations which have come under the writer's observation. Recently Esty and Cathcart [1] have presented data showing the variations in H-ion concentration of unbuffered solutions sterilized in hard and soft glass. They tested the variations in 0.85% sodium chloride solution, distilled water, and in weak solutions of hydrochloric acid and sodium hydroxide. Their results show an increase in alkalinity as the heating is prolonged in soft glass tubes, whereas an increase in acidity was observed in hard glass tubes.

The influence of variation in H-ion concentration of the medium has not been determined for certain serologic reactions used commonly for test purposes. But there is a general recognition of a relationship between H-ion concentration and agglutination. For theoretical considerations the reader is referred to a recent paper by Coulter.[2] A single illustration of the influence of H-ion concentration on agglutination is given in table 1.

Received for publication Aug. 30, 1921.

[1] J. Infect. Dis., 1921, 29, p. 29.
[2] J. Gen'l Phys., 1921, 3, p. 309.

The tests for which the data are given in table 1 were made with monovalent meningococcus rabbit serum. The immunizing strain and test strain belonged to type 2. The antigen was killed by heat and made up to a standard density so that the final suspension contained the equivalent of 500 part per million of silica standard. Antigen suspensions and serum dilutions were made up in salt solutions varying in H-ion concentration. They were held at the desired P_H values by the use of buffer mixtures, as described further on. For the tests the various antigen suspensions were added to the corresponding serum dilutions. Incubation took place over night in a water bath at 56 C.

TABLE 1

INFLUENCE OF H-ION CONCENTRATION ON AGGLUTINATION OF MENINGOCOCCI

H ion Concentration	Salt Solution Alone	Normal Serum 1:50	Immune Serum Diluted 1 Part in:					
			50	100	200	400	800	1600
P_H 5.6	0	0	4	4	4	4	4	3
P_H 6.0	0	0	4	4	4	4	4	3
P_H 6.4	0	0	4	4	4	4	3	2
P_H 6.8	0	0	4	4	4	4	3	2
P_H 7.0	0	0	4	4	4	3	3	1
P_H 7.4	0	0	4	4	4	3	2	1
P_H 7.7	0	0	3	4	4	3	2	1
P_H 8.0	0	0	3	4	4	3	2	1
P_H 8.6	0	0	4	4	4	3	2	1

4 = complete agglutination; 3 = turbidity in a control tube containing 75% as much antigen as in the tubes in which the test was carried out; 2 = turbidity in a control tube containing 50% of the antigen; 1 = turbidity in a control tube containing 25% of the anitigen.

According to the method used for reading the results of routine tests at the Hygienic Laboratory, by which reactions expressed by 4 and 3 are considered positive, and those expressed by 2 and 1 are considered negative, this serum had a titer of 1:400 when the reaction was P_H 7.4; a titer of 1:800 when the reaction was P_H 7; and a titer of 1:1,600 when the reaction was P_H 6.

Russell, Nichols and Stimmel[3] found that there was a wide variation in the reaction of typhoid vaccines, and they devised a method by which variations in either direction could be controlled. A solution of 8.7 gm. KH_2PO_4 and 165 gm. K_2HPO_4 in one liter of distilled water was prepared. Two c c of this solution added to each liter of 0.85% NaC1 solution used in making the vaccine was found to hold the reaction at about P_H 7.4. The reaction of the buffer solution was about P_H 8, that of the buffered salt solution P_H 7.4.

[3] Milit. Surgeon, 1920, 47, p. 359.

The simple formula here proposed for a buffered salt solution would be applicable to the preparation of a salt solution with a controlled H-ion concentration for any biologic use except when it is desirable to have calcium in the solution. (The calcium would combine with the phosphates to form an insoluble precipitate.)

The controlling agent in the buffered salt solution is a phosphate mixture prepared according to Sørenson. The $\frac{m}{15}$ primary (KH_2PO_4) and secondary ($Na_2HPO_4 \cdot 2\,H_2O$) phosphates are mixed together in the proportions given in Sørensen's tables to obtain any desired P_H value between 5.3 and 8.

In practice the procedure is as follows: A $\frac{m}{15}$ solution of primary phosphate is prepared by adding 9.078 gm. KH_2PO_4 to 1 liter of distilled water. A $\frac{m}{15}$ solution of secondary phosphate is prepared by adding 11.876 gm. $Na_2HPO_4 \cdot 2\,H_2O$ to 1 liter of distilled water. A mixture of 6 c c of the secondary solution and 4 c c of the primary solution has a P_H value very near 7. A mixture of 8 c c of the secondary solution and 2 c c of the primary solution has a P_H value very near 7.4. A solution of any other desired concentration within the range of the phosphate mixture can be obtained by altering the proportions of primary and secondary solutions.

In ordinary routine work commercial chemicals and a rough balance can be used. The mixtures should be controlled by comparing with standard buffer solutions, adjusting to the desired H-ion concentration by adding a little more of the acid or alkaline solution as required. It should be borne in mind that the commercial secondary phosphate contains 12 mols of water of crystallization, and if used in the buffer mixtures the $\frac{m}{15}$ solution should be calculated accordingly. The salt containing 2 mols of water of crystallization is prepared by exposing to the ordinary atmosphere the crystals containing the 12 mols of water. About 2 weeks' exposure is sufficient. For further information regarding Sørensen's standard buffer solutions the reader is referred to Clark, "The Determination of Hydrogen Ions," from which this information was obtained.

For the preparation of the isotonic buffered salt solution 1 part of phosphate mixture of the desired H-ion concentration is added to 9 parts of 0.9% NaCl solution.

The efficacy of the buffered salt solution to maintain the desired H-ion concentration, by taking care of the variations in reaction to which laboratory solutions treated with due care are subject, was tested. Unbuffered salt solution was rendered acid or alkaline by the addition of HCl or NaOh. To 9 parts of these salt solutions 1 part of phosphate mixture P_H 7 was added. The salt solutions with H-ion concentrations up to P_H 3.8 were completely neutralized by the buffer. Those with P_H values of 3.4 and 3.6 had a P_H value of 6.9 and the P_H 3 solution had a P_H value of 6.8 after the addition of the buffer. The alkaline solutions with P_H values up to 10 were completely neutralized by the buffer. But the buffer was not capable of controlling perfectly the alkali in a sample of water, said to be distilled, which had been sterilized in a soft glass container. The water had a P_H value of 8.8. When the buffer was added the solution had a H-ion concentration of 7.2. This illustrates how the efficiency of the buffer depends on the nature of the solution to which it is added.

The P_H values recorded in this paper were determined by the use of the colorimetric method. There are certain errors which would be detected by the electrometric method, but these are negligible from a practical point of view when buffered solutions are used in serologic tests.

INFECTION OF THE MENINGES AND LUNGS BY A SPECIES OF ACTINOMYCES

Howard H. Bell

From the Department of Pathology, Washington University School of Medicine, St. Louis

Infection of the central nervous system by branching threadlike organisms is rare. I have studied a case of primary meningeal infection with pulmonary embolic abscesses, and comparison of this case with those in the literature reveals many interesting features. I have found records of 46 instances of infection of the central nervous system by this type of organism; in 15 instances the infection was probably primary in the nervous system and in 31 the infection obviously was secondary to a chronic focus, or foci, elsewhere in the body.

Musgrave, Clegg and Polk [1] cite a series of 257 cases of infection by these organisms studied by Duvan, in which 19 showed infection of the nervous system, and a series of 109 cases studied by Ackland in which 5 showed infection of the nervous system.

Abstract of History

A white adult male, 44 years old, traveling salesman, was admitted to Barnes Hospital, Dec. 14, 1920, complaining of headache and high fever. The patient gave a history of furunculosis for the past 4 or 5 months and of having had a small pimple on the outside of his nose about 2 weeks before admission. The illness commenced Dec. 6, 1920, with a chill. Dec. 8, the patient complained of cold in the head and fever. Dec. 9 severe headache developed, with chills, and the temperature rose to 100 to 104 F. and continued until admission.

Symptoms of meningitis became more and more evident. The cerebrospinal fluid was turbid and under increased pressure. The cell count was 2,300, 88% were polymorphonuclears. Globulin and albumin were increased. The patient died Dec. 20.

Necropsy Report (F. A. McJunkin).—The body was that of a well developed and well nourished man. Both eyes protruded slightly; the conjunctivae were swollen and ecchymotic.

On the pleural surface of the left lung were about two dozen raised areas from 2 mm. to 2 cm. in diameter, which were firm and rather sharply circumscribed; the peripheries were dark red, and the centers were yellowish white, and purulent. A small amount of gas was present in a few. The pus was viscid and tenacious and brownish gray. The right lung contained about half a dozen similar nodules.

A smaller vessel at the periphery of one of the consolidated areas was occluded.

Received for publication, Sept. 10, 1921.

[1] Philippine Jour. Sc., 3 Sec., B, 1908, p. 483.

On cutting the dura over the right temporal lobe a small amount of grayish pus escaped. The hypophysis was surrounded by a purulent exudate and both cavernous sinuses were completely filled with pus. In the anterior part of the middle fossa on the right side was a mass of exudate 1 cm. thick, which was adherent to the skull where the abducens and oculomotor entered. The entire base of the brain was covered with yellowish pus which extended over the right temporal lobe and to a less extent over the right frontal and occipital lobes. The involvement on the left side of the brain was less.

The vessels over the spinal cord were injected but no distinct inflammatory exudate was present.

Microscopic Examination.—The lesions in the lungs were strikingly focal; at the periphery of the areas the vessels were much distended and there was hemorrhage into the alveoli. In the centers of some areas appeared vacuoles around which were leukocytes chiefly of the neutrophilic variety, and also, a considerable number of mononuclear lekocytes some of which had ingested the neutrophils and other material. In the centers the alveolar septums had disappeared although toward the peripheries they could be recognized and contained polymorphonuclear and mononuclear cells. In the inner part of the abscess walls appeared bluish masses of bacillary forms and delicate filaments. In one section a vessel at the site of branching was completely filled with masses of organisms and granular débris; other smaller vessels in that vicinity were filled with the same material.

The entire cortex of the brain toward the base was covered with an exudate which was thickest in the sulci. Neutrophils and large mononuclear leukocytes were present in varying proportions. There were circumscribed foci consisting entirely of neutrophils and in places there were areas of large mononuclear leukocytes containing large vacuoles. In many places the distended vessels were filled with exudate, and in some of these appeared a yellowish pigment resembling disintegrated hemoglobin. Masses of organisms were present in all of these localities.

The entire pituitary body was covered with a fibrinopurulent exudate; the anterior part showed necrosis for a distance of 2 mm. The sections included the cavernous sinus which contained cellular exudate and masses of bacillary forms and what appeared to be branching organisms.

There were a few sclerotic glomeruli in the cortex near the capsule which were infiltrated with lymphocytes. Some of the tubules showed hyaline casts. In other places there was a small amount of perivascular infiltration with lymphocytes. In one small vessel was a fibrinous clot containing numerous leukocytes but no micro-organisms could be found.

In the cortex of the suprarenals were scattered suprarenal cells and foci of cells undergoing necrosis, some of which contained globules of fat. The necrotic areas were invaded by large mononuclear leukocytes.

No abnormalities were observed in the other organs.

Anatomic Diagnosis.—Septic thrombosis of cavernous sinuses; purulent meningitis; septic emboli of lungs; edema and ecchymosis of conjunctivae were diagnosed.

DESCRIPTION OF THE ACTINOMYCES

Films of pus from the lesions in the meninges and lungs stained by Gram's method showed many fairly long bacillary forms, often slightly curved with bluntly pointed, occasionally square, ends. Several bacillary forms often appeared to be in chains. Curved or comma forms and coccoid forms were not infrequent. Occasionally there was a fairly long bacillary form with spherical bodies at short intervals which were gram-positive, while the rod was slightly or not at all gram-positive. The film gave the appearance of a mixed infection. Branching was infrequent, but after long search could be found. Stained with carbolfuchsin, the picture was slightly different. The mycelia were stained as well as the disintegration products and fairly long filaments could be recognized; short bacillary and coccoid forms were also recognized. Branching appeared only slightly more frequently.

Cultures were made on blood agar in tube slants and in Petri dishes, on brown blood agar, on milk, deep gelatin, potato, deep glucose agar and on meat mediums. The meat medium was identical with that used by the Royal Medical Corps in France for growing anaerobes associated with war wounds; it was made by boiling finely ground muscle with an equal weight of tap water, made alkaline with sodium hydroxide and tubed so that about 5 c.mm. finely ground meat would be covered with 1 c.mm. of fluid in which the meat was boiled; the medium was then autoclaved.

About 30 inoculations were made in all. After 2 weeks' inoculation growth was found in one meat tube which was gradually digested as growth proceeded. The morphology of the organism in the primary culture was identical with that of the organism in the lesion. Primary subsequent inoculations from this meat tube showed no growth. Some inoculations were incubated 3 weeks in anaerobic jars and no growth took place. After inoculation of about 8 tubes each of plain broth, dextrose broth, plain broth containing hydrocele fluid, plain agar slants, glucose agar slant, plain deep agar, blood agar slant, Bordet-Gengou potato medium, milk, gelatin, potato, glycerol potato, Lubenau's egg medium, Petroff's egg medium, meat mediums and Loeffler's serum, growth was obtained on one blood agar slant. The morphology of the organism in secondary culture was identical with that observed in the primary culture. Subinoculations from this second generation grew readily on all mediums, and better aerobically than anaerobically. Young generations showed many long filaments with a few bacillary and coccoid forms. On longer incubation these same cultures showed a marked tendency toward disintegration with chain sporulation producing many bacillary and coccoid forms. No stained filaments appeared in cultures 3 months old, and all forms appeared as very short bacilli or cocci, often in chains. The formation of true spores and the presence of motility have not been observed.

The colonies were umbilicated and yellowish gray; on potato the color was frequently more yellowish. The colonies coalesced and the growth wrinkled on the surface of the medium. On an agar slant the growth penetrated the medium slightly, although it crumbled easily and particles of growth could be readily removed. On Bordet-Gengou potato medium the growth was blackish and had a metallic luster. Gelatin and Loeffler's medium were slowly liquefied. Litmus milk was slowly turned deep blue and often showed a slight coagulation which was rather soft in consistency but firm enough to remain at the bottom in a tilted tube; the lower part of the medium was gradually bleached toward a violet brown color, and evidence of digestion appeared. After a period of 3 or 4 weeks digestion was apparently complete and the fluid remaining was a muddy brownish color.

The growth over a period of three months was not alcohol-fast and not acid-alcohol-fast; however, it was not entirely decolorized by aqueous acid solution and the filaments often showed a slight brownish color when counterstained with Loeffler's methylene blue.

Intrapulmonary, intraperitoneal and subcutaneous inoculations of the pus into guinea-pigs gave negative results. Intratracheal, intravenous, intrapulmonary, intraperitoneal and subcutaneous inoculations of the pus into rabbits likewise gave negative results. Similar inoculations of the culture were negative. Intracerebral inoculations of the culture into a rabbit produced no symptoms or recognizable pathologic change.

CASES IN THE LITERATURE RESEMBLING IN SOME RESPECTS THE ONE REPORTED

Infections, probably primary in the nervous system, were described by Bollinger,[2] Musser, Pearce and Gwyn,[3] and Howard.[4] The infecting organisms were not recovered in culture and therefore only limited comparison can be made with other organisms. The morphology in each instance as shown in stained preparations was similar to the one I have described.

Naunyn[5] observed meningeal infection associated with excresences on the mitral valve; threadlike branching organisms were present in both situations. No mention of cultures was made.

Sabrazés et Rivière[6] described infection of the brain associated with lesions in the apexes of the lungs and infarct of one kidney. In stained preparations were long branching filamentous organisms some of which showed unstained areas; chains of irregular coccoid forms were occasionally seen. No filaments were found in the lesions of the lungs. All cultures were negative except for one colony which grew in deep gelatin. Subcultures failed to grow.

Almquist[7] described a case of meningeal infection unassociated with demonstrable lesions elsewhere. A large micrococcus, B. proteus, and one colony of a "streptothrix" were grown in cultures. No mention was made of finding this organism in the pus or in the sections. The source of this organism consequently is questionable. It grew luxuriantly in cultures, liquefied gelatin and produced aerial hyphae. It stained lightly with anilin dyes and showed frequent branching.

Ferré et Faguet[8] reported a case in which the infection was apparently primary in the brain. A "streptothrix" was obtained in pure culture which grew well on ordinary mediums but best on potato. It showed knoblike terminations. It was gram-positive and nopathogenic for guinea-pigs. On subdural injections in rabbits, the organisms were found in other organs but without reaction.

Eppinger[9] described an infection of the meninges associated with lesions of the lungs, pleurae, and peribronchial, mediastinal and right supraclavicular lymph nodes. A branching threadlike organism was found in the pus of the lesions and was described by Eppinger as Cladothrix asteroides. Later MacCallum[10] isolated a similar organism from a case of peritonitis and classified it as Actinomyces asteroides. This organism grew well on artificial mediums and produced a buff colored pigment. The filaments were fairly short and moderately acid-fast. Gelatin was not liquefied. It was relatively very pathogenic for laboratory animals.

From four of the cases already mentioned organisms have been cultured from the cerebral lesions. The organism isolated by Almquist, Ferré et Faguet, Eppinger and from the case here reported, were truly branching organisms which grew aerobically at room and incubator temperatures. In suppurative lesions produced by them they have

[2] München. med. Wchnschr., 1887, 34, p. 789.
[3] Trans. Assn. Am. Phys., 1901, 16, p. 208.
[4] Jour. Med. Research, 1903, 9, p. 301.
[5] Mitt. a. d. Med. Klinik zu Königsberg, 1888.
[6] Presse méd., 1894, 2, p. 302.
[7] Ztschr. f. Hyg. u. Infectionskrankh., 1890, 8, p. 193.
[8] Mercredi Méd., 1895, 6. 441.
[9] Beitr. f. path. Anat. u. z. allg. Path. 1891, 9, p. 287.
[10] Centralbl. f. Bakt., O., I. 1902, 31, p. 529.

appeared as interlacing masses of mycelia and not as compact colonies. They differed from one another in certain details as follows:

The strain described by Almquist showed aerial hyphae and liquefied gelatin.

The one described by Ferré et Faguet showed knoblike terminations and grew best on potato.

The one isolated by Eppinger showed fairly short branching filaments which were moderately acid-fast. It did not liquefy gelatin.

The one isolated from our case did not produce aerial hyphae or knoblike terminations of the filaments, and liquefied gelatin.

INFECTIONS OF THE NERVOUS SYSTEM BY BRANCHING ORGANISMS DISSIMILAR TO THE ONE NOW REPORTED

The terms actinomycosis bovis and actinomycosis hominis are used to designate chronic granulating and suppurating lesions, the pus of which contains the characteristic yellowish granules composed of dense aggregates of branching threads and their products including the characteristic refringent club-shaped bodies radially displaced at the periphery. Some variation in the organism causing typical actinomycosis has occurred.

In the case described by O. Israel,[11] the part of the process involving the vertebrae showed only leptothrix forms while the lesions elsewhere in the body showed the characteristic yellowish granules with club formation. The case described by Gangee[12] showed chronic "actinomycosis" of the trunk with secondary cerebral involvement; the pus contained interlacing masses of mycelia without club formation in any lesion. Nevertheless, it is accepted by many that true actinomycosis is caused by gram-positive organisms of the type described by Wolf and Israel in 1891. The organism described by them grew reluctantly, preferably under anaerobic conditions and at incubator temperature. Cerebral infection was preceded by actinomycosis elsewhere in the body. Infections probably occurred by contiguity of structure in some instances and in others was transmitted by the blood stream. Many of the cases of cerebral infections of this type are reviewed by Askanazy.[13]

DISCUSSION OF GRAM-POSITIVE THREADLIKE BRANCHING ORGANISMS

These organisms have been described under at least five generic names: Actinomyces, Clodothrix, Nocardia, Oospora and Streptothrix.[14] Claypole[15] considered these organisms as belonging to one genus and

[11] Berl. klin. Wchnschr., 1884, 21, S. 360.
[12] Brit. Med. Jour., 1889, 1, p. 1172.
[13] Rev. méd. de la Suisse romande, 1919, 39, p. 515.
[14] Lancet, 1910, 1, p. 551.
[15] Jour. Exper. Med., 1913, 17, p. 99.

urged the use of streptothrix as the generic name. Wright[16] regarded Actinomyces and the organism described by Nocard as two distinct genera. He opposed the use of the names Streptothrix, Clodothrix and Oospora because they have been used previously for plant genera to which these organisms do not belong. Actinomyces was accepted by him as the generic name for the organisms causing Actinomycosis bovis and Actinomycosis hominis, and Nocardia as the generic name for the organisms similar to the one described by Nocard, which was truly branching filamentous and grew best aerobically and well at room temperature.

The committee on the Society of American Bacteriologists on characterization and classification of bacterial types[17] recommended the generic name Actinomyces for the entire group with Actinomyces bovis as a type species.

Acitinomyces shows some variation in the oxygen tension requirements and in growth in gelatin. Silberschmidt[18] advanced a classification based on these cultural differences. After comparing his own strains with others obtained elsewhere he recognized the following groups:

1. Growth aerobic and at room temperature. Colonies on agar and blood serum adherent and send out numerous mycelial outgrowths into the mediums.
(a) Liquefies gelatin; threads long; interlaced and unbroken, includes Actinomyces hominis and bovis (Boström and others) and Actinomadurae.
(b) Does not liquefy gelatin, threads broken and often appearing in short forms, Actinomyces asteroides (Eppinger) Actinomyces caprae (Silberschmidt).
2. Colonies not adherent to mediums, gelatin not liquified, threads mostly short and many bacillary forms, "Actinomyces farcinic," and the organism obtained in Silberschmidt's Case 3.
3. Growth preferably anaerobic, colonies show no mycelial projections, and on solid medium are usually small and sharply circumscribed. No growth on gelatin or at room temperature; colonies are readily crushed and broken up. The organism does not survive as long as those of Groups 1 and 2 on artificial mediums. To this group belong the cultures from 7 of his human cases as well as those from actinomycosis of cattle.

I have found record of 8 cases of infection of the nervous system by branching threadlike organisms which were gram-negative.

Rutelli[19] reported a case of primary infection of the meninges by a "streptothrix" in a child who died 8 days after the onset of the illness. The patient had fever, vomited and developed diarrhea. The leukocyte count was

[16] Jour. Med. Research, 1905, 13, p. 349.
[17] Jour. Bacteriol., 1920, 5, p. 191.
[18] Ztschr. f. Hyg. U. Infectionskrankh., 1901, 37, p. 345.
[19] La Pediatria, 1915, 23, p. 712.

15,000 (48% polymorphonuclear, 31% lymphocytes, 13% mononuclear and 8% other cells). In the cerebrospinal fluid were organisms in filaments which at times showed granules. This organism grew readily on Bordet-Gengou medium aerobically and showed short filaments, streptobacilli and large coccoid forms which were a little elongated. Branching was present. The organism was gram-negative, and was neither alcohol-fast nor acid-fast. Intraperitoneal injections into guinea-pigs produced a purulent peritonitis which was fatal in 3 days. The patient's blood did not contain agglutinins.

Sindoni[20] reported six cases of primary infection of the meninges in children. These occurred during an epidemic of acute cerebrospinal meningitis and all showed the symptoms of acute meningitis.

1.—A "streptothrix" occurred in pure culture from the cerebrospinal fluid.

2.—After the administration of antimeningococcus serum there was some temporary improvement in the condition. On the twelfth day after the onset a "streptothrix" was grown in pure culture from the cerebrospinal fluid.

3.—Early cultures from the cerebrospinal fluid showed the presence of the meningococcus in pure growth. Later cultures showed also the presence of a "streptothrix."

4.—Cultures from the cerebrospinal fluid showed both the meningococcus and a "streptothrix."

5.—Cultures from the cerebrospinal fluid showed the meningococcus. Some temporary improvement in the condition followed the administration of antimeningococcus serum. Later cultures gave a "streptothrix."

6.—A "streptothrix" was grown in pure culture from the cerebrospinal fluid.

Five cases were fatal. In the remaining case the outcome was not known. Sindoni considered that the meningococcus infection diminished the resistance of the patients and favored secondary infection by "streptothrix." The organisms were apperently identical with the one described by Rutelli.

Khárina-Marinucci[21] described a case of acute suppurative meningitis in a child caused by "streptothrix." The patient developed slight bronchopneumonia the cause of which was not determined. The possibility of an acute primary pulmonary infection cannot be excluded in this case. The organism was apparently identical with the ones described by Rutelli and Sindoni.

In the "Final Report of the Committee of the Society of American Bacteriologists on the Characterization and Classification of Bacterial Types," consideration is given to "Actinobacillus Brumpt," which resembles the gram-negative organisms described by Rutelli, Sindoni and Khárina-Marinucci.

SUMMARY

The gram-positive micro-organism isolated from my case grows best aerobically and well at room temperature. Under the classification given by Silberschmidt, it resembles 1a, although his description is insufficient in detail to attach it definitely to his classification. It differs from Actinomyces bovis in that it grows better under aerobic conditions and well at room temperature; from Actinomyces asteroides of Eppinger in that it liquefies gelatin; from the actinomyces of Almquist in that it does not possess arerial hyphae, and from the actinomyces of

[20] Ibid., 1916, 24, p. 530.
[21] Ibid., 1918, 26, p. 536.

Ferré et Faguet in that it does not show knoblike terminations of the mycelia. It furthermore differs in other details.

The organisms described by Rutelli, Sindoni and Khárina-Marinucci in association with acute primary meningitis were gram-negative and distinct from the ones described by Wolf and Israel, Eppinger, Almquist Ferré et Faguet and the one from the case reported.

Six fairly distinct types of filamentous branching organisms have been isolated from infections of the nervous system. (1) Actinomyces bovis and Actinomyces hominis (doubtless identical), (2) actinomyces of Eppinger, (3) actinomyces of Almquist, (4) actinomyces of Ferré et Faguet, (5) actinomyces from the case reported, and (6) the gram-negative micro-organism described by Rutelli, Sindoni and Khárina-Marinucci.

The infection of the nervous system usually ran an acute clinical course and was fatal in all instances in which the disease was recognized (except in one case in which the outcome was not known) usually within 2 to 14 days after the onset of cerebral manifestations, although the development of the disease in several instances was apparently more insidious. The patients with actinomycosis observed by Enriquez and Sicard and Keller were benefited by decompression operations. Enriquez and Sicard's patient lived several weeks after the operation and died from acute suppurative meningitis caused by a staphylococcus. Keller evacuated the Actinomycosis abscess of the brain, and the patient was temporarily relieved. The symptoms returned in about one year and a second operation was performed, the patient dying soon after.

The lesions in the brain usually were represented by single or multiple abscess formation associated with more or less purulent meningitis, and in several instances by purulent meningitis without abscess formation. There is a record of thrombosis of the larger venous channels in one case described by Ponfick,[22] in one by Moosbrugger,[23] and in two cases by Askanazy,[13] to which our case may be added.

[22] Die Actinomykose des Menschen, 1882.
[23] Beitr. z. klin. Chir., 1886, 2, p. 339.

ANAPHYLATOXIN AND ANAPHYLAXIS

XII. STUDIES ON THE CHEMISTRY OF THE BLOOD

W. M. German

From the Hygienic Laboratory of the University of Michigan, Ann Arbor

Since the phenomenon of anaphylaxis was first observed many attempts have been made to explain it. Most of these attempts have been purely theoretical, based on biologic data and when any chemical investigation has been made it has involved the antigen primarily, giving the chemistry of the animal tissues and body fluids secondary importance. Conclusions have been reached, therefore, explaining the mechanism of anaphylaxis from observations made on the nature of the antigen and its biochemical possibilities when injected, assuming that the source of the poison (if such) was the antigen.

A more recent view [1, 2] is in favor of considering the constituents of the serum and tissues of the animal body as the source or matrix of the poison or toxic body responsible for the anaphylactic phenomena; and that the toxic body (anaphylatoxin) produced in vitro is identical with that produced in the sensitized animal body by the injection of a suitable antigen. It should be stated, however, that Besredka does not consider anaphylatoxin as having any relation to anaphylactic shock.

In a previous paper [3] it has been shown that amino nitrogen determinations in toxic and control normal serums do not lend support to the theory of proteolysis.

It seemed desirable to follow up this work with a study of the effect, if there is any, produced on the alkaline reserve in the process of poison production and thus to determine whether acidosis has any bearing on anaphylatoxin production or anaphylaxis.

ALKALINE RESERVE AND ANAPHYLATOXIN

In the first series of experiments, anaphylatoxin was prepared with the aid of inulin, following the procedure heretofore employed.[3]

Received for publication Aug. 1, 1921.

[1] Bordet and Zunz: Ztschr. f. Immunitätsf., 1914, 23, p. 49.

[2] Novy and DeKruif: "Anaphylatoxin and Anaphylaxis," Jour. Infect. Dis., 1917, 20, p. 499; Jour. Am. Med. Assn., 1917, 68, p. 1524.

[3] De Kruif, P. H., and German, W. M.: Jour. Infect. Dis., 1917, 20, p. 833.

Experiments with Inulin Anaphylatoxin.—Six normal white rats were bled from the heart by means of the usual pipet;[4] the blood was defibrinated, pooled and centrifugated. The supernatant serum was pipetted off and treated as follows:

A. To 5 c c of the serum, 1 c c of 5% inulin suspension (in 0.85% salt solution) was added and the well shaken mixture was then incubated at 38 C. for 15 minutes. It was then centrifugated at 3000 r.p.m. for 15 minutes and the supernatant serum was pipetted off. This was then tested: (1) for toxicity, 1 c c being injected intravenously into a guinea-pig of about 200 gm.; (2) 1 c c was subjected to the Van Slyke method for the determination of plasma bicarbonate, the gasometric CO_2 apparatus being employed.[5]

B. The other portion of 5 c c serum served for control purposes. After adding 1 c c of 0.85% NaCl solution, corresponding to the amount of inulin suspension used in A, the mixture was incubated and centrifugated the same as portion A and at the same time. The clear supernatant serum was then tested (1) for toxicity, and (2) for CO_2 capacity. For each test 1 c c was used, the same as in portion A.

TABLE 1

CARBON DIOXIDE CAPACITY AND ANAPHYLATOXIN IN RAT SERUM TREATED WITH INULIN

Experiment	Percentage CO_2 in		Difference	Intravenous Injection* of 1 C c of	
	Toxic Serum	Control Serum		Toxic Serum	Control Serum
12	43.3	42.9	0.4	Shock and death in 3 min.........	Nil
13	47.3	46.4	0.9	Severe shock........................	Nil
20	39.9	38.1	1.8	Severe shock........................	Nil
21	43.5	41.5	2.0	Shock and death in 3.5 min........	Nil

* The toxicity tests were made on guinea-pigs of 200-250 gm. in this and all subsequent experiments.

It will be seen from Table 1 that the CO_2 capacity of the anaphylatoxic serum is in each instance greater than that of the normal control serum, the average difference being only 1.2%. Clearly, the results show no decrease in the alkaline reserve in the toxic serums as compared with the corresponding control serums.

Experiments with Agar Anaphylatoxin.—A second set of experiments with essentially the same technic throughout but using agar-agar as the anaphylatoxin inducing agent is outlined.

Seven normal white rats were bled from the heart by means of the usual heart pipet, the blood was defibrinated, pooled and centrifugated. The supernatant serum was pipetted off and treated as follows:

A. Seven c c of the serum were treated by the agar sol-gel method. (For this purpose 1.7 c c of the 0.5% agar solution was added to the serum, mixed and iced for 1 hour.) The well shaken mixture was then incubated at 38 C. for 10 minutes. It was then centrifugated at 3,000 r.p.m. for 15 minutes and the supernatant serum was pipetted off. This was then tested: (1) for toxicity, 1 c c being injected intravenously into a guinea-pig of about 200 gm.; and

[4] Novy and De Kruif: Ibid., 1917, 20, p. 502.
[5] Jour. Biol. Chem., 1917, 30, p. 347.

(2) for CO_2 capacity, 6 c c being subjected to the Van Slyke bicarbonate determination, 1 c c samples being used for each determination.

B. The other portion of 7 c c serum served for control purposes. After adding 1.7 c c of 0.85% salt solution, corresponding to the amount of agar solution used in A, the well shaken mixture was iced for 1 hour and then incubated at 38 C. for 10 minutes. It was then centrifugated at 3,000 r.p.m. for 15 minutes, the same as portion A and at the same time. The clear supernatant serum was then tested for (1) toxicity and (2) for CO_2 capacity. For each test 1 c c was used, the same as in portion A. The results of 4 experiments as outlined are given in table 2.

TABLE 2

CARBON DIOXIDE CAPACITY AND ANAPHYLATOXIN IN RAT SERUM TREATED WITH AGAR

Experiment	Percentage CO_2 in		Difference	Intravenous Injection of 1 C c of	
	Toxic Serum	Control Serum		Toxic Serum	Control Serum
16	43.6	41.6	2.0	Typical death	Nil
3a	26.9	27.9	—1.0	Severe shock	Nil
17	43.3	42.4	0.9	Typical death	Nil
2a	37.1	30.4	6.7	Typical death	Nil

Experiments with Distilled Water Anaphylatoxin.—In a third set of experiments distilled water was used as the anaphylatoxin inducing agent by the method described by Novy and De Kruif.[6]

Three normal white rats were bled from the heart by means of the usual pipet; the blood was defibrinated, pooled and centrifugated. The supernatant serum was pipetted off and treated thus:

A. To 2 c c of serum were added 12 c c of distilled water. After thorough shaking this mixture was incubated at 38 C. for 30 minutes. This was then tested for (1) toxicity, 7 c c or the equivalent of 1 c c of serum being injected intravenously into a guinea-pig of about 200 gm.; and (2) for CO_2 capacity, the Van Slyke plasma bicarbonate method being used as before.

B. For purposes of control, to 2 c c of serum were added 12 c c distilled water, and, after being thoroughly shaken, the mixture was iced for 30 minutes at the same time that A was being incubated. This was then tested (1) for toxicity, 7 c c (or the equivalent of 1 c c of serum) being injected intravenously into a guinea-pig of about 200 gm.; and (2) for CO_2 capacity, the Van Slyke plasma bicarbonate method being used as before.

C. As a further control 5 c c distilled water were incubated as in the preceding and portions of 1 c c were subjected to the Van Slyke plasma bicarbonate method. The result was subtracted from the results obtained in A and B to correct for the dilution resulting from the addition of distilled water and to put the results on the basis of incubated serum.

In both of the experiments given in table 3, the carbon dioxide of the anaphylatoxic serum is slightly greater than that of the control, the average difference being 1.75%, which is practically the same as noted in table 1.

[6] Jour. Infect. Dis., 1917, 20, p. 807.

TABLE 3

CARBON DIOXIDE CAPACITY AND ANAPHYLATOXIN IN RAT SERUM TREATED WITH DISTILLED WATER

Experiment	Percentage CO_2 in		Difference	Intravenous Injection of 1 C c of	
	Toxic Serum	Control Serum		Toxic Serum	Control Serum
23	22.0	19.5	2.5	Typical shock and death...........	Nil
25	11.0	10.0	1.0	Typical shock and death...........	Nil

Experiments with Inulin Anaphylatoxin in Guinea-Pig Serum.—A fourth set of experiments, observing the same procedure and technic, but using guinea-pig serum instead of rat serum, yielded results which are given in Table 4.

For each experiment a guinea-pig was bled from the heart by means of a blood pipet; the blood was defibrinated, centrifugated and the supernatant serum was pipetted off. It was then treated as follows:

A. To 5 c c of the serum 1 c c of 5% inulin suspension in 0.85% salt solution was added and the well shaken mixture was then incubated at 38 C. for 20 minutes. It was then centrifugated at 3,000 r.p.m. for 15 minutes and the supernatant serum was pipetted off. This was then tested (1) for toxicity, 2.5 c c being injected intravenously into a guinea-pig of about 200 gm.; and (2) for CO_2 capacity, being subjected to the Van Slyke plasma bicarbonate method as before.

B. For purposes of control, to another portion of 5 c c of the serum was added 1 c c of 0.85% salt solution. After thorough shaking the mixture was incubated at 38 C. for 20 minutes at the same time as A; was centrifugated at 3,000 r.p.m. for 15 minutes and the clear supernatant serum pipetted off. This was then tested (1) for toxicity, 2.5 c c being injected intravenously into a guinea-pig of about 200 gm.; and (2) for CO_2 capacity, the Van Slyke plasma bicarbonate method being used as before.

TABLE 4

CARBON DIOXIDE CAPACITY AND ANAPHYLATOXIN IN GUINEA-PIG SERUM TREATED WITH INULIN, AGAR AND DISTILLED WATER

	Experiment	Percentage CO_2 in		Difference	Intravenous Injection of 1 C c of	
		Toxic Serum	Control Serum		Toxic Serum	Control Serum
Inulin............	14b	31.2	32.1	0.9	Nil.......................	Nil
Inulin............	15	36.6	35.7	0.9	Severe shock.............	Nil
Agar.............	14a	44.4	41.7	2.7	Typical shock and death.	Nil
Distilled water....	22	37.1	30.4	6.7	Nil.......................	Nil

The fact that guinea-pig serum is less easily made toxic explains the poor grade of anaphylatoxin produced. The average difference between the normal control and anaphylatoxic serum in CO_2 capacity is here only 0.9%, which is small enough to be within the limits of experimental error.

Experiments with Rat Plasma Inulin Anaphylatoxin.—For each experiment 5 or 6 normal white rats were bled from the heart, the blood being received directly into a centrifuge tube containing a few milligrams of powdered potassium oxalate. After being centrifugated, the supernatant plasma was pipetted off and pooled. This was divided into two equal portions:

A. To 3 c c of plasma was added 0.5 c c of 5% inulin suspension (in 0.85% salt solution). The well shaken mixture was incubated at 38 C. for 15 minutes. It was then centrifugated at 3,000 r.p.m. for 15 minutes and the supernatant plasma was pipetted off. This was then tested (1) for toxicity, 1 c c being injected intravenously into a guinea-pig of about 200 gm.; and (2) for CO_2 capacity, being subjected to the Van Slyke plasma bicarbonate method in 1 c c portions.

B. For control purposes, to 3 c c of the plasma was added 0.5 c c of 0.85% salt solution and the mixture was incubated at 38 C. for 15 minutes at the same time as A. After being centrifugated for 15 minutes at 3,000 r.p.m. the supernatant plasma was pipetted off and tested (1) for toxicity, 1 c c being injected intravenously into a guinea-pig of about 200 gm.; and (2) for CO_2 capacity, being subjected to the Van Slyke plasma bicarbonate method as usual. The results of 5 such experiments are given in table 5, all carried out under exactly the same conditions throughout.

TABLE 5

CARBON DIOXIDE CAPACITY AND ANAPHYLATOXIN IN RAT PLASMA TREATED WITH INULIN

Experiment	Percentage CO_2 in		Difference	Intravenous Injection of 1 C c of	
	Toxic Serum	Control Serum		Toxic Serum	Control Serum
1	23.9	24.2	0.3	Typical shock and death............	Nil
2	29.3	28.5	0.8	Typical shock and death............	Nil
3	24.7	25.6	0.9	Severe shock........................	Nil
4	29.4	27.5	1.9	Typical shock and death............	Nil
5	39.8	37.9	0.9	Severe shock........................	Nil

Here again it can be seen that the average difference in the CO_2 capacity between the anaphylatoxic and normal control plasma is 0.9%, a figure that is sufficiently small to be within the range of experimental error. In every case the plasma was made toxic by incubation while no change in the plasma alkaline reserve kept pace with it.

Experiments with Rat Plasma-Distilled Water Anaphylatoxin.—Finally, rat plasma was made toxic by the use of distilled water, the procedure being the same as that employed with rat serum (Table 3).

For each experiment 5 or more normal rats were bled from the heart, the blood being oxalated by the addition of powdered potassium oxalate, as given in the foregoing, and centrifugated. The supernatant plasma was pipetted off and pooled. This was divided into two portions.

A. To 2 c c plasma were added 10 c c of distilled water. This mixture was shaken for one minute and incubated for 20 minutes at 38 C. It was then tested (1) for toxicity, 6 c c (or the equivalent of 1 c c of plasma) being injected intravenously into a guinea-pig of about 200 gm., and (2) for CO_2 capacity, being subjected in 2 c c samples to the Van Slyke plasma bicarbonate method.

B. For purposes of control, to 2 c c of plasma were added 10 c c distilled water and after being shaken thoroughly the mixture was iced for 30 minutes at the same time that A was being incubated. This was then tested (1) for toxicity, 6 c c (or the equivalent of 1 c c of serum) being injected intravenously into a guinea-pig of about 200 gm.; and (2) for CO_2 capacity, being subjected to the Van Slyke plasma bicarbonate method in 2 c c samples.

C. As a further control, 5 c c of distilled water were subjected to the Van Slyke plasma bicarbonate method. The result was deducted from results obtained in A and B to correct for the addition of distilled water and to put the results on the basis of undiluted plasma.

The results of 6 such experiments, all carried out under exactly the same conditions, are given in Table 6.

TABLE 6

CARBON DIOXIDE CAPACITY AND ANAPHYLATOXIN IN RAT PLASMA TREATED WITH DISTILLED WATER

Experiment	Percentage CO_2 in		Difference	Intravenous Injection of 1 C c of	
	Toxic Serum	Control Serum		Toxic Serum	Control Serum
6	35.9	38.7	2.8	Typical shock and death	Nil
7	24.4	57.0	32.6	Typical shock and death	Nil
8	53.7	53.7	0.0	Severe shock	Nil
9	47.3	47.3	0.0	Severe shock	Nil
10	48.1	50.0	1.9	Severe shock	Nil
11	66.2	55.7	10.5	Typical shock and death	Nil

In this series of experiments there is an average difference of 7.8% in the CO_2 capacity between the anaphylatoxic and control plasma. Such a discrepancy can be accounted for by the fact that CO_2 determinations on 2 c c of the experimental unknown which represents only 0.2 c c of plasma are rendered more liable to error by the factors, dilution and extremely small quantities. The experimental error is therefore large.

Briefly, the results of comparison of CO_2 capacity of anaphylatoxic and normal control serum and plasma are summed up as follows:

Of 25 experiments, in 16 the percentage of bound CO_2 was greater in the anaphylatoxic serum as compared with the normal control; and was less in 7 instances, and in 2, was equal to the controls.

The small differences in percentage of CO_2 which were obtained can easily be within the limits of experimental error.

These facts point to the exclusion of the alkaline reserve as a factor in the mechanism of anaphylatoxin production in serum or plasma.

BLOOD AMMONIA AND ANAPHYLATOXIN

Since, in acidosis there is an increase in blood ammonia as a compensatory attempt to protect the alkaline reserve, a series of blood ammonia determinations were carried out as a check on the foregoing determinations of CO_2 capacity of serum and plasma.

Experiments with Rat Serum-Agar Anaphylatoxin, Inulin Anaphylatoxin, and Distilled Water Anaphylatoxin.—Six normal white rats were bled from the heart by means of a heart pipet, the blood was defibrinated and pooled. This was divided into two portions, A and B.

A. Four and one-half c c serum were treated with agar by the sol-gel method (1 c c of 0.5% agar solution being added, the whole being shaken for 1 minute, then iced for 1 hour and incubated for 10 minutes at 38 C. It was then centrifugated at 3,000 r.p.m. for 15 minutes and the supernatant serum pipetted off. This was then tested (1) for toxicity, 1 c c being injected intravenously into a guinea-pig of about 200 gm., and (2) for ammonia content, being subjected to Folin's method for the determination of blood ammonia.

B. For control purposes 4.5 c c serum were treated with 0.1 c c physiologic salt solution, the mixture shaken for 1 minute, iced for 1 hour at the same time as A, then incubated for 10 minutes at 38 C. It was then centrifugated at 3,000 r.p.m. and the supernatant serum pipetted off. This was then tested (1) for toxicity, 1 c c being injected intravenously into a guinea-pig of about 200 gm., and (2) for ammonia content, being subjected to Folin's method.

Eight such experiments were carried out using agar, inulin and distilled water as inducing agents. The plan and technic in each case were essentially the same. The results of these experiments can be seen and compared in table 7. Separate pooled rat serums were used in each experiment, except in experiment 2a in which guinea-pig serum was used.

TABLE 7

BLOOD AMMONIA AND ANAPHYLATOXIN

	Experiment	Mg. NH_3 per 100 C c Blood in		Difference	Intravenous Injection of 1 C c of	
		Toxic Serum	Control Serum		Toxic Serum	Control Serum
Agar	3a	0.20	0.20	0.0	Typical shock and death	Nil
Agar	22	2.5	2.5	0.0	Typical shock and death	Nil
Agar	2a	0.75	0.75	0.0	Typical shock and death	Nil
Inulin	4a	0.60	1.0	0.4	Typical shock and death	Nil
Inulin	20	1.0	1.0	0.0	Typical shock and death	Nil
Inulin	21	1.0	1.0	0.0	Typical shock and death	Nil
Distilled water	23	1.0	1.5	0.5	Typical shock and death	Nil
Distilled water	25	1.0	1.0	0.0	Typical shock and death	Nil

It will be seen from table 7 that there is practically no change in the ammonia content of toxic serums as compared with corresponding controls and hence the conclusion is justified that the mechanism of anaphylatoxin production in serum does not involve any alteration in the amount of ammonia.

ALKALINE RESERVE AND SPECIFIC ANAPHYLAXIS

Since no alteration can be detected in the alkaline reserve in vitro, it appeared desirable to determine whether any such change took place in the animal body. Here a difference, notably a decrease, in the plasma bicarbonate content during or after acute anaphylactic shock would point to acidosis, if such a condition were concerned with the phenomenon of shock. With this in view, two series of experiments were carried out, the first series in rabbits which had been sensitized against a protein antigen (specific anaphylaxis). The second set was carried out on normal rabbits in which anaphylactic symptoms were induced by the injection of a nonspecific antigen as agar (nonspecific anaphylaxis). Rabbits were selected as experimental animals even though they responded with difficulty to attempts to induce anaphylaxis because the volume of blood required for plasma determinations did not permit the use of the smaller laboratory animals.

Outline of Experiment.—Specific Anaphylactic Shock.—A normal Belgian rabbit received intravenously 10 c c normal rat serum every 4 days for 3 weeks. Seven days were allowed to elapse, at the end of which an excellent precipitin reaction was obtained against normal rat serum. The sensitized rabbit was attached to a Latapie board and with aseptic technic the left carotid artery was exposed. In this a sterile paraffined cannula was introduced and secured by means of a ligature.

A. Ten c c blood were withdrawn through the cannula and received in a centrifuge tube containing 10 mg. powdered potassium oxalate. The oxalated blood was then centrifugated at 3,000 r.p.m. for 15 minutes and the supernatant plasma pipetted off. This was subjected to the Van Slyke bicarbonate determination.

Twenty-five c c normal rat serum were then injected slowly into the ear vein. This was followed in 3½ minutes by a profound anaphylactic shock. When the symptoms of shock had nearly subsided and immediately before death:

B. Ten c c blood were withdrawn through the cannula and received in a centrifuge tube containing 10 mg. powdered potassium oxalate. The oxalated blood was then centrifugated at 3,000 r.p.m. for 15 minutes and the supernatant plasma pipetted off. This was then subjected to the Van Slyke plasma bicarbonate determination. Necropsy showed delayed coagulation (25 minutes); no thrombi were found in the heart or great vessels.

Six such experiments on specific anaphylactic shock were carried out. The sensitizing was done in the same manner in every case. In 3 instances rat serum was used as antigen, in 2 experiments guinea-pig serum was used and in one case guinea-pig whole blood was used. The results of this series are outlined in table 8.

TABLE 8

ALKALINE RESERVE AND SPECIFIC ANAPHYLACTIC SHOCK IN RABBITS

Experiment	Percentage CO_2 in Serum		Sensitized to	Difference	Result
	Before Shock	After Shock			
18	14.2	16.0	Rat serum..............	1.8	Typical shock and death
18b	22.1	18.3	Rat serum..............	3.8	Typical shock
19	46.5	33.0	Rat serum..............	13.5	Typical shock and death
24	35.4	36.1	Guinea-pig serum.......	0.7	Typical shock
26	48.5	49.8	Guinea-pig serum.......	1.3	Typical shock and death
27	42.2	41.9	Guinea-pig whole blood	0.3	Typical shock and death

In every case an intense shock was produced. In two instances recovery followed, but this is not unusual in anaphylaxis in rabbits. In this series the average difference in plasma bicarbonate content before and after shock is not only very small but inconstant, frequently being greater after shock than before. Both of these facts are incompatible with the idea that the alkaline reserve is involved.

ALKALINE RESERVE AND NON-SPECIFIC ANAPHYLACTIC SHOCK

Since anaphylactic shock can be induced in normal animals by the injection of suitable substances, a series of experiments were carried out on normal rabbits using agar as the inducing agent. This was prepared according to the method of Novy and De Kruif.[7] The routine of procedure was essentially the same as in the experiments with sensitized animals except that no preliminary sensitization was required.

Outline of Experiment—Nonspecific Anaphylactic Shock.—A normal Belgian rabbit of about 2 kg. weight was attached to a Latapie board. With aseptic technic, 10 c c blood were withdrawn by heart puncture and transferred to a centrifuge tube containing 10 mg. powdered potassium oxalate. The oxalated blood was centrifugated at 3,000 r.p.m. for 15 minutes and the supernatant plasma was pipetted off. This was subjected to the Van Slyke plasma bicarbonate determination.

Twenty-five c c agar sol-gel was injected slowly into the ear vein. This was followed in 3 minutes by a profound anaphylactic shock. When the symptoms had subsided and immediately before death 10 c c blood were withdrawn by heart puncture and transferred to a centrifuge tube containing 10 mg. powdered potassium oxalate. The oxalated blood was then centrifugated at 3,000 r.p.m. for 15 minutes and the supernatant plasma pipetted off. This was then subjected to the Van Slyke plasma bicarbonate method.

Necropsy showed fluid blood, a very small pericardial hemorrhage and no thrombi in the heart or the great vessels.

[7] Jour. Infect. Dis., 1917, 20, p. 631.

The difference in plasma bicarbonate content before and after shock was in this case 1%. A series of 4 such experiments, identical in detail and technic are given in table 9.

TABLE 9

ALKALINE RESERVE AND NONSPECIFIC ANAPHYLAXIS IN NORMAL RABBITS AFTER AGAR INJECTION

Experiment	Percentage CO_2 in Plasma		Difference	Result of Injection
	Before Injection	After Injection		
28	40.0	40.0	0.0	Typical shock and death
29	32.5	30.8	1.7	Typical shock and death
30	32.5	31.5	1.0	Typical shock and death
31	27.0	28.0	1.0	Typical shock and death

In this series with an average difference in plasma bicarbonate content of 0.9%, before and after shock, and with one instance in the 4 in which the percentage is greater after than before, the obvious conclusion to make is that the alkaline reserve is not involved in the phenomenon.

BLOOD AMMONIA AND SPECIFIC ANAPHYLAXIS

Again as a check on the plasma bicarbonate determinations, in anaphylaxis before and after shock, micro determinations of ammonia [8] were carried out. The technic employed was essentially the same as that used for specific anaphylaxis except that ammonia determinations were made instead of those for carbon dioxide. Four such experiments are outlined in table 10.

TABLE 10

BLOOD AMMONIA AND SPECIFIC ANAPHYLACTIC SHOCK IN RABBITS

Experiment	Mg. NH_3 per 100 C c in Blood		Difference	Sensitized to	Result of Injection
	Before Injection	After Injection			
19	0.5	0.45	0.05	Rat serum..............	Typical shock
24	0.8	0.8	0.00	Guinea-pig serum.......	Typical shock
26	0.32	0.30	0.02	Guinea-pig serum........	Typical shock and death
27	0.4	0.5	0.10	Guinea-pig whole blood..	Typical shock and death

The average difference is seen to be 0.64 mg. ammonia per 100 c c blood. This again points to the same conclusion as was reached in anaphylatoxin and ammonia content, namely, that the blood ammonia is not in any way disturbed in the process.

[8] Folin and Macallum: Jour. Biol. Chem., 1912, 11, p. 523.

SUMMARY AND CONCLUSIONS

In the production of anaphylatoxin in vitro in serum or in plasma there is no demonstrable disturbance in the alkaline reserve as shown by the Van Slyke plasma bicarbonate method.

Likewise micro determinations of blood ammonia showed no variations in this constituent in anaphylatoxic serums as compared with normal serums.

In experimental anaphylaxis, either specific or nonspecific, no disturbance in the alkaline reserve could be demonstrated. Further, in these conditions, no variations in the blood ammonia could be detected. The conclusion that suggests itself is that the alkaline reserve is not involved in any demonstrable manner in the phenomenon of anaphylatoxin production and anaphylaxis.

These results are corroborative of those obtained in the study of amino nitrogen in relation to anaphylatoxin.[3] Therefore, the general conclusion to be drawn is that anaphylatoxin production is not accompanied by changes in amino nitrogen, in blood ammonia, or in the alkaline reserve.

THE PATHOGENICITY OF BACILLUS BOTULINUS *

Paul F. Orr

From the Department of Preventive Medicine and Hygiene, Harvard University Medical School, Boston, Mass.

The early work of van Ermengem [1] indicated that B. botulinus or its spores are not pathogenic in themselves. This view was soon confirmed by others and emphasized by the statements that this organism does not thrive at the body temperature and therefore could not produce toxin within the body of warm blooded animals. In other words, it is commonly asserted that botulism is always due to toxin preformed in the food. It has, however, been recently shown that B. botulinus may grow and produce toxin in vitro at 37 C. In fact this is the optimum temperature for most strains of this organism. The question naturally arises, can the spores germinate in the body? Have they invasive power? Can toxin be formed within the body? In short, is B. botulinus pathogenic? The answers to these questions have practical as well as theoretical importance.

Optimum Temperature for Growth of B. Botulinus

Van Ermengem,[2] who first described B. botulinus, stated that "it grows within a rather wide range of temperature: below 18 C. the growth is slow and restricted; at 20 C. it develops quickly and abundantly, and will usually liquefy a layer of gelatin 15 to 18 cm. thick in 8 days. The optimum appears to lie between 20 and 30 C. In an incubator regulated to exactly 38.5 C., colonies in sugar agar are moderately numerous; however, the growth is meagre in comparison with that at 35 C. The solid medium is not fragmented; after 24 to 36 hours growth ceases. If the tubes are then brought to 20 C., an abundant gas formation often begins. On the other hand, it is usually not possible to obtain a perceptible growth in dextrose broth at 38.5 C. if the tubes are hermetically sealed. When taken out of the incubator and placed at the ordinary temperature, they show heavy clouding and gas formation within 48 hours. A few tubes, however, become clouded at 38.5 C.; a satisfactory reason for the growth could not be found. The organisms grown at from 37 to 38.5 C. have taken on an abnormal form and exhibit very long threads with irregular granules and occasional thickening. Spores are not present and the cultures with these involution forms are only slightly active and soon lose their vitality. One observes a moderate growth in glucose bouillon at a higher temperature, as 38 C., if care is taken to allow the gas which is produced to escape freely. Nevertheless, the bacilli assume the forms of threads and the growth ceases after a few hours.

Received for publication, Aug. 3, 1921.

* This is part of an extensive investigation on food poisoning, with special reference to botulism, that is being done under the auspices of the Advisory Committee on the Toxicity of Preserved Foods of the National Research Council under a grant from the National Canners' Association.

[1] Ztschr. f. Hyg. u. Infekhonskr., 1897, 1, p. 26.

[2] Loc. cit.

"From these experiments, the conclusion may be drawn that the body temperature of warm blooded animals is unfavorable for the normal development, and that the temperature of 35 C. and above is to be considered as dysgenetic (*dysgenetisch*)."

Romer[3] found the optimum temperature for growth of a strain of B. botulinus which he had isolated from pork to be about 22 C. Spores were soon found at this temperature while at higher temperatures they were not formed and many involution forms appeared. At 37 C. growth was scant, and the cultures remained alive only a short time.

Dickson,[4] who has isolated several strains of B. botulinus in connection with different outbreaks of botulism on the Pacific Coast, states that the optimum temperature for the growth of the bacillus and for the development of toxin lies between 20 and 30 C.

Graham and Brueckner[5] isolated a strain of B. botulinus from some ensilage involved in a forage poisoning outbreak among horses in Illinois. They state that the optimum temperature for growth of this organism was from 22 to 25 C.

With the exception of these four observations, most of the reports indicate that B. botulinus not only grows at 37 C. but actually prefers the body temperature for its development, yet the accepted view has been that this organism is a strict saprophyte unable to grow at body temperature.

In a preliminary report[6] I have stated that, contrary to the general view, the optimum temperature for growth of B. botulinus is that of the body temperature, 37 C., and this was found to be most favorable for the growth and spore production of all of the 16 strains studied, including the strains of Dickson and Graham and Brueckner. Toxin is readily formed at this temperature. I have since obtained similar observations on 8 more strains of this organism.

Matzuschita,[7] in a study of the growth and spore formation of a number of anaerobes, found that the optimum temperature for growth for B. botulinus was from 34 to 38 C., and the maximum temperature was about 45.5 C., while 38 C. was most favorable for spore production, and the maximum was about 45.5 C.

Landman,[8] in describing a strain of B. botulinus which was isolated from a bean salad, states that it grows as well at 37 C. as at 24 C., differing thereby from the van Ermengem strain which showed only a very slight growth at 37 C. He was unable to observe any thread formation in old cultures of his strain as had been described by van Ermengem. Spores were formed more quickly at 37 C. than at lower temperatures; however, a stronger toxin was produced at the lower temperatures. Of the toxin produced at 24 C., 0.00003 c c was fatal for white mice and 0.0003 c c was fatal for guinea-pigs, while of the toxin produced at 37 C., 0.01 c c was fatal for mice and 0.1 c c for guinea-pigs.

Schumacher[9] states that the strain of B. botulinus which he isolated from ham grows at 18 C. and tolerates also higher temperatures, even up to 37 C.

Konstansoff,[10] in a study of fish poisoning in Russia, states that he isolated an anaerobic organism, B. ichthyismi, which, if not identical with, is very closely related to, B. botulinus. The optimum temperature for growth of

[3] Centralbl. f. Bakteriol. I, 1900, 27, p. 857.
[4] Monograph 8, Rockefeller Institute, 1918.
[5] J. Bacteriol., 1919, 4, p. 1.
[6] Proc. Soc. Exper. Biol. & Med., 1919, 17, p. 47.
[7] Zur Phys. d. Sporenbildung der Bacillen, etc., Diss., 1902.
[8] Hyg. Rundschau, 1904, 14, p. 449.
[9] München. med. Wchnschr., 1913, 60, p. 124.
[10] Vestnik Abshtchestvenney Higieni, 1915, 51, p. 766.

B. ichthyismi was found to be about 35 to 37 C., while at 20 C. the organism does not grow. In working with several atoxic strains of B. botulinus, this investigator found that the optimum temperature for growth was from 20 to 37 C.

Nevin[11] succeeded in isolating a strain of B. botulinus from some home-made cottage cheese which had caused botulism poisoning in 3 persons. This strain grew and produced toxin readily at 37 C. in the hands of Nevin as well as Shippen.[12]

Similar results are reported by Burke,[13] who has been working with the strains obtained from Dickson as well as with some isolated by herself. She states that as originally recorded, the optimum temperature was from 22 to 28 C.; however, the pure strains isolated at Stanford grow more rapidly at 37.5 C. Agar shake cultures showed a well defined and typical growth in 24 hours at 37.5 C., while at 28 C. from 36 to 40 hours were required for the same growth, and at lower temperatures the growth was still slower. She found that toxin was produced at 37.5 C. as well as at 28 C.

Thom, Edmondson and Giltner[14] describe a strain of B. botulinus which they isolated from asparagus salad in a case of food poisoning. They state that "The organism grows best at 37 C. contrary to the findings of van Ermengem with respect to his strain, but in harmony with other workers in this laboratory with cultures of the Nevin strain." It is interesting to note that the strongest toxin obtained by Thom and his co-workers was from a culture which was incubated at 35 C. for a period of 28 days, the minimum lethal dose for guinea-pigs being 0.0001 c c.

Armstrong, Story and Scott[15] state that the strain of B. botulinus which they isolated from ripe olives, the causative factor of an outbreak of botulism, grows best at 37 C.; however, growth occurs also at room temperature but only after several days. Toxin was also produced more rapidly at 37 C., a 9-day-old culture developing a toxin approximately 200 times as strong as an 11-day-old culture grown at room temperature.

This brief review of the observations regarding the temperature relations of B. botulinus shows that at least some strains of this organism develop readily and produce toxin at body temperature. This brings up the question of the ability of the organism to grow and elaborate toxin within the body.

GROWTH AND TOXIN PRODUCTION OF B. BOTULINUS WITHIN THE BODY

As stated, B. botulinus is considered to be a saprophyte, lacking power for harm in the body, except through its toxin preformed in the food. However, in several instances B. botulinus or its spores have been recovered from the organs of man and animals dead of botulism, suggesting that under favorable conditions, it may invade the tissues. It is interesting to note, however, that in practically every case in which

[11] J. Infect. Dis., 1921, 28, p. 226.
[12] Arch. Int. Med., 1919, 23, p. 346.
[13] J. Bacteriol., 1919, 4, p. 555.
[14] Jour. Am. Med. Assn., 1919, 73, p. 907.
[15] Public Health Reports, 1919, 34, p. 2877.

the organism was recovered from the tissue in experimental botulism, it was from animals infected by injection of cultures rather than by feeding. Thus, Romer recovered the bacillus in one case from the spleen of a mouse which was killed 12 hours after the injection of 0.5 c c of a broth culture, indicating that we are not dealing with a terminal invasion. Van Ermengem [16] stated that the organism could be recovered from the liver, spleen, etc., only in cases in which large quantities of spore-containing material was injected intravenously, and even then the number of bacteria in the organs is so small that they cannot be readily identified by microscopic examination.

TABLE 1

RECOVERY OF B. BOTULINUS FROM THE TISSUES OF GUINEA-PIGS AFTER THE DEATH OF THESE ANIMALS FOLLOWING THE ADMINISTRATION OF TOXIN-FREE SPORES

Exper.	Botulinus Strain No.	Type	Number of Toxin-Free Spores Administered	Mode of Administration	Results as to Recovery of B. botulinus
1	11	B	50,000,000	Subcutaneous	Negative
	11	B	50,000,000	Subcutaneous	Negative
	15	A	50,000,000	Subcutaneous	From liver and spleen
	15	A	50,000,000	Subcutaneous	From spleen
	16	A	50,000,000	Subcutaneous	Negative
	16	A	50,000,000	Subcutaneous	From liver and spleen
2	11	B	2 c c No. spores not determined	Per os	From liver
	11	B	1 c c	Per os	Negative
	11	B	0.25 c c	Subcutaneous	Negative
	11	B	0.25 c c	Subcutaneous	Negative
3	11	B	125,000,000	Per os	From liver and spleen
	11	B	125,000,000	Per os	Negative
	11	B	125,000,000	Per os	Negative
4	11	B	45,000,000	Subcutaneous	From liver and spleen
	11	B	45,000,000	Subcutaneous	From spleen
	11	B	90,000,000	Per os	From liver and spleen
5	11	B	200,000,000	Per os	From liver and spleen
	11	B	100,000,000	Per os	Negative

I have been able to recover B. botulinus from the organs of animals which have died following the administration of toxin-free spores either subcutaneously or by the mouth. In 4 of 8 guinea-pigs the organism was recovered from the liver or spleen after feeding experiments; and in 5 of 10 guinea-pigs after subcutaneous inoculation (table 1).

Necropsy examination was made either at the time of death of the animals or shortly thereafter. Bits of tissue were removed with bacteriologic precaution and cultivated in minced meat and dextrose agar medium. Failure to recover B. botulinus by cultural methods does not

[16] Kolle u. Wassermann, Handbuch d. path. Organismen, 1912, 4, p. 909.

necessarily mean that the organism was absent. Microscopic examination of sections of the various organs was not made.

The question of pathogenicity of the toxin-free spores and bacilli when fed or injected has received little attention since the work of van Ermengem. The following quotation is from his classic paper.[1]

"We repeat briefly the experiments which demonstrate that B. botulinus is absolutely incapable of reproducing itself in the animal body. After we convinced ourselves of the potency of the cultures filtered through porcelain and further had seen that they were active in the same minimum lethal doses as the cultures containing the bacteria, we undertook numerous microscopical and cultural experiments, which all showed that B. botulinus does not multiply either in the exudate, liver, spleen, kidneys, salivary glands, nervous system, or in the intestinal tract. It disappears quickly after subcutaneous, intravenous and intraperitoneal injections, and induces a considerable phagocytosis, even as much as is the case with B. subtilis, one of the most harmless saprophytes. These facts do not, however, justify us in denying any infectiousness to B. botulinus. It is possible that we cannot imitate the local or the general conditions in the animal experiments, which would permit the growth of the bacillus in the animal body. Apart from the high potency of the toxin, transitory multiplication in the organism, that is, in the digestive tract, etc., might take place, which, even without demonstrable proof, might be sufficient to cause a fatal infection.

"With this object in mind, we attempted to free the cultures of their toxic principles, without injuring the vegetative properties of the bacteria, by washing, addition of alkali and high temperature (70 C.). Further, we attempted to protect the bacteria against phagocytosis by enveloping them in agar, or adding substances which injure the tissues and ward off the leucocytes, etc. Repeated experiments of this type gave negative results.

"On the contrary, Vaillard and Rouget,[17] using the tetanus bacillus and Besson[18] using the edema bacillus, have produced true infection of animals in similar experiments.

"Consequently, a basic difference exists between the B. botulinus and the above pathogenic species. The first is an organism which lacks any virulence in the sense that it does not possess the ability to develop in the living animal body. It belongs therefore to the well characterized but small group of pathogenic saprophytes, which one may call *'toxicogenic,'* in contrast to the pathogenic infectious micro-organism."

Similar negative results were obtained by Romer[3] and Landmann[8] and more recently by Dickson,[19] who states that "the toxin is never formed within the body as the optimum temperature of B. botulinus is from 24 to 28 C. and the toxin will not form at a temperature of 37.5 C., the normal temperature of the body."

Shippen[12] found that the spores of the Nevin strain of B. botulinus were not pathogenic when administered to a rabbit subcutaneously or per os. His experimental work on this point, however, was meager. Shippen infers that, since this organism can produce toxin at body temperature and in an acid medium under aerobic conditions (symbiotically), it might develop in the human intestine.

[17] Ann. de l'Inst. Pasteur, 1892, 6, p. 385; 1893, 7, p. 755.
[18] Ibid., 1895, 9, p. 179.
[19] Can. Med. Assoc. Jour., 1918, p. 2.

Thom, Edmondson and Giltner[14] conclude from their work that B. botulinus when freed of its toxin by washing, or the spores freed from toxin by heating do not produce symptoms of poisoning when fed or injected. It is to be noted that several of their animals injected with washed organisms died in from 3 to 4 days, but they infer that the bacteria were not sufficiently washed free of toxin as the heated spores proved noninfectious. Recently these investigators[20] report that they have succeeded in producing the specific disease in guinea-pigs by feeding massive doses of toxin-free spores of B. botulinus.

Armstrong, Story and Scott[15] undertook some experiments dealing with the growth and toxin formation of B. botulinus in animals. On the whole, negative results were obtained by these authors. A few of the guinea-pigs died, but this was attributed to the fact that the organisms were not entirely freed of toxin.

Some time ago, I reported[21] that it had been possible in this laboratory to produce symptoms of botulism in guinea-pigs by feeding or injecting toxin-free spores of B. botulinus (Nevin strain). This observation has been confirmed and extended in the following experiments.

The toxin-free spores of 3 different strains of B. botulinus were used; No. 11, a type B. strain, and Nos. 15 and 16, type A strains. Spores were obtained from minced meat cultures, which were from 4 weeks to 6 months old. The cultures were centrifugalized, the supernatant liquid removed, passed through a Berkefeld filter and from 0.5 to 1 c c of this filtrate, as a control, was fed to guinea-pigs. These animals died in from 20 to 30 hours. The sedimented spores were washed 3 times, suspended in salt solution and heated in a water bath at 80 C. for 30 minutes side by side with another tube containing some of the filtered toxin. In every case guinea-pigs fed or injected with this heated filtered toxin remained normal, showing that the heating was sufficient to destroy the toxin. The approximate number of spores in the various suspensions were determined by a series of dilutions in agar shake cultures.

The spores were administered to some animals subcutaneously and to others by the mouth. With the latter mode of administration, some of the guinea-pigs were given the spores through a stomach tube, while others were fed the spores on pieces of bread (table 2). It is to be observed that botulism occurred quite regularly in the guinea-pigs which were fed or injected with toxin-free spores. That death was due to botulism is shown by the fact that control animals (guinea-pigs 234, 280 and 290), which received specific antitoxin as well as the spores, remained alive.

[20] Arch. Int. Med., 1920, 26, p. 356.
[21] Abstr. Bacteriol., 1920, 4, p. 10.

Death in the guinea-pigs following the administration of botulinus spores must have resulted from the elaboration of toxin within the animal's body, as it was shown by control guinea-pigs (104, 142, 143, 144 and 400) that the heat to which the spores were subjected was sufficient to destroy the toxin.

TABLE 2

PRODUCTION OF BOTULISM IN GUINEA-PIGS BY THE ADMINISTRATION OF TOXIN-FREE SPORES OF B. BOTULINUS

Guinea-Pigs	Amount Heated Toxic Filtrate	Number Toxin-Free Spores	Age of Spores	Method of Introduction	Amount Specific Antitoxin Injected	Strain No.	Type	Results
324	......	50,000,000	6 mos.	Subcutaneous	....	11	B	Died after 90 hours
328	......	50,000,000	6 mos.	Subcutaneous	....	11	B	Died after 76 hours
321	......	50,000,000	6 mos.	Subcutaneous	....	15	A	Died after 90 hours
330	......	50,000,000	6 mos.	Subcutaneous	....	15	A	Died after 106 hours
322	......	50,000,000	6 mos.	Subcutaneous	....	16	A	Died after 50 hours
326	......	50,000,000	6 mos.	Subcutaneous	....	16	A	Died after 90 hours
104	1.0 c c	....	......	Per os	....	11	B	Remained normal
108	......	125,000,000	4 wks.	Per os	....	11	B	Died after 84 hours
109	......	125,000,000	4 wks.	Per os	....	11	B	Died after 143 hours
110	......	125,000,000	4 wks.	Per os	....	11	B	Died after 93 hours
142	1.0 c c	....	......	Per os	....	11	B	Remained normal
143	1.0 c c	....	......	Per os	....	11	B	Remained normal
144	0.5 c c	....	......	Subcutaneous	....	11	B	Remained normal
145	......	45,000,000	4 wks.	Subcutaneous	....	11	B	Died after 249 hours
146	......	45,000,000	4 wks.	Subcutaneous	....	11	B	Died after 96 hours
147	......	90,000,000	4 wks.	Per os	....	11	B	Died after 120 hours
148	......	90,000,000	4 wks.	Per os	....	11	B	Developed weakness after 2 weeks. Finally recovered
400	1.0 c c	....	......	Per os	....	11	B	Remained normal
250	......	200,000,000	4 wks.	Per os	....	11	B	Died after 33½ hours
286	......	100,000,000	4 wks.	Per os	....	11	B	Died after 66 hours
234	......	200,000,000	4 wks.	Per os	50 units	11	B	Survived
280	......	200,000,000	4 wks.	Per os	500 units	11	B	Survived
290	......	200,000,000	4 wks.	Per os	5000 units	11	B	Survived
257	......	....	......	....	5000 units	11	B	Survived

The results from the subcutaneous injection of guinea-pigs of strains 11, 15 and 16 were quite comparable; in fact, there were no striking differences either in the symptoms or the course of the illness. Death resulted usually on the third or fourth day.

Guinea-pig 145, injected subcutaneously with 45 million spores, did not die until the tenth day, having developed symptoms on the sixth day, indicating that the number of spores may play an important rôle in producing botulinus infection. Of guinea-pigs 147 and 148, which were given 90 million spores per os, one animal died on the fifth day and the other, although developing weakness, survived. Guinea-pigs 250 and 256, given 200 million and 100 million spores, respectively, in the same manner, died on the second and fourth day.

Similarly, a series of white mice were injected with toxin-free spores of strains 11, 15 and 16, prepared as indicated. Some of the mice were given protective doses of specific antitoxin to serve as controls (table 3).

All of the mice inoculated with the spores of strain 15 and some of the mice inoculated with strain 11 survived as well as those injected with the strain 16, but which were given antitoxin. On the other hand, all of the mice injected with spores of strain 16 and not receiving antitoxin died. Whether or not these differences in results are due to differences in virulence of the strain cannot be definitely stated.

TABLE 3

RESULTS OF INOCULATION OF WHITE MICE WITH THE TOXIN-FREE SPORES OF B. BOTULINUS

No. of Mice	Method of Inoculation	No. Spores Injected	Strain B. Botulinus	Type	Antitoxin Injected	Results
4	Subcutaneous	10,000,000	11	B	......	1 died 70 hours, 3 survived
1	Subcutaneous	10,000,000	11	B	0.1 c c	Survived
4	Intraperitoneal	10,000,000	11	B	......	1 died 58 hours, 3 survived
1	Intraperitoneal	10,000,000	11	B	0.1 c c	Survived
4	Subcutaneous	10,000,000	15	A	......	All survived
1	Subcutaneous	10,000,000	15	A	0.1 c c	Survived
4	Intraperitoneal	10,000,000	15	A	......	All survived
1	Intraperitoneal	10,000,000	15	A	0.1 c c	Survived
4	Subcutaneous	10,000,000	16	A	......	All died in 44 hours
1	Subcutaneous	10,000,000	16	A	0.1 c c	Survived
4	Intraperitoneal	10,000,000	16	A	......	2 died 24 hours, 2 died 27 hours
1	Intraperitoneal	40,000,000	11	B	......	Survived
1	Intraperitoneal	40,000,000	11	B	......	Survived
1	Intraperitoneal	40,000,000	11	B	0.1 c c	Survived
1	Subcutaneous	20,000,000	11	B	......	Died 120 hours
1	Subcutaneous	20,000,000	11	B	......	Died 120 hours
1	Subcutaneous	20,000,000	11	B	0.1 c c	Survived

With strain 11, the mice which were injected subcutaneously with 20 million spores died in about 120 hours, while those injected intraperitoneally with 40 million survived, the variations in results of which may be attributed to differences in phagocytic action. The results of this series of inoculations indicate that, in mice, toxin-free spores of B. botulinus may occasionally produce an infection, when enormous numbers are injected intraperitoneally or subcutaneously.

TOXIN PRODUCTION IN VITRO

As a supplementary experiment, a tube containing 10 c c of 0.85% sterile salt solution, a tube containing 10 c c of sterile defibrinated normal guinea-pig blood, and a tube containing 10 c c of minced meat medium were each inoculated with 200 million of the same toxin-free spores as were fed to the guinea-pigs. These tubes were incubated at 37 C. and at the first appearance of symptoms of botulism in guinea-pigs 250 and 286, these 3 cultures were filtered through Berkefeld filters (the blood, however, was centrifuged) and 4 c c of each of the resulting filtrates were fed to normal guinea-pigs. The guinea-pig fed 4 c c of the filtrate from the salt solution culture remained normal, thus showing no toxin production in this medium. The guinea-pig fed 4 c c of centrifugalized blood culture died 11 hours later. The guinea-pig fed 5 c c of the filtrate from the minced meat culture died 5 hours later, or a total time of 35 hours from the inoculation of the meat culture, whereas in the experiment showing the possibility of development of spores in vivo, the guinea-pig (250) died in 33½ hours, a fairly close correlation.

As a direct proof of the actual production of toxin in the body, the brain and heart blood were taken from the guinea-pigs which died following the ingestion of toxin-free spores and used to prepare an antigen for precipitation tests according to the method of Bronfenbrenner and Schlesinger.[22] The antigen prepared from the brain of the guinea-pig (286) which died after 66 hours gave a positive precipitin test for botulinus toxin. The antigen prepared from the blood of this guinea-pig, as well as a similar antigen prepared from the brain and blood of the guinea-pig (250) which died in 33 hours, gave negative precipitin tests. In addition, to test further for the presence of toxin in these tissues some of the solutions containing the triturated brain and blood of the animals which died were injected into white mice. The mouse injected with the triturated brain which gave the positive precipitin test died after 4 days, others remained alive, thus fully confirming the results of the precipitin test.

The results of these experiments indicate that feeding massive doses of toxin-free spores to guinea-pigs may produce botulinus infection. That death of the animals used in these experiments was due to botulism is shown by the fact that those animals given specific antitoxin were protected. The recovery of B. botulinus from the internal organs as well as the identification of botulinus toxin in the brain of one of the animals would seem to indicate an infection with resulting elaboration of toxin in the body.

It was found that the inoculation of 200 million spores into defibrinated guinea-pig blood and into minced meat would produce enough toxin in 30 hours at 37 C. to kill a guinea-pig in from 5 to 11 hours.

[22] Proc. Soc. Exp. Biol. and Med., 1919, 17, p. 24.

The results of the inoculation of mice with toxin-free spores would indicate that infection was more likely to occur as a result of subcutaneous injection than of intraperitoneal injections, probably due to inferior phagocytic action in the former case.

On the whole, it has been possible to produce botulinus infection by feeding and injecting massive doses of toxin-free spores of B. botulinus. Whether botulinus infection ever occurs is a matter of conjecture. It seems that under certain conditions this might occur, especially as a combined intoxication and infection. Botulism due solely to an initial infection with B. botulinus is probably exceedingly rare, as it would be quite unusual for a person to ingest a massive quantity of spores without getting a relatively large amount of toxin also.

In connection with this work, it is interesting to note that Ronca,[23] who has been studying the possibility of blackleg infection through the ingestion of the causative organism, one of the pathogenic anaerobes, has found that experimental blackleg infection of guinea-pigs was successful only when massive doses of the organism were ingested. Ronca concludes that under certain favorable conditions blackleg infection may be brought about by ingestion of B. chauvaei, which, unaltered by the passage through the stomach, may gain access to the circulation through some vulnerable point in the intestinal walls.

CONCLUSIONS

The optimum temperature for growth and elaboration of toxin by B. botulinus is that of the body temperature, 37 C.

B. botulinus can be recovered from the internal organs of animals which have been fed or injected with toxic cultures and also with toxin-free spores of this organism.

B. botulinus, under certain conditions, will grow and produce toxin in the body of the guinea-pig.

Experimental botulism can be produced in laboratory animals by the feeding or injection of massive quantities of toxin-free spores of B. botulinus.

The presence of toxin produced in the body as a result of growth of toxin-free spores in the body can be demonstrated by the precipitin test as well as by direct toxicity tests.

Botulism poisoning in man due to the ingestion of spores is probably very rare, if it occurs at all. The possibility of such occurrence must, however, be considered.

[23] Clin. Vet. Ross. Polyea Sanit. e Sg., 1920, 43, p. 195.

STUDY ON THE CLASSIFICATION OF STREPTOCOCCI

Etta Fisk and Earl L. Burky

From the Laboratory of Hygiene, University of Pennsylvania, Philadelphia

The purpose of this study is the classification of streptococci by the appearance of deep colonies in blood agar plates of uniform composition and thickness; and a further classification by the fermentation reactions in inulin, lactose, mannite, raffinose, saccharose and salicin; and last, by a study of the agglutination reactions in serum of immunized animals. Lastly an attempt is made to show the relationship of the serologic groups to the blood agar and sugar reaction groups. Some additional properties have been investigated and the general results noted in their bearing on the main issues.

Brown [1] classifies the streptococci, by the growth and action of deep colonies in blood agar, into three main groups: alpha, beta and gamma and a subgroup, alpha prime.

Alpha colonies are those which in other classifications are called "viridans" or "green" and which in deep colonies produce a 0.8-1.0 mm. double-convex, oval, or complex colony, surrounded by a small zone of green colored red cells at the end of 48 hours' incubation. The complex colony is not definitely double-convex or oval, but a seeming combination of two such colonies. It appears at first as if there are two colonies lying at right angles to each other, one superimposed on the other. When placed in the icebox for from 24-48 hours, there appears surrounding the area of green coloration a zone of hemolysis, wherein no red cells or color is visible. Further incubation produces a second ring of green formation and a secondary zone of hemolysis occurs if it is placed again in the icebox. There are, then, alternating concentric zones of hemolysis with the first zone of green immediately surrounding the colony. The number of zones possible seems in the main limited to the number of incubations and refrigerations, although the drying of the medium and the lack of available food supply serves as a check on the growth. This description in the main fits all the alpha streptococci. Many of them, however, are apparently limited to smaller

Received for publication, Aug. 1, 1921.

[1] Monograph 9, Rockefeller Institute, 1919.

colonies and proportionately smaller zones, and some do not elaborate as clear-cut zones as others. Most of these differences, however, seem to be one of degree and not of kind, so that a further differentiation would lead to confusion rather than clarity.

Brown, however, does make one further differentiation—alpha prime—in the alpha group. This he describes as a colony in which the zone of hemolysis is not clear-cut macroscopically. This is accounted for, when examined microscopically, by finding in the hemolytic zones scattered green-colored red cells which are the survivors of the hemolytic action which destroyed the larger number of the cells. Next to the colony the number of cells is slightly greater than in the more distant portions of the agar. We have never seen any colonies to fit this description.

In the beta group fall those streptococci which in other classifications have been described as "hemolytic." The deep colonies, in size and shape resembling the alpha type, surround themselves on the plate with a zone of clear agar containing no visible cells or hemoglobin. This zone varies in size from 3-8 mm. at the end of 48 hours' incubation. Further incubation or cultivation in the icebox produces no change in the type of hemolysis. The diameter of the zone of hemolysis increases in most cases on further incubation at body or refrigerator temperature.

Those streptococci which produce no change in the blood agar medium and which are known in the older groupings as "nonhemolytic" constitute the gamma group.

Since the terms alpha and beta are nondescriptive and the general tendency has been recently to use the more descriptive terms "green" and "hemolytic," we shall hereafter refer to the groups by the latter terms.

The numerical classification used in this study for the grouping of the sugar reactions is Brown's,[1] as shown in table 1.

About 90 organisms were isolated. The sources of the cultures are given in table 2. They were personally collected, with the exception of those which came from the laboratory of the University Hospital. All of the cultures were fished from surface platings on blood agar and isolated as hemolytic streptococci; and some were classified on the basis of their reaction in sugar mediums, as suggested by Holman,[2] using Hiss serum water medium with 1% of inulin, lactose, mannite and salicin.

[2] Jour. Med. Res., 1916, 34, p. 315.

Mediums.—The agar medium used in this study was composed of 2 gm. of Liebig's extract of beef, 10 gm. of Witte's peptone and 15 gm. of Difco agar-standardized to the liter. This medium was made by dissolving the agar in boiling water and adding the other ingredients, while the medium was cooling to 60 C., securing thorough solution by rapid stirring. When cool enough, one beaten egg per liter was added and the whole again brought to the boiling point, filtered and the reaction adjusted to P_H 7.4. When sterilized at 15 lbs. for 15 minutes, the final reaction which was tested on several occasions never fell below P_H 7. The medium was tubed—12 c c to the tube—or placed in small flasks — 75 c c to the flask — and stored in the icebox until used. Evaporation and shrinkage were slight.

TABLE 1

Tabulation of Streptococci (After Brown[1])

Mannite	Lactose	Salicin	Groups	Type in Blood Agar Green, hemolytic or nonhemolytic	
−	+	+	1	S. mitis	Green
−	+	+	1	S. pyogenes	Hemolytic
−	+	−	2	S. salivarius	Green
−	+	−	2	S. anginosus	Hemolytic
−	−	+	3	S. equinus	Green
−	−	+	3	S. equi	Hemolytic
−	−	−	4	S. ignavus	Green
−	−	−	4	S. subacidus	Hemolytic
+	+	+	5	S. faecalis	Green
+	+	+	5	S. infrequens	Hemolytic
+	+	−	6		
+	−	+	7	S. alactosus	Hemolytic
+	−	−	8		

	.1	.2	.3	.4	.5	.6	.7	.8
Raffinose	−	+	−	+	−	+	−	+
Inulin	−		+		−		+	
Saccharose	+				−			

The blood was secured in a sterile Erlenmyer flask—250 c c—fitted as an aspirating bottle. The needle was capped with a glass tube before sterilization in the autoclave. The blood was taken from the jugular vein of the sheep. It was then defibrinated in the bottle and pipetted to sterile test tubes, where, if no contamination occurred, it gave satisfactory results for a period of at least one week.

The blood was added to the agar, 0.6 c c to a 12 c c tube, just before pouring the plates; 4 c c to a 75 c c flask of agar. This flask agar was poured into sterile tubes and used for stock cultures and other work requiring blood agar.

An attempt was made to secure the blood from the same sheep at each bleeding, but this was not always possible. On several occasions an animal was used, whose blood at each bleeding was grossly contaminated with green streptococci of the 1.1, 1.2 and 2.2 varieties. This contamination was observed on one occasion when the technic of securing the blood was the same as usual. The contamination, however, was laid to faulty technic. A second contamination occurred using the same sheep. Blood agar slants made from this bleeding were so grossly contaminated as apparently to preclude any other source than that of the blood. A special bleeding was now carried out and the same type of organisms isolated. No attempt was made to identify them again individually, but they were distinctly green streptococci with an extremely long chain formation in broth.

This particular occurrence is stressed because of the oft-repeated statements that the green and hemolytic organisms are capable of two appearances or rather of mutation. It seems possible that a green contamination in a tube might be the source of a so-called mutation. Green organisms, furthermore, develop but slowly and blood agar mediums should be incubated at least 72 hours—48 hours in the incubator and 24 hours at room temperature—before it is accepted for use.

Sugar Mediums.—At the beginning of this work, Hiss serum water medium was used and made on the standard formula: 1 part serum, 3 parts water, 1% sugar and litmus to color a satisfactory blue. This was found difficult to sterilize and in some of the sugars, particularly mannite, an odd shade of purple was observed that was confusing. Some of the organisms, however, were satisfactorily identified on this medium.

Trypsinized peptone water was then tried. This is a simple peptone water, treated in the incubator for three hours with trypsin—1 gm. to the liter of broth. At the end of this time it was brought to the boiling point and 2 gm. of meat extract added and the product filtered. The reaction is adjusted to P_H 7.2, 1% sugar and Andrade's indicator added. It was then sterilized at 15 pounds of pressure for 15 minutes. This medium when used with the cultures identified on the serum water medium produced the same results.

This medium had the advantage of being easy to prepare as the securing of suitable serum in large amounts was difficult; it was easier to sterilize, and the Andrade indicator gave a more delicate indication of the amount of acid production. The serum water medium coagulated in the presence of much acid, but a comparison of results on both mediums would indicate that a pronounced shade of red in the medium with the Andrade indicator is the equivalent of coagulation in the serum water medium. It also possessed the great advantage of showing growth by turbidity or sediment formation in tubes showing no acid formation.

Broth, plain, trypsinized, was made in the same way as the carbohydrate mediums, eliminating the fermentable substances. This, with the exception of one culture, produced a suitable growth for staining and sugar tube inoculation.

Broth, hormone, was prepared as follows: To 3 liters of water warmed to 60 C., were added 3 beaten eggs and 5 pounds of ground beef heart. To this warm mixture were added 2 liters of water containing the following dissolved materials: 50 gm. of peptone, 12.5 gm. of salt, 12.5 gm. of trypsinized peptone and 50 gm. of gelatin. The entire mixture was gradually raised to the boiling point without stirring after the beef has started to coagulate. It was boiled from 15-20 minutes. A small portion was filtered through filter paper and to the measured filtrate was added enough 10% HCl to cause the maximum precipitation.. HCl was added to the unfiltered portion of the mixture in the same proportion. It was boiled for a few minutes. The precipitation with HCl was repeated until no further precipitation occurred. When there was no further precipitate, the liquid was drawn from the coagulum and sterilized at 12 pounds of pressure for 15 minutes.

The next day the supernatant fluid was siphoned from the sediment. The reaction was adjusted to P_H 7.8-8 in the cold; 0.25% dextrose was dissolved in the mixture by boiling. It was poured into tall jars and allowed to settle until the supernatant fluid was perfectly clear, when it was tubed and sterilized. We sterilized in the autoclave and had apparently no disastrous results. This medium allows streptococci to grow luxuriantly.

Milk.—Certified milk was suitably colored with litmus, tubed and sterilized by raising the pressure to 15 pounds slowly, maintaining for 15 minutes and then allowing the autoclave to return to normal pressure by simply turning off the heat.

All of the mediums requiring peptone and meat extract were made from a 1 lb. jar of Liebig's extract and a 1 kg. bottle of Witte's peptone, both of which were from prewar stock.

Method of Study.—The cultures were studied as follows: A loopful of stock culture was inoculated into a series of 4 tubes by the usual serial tube method. The first 2 tubes of the series contained salt solution, the last 2, liquid blood agar, as many platings have shown the most successful plates to be those from the third and fourth dilutions. The plates were then incubated for 48 hours when the kind of hemolysis was recorded. If the plates all showed the same general kind of hemolysis and colony, two deep colonies were fished to broth by cutting out the surrounding agar in a small block; this block was then macerated on the wall of a broth tube and washed into the fluid portion of the broth. This method is mentioned because in a great many cases the ordinary stabbing of a deep colony seems insufficient to produce growth. The broth tubes were then incubated for 24 hours when the macroscopic appearance was noted and the stained preparations examined. A stock culture was made on blood agar and plants to sugar tubes by adding 0.5 c c of the broth culture to each sugar tube. Fermentations were noted at the end of 1, 3 and 7 days. Streptococci reach their full powers of fermentation at the end of 3 days if the sugar tubes receive a moderately heavy inoculation to overcome the initial lag. If the two fishings agreed in their sugar reactions, one stock culture was discarded.

If on the original plate there was present more than one kind of hemolysis or if the appearance of the two colonies varied materially in size or shape, two fishings of each general type were made and the procedure as given followed.

If the two sugar fermentations from the same type of colony did not agree, the two blood agar stock cultures were checked from the beginning by replating.

When the sugar reactions had been determined and agreed, one stock culture was again replated and put through the same procedure as a check.

The following standard was adopted: That on the original agar plate they agree in hemolysis; that the two fishings agree in sugar reactions; that one of the fishings when replated produce the same type of hemolysis; that this replating produce the same sugar fermentations from the two fishings as the original fishing. Later on, this was modified so that a culture yielding two colonies, alike on blood agar and in sugar reactions, was considered as determined.

Preparation of Antigens.—The first antigens used were blood-agar cultures suspended in salt solution. These, as a rule, were not smooth and tended to spontaneous clumping. Varying results were obtained with them. On occasions they were apparently agglutinated and again the same lot of antiserum produced no effect. Heat killed antigens were more satisfactory than live antigens.

Broth cultures were then tried. The majority of these, when the growth was heavy, were granular and unsatisfactory for that reason.

Hormone broth caused a heavy growth, which, if centrifuged and washed in Locke's solution (0.01% $CaCl_2$, 0.02% KCl in salt solution) within 18 hours after inoculation, produced a satisfactory product. The centrifuged and washed antigen was diluted with Locke's solution to a strength of 2 billion per c c and preserved with phenol to a strength of 0.5%.

Preparation of Antiserums.—In the preparation of antiserums, various methods were used, no one of which produced a very high titer in all of the animals used. In the first method we injected subcutaneously killed, blood agar cultures suspended in salt solution, followed by live cultures. Three doses were given on 3 successive days followed by an interval of 3 more days before resuming the injections. In most cases the animals developed open abscesses at the site of inoculation when large doses were given. This method produced low titers. These serums were titrated against blood agar antigens and the low titers may have been caused by unsatisfactory antigens.

Intravenous injections were then tried with antigens grown both in blood agar and broth. The most satisfactory results were obtained by using serum broth cultures in increasing doses every third day, using killed cultures for the first 3 injections. It was noticed on 3 occasions that after the inoculation of killed organisms, the first injection of a live broth culture of hemolytic organism caused the death of the rabbit no matter how small the dose. When these same organisms were centrifuged and resuspended in salt solution, there was no noticeable effect on the rabbits while some immunity was obtained. This disagrees with Kinsella[3] who found that washed streptococci produced no immunity.

The green organisms produced a much higher immunity than did the hemolytic type in the same number of injections. Some hemolytic cultures seem incapable of producing agglutinins. Several of the hemolytic type produced no measurable agglutinins after as many as 15 injections. The one hemolytic culture which has produced agglutinins had a titer of only 400, whereas titers as high as 3,000 were obtained in the green group. This seems to point to some fundamental difference between the two groups.

Chickens were used for the production of immune serums. They were immunized by our earlier methods and the titers were about the same as in the rabbit serums. It was thought possible that the chickens would be capable of producing high titers because of their protective substances against pneumococci.

Serologic Tests.—In making the agglutinations, 3 dilutions of each immune serum were used. The lowest dilution in each case was 1:50, the highest was one-half the titer of the serum with its homologous antigen and the third was a dilution halfway between the low and the high. Each agglutination was controlled by a plain antigen suspension in Locke's solution for the occurrence of spontaneous agglutination and by a normal rabbit serum in dilution of 1:50. The tubes were incubated in a water bath at 56 C. for 3 hours when readings were made. Agglutinations were read as positive if the controls showed no agglutination.

[3] Jour. Exper. Med., 1918, 28, p. 151.

TABLE 2

CULTURAL AND AGGLUTINATIVE CHARACTERISTICS OF STREPTOCOCCI *

Classification Green	Classification Brown	Serial Number	Source	Milk Reaction	Milk Coagulation	Milk Reduction	Agglutination Serums 14	19	22	M4	M9	Remarks
S. mitis	1.1	22	Tuberculosis sputum........	A	P	+	100	—	800	—	—	Nonpathogenic
	1.1	31	Influenza....................	A	+	+	100	—	400	—	—	
	1.1	35	Influenza....................	A	+	+	100	—	100	—	—	
	1.1	37	Influenza....................	A	+	+	400	—	400	—	—	
	1.1	43	Tuberculosis sputum........	A	+	+	400	—	400	—	—	
	1.1	48	Tuberculosis sputum........	A	+	+	50	—	—	—	—	
	1.1	128	Normal throat..............	A	+	+	400	—	400	—	—	
	1.1	UN/C	Contaminated blood agar...	A	+	+	100	—	100	—	—	
....	1.2	14	Peritonsillar abscess.........	A	+	+	1600	—	—	—	—	Nonpathogenic
	1.2	51	Tuberculosis sputum........	A	+	+	400	—	100	—	—	
	1.2	78	Empyema..................	A	P	—	—	—	—	—	—	Described by Smith and Brown, Hartzell and Henrici, Kligler, Broadhurst. Suggested name, S. secundomitis
	1.2	Fec 1	Sheep feces..................	A	+	+	—	—	—	—	—	
	1.2	Fec 4	Sheep feces..................	A	+	+	—	—	—	—	—	
	1.2	UN/B	Contaminated blood agar...	A	+	+	100	—	—	—	—	
....	1.3	52	Tuberculosis sputum.......	—	—	—	—	—	—	—	—	
	1.3	61	Normal throat..............	—	—	—	—	—	—	—	—	Acid production slight in sugars. Described by Smith and Brown, Broadhurst. Suggested name, S. tertiomoitis
	1.3	SH/D	Slaughter house blood.......	—	—	—	—	—	—	—	—	
....	1.4	23	Tuberculosis sputum........	A	—	—	—	—	—	—	—	Nonpathogenic
	1.4	65	Contaminated blood agar...	A	—	—	—	—	—	—	—	
	1.4	88	Influenza pneumonia........	a	—	—	—	—	—	—	—	Described by Kligler, Broadhurst. Suggested name, S. quartomitis. Acid production slight in sugars
	1.4	168	Tuberculosis sputum........	A	—	—	—	—	—	—	—	
	1.4	SH/B	Slaughter house blood.......	—	—	—	—	—	—	—	—	
....	2.2	100	Tuberculosis sputum........	A	—	—	—	—	—	—	—	Nonpathogenic
	2.2	101	Tuberculosis sputum........	A	—	—	—	—	—	—	—	
	2.2	UN/A	Contaminated blood agar...	A	+	+	100	—	—	—	—	Described by Smith and Brown, Hartzell and Henrici, Kligler, Broadhurst. Suggested name, S. secundosalivarius
S. equinus	3.1	62	Tuberculosis sputum........	—	—	—	—	—	—	—	—	
S. faecalis	5.1	35a	Contaminated blood agar...	—	—	—	—	—	—	—	—	Nonpathogenic
	5.1	54	Contaminated blood agar...	a	—	—	—	—	—	—	—	Acid production slight in sugars
	5.1	SH/A	Slaughter house blood.......	—	—	—	—	—	—	—	—	

....	5.3	67	Contaminated blood agar...	—	—	—	—	—	—	—	—	Acid production slight in sugars
	5.3	68	Like 67	a	—	—	—	—	—	—	—	Described by Broadhurst
	5.3	70	Like 67	—	—	—	—	—	—	—	—	Suggested name, S. tertiofaecalis
....	5.4	50	Tuberculosis sputum	A	+	+	—	—	—	—	—	Described by Broadhurst. Suggested name, S. quartofaecalis. Diplococcus; no chains; no capsule; not bile-soluble
Hemolytic S. pyogenes	1.1	11	Tuberculosis sputum	A	—	—	—	—	—	—	—	Pathogenic
	1.1	15	Boil	A	—	—	—	—	—	—	—	
	1.1	16	Impetigo	A	—	—	—	—	—	—	—	
	1.1	17	Impetigo	A	—	—	—	—	—	—	—	
	1.1	19	Impetigo	A	—	—	—	300	—	—	400	Pathogenic
	1.1	20	Impetigo	A	—	—	—	—	—	—	—	
	1.1	21	Impetigo	A	—	—	—	—	—	—	—	
	1.1	26	Maternity case	a	—	—	—	—	—	—	—	
	1.1	27	Septicemia	a	—	—	—	—	—	—	—	
	1.1	28	Tuberculosis sputum	A	—	—	—	—	—	—	—	
	1.1	57	Arm infection after vein removal	A	—	—	—	—	—	—	—	
	1.1	79	Maternity case	A	—	—	—	—	—	—	—	
	1.1	114	Tuberculosis sputum	A	—	—	—	—	—	800	—	
	1.1	117	Tuberculosis sputum	A	—	—	—	—	—	—	—	
	1.1	150	Bott's disease abscess	A	—	—	—	—	—	—	—	
	1.1	172	Tuberculosis sputum	A	+	+	—	—	—	—	—	
	1.1	174	Empyema	A	—	—	—	—	—	800	—	
	1.1	177	Impetigo	A	—	—	—	—	—	—	—	
	1.1	178	Impetigo	A	—	—	—	—	—	—	—	
	1.1	184	Impetigo	A	—	—	—	—	—	—	—	
	1.1	P	Abscess of axilla	A	—	—	—	—	—	—	—	
	1.1	X	Cellulitis of hand	A	—	—	—	—	—	—	—	
....	1.5	173	Empyema	A	—	—	—	—	—	—	—	
	1.5	M12	Pasteurized 'A' milk	A	+	+	—	—	—	—	—	S. lacticus (Salter)
	1.5	M15	Pasteurized 'A' milk	A	+	+	—	—	—	—	—	S. lacticus (Salter)
S. anginosus	2.1	58	Tuberculosis sputum	a	—	—	—	—	—	—	—	Pathogenic
S. subacidus	4.1	123	Medical ward	—	—	—	—	—	—	—	—	
S. infrequens	5.1	24	Septicemia	a	—	—	—	—	—	—	—	
	5.1	151	Pericardial fluid, pneumonia	a	—	—	—	—	—	—	—	
	5.1	175	Empyema	a	—	—	—	—	—	—	400	
....	5.5	M11	Pasteurized 'A' milk	A	+	+	—	—	—	—	—	Suggested name, S. quilacticus

* The readings of the milk reactions were made at the end of 7 days. "a" indicates slight acid production. Antiserums 14, 19 and 22 were made from the corresponding cultures; M4 and M9 were secured from the H. K. Mulford Co. and reprecent Dochez types of streptococci I (S3) and III (S60), respectively. The numbers in the agglutination columns represent the highest dilution in which satisfactory and constant agglutinations were secured. The negative signs indicate no agglutination in a dilution of 1 : 50 or higher.

Absorption tests were made with all antigens, whose agglutinations were positive, by adding to a 1:5 dilution of the serum, four times its volume of antigen. The mixtures were incubated for 3 hours at 56 C. and allowed to stand over night in the icebox. The next morning they were centrifuged and the supernatant fluid used in agglutination tests with the homologous culture. If the serum showed an appreciable decline in its agglutinating powers with its homologous culture the original agglutination was considered positive.

Complement-fixation tests were made using cultures which represented the cultural groups. The antigens were heavy salt solution suspensions of broth cultures. Homologous culture and serum were used to determine the amboceptor dosage. The same quantity of antigen was used with all cultures after the proper dosage had been determined in homologous culture and serum. Complement fixation occurred indiscriminately; there was no relation between the power of fixing complement and the cultural groups. This agrees with the results of Kinsella and Swift,[4] Howell and Hitchens,[5] and others.

Bactericidal tests were carried out with the technic of Havens.[6] No relation exists between the bactericidal powers and the cultural groups, except that green serum has no effect on the hemolytic group and vice versa.

SUMMARY OF TABLE 2

The growth in broth is not recorded because of the variations in growth and morphology in the same culture at various times.

None of the organisms resembling pneumococci were bile-soluble.

Green types, as compared with hemolytic types in source, are apparently less pathogenic and in many cases purely saphrophytic in nature.

The reaction in milk seems the most distinctive single reaction we have. Green 1.1 cultures without a single exception produce acid, coagulation and reduction, while the hemolytic 1.1 cultures agree, with one exception, in their inability to coagulate and reduce milk. This one exception is from a questionable pathogenic source. On this basis we may assume that the more pathogenic have less power to affect milk than the saphrophytic. We have a specific example of this in comparing hemolytic 1.5 cultures. Those from milk are powerful in their action on milk while the one from a pathogenic source produces a moderate amount of acid in comparison with acid and coagulation in the others.

The green 1.2 cultures which the serologic reactions show to be closley related to the 1.1 group act much in the same way on milk. This group, which has its main distinction in the ability to ferment raffinose, is otherwise morphologically and culturally like the green 1.1 group.

[4] Jour. Exper. Med., 1917, 15, p. 877.
[5] Jour. Infect. Dis., 1918, 12, p. 230.
[6] Ibid., 1919, 15, p. 315.

Serologically there seems to be no great difference between the green 1.1 and 1.2 groups. Green 1.2 serum agglutinates as many green 1.1 cultures as does a 1.1 serum, but one of the green 1.2 cultures is agglutinated by a 1.1 serum and that in a comparatively low dilution. Not all of either group are agglutinated by their culturally homologous serum. Therefore, it would seem that raffinose fermentation is not a distinctive reaction, although an antiserum from a raffinose fermenting strain has a wider range of agglutination than antiserum from a strain not fermenting raffinose.

Should Brown's sugar grouping be proved of value, the use of some system of nomenclature in connection with this chart would be advisable. The addition of the proper Roman ordinal—to represent the second half of the number—to the name already assigned which represents the first half of the number would orient the name to the number without the addition of entirely new names. It is in accordance with such a system that we suggest the name—S. secundomitis for the green 1.2 group. We have not included with the suggested names, the writers who have previously reported these organisms, as their names are listed in the chart. Nor are the morphologic characteristics included as they vary within the limits of streptococcal growth both as to individual size and length of chain.

Green 1.3 and 1.4 organisms which ferment inulin have but little power to affect milk. They produce no coagulation, and some of them are barely able to produce a trace of acidity; few produce a strong acid reaction. This inability to react on milk gives us another method of differentiating questionable streptococci from pneumococci.

These organisms are also slight acid producers in other sugar mediums. With Andrade's indicator the end-point is a faint pink. This may account for the slight reaction in milk. Otherwise, culturally, they are like S. mitis. Serologically, these two groups are distinct and separate from green 1.1 and 1.2. There have been no agglutinations in any one of them by serums from the 1.1 and 1.2 groups. Suggested names are: S. tertiomitis and S. quartomitis.

The next group, green 2.2, has its main distinction from the preceding organisms in its inability to ferment salicin. Here, again, we have two organisms from a possible pathogenic source with but little action on milk. The third from an apparently saphrophytic source is vigorous in its action on milk. The same saphrophytic organism is agglutinated by a green 1.2 serum. The best explanation for this is that the raffinose fermenters are closely related serologically. The agglutination of this nonfermenter of salicin by a salicin fermenting antiserum discards salicin from an important place in the cultural grouping. Culturally these organisms present no other distinctive reactions. S. secundosalivarius is the suggested name.

S. faecalis, green 5.1 ferments mannite and has little action on milk. These organisms attack the sugars only slightly and are not agglutinated by our serums. The green 5.3 group has the same general characteristics as green 5.1 but in addition ferments inulin. They are like the other inulin fermenters in their action on milk. S. tertiofaecalis is the suggested name.

Culture 50 represents the green 5.4 group. Morphologically it is a diplococcus, never appearing in chains. No capsule, however, can be demonstrated nor is it bile-soluble. Its reaction in milk is like that of the pneumococcus, and in addition it ferments inulin. None of our serums agglutinate it, although both green and hemolytic serums are capable of fixing complement in its presence. S. quartofaecalis is the suggested name.

In the entire hemolytic group of organisms we find 4 of them capable of producing acid, coagulation and reduction in milk. Three of these are from milk sources and 2 are typical of the S. lacticus group, while the third has the additional property of fermenting mannite. Only one hemolytic organism from a source which is likely to be pathogenic is capable of causing coagulation in milk. The agglutination positives are so few as to prevent any sweeping conclusions, but they point to the fact that the sugar fermentations are not an indication of the serologic relations.

Organism M11 ferments mannite in addition to lactose and salicin and in considering that its source is milk we may assume that it is but a variation of the S. lacticus group. S. quilacticus is the suggested name.

A summary of all the agglutination reactions places the green and hemolytic organisms in two distinct serologic groups. In no case has there been any cross agglutination between the green cultures and hemolytic serums, and the converse is equally true. The number of positive results recorded in the green group, and the way in which they arrange themselves indicates that the fundamental differences in addition to the blood reactions are those of inulin and mannite fermentation.

The pathogenesis of some of these cultures has been tested directly. They were picked at random for the test but included most of the cultural groups. None of the green cultures was able to produce death in long or short periods of time and return the organism in pure culture. In the hemolytic group 3 cultures out of five killed guinea-pigs in 24 hours, the organism being recovered in pure culture. In these tests guinea-pigs were injected intraperitoneally with 2 c c of a 24-hour broth culture.

DISCUSSION

Brown[1] states that in his studies the types previously outlined have their various characteristics in blood agar fixed and unchanging; that is, on standard culture mediums, hemolytic types do not revert to green or green to hemolytic. Havens,[6] on the contrary, states that streptococci grown on culture mediums for a few weeks after isolation lose their hemolytic powers in blood broth and become avirulent. This differs with the results in this study. Streptococci kept on blood agar for over a year now produce zones of hemolysis from 6-8 mm. in diameter in 24 hours. The same cultures when planted in blood broth still have power to cause diffusion of hemoglobin. This is not true of all cultures isolated, but, as was previously stated, these cultures were classified as hemolytic from surface platings and subsequently found not to be of the hemolytic type.

Surface plating seems responsible for a great deal of this confusion. A green organism planted on the surface of a blood-agar plate elaborates its first growth with the production of the green zone. Its secondary zone of hemolysis starts forming as in the deep colonies. The colony spreads, in its growth covering the green zone, leaving the colony in an apparent zone of hemolysis. Brown states that the secondary zone forms in the icebox or at temperatures lower that that of the incubator. This is not always true. Plates have been taken directly from the incubator to the microscope and in many cases the secondary ring is well formed. If observed within from 2-3 minutes after leaving the incubator, it seems hardly possible that the secondary ring of hemolysis could form because of the slight change in temperature in so short a time.

On this basis an investigator, using the surface method, might easily fish a green type on observing the secondary zone of hemolysis, supposing it to be a hemolytic colony. He plants it in a blood agar medium as a stock culture. In most cases that green type will color the entire tube green in a few days. Further platings, after this green has been noted, will in all likelihood class the organism as a green type. The investigator then having two results at variance with each other might be led to assume that a hemolytic organism has become a green type.

With the foregoing in mind we are adding at this point a rather detailed history of culture 19. This culture, having been roughly determined as hemolytic 1.1, was selected to immunize a pair of rabbits. Because of the necessity of having a strain of undoubted purity for the source of the antiserum, the checking which follows was done with great care and detail. On its second plating, a typical hemolytic colony grew in the depths, but on the surface there appeared a wrinkled, 2-3 mm. colony, surrounded by a greenish zone which looked neither green nor hemolytic hemolysis, but more like a green pigmentation independent of the blood itself. There was no noticeable formation of the secondary ring of hemolysis which surrounds the green formation in typical green hemolysis. This was proved a variation by fishing and finding the sugar reactions to be 1.1, replating it and finding both the new-formed wrinkled colonies and deep colonies—which were again typical—and confirming on the sugars as 1.1. On one of the secondary platings, the blood was contaminated by a green type—mentioned under Blood in the section on media—which further complicated the determination. Not all hemolytic cultures produce this type of surface growth, nor does every surface colony of this culture produce this reaction.

This type of growth corresponds closely with S. metachromatos (Brown). The following is a condensed description of the organism in a letter from Dr. Brown, "The colony on defibrinated blood agar is conical in shape, the edges irregularly serrated. The colony itself becomes brownish and has a granular appearance, with the greenish pigmentation surrounding it. When the colony is lifted, it frequently comes away in its entirety and shows the agar more or less pitted. In serum bouillon, the culture settles to the bottom and is fluffy."

These results and conjectures are inserted here because throughout the literature, there are constantly recurring statements that streptococci of various types lose or gain some of the powers of hemolysis, when grown on culture mediums for long periods of time. Our results disagree with such conclusions.

SUMMARY

Green and hemolytic types of streptococci are distinct culturally and serologically, the last measured by the agglutination reactions.

The sugar reactions are not indicators of serologic groupings, but possibly inulin fermentation and the reaction in milk may be used as of value in group determination in conjunction with the blood type.

METABOLISM OF B. WELCHII, VIBRION SEPTIQUE, B. FALLAX, B. TERTIUS, B. TETANI, B. PSEUDOTETANI, B. BOTULINUS, B. BIFERMENTANS, B. OEDEMATIENS, B. AEROFOETIDUS, B. SPOROGENES, B. HISTOLYTICUS, AND B. PUTRIFICUS

STUDIES IN BACTERIAL METABOLISM, XLIV-LV

Arthur Isaac Kendall; Alexander Alfred Day, and Arthur William Walker

From the Department of Bacteriology, Northwestern University Medical School, Chicago, Ill.

BACILLUS WELCHII

STUDY XLIV

Bacillus welchii, also known as Bacillus perfringens, Bacillus aerogenes capsulatus, the "gas bacillus," and by several other names,[1] is an anaerobic bacillus, originally isolated and described by Welch and Nuttall[2] as a "gas-producing organism capable of rapid development in the body after death." Welch[3] has previously published a preliminary report on the bacillus, announcing its occurrence in the blood and emphysematous tissues of a patient who had died as the result of the rupture of an aortic aneurysm. About the same time Fraenkel[4] had described in rather general terms his Bacillus phlegmones-emphysematosae, and called attention to a probable causal relation of it to gas phlegmon (emphysematous-cellulitis or emphysematous-gangrene).

It seems probable that the Welch bacillus is the type member of either a group of closely related organisms, or of a series of identifiable variants of the same bacillus. A voluminous literature has grown up around the "gas bacillus," or Welch bacillus group, not only with reference to pathogenicity but also in regard to distribution in soil, dust, water, sewage and in the intestinal tract of man.[1] During the Great War it achieved conspicuous notoriety as the chief incitant of gas gangrene.[5] The resulting intense scrutiny to which the Welch bacillus

Received for publication Oct. 12, 1921.

[1] Simonds, Monograph 8, Rockefeller Institute, 1915.
[2] Johns Hopkins Hosp. Bull., 1892, 3, p. 81.
[3] Jour. Exper. Med., 1896, I, p. 5.
[4] Centralbl. f. Bakteriol., 1893, 13, p. 13; Ueber Gas Phlegmon, 1893.
[5] Weinberg and Séguin: La Gangrène Gazeuse, 1917. Also, Report 39, Medical Research Committee, 1919.

has been subjected, both culturally, pathologically and serologically, has cleared up many of the extraordinary and extravagant claims of its "polymorphism" and other unusual departures from bacterial stability, and it is now apparently a well-defined entity whose salient characteristics are those described in the comprehensive monograph of Simonds.[1]

The biochemistry of this bacillus has received comparatively little attention, although it possesses some inherent features which are noteworthy, both with respect to the organism itself, and in contrast to or comparison with, closely related anaerobic bacteria. The observations on this aspect of the life history of the gas bacillus prior to the publication of Simonds' study are unreliable, because the earlier published descriptions convey almost conclusive evidence of contamination of the cultures studied with proteolytic anaerobic organisms, or even with aerobic microbes. Thus, Klein,[6] Tissier and Martelly,[7] and Grassberger and Schattenfroh,[8] described protein digestive powers, proteolytic enzymes, or even in the latter instance [9] a "dimorphism," one phase of which was proteoclastic, to the Welch organism. Rosenthal [10] mentions an aerobic state, in which the morphology and characteristics of the organism change with increasing aerobic tolerance to the final acquisition of an oval, coccoid form, indistinguishable from that of Micrococcus ovalis.

The original studies of Welch and Nuttall [2] were quite clear with reference to evidence of proteolysis in gelatin. They state, "The bacillus is best classed among the non-liquefiers of gelatin, although in anaerobic cultures of 5 per cent. of sugar gelatin there may be a slight softening due to peptonization of the gelatin over a limited area, as is made manifest by the settling of the growth toward the bottom of the line of puncture in stab cultures, and by a slight displacement of the gas bacillus in changing the position of the tube. Cultures in gelatin which have developed at 35-37° C. become solid upon cooling the tube."

Simonds [1] was apparently the first observer actually to measure the chemical changes induced by Welch bacillus in mediums of known composition. His analytic figures show clearly that its action on protein (nutrient broth) is very small indeed. Carbohydrates (glucose, lactose, saccharose, starch and glycerol), on the contrary, are energetically attacked with the formation of much gas, considerable acid,

[6] Centralbl. f. Bakteriol., 1895, 18, p. 737.
[7] Ann. Inst. Past., 1902, 16, p. 865.
[8] Arch. f. Hyg., 1902, 42, p. 219.
[9] Arch. f. Hyg., 1904, 48, p. 1.
[10] L'Aerobisation des microbes anaérobies, 1908. Compt. rend. Soc. de Biol., 1906, 58, p. 828.

and with minimal effect on the protein constituents of these fermentation mediums.

Wolf and Harris [11] carried out an elaborate series of metabolism studies on an anaerobic organism identified as B. welchii. A variety of mediums were used and observations during various periods of growth were made on the nitrogenous changes induced in these mediums, together with the rate and amount of gas formation. They found that the gas production by their organism in milk was quite variable, although in each instance a large volume was formed. Their actual figures of gas production per liter of medium at the end of approximately 24 hours varied from about 1,650 c c to as much as 3,820 c c. This large liberation of gas is in accord with the most prominent feature of milk cultures of the gas bacillus, the so-called "stormy fermentation." The gas was found to be approximately two-thirds hydrogen, the remainder practically entirely carbon dioxide. These figures are in close accord with those of Theobald Smith.[12] The titratable acidity of the cultures rose from about 20 to 62 c c of normal acid per liter during the period of intense fermentative activity. The hydrogen-ion value in one experiment appears to have increased from P_H 6.0 to approximately P_H 4.58.

The nitrogenous changes observed by them were significant. In one experiment, which seems to be representative, the amino nitrogen increased from an initial content of 3.8 mg. per 100 c c of milk to 26.5 mg. in 100 c c of milk within an incubation period of 35 hours. The ammonia change during the same interval was very small. At the start the milk contained 4.0 mg. of ammonia per 100 c c, and at the end of 33 hours' incubation the increase was only 1.6 mg. in the same volume. Somewhat more than 3 gm. of lactose per liter were changed to carbon dioxide and hydrogen, and organic acids, during this period.

The pressure generated by the rapid evolution of gas in the milk was very considerable. In one experiment the culture generated gas to the extent of 1.5 times the entire initial volume of the medium, and the pressure in a mercury manometer rose to the astonishing height of 1,520 mm. of mercury—about 2 atmospheres. It will be remembered that Taylor [13] has previously shown that a pressure of gas exceeding 1.5 atmosphere was generated in one of his cultures of the gas bacillus within 5 hours, and the exact pressure was unrecorded because the

[11] Jour. Path. & Bacteriol., 1917, 21, p. 386.
[12] Ztschr. f. Infektionskrankh. d. Haustiere, 1906, I, p. 26. Jour. Med. Res., 1905, 14, p. 193.
[13] Lancet, 1916, 1, p. 123.

manometer became disarranged at this time. Taylor believed that the pressure exerted in muscular tissues by the generation of gas might be a potent factor both in spreading the infection of the Welch bacillus through the tissues by forcing apart the muscle fibers, and by actually causing serious mechanical damage to the muscular tissues through intramuscular gas pressure.

Wolf and Harris [11] also performed metabolism experiments in sugar-free broth, using a tryptic digest of casein carefully freed from sugar as a medium. It was found that about 20 mg. of amino-nitrogen and 42.5 mg. of ammonia were formed per 100 c c of medium in 27 hours. The reaction underwent very little change, from P_H 7.68 to P_H 7.49. Wolf and Harris emphasize the rise in amino nitrogen in their cultures, in contrast to the negligible amount of ammonia produced simultaneously. The reverse appears to have been observed in cultures of Vibrion septique.[14] They state that an odor suggestive of cultures of B. sporogenes was detected at the end of the experiment, but were apparently unable to detect a contaminant, if such existed. They very properly state that the results are not suggestive of contamination with B. sporogenes, which would undoubtedly have formed much more ammonia than that found in this experiment.

A study of the analytic figures of Wolf and Harris reveals clearly the sparing action which utilizable carbohydrate exerts for protein in cultures of the organism containing both sugar and protein available as sources of energy. These studies emphasize particularly the rapidity of growth of the organism they identified as the Welch bacillus and indicate clearly that the bacillus is carbohydrophilic rather than proteophilic. Action on protein and protein derivatives, in fact, was found to be minimal, even in the absence of utilizable carbohydrate, which is wholly in accord with the observations of Simonds.[1]

A peculiar and striking feature of the growth of the Welch bacillus is the formation of a soluble poison, reminiscent in many respects of the soluble toxins of organisms like B. diphtheriae. Bull and Pritchett [15] discovered that filtrates of 18-24 hour cultures of B. welchii [16] contain a soluble poison which incites many of the signs and symptoms of gas gangrene in experimental animals. A striking peculiarity of this poisonous substance is its diminution in potency as the culture becomes older. Indeed, after 48 hours' incubation the

[14] Jour. Path. & Bacteriol., 1918, 22, p. 115.
[15] Jour. Exper. Med., 1917, 26, p. 119.
[16] Culture 617 D, of Simonds.

poisonous properties of the filtrate may be practically negligible, even though 18-24 hour samples of the same culture, freed from organisms, were powerfully toxic. The presence of utilizable sugars has little or no apparent influence in reducing the production of this poison, contrasting in this respect sharply with the formation of soluble toxin in cultures of the diphtheria bacillus.[17] It will be remembered that diphtheria toxin is formed relatively slowly in protein mediums, reaching the maximum about the eighth or tenth day of incubation; also the presence of more than small amounts of utilizable carbohydrate prevents the formation of soluble toxin in cultures of the diphtheria bacillus. The genesis of the gas bacillus poison, therefore, differs from the formation of the soluble toxin of the diphtheria bacillus in at least two particulars. First, it appears early in the life history of the culture when the multiplication of the organisms—the birth rate, in other words—is maximal, and before the accumulation of products indicative of the energy phase of large numbers of mature bacilli becomes manifest. Secondly, the soluble poison of the Welch bacillus decreases rapidly in potency during the period when the energy phase of the life history of the culture has become dominant, and has succeeded the initial phase of rapid multiplication. It may be surmised that the soluble poison of the gas bacillus, therefore, is a substance or substances produced incidentally during the reproductive process of the organism. It is a waste product of structure rather than of energy. The rapid diminution in potency may be due to lability of the poison, or to its actual neutralization, disintegration or destruction, as the energy phase of the culture with its resulting products becomes prominent. Filtrates of cultures at the height of poison production, freed from bacteria, appear to be relatively stable, however, again suggesting that the phenomena attending the energy phase of the culture are destructive of the poisonous substance.

The gas bacillus poison, injected into suitable animals in properly spaced and measured amounts, incites the formation of specific antibodies, or at least of substances capable of neutralizing this poisonous substance. In this respect, the soluble, poisonous substance is analogous to the known soluble toxins in that both incite specific reactions in suitable hosts.

The experiments on the metabolism of the Welch bacillus, recorded in the following, and those in succeeding contributions, were under-

[17] Theobald Smith, Jour. Exper. Med., 1899, 4, p. 373.

taken on a request from the Medical Section of the National Research Council that a study be made of the biochemistry of the anaerobic bacteria which are associated with wounds of warfare. This work has been pursued for more than four years. A part of this time, however, was spent in searching for methods of isolation and culture of anaerobic organisms of greater precision than those available at the beginning of the investigation. The greatest problem encountered was that of securing cultures of undoubted purity. Isolation of single spores has been found extremely tedious, but reliable; hence, all cultures of the anaerobic bacteria studied were purified thrice by the modified Barber single cell method, previously described.[18] The cultures intended for metabolic study were grown in specifically designed flasks, each holding about 110 c c of medium. An individual flask was inoculated for each kind of medium for each day of observation. A set of 60 flasks, therefore, was required for each organism, including of course suitable controls. It is believed that this procedure of single flasks for each medium each day far exceeds in accuracy the alternate plan of removing samples at stated intervals from the same flask. The smoothness of the "growth curves" charted from the analyses is indicative of the precision of the entire process.

The several kinds of mediums (shown in the analytic tables) were seeded at the same time with two drops of an active meat-liver medium culture of the organism under consideration. Incubation was practiced at 37 C. for the various times indicated in the tables.

The analytic methods employed were those described in previous communications.[19] The determinations included the change in titratable acidity,[20] the measurement of changes in the nitrogenous constituents of the mediums—ammonia formation, amino acid liberation and utilization—the total nitrogen content, and attempts to demonstrate soluble proteolytic enzymes. In other words, the nitrogenous metabolism of the culture was followed, precisely as the nitrogenous metabolism of the body is followed through the measurement of the nitrogenous constituents of the blood and the urine.

Previous studies on the metabolism of aerobic and facultatively anaerobic organisms [19, 21] have shown material differences between the

[18] Kendall, Ryan and Cook: Jour. Infect. Dis., 1921, 29, p. 227.

[19] Kendall and Farmer: Jour. Biol. Chem., 1912, 12, p. 13. Kendall, Day and Walker: Jour. Am. Chem. Soc., 1913, 35, p. 1201. Kendall and Walker: Jour. Infect. Dis., 1915, 17, p. 442.

[20] These studies were started before the indicator method for hydrogen-ion measurement was developed to a satisfactory degree.

[21] Sears: Jour. Infect. Dis., 1916, 19, p. 105.

TABLE 1

BACILLUS WELCHII, 617D

	Day	Plain: Reaction	Plain: Ammonia Nitrogen	Plain: Amino Nitrogen	Plain: Percentage Ammonia to Total Nitrogen	Gelatin: Reaction	Gelatin: Ammonia Nitrogen	Gelatin: Amino Nitrogen	Gelatin: Percentage Ammonia to Total Nitrogen	Glucose: Reaction	Glucose: Ammonia Nitrogen	Glucose: Amino Nitrogen	Glucose: Percentage Ammonia to Total Nitrogen
Control April, 1917	..	—0.60	4.2	21.0	2.14	—0.90	4.2	43.4	0.47	—0.20	4.2	21.0	2.14
	1	—0.60	12.6	35.7	6.42	+0.10	11.9	46.9	1.35	+2.90	4.9	25.9	2.50
	3	—0.70	16.8	40.6	8.58	+0.10	16.8	49.0	1.91	+2.90	4.9	25.9	2.50
	6	—0.70	18.2	50.4	9.30	+0.10	18.2	56.0	7.05	+2.70	4.9	23.8	2.50
	13	—0.70	19.6	52.5	10.00	+0.10	23.8	78.4	2.70	+2.30	5.6	25.2	2.85
Control April, 1918	..	—0.40	4.9	23.8	2.46	—0.70	5.6	46.2	0.59	—0.40	4.9	23.8	2.46
	1	—0.40	12.6	26.6	6.64	—0.30	10.5	50.4	1.10	+2.20	4.2	21.7	2.22
	3	—0.80	16.8	50.4	8.90	0.00	13.3	52.5	1.39	+2.20	4.9	23.8	2.46
	6	—0.70	17.5	58.8	9.28	+0.10	15.4	53.9	1.62	+2.20	5.6	25.2	2.95
	14	—0.70	20.3	58.1	10.06	+0.15	20.3	65.1	2.13	+2.00	5.6	25.2	2.95
Control March, 1920	..	—0.60	17.5	20.3	7.81	—0.70	4.2	36.4	0.62	—0.60	18.9	21.7	8.43
	1	—0.80	25.9	30.1	11.55	—0.80	3.5	39.2	0.52	+4.70	21.0	32.2	9.38
	3	—0.70	28.7	49.7	12.81	—0.50	11.9	42.0	1.77	+4.80	21.7	32.9	9.70
	6	—0.70	28.7	49.7	12.81	—0.40	11.2	46.9	1.67	+4.90	23.1	35.0	10.03
	9	—0.80	34.3	53.9	15.26	—0.50	3.5	56.7	0.52	+5.00	22.4	35.0	10.00
	14	—0.90	36.4	58.1	16.24	+0.20	21.0	56.7	3.13	+5.10	22.4	35.7	10.00

	Day	Mannitol: Reaction	Mannitol: Ammonia Nitrogen	Mannitol: Amino Nitrogen	Mannitol: Percentage Ammonia to Total Nitrogen	Glycerol: Reaction	Glycerol: Ammonia Nitrogen	Glycerol: Amino Nitrogen	Glycerol: Percentage Ammonia to Total Nitrogen	Lactose: Reaction	Lactose: Ammonia Nitrogen	Lactose: Amino Nitrogen	Lactose: Percentage Ammonia to Total Nitrogen
Control April, 1917	..	—0.70	3.5	23.1	1.77	—0.70	3.5	23.1	1.77	—0.50	4.2	21.0	2.14
	1	—0.80	10.5	33.1	5.36	+1.10	11.2	26.6	5.70	+2.40	5.6	29.4	2.86
	3	—0.80	15.4	43.4	7.88	+1.50	11.2	26.6	5.70	+2.40	5.6	28.7	2.86
	6	—0.90	16.8	51.8	8.58	.....	....	....	.....	+2.20	5.6	28.0	2.86
	13	—1.00	18.2	55.3	9.40	+1.50	11.2	26.6	5.70	+2.20	5.6	28.0	2.86
Control April, 1918	..	—0.50	5.6	23.8	2.95	—0.60	4.9	22.4	2.46	—0.40	5.6	23.8	2.95
	1	—0.70	12.6	24.5	6.64	+1.90	10.5	25.9	5.55	+2.20	5.6	25.2	2.95
	3	—0.70	16.1	39.9	8.52	+1.90	11.9	25.9	6.30	+2.40	15.4	43.4	8.16
	6	—0.80	16.8	43.4	8.90	+2.00	10.5	25.2	5.55	+2.30	5.6	30.1	2.95
	14	—0.80	19.6	57.4	10.03	+2.00	11.9	28.7	6.30	+2.00	7.7	30.1	4.07
Control March, 1920	..	—0.70	18.2	21.0	8.13	—0.60	17.5	21.7	7.81	—0.60	18.2	21.0	8.12
	1	—0.80	27.3	31.5	12.20	+3.00	23.1	28.0	10.03	+3.40	23.1	28.7	12.80
	3	—0.90	32.2	37.8	14.30	+3.20	25.2	30.8	11.20	+3.40	25.2	29.4	11.20
	6	—0.80	35.0	42.7	15.70	+4.00	24.5	30.1	10.90	+3.60	25.9	32.9	11.55
	9	—0.80	35.0	49.7	15.70	+3.80	24.5	30.1	10.90	+3.60	25.9	35.7	11.55
	14	—0.90	34.3	53.9	15.30	+3.50	24.5	30.1	10.90	+3.40	25.2	35.7	11.20

	Day	Saccharose: Reaction	Saccharose: Ammonia Nitrogen	Saccharose: Amino Nitrogen	Saccharose: Percentage Ammonia to Total Nitrogen	Starch: Reaction	Starch: Ammonia Nitrogen	Starch: Amino Nitrogen	Starch: Percentage Ammonia to Total Nitrogen	Milk: Reaction	Milk: Ammonia Nitrogen	Milk: Amino Nitrogen	Milk: Percentage Ammonia to Total Nitrogen
Control April, 1917	..	—0.60	4.2	22.4	2.14	—0.70	2.8	22.4	1.42	+1.40	4.2	22.4	4.84
	1	+2.50	7.0	28.0	3.58	+2.00	10.5	31.5	5.36	+3.70	7.0	11.9	2.58
	3	+2.50	7.0	28.0	3.58	+2.00	11.2	30.8	5.70	+4.00	8.4	12.6	2.73
	6	+2.20	7.0	28.0	3.58	+2.00	11.2	30.8	5.70	+4.00	8.4	14.7	3.19
	13	+2.00	7.7	28.7	3.93	+1.90	11.9	31.5	6.01	+4.30	8.4	14.7	3.19
Control April, 1918	..	—0.40	5.6	22.4	2.95	—0.55	5.6	23.1	2.95	+1.10	5.6	14.7	2.96
	1	+2.80	6.3	22.4	3.33	+3.20	11.9	28.7	6.30	+3.60	8.4	9.1	1.97
	3	+2.80	8.4	30.1	4.44	+3.00	11.9	28.7	6.30	+4.00	9.1	11.9	2.40
	6	+2.70	7.7	30.1	4.07	+2.90	11.9	28.7	6.30	+3.80	9.1	11.9	2.40
	14	+2.00	8.4	30.1	4.41	+2.30	12.6	30.8	6.64	+4.00	11.2	16.1	3.24
Control March, 1920	..	—0.60	18.2	21.0	.....	—0.50	17.5	21.7	.....	+1.70	4.2	25.2	5.46
	1	+4.40	25.9	30.8	11.55	+4.30	24.5	34.3	10.90	+3.50	4.2	9.1	2.51
	3	+4.40	25.9	30.8	11.55	+4.60	25.9	34.4	11.55	+3.60	6.3	12.6	2.73
	6	+4.40	25.9	32.9	11.55	+4.90	26.6	35.0	11.80	+3.60	7.0	13.3	2.88
	9	+4.50	26.6	32.9	11.80	+5.10	26.6	36.4	11.80	+4.00	7.7	16.8	3.64
	14	+4.60	25.2	33.6	11.20	+5.10	27.3	37.1	12.20	+4.00	7.7	18.2	3.94

Reaction: — = alkaline to neutral red; + = acid to neutral red; c c normal acid or alkali per 100 c c of medium.
Ammonia and amino nitrogen expressed in milligrams per 100 c c of culture medium.
Control indicates initial composition of medium. Net results may be obtained by subtracting the control from the day's analysis.
Amino nitrogen is corrected in each instance for ammonia.

TABLE 2

BACILLUS WELCHII

	Day	Plain: Reaction	Plain: Ammonia Nitrogen	Plain: Amino Nitrogen	Plain: Percentage Ammonia to Total Nitrogen	Gelatin: Reaction	Gelatin: Ammonia Nitrogen	Gelatin: Amino Nitrogen	Gelatin: Percentage Ammonia to Total Nitrogen	Glucose: Reaction	Glucose: Ammonia Nitrogen	Glucose: Amino Nitrogen	Glucose: Percentage Ammonia to Total Nitrogen	Mannitol: Reaction	Mannitol: Ammonia Nitrogen	Mannitol: Amino Nitrogen	Mannitol: Percentage Ammonia to Total Nitrogen
Control	..	—0.50	3.5	23.1	2.00	—0.50	4.2	42.0	0.47	—0.20	3.5	20.3	2.00	—0.50	3.5	23.1	2.00
B. welchii "A"	1	—0.60	12.6	23.8	7.20	—0.60	4.2	42.0	0.47	+2.70	4.2	21.0	2.40	—0.50	11.9	27.3	6.80
	3	—0.60	14.7	23.8	8.40	—0.60	7.0	49.0	0.78	+2.60	4.2	21.0	2.40	—0.50	14.0	33.6	8.00
	6	—0.50	16.1	28.0	9.20	—0.30	9.8	52.5	1.11	+2.50	4.2	21.0	2.40	—0.50	15.4	41.3	8.80
	13	—0.50	16.8	28.0	9.51	—0.35	12.6	68.1	1.41	+2.40	4.2	21.0	2.40	—0.50	15.4	41.3	9.20
	20	—0.50	18.2	35.0	10.40	—0.40	14.7	63.7	1.64	+2.70	4.2	21.0	2.40	—0.50	16.8	46.9	10.00
Control	..	—0.50	3.5	21.7	1.92	—0.90	2.8	42.0	0.33	—0.20	2.8	20.3	1.54	—0.60	2.8	22.4	1.54
B. welchii "B"	1	—0.60	9.1	30.8	5.00	—0.80	4.2	46.9	0.49	+2.40	3.5	21.7	1.92	—0.40	9.8	22.4	5.38
	3	—0.50	10.5	35.7	5.58	—0.60	7.7	49.0	0.91	+2.40	4.2	21.7	2.31	—0.60	11.2	28.0	6.16
	6	—0.50	11.9	35.7	6.54	—0.60	11.6	56.7	1.35	+2.20	4.9	23.1	2.69	—0.50	13.3	30.8	7.30
	13	—0.50	16.1	35.7	8.84	—0.80	15.4	61.6	1.80	+2.20	4.9	25.9	2.69	—0.50	16.1	35.7	8.84
Control	..	—0.60	4.2	21.0	2.14	—0.90	3.5	43.4	0.39	—0.20	4.2	21.0	2.14	—0.70	3.5	23.1	1.79
B. welchii "C"	1	—0.50	4.2	30.1	2.14	—0.80	8.4	49.7	0.95	+2.80	4.9	24.5	2.50	—0.60	2.8	30.1	1.43
	3	—0.60	11.2	42.7	5.72	—0.80	12.6	54.6	1.43	+2.60	4.9	25.9	2.50	—0.80	9.8	32.9	5.00
	6	—0.70	12.6	42.7	6.43	—0.80	14.7	59.5	1.67	+2.50	4.9	25.9	2.50	—0.90	11.2	41.3	5.72
	13	—0.80	13.3	48.3	6.78	—0.80	16.1	59.5	1.83	+2.50	5.6	28.0	2.86	—0.80	14.7	56.7	7.50
Control	..	—0.50	3.5	23.1	2.00	—0.90	4.2	40.6	0.47	+0.10	3.5	20.3	2.00	—0.60	3.5	21.7	2.00
B. welchii "D"	1	—0.50	7.0	25.9	4.00	—0.80	7.0	40.6	0.78	+2.40	4.9	23.1	2.80	—0.50	7.0	26.6	4.00
	3	—0.50	10.5	34.8	6.00	—0.80	9.1	44.8	1.02	+2.40	4.9	23.1	2.80	—0.60	8.4	31.5	4.80
	6	—0.60	10.5	39.2	6.00	—0.60	11.9	56.0	1.33	+2.20	4.9	23.1	2.80	—0.60	9.8	34.3	5.60
	13	—0.60	13.3	39.2	7.60	—0.60	14.7	56.0	1.72	+2.00	4.9	23.1	2.80	—0.60	14.0	39.9	8.00
Control	..	—0.50	3.5	23.1	2.00	—0.90	4.2	40.6	0.47	+0.10	3.5	20.3	2.00	—0.60	3.5	21.7	2.00
B. welchii "E"	1	—0.50	7.0	26.6	4.00	—0.80	6.3	43.4	0.69	+2.30	4.2	22.4	2.40	—0.50	6.3	27.3	3.60
	3	—0.60	10.5	37.1	6.00	—0.80	14.0	48.3	1.56	+2.20	4.2	22.4	2.40	—0.60	10.5	37.1	6.00
	6	—0.60	10.5	37.1	6.00	—0.70	14.0	53.2	1.56	+2.40	4.2	22.4	2.40	—0.60	7.7	29.4	4.40
	13	—0.60	13.3	39.2	7.61	—0.70	19.6	56.7	2.19	+2.20	4.2	22.4	2.40	—0.60	13.3	42.0	7.61

	Day	Glycerol: Reaction	Glycerol: Ammonia Nitrogen	Glycerol: Amino Nitrogen	Glycerol: Percentage Ammonia to Total Nitrogen	Lactose: Reaction	Lactose: Ammonia Nitrogen	Lactose: Amino Nitrogen	Lactose: Percentage Ammonia to Total Nitrogen	Saccharose: Reaction	Saccharose: Ammonia Nitrogen	Saccharose: Amino Nitrogen	Saccharose: Percentage Ammonia to Total Nitrogen	Starch: Reaction	Starch: Ammonia Nitrogen	Starch: Amino Nitrogen	Starch: Percentage Ammonia to Total Nitrogen	Milk: Reaction	Milk: Ammonia Nitrogen	Milk: Amino Nitrogen	Milk: Percentage Ammonia to Total Nitrogen
Control	..	—0.60	3.5	23.1	2.00	—0.60	3.5	23.1	2.00	—0.60	3.5	23.1	2.00	—0.60	3.5	23.1	2.00	+1.29	7.0	21.0	1.41
B. welchii "A"	1	+1.80	10.5	23.1	6.00	+2.30	4.2	27.3	2.40	+2.20	4.9	25.2	2.80	+2.80	10.5	31.5	6.00	+3.60	11.2	11.2	2.25
	3	+1.60	10.5	23.1	6.00	+2.40	4.9	27.3	2.80	+2.40	4.9	25.2	2.80	+2.80	10.5	31.5	6.00	+3.80	11.2	11.9	2.25
	6	+1.70	10.5	23.1	6.00	+2.00	5.6	28.0	3.20	+2.20	5.6	25.2	3.20	+2.60	11.2	32.2	6.40	+4.20	11.2	14.0	2.25
	13	+1.40	9.8	24.5	5.60	+2.20	5.6	28.0	3.20	+2.10	5.6	25.2	3.20	+2.50	11.2	32.2	6.40	+4.00	11.9	14.7	2.40
	20	+1.30	11.2	26.6	6.60	+1.80	5.6	30.1	3.20	+1.80	4.9	28.7	2.80	+2.50	11.9	32.2	6.80	+3.90	12.6	18.2	2.54
Control	..	—0.50	2.8	22.4	1.54	—0.50	2.8	22.4	1.54	—0.40	2.8	22.4	1.54	—0.40	2.8	22.4	1.54	+1.40	2.8	22.4	0.59
B. welchii "B"	1	+1.40	7.0	23.1	3.88	+2.80	1.4	26.6	0.77	+2.80	1.4	28.0	0.77	+2.60	9.1	26.6	5.00	+3.60	4.2	19.6	0.88
	3	+1.70	7.7	24.5	4.23	+2.00	2.8	26.6	1.54	+2.40	2.1	32.2	1.15	+2.60	9.1	26.6	5.00	+4.50	7.0	29.4	1.47
	6	+1.60	7.7	25.9	4.23	+2.00	3.5	28.7	1.92	+2.10	2.1	39.2	1.15	+2.60	9.1	26.6	5.00	+4.90	8.4	33.6	1.71
	13	+1.50	8.4	28.0	4.61	+2.00	4.2	28.7	2.32	+2.00	2.8	42.7	1.54	+2.60	9.8	29.4	5.38	+4.50	9.8	36.4	2.03
Control	..	—0.70	3.5	23.1	1.79	—0.50	4.2	21.0	2.14	—0.60	4.2	22.4	2.14	—0.70	2.8	22.4	1.42	+1.40	4.2	22.4	0.91
B. welchii "C"	1	+0.70	7.7	25.2	3.93	+3.00	4.9	30.1	2.50	+2.80	4.2	29.4	2.14	+2.20	8.4	30.1	4.28	+2.20	3.5	16.1	0.76
	3	+0.70	8.4	25.9	4.28	+2.80	4.9	30.1	2.50	+3.00	4.2	29.4	2.14	+2.20	9.8	29.4	5.00	+4.40	4.9	16.1	1.06
	6	+0.60	8.4	25.9	4.28	+2.20	5.6	42.2	2.80	+3.00	4.9	31.5	2.50	+2.00	9.1	30.8	4.64	+4.90	5.6	15.4	1.21
	13	+0.60	8.4	25.9	4.28	+2.10	5.6	32.2	2.86	+2.20	5.6	32.2	2.86	+2.00	8.4	33.6	4.28	+4.90	5.6	15.4	1.21
Control	..	—0.50	2.8	22.4	1.60	—0.50	3.5	21.7	2.00	—0.50	3.5	21.7	2.00	—0.50	2.8	22.4	1.60	+1.40	4.2	21.0	0.86
B. welchii "D"	1	+0.50	7.0	23.8	4.00	+2.40	4.9	28.0	2.80	+2.50	4.2	27.3	2.40	+2.80	7.7	30.1	4.40	+3.20	3.5	12.6	0.72
	3	+1.00	7.0	25.9	4.00	+2.00	5.6	29.4	3.20	+2.60	4.2	27.3	2.40	+3.00	7.7	30.8	4.40	+3.30	4.2	16.8	0.85
	6	+0.70	8.4	28.0	4.80	+1.80	5.6	32.2	3.20	+2.00	4.2	27.3	2.40	+2.60	7.7	30.8	4.40	+3.40	4.2	19.6	0.86
	13	+0.60	8.4	26.6	4.80	+1.60	5.6	30.8	3.20	+2.00	4.9	29.4	2.80	+2.20	7.7	32.2	4.40	+3.60	4.9	21.7	1.00
Control	..	—0.50	2.8	22.4	1.60	—0.50	3.5	21.7	2.00	—0.50	3.5	21.7	2.00	—0.50	2.8	22.4	1.60	+1.40	4.2	21.0	0.87
B. welchii "E"	1	+0.60	7.0	25.9	4.0	+1.80	4.2	24.5	2.40	+2.20	4.2	25.2	2.40	+2.20	7.0	28.0	4.00	+3.70	6.3	10.5	1.30
	3	+1.00	7.0	28.0	4.0	+1.90	4.2	26.6	2.40	+2.00	4.2	25.9	2.40	+2,10	7.0	29.4	4.00	+4.00	6.3	13.3	1.30
	6	+0.90	7.0	28.0	4.0	+1.80	4.2	26.6	2.40	+2.00	4.2	25.2	2.40	+2.20	7.7	29.4	4.40	+4.20	7.0	14.0	1.44
	13	+0.80	7.7	28.0	4.40	+1.70	4.2	28.0	2.40	+1.90	4.2	25.2	2.40	+2.20	8.4	30.1	4.80	+4.00	7.0	11.2	1.44

Control	..	—0.60	3.5	23.1	1.79	—0.50	3.5	39.9	0.40	—0.20	3.5	18.9	1.79
B. welchii "F"	1	—0.70	9.1	32.2	4.64	—0.60	3.5	41.3	0.40	+2.50	4.2	25.2	2.15
	3	—0.70	10.5	35.7	5.36	—0.60	7.0	49.0	0.80	+2.40	4.2	25.2	2.15
	6	—0.80	11.2	39.2	5.71	—0.40	9.8	53.7	1.10	+2.30	4.2	25.2	2.15
	13	—0.80	14.0	49.7	7.14	—0.20	13.3	58.8	1.49	+2.20	4.2	25.2	2.15
	20	—0.70	14.7	49.7	7.50	—0.10	14.7	65.1	1.66	+2.40	4.9	25.9	2.51
Control	..	—0.60	4.2	21.0	2.14	—0.90	14.2	43.4	0.48	—0.20	4.2	21.0	2.14
B. welchii "G"	1	—0.80	8.4	32.2	4.28	—1.10	8.4	42.0	0.95	+2.60	5.6	22.4	2.96
	3	—0.80	11.9	46.9	6.08	—1.20	10.5	51.1	1.19	+2.80	5.6	24.5	2.96
	6	—0.90	11.9	52.5	6.08	—1.20	10.5	56.7	1.19	+2.80	5.6	25.2	2.96
	13	—0.80	11.9	52.5	6.08	—1.30	15.4	66.5	1.75	+2.60	5.6	25.2	2.96
Control	..	—0.60	4.2	21.0	2.14	—0.90	4.2	43.4	0.48	—0.20	4.2	21.0	2.14
B. welchii "H"	1	—0.80	8.4	28.0	4.28	—1.00	8.4	42.0	0.95	+2.50	5.6	23.8	2.86
	3	—.080	11.2	40.6	5.72	—1.00	10.5	51.1	1.15	+3.00	5.6	23.8	2.86
	6	—0.80	11.9	49.7	6.08	—0.90	10.5	56.7	1.15	+2.80	5.6	23.8	2.86
	13	—0.70	13.3	58.1	6.79	—0.80	15.4	66.5	1.74	+2.60	5.6	23.8	2.86
Control	..	—0.60	17.5	20.3	7.81	—0.70	4.2	36.4	0.15	—0.60	19.6	21.7	8.74
B. welchii "I"	1	—0.90	28.7	29.4	12.80	—0.80	5.6	36.4	0.21	+4.00	24.5	30.8	10.90
	3	—0.80	34.3	31.5	15.30	—1.00	5.6	36.4	0.21	+4.00	25.2	30.8	11.25
	6	—0.80	33.6	36.4	14.90	—0.80	16.1	41.3	1.92	+4.20	25.2	35.7	11.25
	9	—0.90	35.0	41.3	15.68	—0.80	13.3	47.6	1.50	+4.30	25.9	32.9	11.55
	14	—1.00	36.4	46.9	16.20	—0.60	14.0	47.6	1.61	+3.80	25.9	33.6	11.55
Control	..	—0.50	3.5	23.1	1.85	—0.80	4.9	44.1	0.54	—0.20	3.5	21.7	1.85
B. welchii "J"	1	—0.60	9.8	32.9	5.18	—0.60	4.9	47.6	0.54	+2.40	5.6	25.2	2.96
	3	—0.60	10.5	39.2	5.55	—0.70	9.1	51.8	1.01	+2.30	4.9	25.9	2.59
	6	—0.70	11.2	46.7	5.94	—0.60	12.6	60.2	1.39	+2.50	4.9	25.9	2.59
	13	—0.70	14.7	58.8	7.78	—0.70	16.1	77.0	1.79	+2.30	4.9	25.9	2.59
	21	—0.70	14.0	58.1	7.41	—0.70	16.1	77.7	1.79	+2.00	7.7	30.1	4.07
Control	..	—0.50	3.5	23.1	1.98	—0.90	4.2	40.6	0.47	+0.10	3.5	20.3	1.98
B. welchii "K"	1	—0.50	7.7	29.4	4.40	—0.80	4.2	42.0	0.47	+2.50	4.9	23.1	2.78
	3	—0.60	10.5	32.2	6.00	—0.90	6.3	44.1	0.70	+2.20	4.9	23.1	2.78
	6	—.070	12.6	44.1	7.20	—0.90	11.9	53.2	1.33	+2.20	4.9	24.5	2.78
	13	—0.70	13.3	46.9	7.60	—1.00	14.7	65.8	1.64	+2.00	4.9	24.5	2.78
Control	..	—0.60	4.2	21.0	2.14	—0.90	4.2	43.4	0.48	—0.20	4.2	21.0	2.14
B. welchii "L"	1	—0.60	9.1	34.3	4.65	—0.90	4.9	46.2	0.56	+2.60	4.9	23.1	2.50
	3	—0.80	12.6	46.2	6.43	—0.70	9.8	49.0	1.11	+2.70	4.9	23.1	2.50
	6	—0.80	15.4	56.0	7.86	—0.60	13.3	54.6	1.51	+2.30	5.6	25.2	2.86
	13	—0.70	13.3	53 9	6.78	—0.80	16.1	67.2	1.83	+2.20	5.6	25.2	2.86

Control	..	—0.60	3.5	21.7	1.79	—0.40	2.8	22.4	1.44	—0.50	3.5	21.7	1.79
B. welchii "F"	1	—0.70	8.4	28.0	4.29	+0.20	4.2	22.4	2.14	+1.90	5:6	28.0	2.86
	3	—0.70	10.5	35.0	5.36	+0.20	4.9	25.2	2.50	+1.90	5.6	28.0	2.86
	6	—0.70	10.5	39.9	5.36	+0.20	4.9	24.5	2.50	+1.60	5.6	28.0	2.86
	13	—0.80	12.6	46.2	6.42	+0.30	4.9	25.2	2.50	+1.70	7.0	29.4	3.60
	20	—0.70	10.5	41.3	5.36	+0.30	4.9	28.0	2.50	+1.80	7.0	30.8	3.60
Control	..	—0.70	3.5	23.1	1.79	—0.70	3.5	23.1	1.79	—0.50	4.2	21.0	2.14
B. welchii "G"	1	—0.90	8.4	30.8	4.28	+0.10	7.7	25.9	3.93	+2.50	6.3	30.1	3.22
	3	—0.90	10.5	33.6	5.36	+0.20	9.1	32.3	4.64	+3.40	7.7	32.2	3.93
	6	—0.90	11.2	40.6	5.72	+0.50	10.5	37.1	5.36	+2.70	7.7	32.9	3.93
	13	—1.00	11.9	53.2	6.08	+0.30	9.8	37.8	5.00	+2.40	7.7	32.9	3.93
Control	..	—0.70	3.5	23.1	1.78	—0.70	3.5	23.1	1.78	—0.50	4.2	21.0	2.14
B. welchii "H"	1	—0.90	8.4	24.5	4.28	+1.00	7.7	23.8	3.93	+2.20	7.0	33.6	3.57
	3	—0.90	9.8	41.3	4.99	+0.90	7.7	25.2	3.93	+2.90	7.0	35.0	3.57
	6	—0.90	10.5	43.4	5.46	......	....	....	.....	+2.70	7.0	35.0	3.57
	13	—1.00	13.3	56.0	6.74	+1.10	7.7	28.7	3.93	+2.60	7.0	35.0	3.57
Control	..	—0.70	18.2	21.0	8.12	—0.60	18.9	21.7	8.46	—0.60	18.9	21.0	8.46
B. welchii "I"	1	—0.90	30.1	25.9	13.40	+1.40	28.7	26.6	12.70	+3.50	24.5	28.0	10.90
	3	—0.90	33.6	37.8	15.00	+1.60	30.8	26.6	13.75	+3.80	26.6	32.2	11.90
	6	—1.00	35.0	37.8	15.60	+2.30	32.2	30.8	14.35	+4.00	28.0	35.0	12.50
	9	—1.10	36.4	41.3	16.20	+2.20	32.2	31.5	14.35	+3.90	25.9	35.7	11.57
	14	—1.00	36.4	45.5	16.20	+2.00	31.5	32.9	14.10	+3.80	25.9	35.7	11.57
Control	..	—0.40	3.5	23.1	1.85	—0.40	3.5	23.1	1.85	—0.40	3.5	23.1	1.85
B. welchii "J"	1	—0.60	10.5	30.1	5.55	+1.60	7.0	27.3	3.70	+2.00	5.6	30.8	2.96
	3	—0.60	10.5	35.7	5.55	+1.70	7.0	27.3	3.70	+2.00	5.6	29.4	2.96
	6	—0.40	10.5	47.6	5.55	+1.40	7.0	27.3	3.70	+2.10	5.6	32.9	2.96
	13	—0.70	14.0	47.6	7.41	+1.20	7.7	28.0	4.07	+2.20	8.4	34.3	4.44
	21	......	....	....	.....	+1.30	7.7	28.0	4.07	+2.20	7.7	32.9	4.07
Control	..	—0.60	3.5	21.7	1.98	—0.50	2.8	22.4	1.60	—0.50	3.5	21.7	1.98
B. welchii "K"	1	—0.80	7.7	28.0	4.40	+1.00	7.7	25.9	4.40	+2.20	7.0	31.5	4.00
	3	—0.80	10:5	37.8	6.00	+1.10	7.7	25.9	4.40	+2.20	7.0	30.8	4.00
	6	—0.70	10.5	36.4	6.00	+1.10	8.4	27.3	4.80	+2.10	7.0	32.2	4.00
	13	—0.70	11.9	44.8	6.80	+1.10	9.8	26.6	5.60	+2.00	7.0	32.2	4.00
Control	..	—0.70	3.5	23.1	1.78	—0.70	3.5	23.1	1.78	—0.50	4.2	21.0	2.14
B. welchii "L"	1	—0.70	8.4	30.1	4.28	+1.00	7.7	28.0	3.93	+2.10	4.2	37.6	2.14
	3	—0.70	11.2	30.1	5.72	+1.00	7.7	28.0	3.93	+3.00	7.7	30.1	3.93
	6	—0.90	12.6	51.1	6.43	+1.10	8.4	30.1	4.28	+2.90	8.4	36.4	4.28
	13	—0.90	12.6	51.1	6.43	+1.00	9.8	32.9	5.00	+2.40	7.7	37.1	3.93

Control	..	—0.60	3.5	21.7	1.79	—0.60	3.5	21.7	1.44	+1.20	4.9	22.4	1.06
B. welchii "F"	1	+2.70	5.6	30.8	2.86	+1.10	9.1	36.4	4.64	+3.20	7.7	13.3	1.66
	3	+2.70	5.6	30.8	2.86	+1.10	9.8	37.8	5.00	+2.70	8.4	12.6	1.82
	6	+2.00	5.6	30.8	2.86	+2.30	10.5	37.1	5.36	+3.20	9.8	20.3	2.12
	13	+2.00	7.0	30.8	3.60	+2.00	13.3	39.9	6.86	+3.20	11.9	21.7	2.57
	20	+2.00	7.0	32.9	3.60	+2.10	14.7	42.7	7.50	+3.60	12.6	28.0	2.33
Control	..	—0.60	4.2	22.4	2.14	—0.70	2.8	22.4	1.43	+1.40	4.2	22.4	0.91
B. welchii "G"	1	+3.10	7.0	20.5	3.57	+1.20	9.8	26.6	5.00	+3.00	7.0	21.7	1.52
	3	+3.10	6.3	28.7	3.22	+2.90	10.5	39.9	5.36	+3.60	7.7	28.7	1.67
	6	+3.20	6.3	29.4	3.22	+3.90	11.9	39.2	6.08	+3.50	8.4	37.1	1.84
	13	+3.20	6.3	29.4	3.22	+3.20	11.9	39.2	6.08	+3.70	7.7	37.1	1.67
Control	..	—0.60	4.2	22.4	2.14	—0.70	2.8	22.4	1.43	+1.40	4.2	22.4	0.91
B. welchii "H"	1	+3.70	4.2	30.8	2.16	+1.20	9.8	26.6	4.99	+1.60	7.0	31.5	1.52
	3	+3.40	6.3	30.1	3.23	+2.90	10.5	39.9	5.36	+1.80	7.7	31.5	1.67
	6	+3.50	6.3	31.5	3.23	+3.90	11.9	35.7	6.07	+2.10	8.4	33.6	1.82
	13	+3.10	6.3	33.1	3.23	+3.20	11.9	35.7	6.07	+2.30	8.4	33.6	1.82
Control	..	—0.60	18.2	21.0	8.12	—0.50	18.2	21.7	8.12	+1.30	3.5	20.3	.....
B. welchii "I"	1	+4.30	22.4	26.6	10.00	+5.30	28.7	31.5	12.80	+2.30	6.3	19.6	1.36
	3	+4.20	24.5	30.1	10.90	+5.50	28.0	31.5	12.50	+2.80	9.1	37.8	1.97
	6	+4.50	25.9	32.9	11.55	+5.50	28.7	34.3	12.80	+3.30	9.1	39.2	1.97
	9	+4.60	25.9	32.9	11.55	+5.40	28.0	35.0	12.50	+4.20	9.1	39.2	1.97
	14	+4.50	25.9	32.9	11.55	+5.10	28.7	35.0	12.80	+4.00	9.1	39.2	1.97
Control	..	—0.50	3.5	23.1	1.85	—0.40	3.5	23.1	1.85	+1.40	7.7	23.1	1.47
B. welchii "J"	1	+2.60	4.9	28.7	2.59	+2.40	7.7	29.4	4.07	+2.20	9.1	21.0	1.87
	3	+2.70	4.9	28.7	2.59	+2.80	7.7	29.4	4.07	+2.20	8.4	31.5	1.60
	6	+2.60	4.9	28.7	2.59	+2.80	7.7	30.8	4.07	+2.80	9.8	37.1	1.87
	13	+2.00	4.9	28.7	2.59	+2.70	7.7	30.8	4.07	+2.90	14.7	53.2	2.80
	21	+2.00	5.6	30.1	2.96	......	....	....	.....	+3.00	14.7	53.2	2.80
Control	..	—0.50	3.5	21.7	1.98	—0.50	2.8	22.4	1.60	+1.40	4.2	21.0	0.86
B. welchii "K"	1	+2.60	7.0	28.7	4.00	+2.80	7.7	30.8	4.40	+3.60	7.0	18.2	1.43
	3	+2.70	7.0	28.7	4.00	+2.80	8.4	30.8	4.80	+4.00	6.3	23.1	1.29
	6	+2.70	7.0	30.8	4.00	+2.60	8.4	32.2	4.80	+4.20	7.0	29.4	1.43
	13	+2.70	7.0	31.5	4.00	+2.60	8.4	32.2	4.80	+4.40	8.4	32.2	1.71
Control	..	—0.60	4.2	22.4	2.14	—0.70	2.8	22.4	1.43	+1.40	4.2	22.4	0.91
B. welchii "L"	1	+2.50	6.3	34.3	3.21	+2.60	9.1	32.9	4.64	+3.30	5.6	21.0	1.21
	3	+2.90	7.0	33.6	3.57	+2.80	9.1	32.9	4.64	+3.50	8.4	25.2	1.82
	6	+2.80	7.0	33.6	3.57	+2.80	9.1	32.9	4.64	+4.30	11.9	38.5	2.58
	13	+2.80	7.0	33.6	3.57	+2.60	9.1	34.3	4.64	+4.50	12.6	39.2	2.73

Reaction: — = alkaline to neutral red; + = acid to neutral red; c c normal acid or alkali per 100 c c of medium.
Ammonia and amino nitrogen expressed in milligrams per 100 c c of culture medium.
Control indicates initial composition of medium. Net results may be obtained by subtracting the control from the day's analysis.
Amino nitrogen is corrected in each instance for ammonia.

various groups, and it is confidently expected that the anaerobic bacilli may exhibit more or less characteristic metabolic curves which may be found eventually to possess value in their differentiation.

An important question arises: Will anaerobic bacteria under parallel laboratory conditions produce from year to year metabolic growth curves which are qualitatively and, within reasonable limits, quantitatively alike? It appears to be a fact that aerobic bacteria will react thus.[22] A study of the metabolism of culture 617 D, for the years 1917, 1918, and 1920 (see table 1) reveals the fact that this strain reacted in a very satisfactory manner. The curves are strikingly similar both with respect to daily transformations and cumulative nitrogenous changes in the mediums. It must be admitted that annual studies were not made of the remaining organisms identified as the Welch bacillus;[23] on the other hand, the general features were faithfully reproduced by each strain, and the general impression is that a single chemical type of organism is under consideration.[24]

Origin of Cultures.—Dr. Simonds isolated 617 D from an infected gunshot wound sustained by a Belgian soldier. It was used by Bull [15] for the production of the soluble toxin characteristic of the Welch bacillus. This culture may be regarded as the type organism of the Welch bacillus group.

Culture A was obtained from the National Research Council. The history is unknown except that the organism was isolated from a case of gas gangrene.

Culture B was isolated from an infected wound by Simonds.

Culture C was isolated from the feces of a dog.

Culture D was obtained from the National Research Council. Its origin is similar to that of culture A.

Culture E was obtained from laboratory dust.

Culture F was obtained from an infected tonsil.

Culture G was isolated from a case of gas gangrene, by Simonds.

Culture H was obtained from the feces of a horse.

Culture I was isolated from a gunshot wound.

Culture J was obtained from a case of "gas bacillus diarrhea."

Culture K was from a fatal case of emphysematous gas gangrene.

Culture L was obtained from Dr. Karl Meyer.

[22] Kendall, Day and Walker: Ibid., 1913, 13, p. 425.

[23] Simonds' criteria (footnote 1) were followed as a standard.

[24] In subsequent publications, the chemical identity of the Welch bacillus will be contrasted with that of other anaerobic bacilli.

DISCUSSION

All the cultures agree in the following cultural characteristics:[25] Gas and acid are produced in glucose, lactose, saccharose, glycerol and starch. Those cultures which were inoculated into maltose fermented it energetically. A stormy fermentation developed in milk. Gelatin was softened in every instance. The time required to bring about a chemical change of the gelatin protein of sufficient magnitude to prevent solidification when the medium was placed in the icebox for several hours varied from 2-13 days. As a general rule, the softening was distinct by the end of the third day of incubation, and it is of interest to find that the amino nitrogen content of the medium at the time of complete fluidification is increased only slightly above that of the uninoculated controls in each culture studied.

It would appear that the softening of the gelatin medium, referred to by Welch and Nuttall,[2] and noticed by many investigators, is plausibly associated with a change in the gelatin protein whereby it becomes so changed chemically that the physical property of solidification no longer takes place, but as the titratable acidity does not change materially, no definite conclusions can be drawn at this time of the significance of the phenomenon. It was not possible, however, to demonstrate the presence of a soluble gelatinase.[26] This is in sharp contrast to the parallel cultures of Bacillus sporogenes.

The ammonia formation (deamination) is greater in mediums containing protein and protein derivatives alone than in those containing both protein and utilizable carbohydrate. In this respect, the amino nitrogen and the ammonia nitrogen show a striking parallelism. As the ammonia appears to be a waste product, indicative of the intracellular utilization of protein,[27] by bacteria, it is not surprising to find that the "sparing action of utilizable carbohydrate for protein" is thus clearly indicated by the distinctly lesser formation of ammonia in those cultures containing utilizable carbohydrate.

The toxicity of the cultures studied was found to decrease rapidly after the first 24 hours of growth; this may possibly stand in relation to the gradual change in the protein molecule, but it is rather more probable that the soluble poison is associated with the period of great

[25] The characters referred to are those induced in mediums on which metabolism studies were made. Complete fermentation reactions will be recorded later.

[26] Bacillus sporogenes and other proteolytic anaerobes produce soluble proteolytic enzymes. These will be discussed in a later communication.

[27] Kendall and Walker: Jour. Infect. Dis., 1915, 17, p. 442.

numerical increase of the bacteria, and therefore "a growth product" rather than an "energy product," which would appear of course cumulatively as the culture grows older.

A noteworthy change in titratable acidity takes place in those mediums containing utilizable carbohydrates; the reaction increases markedly in acidity, even during the first 24 hours' growth. In many instances the maximum acidity is reached, or nearly reached, before the end of the third day, at which time the next series of determinations were made. This is in harmony with the almost explosive violence of the fermentation incited during the initial period of growth. The change of reaction in mediums containing no utilizable carbohydrate is little indeed, even in gelatin, in which a distinct but moderate action on protein (as shown by the formol titration) is indicated. Growth languishes in purely protein mediums although those rich in protein, and especially highly organized protein, are more favorable to development than those containing only protein derivatives, as meat extractives and peptones. Bacillus welchii, therefore, is not a proteophilic organism, and its characteristic activity is on utilizable carbohydrate.

Spores were always found in mediums containing no utilizable carbohydrate; they were never discovered in mediums in which active fermentation had taken place.

The organisms of the Welch group studied in this series produced the typical "stormy fermentation" in milk. The reaction is typically almost explosive in its violence. This phenomenon, due to a rapid decomposition of the lactose with the liberation of gas, and the formation of acid, takes place within the first 24 hours' incubation.[28] A large proportion of the milk sugar is transformed into nonfermentable products by this initial period of rapid development and reactivity. Subsequent development is slow and little additional change, aside from a slight increase in acidity, is demonstrable. The casein is rendered insoluble, owing in part at least to the accumulation of acid products of fermentation, and the insoluble mass is riddled with holes, presumably caused by the liberation of gas as the lactose enclosed in the coagulum is decomposed by the organism. The casein coagulum appears small in amount, suggesting at first sight that an actual

[28] If the milk is not freed from oxygen before inoculation, it not infrequently happens that the casein is coagulated while but little or no visible gas is formed. Simonds (footnote 1) was apparently the first observer to call attention to this peculiar behavior under such conditions.

proteolysis has taken place. A consideration of the nitrogenous changes induced in the medium, however, renders this explanation unlikely. The amino nitrogen decreases materially during the first day of incubation, and although the amount of amino acid may subsequently increase to a point above that of the uninoculated controls, it never reaches an amount indicative of a degree of proteolysis sufficient to account for more than minimal amounts of decomposition of casein. It might be assumed, of course, that the gas bacilli utilized the products of degradation of the protein constituents of the milk, thus masking the chemical evidence of digestion; the very small amount of ammonia formed during the process is distinctly against this possibility, and, in addition, the mediums containing no utilizable carbohydrate (plain broth and gelatin) do not exhibit reactions indicative of more than minimal attack upon proteins. It would appear, therefore, that the gas bacillus is an organism characterized by minimal proteolytic powers, but possessed of unusually vigorous fermentative powers.

Available evidence indicates that alcohols of the hexose series, sorbitol, mannitol, and dulcitol, are not attacked by B. welchii.[1, 5] The hexose sugars, glucose, fructose, mannose and galactose, on the contrary, appear to be energetically attacked. This would suggest that the aldose configuration—CHO,—but not the alcohol configuration—CH_2OH—affords a point of attachment, permitting the endo enzymes of the organism to decompose the aldose molecules, but not the corresponding alcohols. Sucrose, which possesses no free aldehyde grouping, is readily fermented, however, but the possibility or even probability of a preliminary hydrolysis of the sucrose molecule to glucose and fructose must be borne in mind in this instance. Many strains ferment glycerol, a triatomic alcohol, without difficulty; hence, judgment must be withheld concerning the relations between aldehyde and alcohol groupings in determining utilizability of the hexoses until much more detailed studies on complete series of hexose sugars and their derivatives can be made. For the present, however, the nonfermentability of the alcohols derived from the more commonly available hexoses is a point of distinction in the cultural reactions of the gas bacillus.

SUMMARY

B. welchii represents a type of widely distributed and closely related anaerobic bacilli which exhibit in common the ability to induce a vigorous fermentation of the commonly used carbohydrates. The alcohols of the hexose sugars are, so far as known, not utilizable as sources of energy by the members of the gas bacillus group. Glycerol is attacked by many strains. Growth is relatively feeble in nonsaccharine mediums. Gelatin, which is a better substrate than plain broth for the development of the organism in the absence of utilizable carbohydrates, is so altered by the microbes that it will no longer solidify. This softening is not due to the action of a soluble proteolytic enzyme, as is the case with B. sporogenes and other strongly proteolytic anaerobes. The nitrogenous changes in the medium measurable by available methods are of insufficient magnitude to afford a clear-cut, satisfactory explanation of the phenomenon on the basis of nitrogenous decomposition. Little free ammonia is formed, indicating little endogenous utilization of protein. There is a distinct, although moderate, increase of amino nitrogen in the gelatin medium incidental to growth, however, and it is by no means impossible that this amino nitrogen increase, representing the resultant of protein cleavage by the organisms and the unused residue of this cleavage, may be so related to the gelatin molecule that the latter no longer possesses the chemical and physical properties necessary to exhibit the characteristic ability to solidify on cooling. The change in titratable acidity, it should be remarked, is small indeed in purely protein mediums.

The sparing action of utilizable carbohydrates for protein is clearly indicated in the analytic tables.

The most characteristic reaction of the gas bacillus group is in milk. The "stormy fermentation," the slightly pink color of the casein coagulum, the riddled appearance of the latter, and the distinct odor of butyric acid are the significant features. No other group of anaerobic bacteria, so far described, exhibits this cultural complex in its entirety. It may be stated that mixed cultures of bacteria inoculated into milk which has been freed from oxygen and heated to 80 C. for 20 minutes prior to incubation, which exhibit the characteristic stormy fermentation within 18 hours, contain members of the B. welchii group. Material from infected tissues does not, except under unusual conditions, contain gas bacillus spores. Hence, the heating to 80 C. must be dispensed with to obtain results with the milk test. In doubtful cases, the Welch-Nuttall rabbit test [2] will almost always yield a positive result. Subcultures from the liver [29] of such animal will furnish active subcultures although not necessarily in a state of purity.

[29] Kendall and Smith: Boston Med. & Surg. Jour., 1910, 158, p. 578; Arch. Pediatrics, 1911, 28, p. 389.

VIBRION SEPTIQUE

STUDY XLV

The first organism belonging to the group of anaerobic bacteria was isolated by Pasteur [1] and described by him under the designation Vibrion septique. A few years later Koch [2] isolated an anaerobic bacillus from garden soil which, on injection into experimental animals, gave rise to marked edema at and near the site of inoculation. Koch pointed out some relatively minor pathologic differences exhibited by his organism in contrast to Vibrion septique, and named it the bacillus of malignant edema; in bacteriologic terminology, Bacillus oedematis maligni. The latter name has supplanted largely the original term Vibrion septique, but the reasons for so doing do not appear to be convincing. From the standpoint of terminology, neither name is correct. Also, these original studies were made under conditions which make it almost certain that pure cultures were unattainable. In spite of these cultural difficulties, however, the characteristics of the organism, and more particularly the nature of the lesions induced in laboratory animals, are of sufficient definiteness to furnish a satisfactory means of comparison of existing strains with those of Pasteur and Koch. There appears to be unequivocal evidence that Vibrion septique and B. oedematis maligni are to be regarded as identical, and also that the same organism is identifiable among current strains.

The name Vibrion septique is preferable, therefore, to B. oedematis maligni, pending the time when bacteriologic etymologists shall confer a final and correct designation on the microbe. Its use recalls the genius of Pasteur who added to the phenomena of living things the conception of anaerobic existence.

Descriptions of Vibrion septique differ markedly. The earlier observers ascribed proteolytic powers of considerable magnitude to the organism, and even at the present time there is confusion on this point. The most carefully controlled work on this organism, however, by Miss Robertson, Meyer, and others has failed to demonstrate any evidence of significant action on protein.[3] On the contrary, carbohydrates are energetically decomposed.

[1] Pasteur and Joubert: Bull. de l'Acad. méd., 1877, 6, p. 781.

[2] Mitt. a. d. kais. Gesundheitsamte, 1881, 1, p. 48.

[3] See Weinberg and Séguin: La Gangrène Gazeuse, Paris, 1917. Medical Research Committee, Report No. 39, London, 1919, contains literature on the subject.

Vibrion septique became conspicuous during the last half decade as the second most important incitant of fulminating gas gangrene. It is chiefly due to the activities of the organism as a dangerous contaminant of wounds of warfare, and of contused wounds in general, that so much study has been expended on it in recent years. The morphologic, cultural and serologic peculiarities have been thoroughly examined[4] and the nature of the poison has received much attention.[3, 5] The biochemistry, however, in connection with that of other anaerobic bacteria, has not been the subject of study, with the exception of the observations of Wolf.[6] Wolf's studies, in essence, emphasize the following peculiarities of the chemistry of Vibrion septique.

1. The organism produces a brilliant red coloration in the cooked meat medium. This is to be contrasted with a paler pink color produced by several anaerobes grown in protein-carbohydrate mediums, as for example, milk.[7]

2. The fermentation reactions of Vibrion septique show points of resemblance to those of B. welchii, especially with reference to intensity. The associated nitrogenous changes, however, are quantitatively different, Vibrion septique producing somewhat less gas than B. welchii, and also the amount of ammonia accumulating in cultures being less. The amino nitrogen, on the contrary, is relatively greater under approximately parallel conditions.

3. Vibrion septique produces much gas in milk. The total volume may exceed the amount of fermented medium 2.5 times. The rate of evolution of the gas, however, is much slower than that of the Welch bacillus.

4. Vibrion septique is carbohydrophilic rather than proteophilic; in this respect it resembles the Welch bacillus very closely. Wolf's experiments disclose the sparing action of utilizable carbohydrate for protein in cultures of the organism containing sugars.

The soluble poison of Vibrion septique, like that of B. welchii, appears to be associated with the growth of the organism rather than with the period when the products of metabolism are at their maximum. Indeed, after the first day of growth the potency of the poison, like that of the Welch bacillus, decreases rapidly. The nature of the soluble

4 Miss Robertson: British Med. Jour., 1918, I, p. 583. Henry: Jour. Path. & Bacteriol., 1916-1917, 21, p. 344. Meyer: Jour. Infect. Dis., 1915, 17, p. 458.

5 Miss Robertson: Jour. Path. & Bacteriol., 1920, 23, p. 153.

6 Ibid., 1918, 22, p. 115.

7 Simonds: Monograph 5, Rockefeller Institute, 1915, p. 40.

poison is wholly unknown, but it appears that specific serums, containing substances capable of neutralizing it, and therefore possessed of some curative value, have been prepared.[3, 5] As this poison, however, is maximal during the early hours of growth of the organism, there is nothing in the ordinary metabolic chemistry of Vibrion septique which would be of significance in elucidating its nature or potency. Admixture with other organisms appears to prevent the formation of specific antibodies for Vibrion septique,[5] and prolonged incubation definitely reduces the content of filtrates of cultures in poisonous substances. Filtrates of young cultures, on the contrary, are relatively stabile with reference to their poisonous properties. These facts suggest not only that the poisonous principle is formed during the period of rapid multiplication of the organisms, and therefore a labile substance formed as a waste product incidental to the transformation of protein (or protein derivatives) for structural purposes rather than a product of the metabolism of protein for energy. It also suggests that the further growth of Vibrion septique, or of contaminating bacteria, destroys the potency of the poisonous substance.

The cultural identification of Vib. septique presents some difficulty. The close resemblance of the organism to the Welch bacillus has undoubtedly led to confusion in the past, and even at the present time authorities are not in complete accord in the points of difference between these microbes.

It is claimed by many [8] that Vibrion septique fails to ferment saccharose, differing in this respect from the Welch bacillus and Bacillus fallax. On the other hand, there are several observers who have apparently found that saccharose is fermented. Of the eight cultures studied in the series presented below, a majority fermented saccharose with the formation of gas and acid, although the amount of gas evolved and the rate of evolution were distinctly slower than was the case with the more readily attacked carbohydrates, as glucose, lactose and maltose. Glycerol and starch were not fermented by any of the strains studied, and the evolution of gas in milk was much slower than that characteristic of cultures of the Welch bacillus. These appear to be points of difference between the two organisms which may possess more than academic value in their cultural recognition. It is by no means impossible, or even improbable, that the saccharose-ferment-

[8] Miss Robertson: British Med. Jour., 1918, I, p. 583. Achalme: Ann. Inst. Past., 1902, 16, p. 633. Distaso and Jungano, Les Anaérobies, 1910, p. 78. Medical Research Committee, Report 39, 1919, p. 23.

TABLE 1

Vibrion Septique

	Day	Plain				Gelatin				Glucose			
		Reaction	Ammonia Nitrogen	Amino Nitrogen	Percentage Ammonia to Total Nitrogen	Reaction	Ammonia Nitrogen	Amino Nitrogen	Percentage Ammonia to Total Nitrogen	Reaction	Ammonia Nitrogen	Amino Nitrogen	Percentage Ammonia to Total Nitrogen
Control	..	—0.60	11.2	21.0	5.33	—0.60	13.3	37.1	1.79	—0.50	18.2	23.8	8.67
V. septique, A	1	—1.00	14.0	19.6	6.67	—1.00	14.7	35.7	1.98	+3.60	22.4	22.4	10.66
	3	—1.00	17.5	20.3	8.43	—0.90	15.4	37.8	2.08	+3.80	23.1	23.1	11.00
	6	—0.80	18.2	22.4	8.67	—0.70	19.9	39.2	2.68	+4.40	25.9	23.8	12.33
	9	—0.70	18.9	22.4	9.14	—0.40	23.1	42.0	3.12	+4.40	25.9	25.9	12.33
	14	—0.70	18.9	24.5	9.14	—0.70	25.9	44.1	3.48	+4.40	25.9	25.9	12.33
Control	..	—.080	19.6	26.6	9.36	—0.60	13.3	37.1	1.79	—0.50	18.2	23.8	8.67
V. septique, B	1	—0.80	21.0	28.0	10.00	—0.80	16.6	38.5	2.17	+4.00	23.1	24.5	11.00
	3	—0.80	24.5	27.3	11.66	—0.70	18.9	39.9	2.55	+4.00	26.6	23.8	12.67
	6	—0.70	25.2	30.8	12.06	—0.50	22.4	39.2	3.08	+4.00	26.6	25.2	12.67
	9	—0.60	27.3	34.3	12.96	—0.50	22.4	39.2	3.08	+4.10	26.6	26.6	12.67
	15	—0.70	27.3	31.5	12.96	—0.20	23.1	39.9	3.12	+4.10	26.6	26.6	12.67
Control	..	—0.70	16.8	26.6	7.50	—0.70	14.0	42.0	1.92	—0.40	16.1	24.5	7.18
V. septique, C	1	—0.60	19.6	26.6	8.77	—0.50	19.6	40.6	2.69	+3.60	20.3	25.9	9.07
	3	—0.60	21.7	30.1	9.70	—0.50	23.8	42.0	3.25	+3.90	22.4	25.2	10.00
	4	—0.50	23.8	30.8	10.63	—0.40	23.8	43.4	3.25	+3.90	22.4	25.2	10.00
	9	—0.60	24.5	32.9	10.92	—0.40	23.8	46.2	3.25	+3.90	23.1	25.9	10.30
	14	—0.40	24.5	34.3	10.92	—0.40	24.5	49.0	3.37	+3.70	23.1	25.9	10.30

	Day	Mannitol				Glycerol				Lactose			
		Reaction	Ammonia Nitrogen	Amino Nitrogen	Percentage Ammonia to Total Nitrogen	Reaction	Ammonia Nitrogen	Amino Nitrogen	Percentage Ammonia to Total Nitrogen	Reaction	Ammonia Nitrogen	Amino Nitrogen	Percentage Ammonia to Total Nitrogen
Control	..	—0.80	18.2	26.6	8.67	—0.80	18.2	23.8	8.67	—0.50	18.2	25.2	8.67
V. septique, A	1	—0.80	19.6	26.6	9.28	—0.70	18.2	24.5	8.67	+2.50	21.7	27.3	10.33
	3	—1.00	23.8	28.0	11.33	—0.80	21.7	25.9	10.03	+3.10	25.2	26.6	12.06
	6	—1.00	25.2	31.5	12.06	—0.60	21.7	26.6	10.03	+4.10	24.5	26.6	11.66
	9	—1.00	27.3	33.6	12.96	—0.50	24.5	28.7	11.66	+3.90	24.5	27.3	11.66
	14	—0.90	28.0	33.6	13.33	—0.30	23.8	28.7	11.33	+4.00	25.2	27.3	12.06
Control	..	—0.80	18.2	26.6	8.67	—0.80	18.2	23.8	8.67	—0.50	18.2	23.8	8.67
V. septique, B	1	—0.90	22.4	28.0	10.66	—0.80	20.3	24.5	9.70	+2.90	20.3	27.3	9.70
	3	—0.90	23.8	30.8	11.33	—0.60	21.7	27.3	10.03	+2.90	21.0	25.9	10.00
	6	—0.90	25.2	32.2	12.06	—0.60	24.5	27.3	11.66	+2.90	21.7	25.9	10.33
	9	—0.70	25.9	32.9	12.33	—0.70	27.3	28.7	12.96	+3.10	24.5	27.3	11.66
	15	—0.50	28.0	33.6	13.33	—0.40	27.3	28.7	12.96	+3.20	24.5	28.0	11.66
Control	..	—0.60	16.8	26.6	7.50	—0.60	16.8	25.2	7.50	—0.50	16.8	25.2	7.50
V. septique, C	1	—0.60	21.0	26.6	9.38	—0.60	20.3	25.9	9.07	+3.00	21.7	23.1	9.70
	3	—0.60	23.1	25.9	10.30	—0.50	23.1	27.3	10.30	+3.00	23.1	25.2	10.30
	4	—0.60	23.8	26.6	10.63	—0.50	23.8	26.6	10.63	+3.20	23.1	26.6	10.30
	9	—0.70	23.8	28.7	10.63	—0.50	23.8	28.0	10.63	+2.80	23.1	26.6	10.30
	14	—0.70	24.5	28.7	10.92	—0.50	24.5	28.0	10.92	+2.70	23.1	27.3	10.30

	Day	Saccharose				Starch				Milk			
		Reaction	Ammonia Nitrogen	Amino Nitrogen	Percentage Ammonia to Total Nitrogen	Reaction	Ammonia Nitrogen	Amino Nitrogen	Percentage Ammonia to Total Nitrogen	Reaction	Ammonia Nitrogen	Amino Nitrogen	Percentage Ammonia to Total Nitrogen
Control	..	—0.40	18.2	25.2	8.67	—0.90	18.2	23.8	8.67	+1.70	6.3	18.9	1.33
V. septique, A	1	+1.70	22.4	26.6	10.66	—0.80	19.6	25.2	12.06	+2.10	6.3	18.9	1.33
	3	+2.00	23.8	25.2	11.33	—0.80	23.8	26.6	12.67	+2.80	7.7	20.3	1.62
	6	+2.50	23.1	25.2	11.00	—0.50	25.2	28.0	12.06	+3.40	8.4	23.8	1.76
	9	+2.20	23.8	26.6	11.33	—0.40	28.0	29.4	13.33	+2.80	9.8	23.8	2.06
	14	+2.00	24.5	26.6	11.63	—0.50	28.7	30.1	13.66	+3.00	9.8	24.5	2.06
Control	..	—0.40	18.2	25.2	8.67	—0.90	18.2	23.8	8.67	+1.70	6.3	18.9	1.33
V. septique, B	1	+2.20	25.2	26.6	12.06	—0.80	20.3	25.9	9.68	+2.00	6.3	18.9	1.33
	3	+1.50	24.5	28.0	11.66	—0.60	25.2	28.0	12.06	+2.20	8.4	19.6	1.76
	6	+1.60	25.2	29.4	12.06	—0.60	26.6	28.0	12.67	+2.30	9.1	20.3	1.91
	9	+1.80	27.3	30.8	12.96	—0.50	28.0	27.3	13.33	+2.60	9.8	19.6	2.06
	15	+2.10	28.7	30.8	13.66	—0.50	29.2	29.4	13.90	+2.90	9.8	19.6	2.06
Control	..	—0.60	16.8	25.2	7.50	—0.60	16.8	25.2	7.50	+1.70	6.3	18.9	1.33
V. septique, C	1	+2.60	21.7	24.5	9.70	—0.50	22.4	23.8	10.00	+1.80	7.7	18.9	1.62
	3	+2.60	22.4	25.2	10.00	—0.40	23.8	26.6	10.63	+2.30	7.7	18.9	1.62
	4	+2.70	22.4	25.2	10.00	—0.40	23.8	28.0	10.63	+1.70	8.4	19.6	1.76
	9	+2.70	23.8	26.6	10.63	—0.40	24.5	28.7	10.92	+3.00	8.4	19.6	1.76
	14	+2.80	23.8	27.3	10.63	—0.40	25.2	29.4	11.24	+3.00	8.4	19.6	1.76

Control	..	—0.60	10.5	21.7	5.00	—0.70	10.5	36.4	1.53	—0.50	9.8	21.0	4.64	—0.70	10.5	20.3	5.00	—0.60	10.5	21.7	5.00	—0.60	10.5	20.5	5.00	—0.60	10.5	21.7	5.00	—0.70	10.5	21.7	5.00	+1.80	5.6	18.2	1.21
V. septique, D	1	—0.90	16.8	21.0	8.00	—0.80	15.4	36.4	2.24	+2.90	14.0	21.0	6.66	—1.10	15.4	21.0	7.31	—0.70	14.7	21.7	7.00	+2.60	14.7	21.7	7.00	+1.70	16.8	23.1	8.00	—0.70	15.4	19.6	7.31	+1.90	6.3	17.5	1.36
	3	—0.80	19.6	21.0	9.36	—0.50	19.6	37.8	2.86	+2.90	14.7	21.7	7.00	—1.00	18.9	21.7	9.00	—1.00	17.5	21.7	8.33	+2.80	17.5	23.1	8.33	+1.80	17.5	23.8	8.33	—0.50	20.3	18.9	9.68	+2.00	7.7	17.5	1.67
	6	—0.80	21.7	21.7	10.30	—0.40	23.8	37.8	3.44	+2.70	15.4	22.4	7.31	—1.00	19.6	22.4	9.36	—1.00	21.0	25.2	10.00	+2.40	18.9	25.2	9.00	+1.70	19.6	22.4	9.00	—0.35	23.1	21.7	11.00	+2.40	7.0	18.2	1.51
	9	—.090	21.7	21.7	10.30	—0.30	25.2	42.0	3.68	+2.90	16.8	23.1	8.00	—0.80	20.3	23.1	9.68	—0.90	21.0	25.2	10.00	+2.60	19.6	25.2	9.36	+1.80	19.6	25.2	9.35	—0.20	23.1	24.5	11.00	+2.50	8.4	18.2	1.83
	14	—1.00	21.7	22.4	10.30	—0.20	25.9	46.2	3.77	+2.70	16.8	23.8	8.00	—0.80	21.0	23.8	10.00	—0.70	21.7	25.2	10.30	+2.50	19.6	25.9	9.36	+2.00	19.6	25.9	9.36	—0.30	23.8	24.5	11.35	+2.60	9.1	18.9	1.97
Control	..	—0.80	11.2	25.9	4.72	—0.70	3.5	41.3	0.49	—0.80	17.5	27.3	7.36	—0.90	17.5	25.9	7.36	—0.60	17.5	24.5	7.36	—0.80	17.5	27.3	7.36	—0.70	17.5	27.3	7.36	—0.60	17.5	27.3	7.36	+1.60	5.6	18.2	1.24
V. septique, E	1	—1.00	12.6	25.9	5.31	—1.10	4.9	42.7	0.68	+3.30	18.9	27.3	7.95	—1.20	21.0	25.2	8.84	—1.00	20.3	25.9	8.54	+2.70	19.6	28.0	8.23	+2.80	20.3	25.9	8.54	—0.90	20.3	25.9	8.54	+1.90	5.6	16.8	1.24
	3	—1.20	16.8	28.7	7.06	—1.00	4.9	42.7	0.68	+3.30	23.1	27.3	9.72	—1.20	24.5	28.7	10.28	—1.00	23.8	25.2	10.00	+2.90	23.8	29.4	10.00	+2.70	23.1	27.3	9.72	—1.00	24.5	25.9	10.28	+1.90	6.3	17.5	1.38
	6	—1.25	16.8	31.5	7.06	—0.70	6.3	42.7	0.88	+3.60	24.0	30.1	10.10	—1.10	25.2	32.2	10.60	—1.10	24.5	31.5	10.28	+2.70	24.5	29.4	10.28	+2.80	23.8	29.4	10.00	—1.10	25.2	26.6	10.60	+2.40	7.7	20.3	1.69
	9	—1.20	17.5	30.8	7.36	—0.70	9.1	46.2	1.26	+3.20	23.1	30.8	9.72	—1.20	25.9	34.3	10.88	—1.00	24.5	33.6	10.28	+2.80	24.5	29.4	10.28	+2.70	23.8	29.4	10.00	—1.10	25.9	28.7	10.88	+2.50	8.4	21.7	1.84
	14	—1.00	17.5	28.0	7.36	—0.40	14.7	52.5	2.04	+3.10	24.0	27.3	10.10	—1.00	25.9	32.2	10.88	—1.00	25.9	33.6	10.88	+2.80	24.5	27.3	10.28	+2.70	23.1	29.4	9.72	—1.10	25.9	30.1	10.88	+2.90	8.4	21.0	1.84
Control	..	—0.90	13.3	25.2	5.30	—0.60	9.8	28.0	1.44	—0.60	11.9	25.9	4.74	—0.80	11.9	27.3	4.74	—0.80	14.0	26.6	5.58	—0.70	11.9	25.9	4.74	—0.80	11.9	27.3	4.74	—0.80	12.6	26.6	5.00	+1.70	4.9	18.9	1.15
V. septique, F	1	—1.00	15.4	29.4	6.12	—0.60	9.8	28.0	1.44	+2.60	16.1	31.5	6.40	—1.00	14.7	30.1	5.81	—0.90	14.0	26.6	5.58	—0.20	16.1	25.9	6.40	+0.70	16.8	29.4	6.67	—0.80	14.7	25.9	5.81	+1.80	5.6	19.6	1.28
	3	—1.20	20.3	25.9	8.08	—0.70	10.5	27.3	1.55	+2.80	16.8	26.6	6.67	—1.20	19.6	28.0	7.80	—1.20	18.9	23.1	7.50	+3.00	20.3	25.9	8.08	+0.70	18.9	28.7	7.50	—1.10	21.0	25.9	8.32	+2.00	6.3	20.3	1.45
	6	—1.20	21.0	26.6	8.32	—0.70	11.2	30.8	1.64	+2.80	16.8	28.0	6.67	—1.15	20.3	28.7	8.08	—1.20	19.6	25.2	7.80	+3.00	20.3	25.9	8.08	+0.90	20.3	30.1	8.08	—1.10	21.7	24.5	8.62	+2.20	7.0	21.0	1.61
	9	—1.20	21.0	28.0	8.32	—0.70	11.9	31.5	1.75	+2.90	17.5	29.4	6.94	—1.25	21.0	29.4	8.32	—1.20	20.3	27.3	8.08	+3.00	20.3	25.9	8.08	+1.20	21.0	30.1	8.32	—1.20	21.7	25.9	8.62	+2.80	7.0	21.0	1.61
	14	—1.20	21.0	30.1	8.32	—0.80	12.6	32.2	1.86	+2.80	17.5	28.7	6.94	—1.20	21.0	29.4	8.32	—1.10	21.0	28.0	11.05	+2.80	21.0	29.4	8.32	+1.30	21.0	30.1	8.32	—1.10	21.7	26.6	8.62	+3.00	7.7	21.7	1.77
Control	..	—0.70	16.8	26.6	7.50	—0.70	14.0	42.0	6.28	—0.40	16.1	24.5	7.20	—0.60	16.8	26.6	7.50	—0.60	16.8	25.2	7.50	—0.50	16.8	25.2	7.50	—0.60	16.8	25.2	7.50	—0.60	16.8	25.2	7.50	+1.70	4.2	21.0	0.88
V. septique, G	1	—0.80	19.6	29.4	8.76	—0.90	18.9	38.5	8.45	+3.60	18.9	25.9	8.45	—0.90	20.3	25.9	9.06	—0.90	21.0	25.2	9.38	+2.80	21.0	26.6	9.38	+2.70	20.3	25.9	10.90	—0.60	21.0	25.2	9.38	+1.70	4.9	20.3	1.03
	3	—0.80	22.4	30.8	10.00	—0.80	22.4	42.0	10.00	+3.60	21.7	25.9	9.68	—1.00	21.7	27.3	9.68	—0.90	23.8	25.2	10.62	+2.70	23.1	27.3	10.30	+2.80	21.0	27.3	9.38	—0.60	25.2	25.2	10.62	+1.80	4.9	20.3	1.03
	6	—0.80	21.7	30.1	9.68	—0.80	23.1	45.5	10.30	+3.40	22.4	25.9	10.00	—0.90	23.1	27.3	10.30	—0.80	24.5	25.9	10.90	+2.70	23.1	27.3	10.30	+2.70	21.7	27.3	9.68	—0.50	25.9	25.2	10.90	+2.30	6.3	20.3	1.32
	9	—0.70	23.1	30.1	10.30	—0.70	23.1	45.5	10.30	+3.60	22.4	25.9	10.00	—0.80	23.8	28.0	10.62	—0.60	24.5	25.9	10.90	+2.70	23.1	27.3	10.30	+2.60	22.4	28.0	10.00	—0.40	25.9	26.6	10.90	+2.50	6.3	21.7	1.32
	14	—0.60	23.1	30.1	10.30	—0.60	22.4	47.6	10.00	+3.80	21.7	25.2	9.68	—0.80	23.8	27.3	10.62	—0.40	24.5	25.9	10.90	+2.80	23.8	28.0	10.62	+2.60	21.7	27.3	9.68	—0.40	25.2	28.0	10.62	+2.50	7.0	20.3	1.47
Control	..	—0.70	12.6	28.0	5.00	—0.70	6.3	35.7	0.86	—0.20	12.6	25.2	5.00	—0.70	11.9	28.7	4.72	—0.70	11.9	28.7	4.72	—0.70	11.9	25.9	4.72	—0.70	11.9	28.7	4.72	—0.70	12.6	28.0	5.00	+1.50	5.6	22.4	1.14
V. septique, H	1	—0.70	14.7	31.5	5.84	—0.70	9.1	35.0	1.24	+2.40	14.0	25.2	5.53	—0.80	16.1	28.7	6.39	—0.85	13.3	28.7	5.23	+2.10	15.4	32.2	6.12	+1.10	14.0	29.4	5.56	—0.70	16.1	28.7	6.39	+2.00	7.7	22.4	1.57
	3	—0.90	21.0	36.4	8.33	—0.90	11.9	36.4	1.62	+3.60	15.4	26.6	6.10	—1.00	21.7	35.0	8.62	—0.90	15.4	30.8	6.12	+3.20	15.4	32.9	6.12	+1.50	15.4	30.8	6.12	—0.90	25.9	30.1	10.30	+2.50	7.7	23.1	1.57
	6	—1.00	25.2	37.1	10.00	—0.90	13.3	37.1	1.80	+3.80	16.1	27.3	6.39	—0.90	23.1	34.3	9.16	—1.00	19.2	31.5	7.62	+3.40	16.1	32.9	6.39	+1.70	16.1	30.8	6.39	—0.95	27.3	30.8	10.80	+2.90	7.0	22.4	1.42
	13	—1.10	25.9	37.1	10.30	—0.80	15.4	37.8	2.10	+3.90	16.8	28.0	6.70	—0.90	24.5	34.3	9.72	—0.95	19.2	31.5	7.62	+3.20	16.8	32.2	6.66	+1.80	16.8	31.5	6.66	—0.90	27.3	32.2	10.80	+2.70	7.7	23.8	1.57
	20	—1.00	26.6	37.8	10.50	—0.90	15.4	37.1	2.10	+3.70	17.5	28.7	6.95	—0.95	24.5	33.6	9.72	—0.90	19.9	31.5	7.92	+3.10	16.8	32.9	6.66	+1.80	16.8	30.8	6.66	—0.85	27.3	32.9	10.80	+2.80	7.7	23.8	1.57

Reaction: — = alkaline to neutral red; + = acid to neutral red; c c normal acid or alkali per 100 c c of medium.
Ammonia and amino nitrogen expressed in milligrams per 100 c c of culture medium.
Control indicates initial composition of medium. Net results may be obtained by subtracting the control from the day's analysis.
Amino nitrogen is corrected in each instance for ammonia.

ing varieties may be of the same general signficance as the corresponding types of the colon bacillus. If such prove to be the case, the bacteriologist of the future will recognize distinct types of Vibrion septique, precisely as the types of the gas bacillus are now recognized.[4, 7]

The cultures studied in this series comprised the following:

Vibrion septique, culture A—from the National Research Council. Obtained originally from an infected wound.

Vibrion septique, culture B—from the same source.

Vibrion septique, culture C—from Dr. Karl Meyer.

Vibrion septique, culture D—from Dr. Karl Meyer.

Vibrion septique, culture E—from the Army Medical School.

Vibrion septique, culture F—from the Army Medical School.

Vibrion septique, culture G—a stock laboratory culture.

Vibrion septique, culture H—from a culture originally in the Pasteur Institute.

The organisms were purified by the method of single cell isolation described previously.[9] The general plan of inoculation and chemical examination will be found in the study of the Welch bacillus.[10]

DISCUSSION

The analytic figures are self-explanatory. The quantitative changes in the nitrogenous constituents of the different mediums are very similar for the eight organisms studied. This suggests that the various strains may be properly regarded as of one general type. Culture H alone failed to ferment saccharose with the production of gas and acid. The possible significance of this characteristic has been commented on in the foregoing. The inability of all of the strains to induce visible signs of fermentation in glycerol and starch, and the relatively slow accumulation of acid and gas in milk cultures, points to a distinct departure, chemically considered, from the corresponding changes induced by the Welch bacillus.[10] Final judgment should be withheld on the validity of these features as points of distinction between Vibrion septique and the Welch bacillus, until a considerable number of independent studies by various observers have been made. The difficulties attending the purification and study of anaerobic bacteria with existing methods make sweeping statements regarding them of precarious value.

[9] Kendall, Ryan and Cook: Jour. Infect. Dis., 1921, 29, p. 227.

[10] Kendall, Day and Walker: Study XLIV, Jour. Infect. Dis., 1922, 30, p. 141.

The ammonia formation indicative of the intracellular utilization of protein or of protein derivatives for energy,[11] is little indeed, even in cultures, such as gelatin, from which the combined energy and structural requirements must be derived from nitrogenous sources. In this respect, the organism resembles the Welch bacillus.[10] The amino nitrogen accumulation also is minimal, both in protein and carbohydrate-protein mediums. This is quantitatively in contrast with the Welch bacillus, where it was found, in the thirteen strains studied, that the amino nitrogen accumulation was somewhat greater than the ammonia nitrogen formation. This observation is in contrast to that of Wolf,[6] who found that his strain identified as the Vibrion septique produced a gradually increasing amount of amino nitrogen, whereas his strain of the Welch bacillus (B. perfringens) produced minimal amounts of amino nitrogen.

As Wolf stresses this difference as distinctive, it would appear either that there is disagreement on the identification of the respective organisms, or that the differences are of such small magnitude as to be subject to environmental influences that would lead to slight variations in the amounts of amino nitrogen consumed by the organism, thus influencing the residual amino nitrogen which is measured in the cultural mediums. In this respect, so far as the published descriptions of Wolf's organisms show, the fundamental distinctions between his B. perfringens and Vibrion septique appear to agree with the criteria presented for B. welchii and Vibrion septique in this series. As the determination of amino nitrogen represents merely free NH_2 groups in protein, peptone or polypeptids, and not the total nonprotein nitrogen, this difference may be of academic value only. A much more valuable determination of nitrogenous changes in cultural mediums, now determined as amino nitrogen, would be a differentiation into protein and polypeptid nitrogen. Unfortunately this is not possible at the present time.

Gelatin was softened by each strain of Vibrion septique studied. The softening, however, was not due to a detectable soluble enzyme, and the slight change in the nitrogenous constituents of the gelatin suggests strongly that the organism induces only slight decomposition of the medium by the organism. Vibrion septique is not an organism with marked proteolytic powers. In this respect it is in perfect accord with the Welch bacillus.

[11] Kendall and Walker: Ibid., 1915, 17, p. 442.

The organisms studied evolved considerable amounts of gas from the lactose of milk, but the generation of gas was slow and entirely different in character from the almost explosive action of the gas bacillus under similar conditions. The casein was not riddled with holes, as is the case with typical Welch bacillus cultures, and the coagulum appears to be more voluminous. The bright red coloration which gradually develops is more striking than the faint, reddish brown color of typical gas bacillus casein coagula. There is no evidence of more than minimal action on the proteins of the milk, as evidenced by ammonia production and amino acid accmulation.

The reaction of purely protein mediums undergoes little change; in mediums containing utilizable carbohydrate, however, the reaction becomes quite strongly acid.

SUMMARY

Vibrion septique is a carbohydrophilic anaerobic bacillus, which decomposes utilizable carbohydrates energetically with the formation of considerable amounts of titratable acid and the evolution of considerable gas.

It softens gelatin, but without visible evidences of energetic action on the protein of the medium. Gas and acid are generated in milk cultures, and the casein coagulum becomes vividly pink. The nitrogenous changes in milk are minimal, suggesting that the principal change (energy change) is at the expense of the lactose. The nature and extent of the visible changes in milk, however, are quantitatively distinctly less than those characteristic of the Welch bacillus.

Vibrion septique possesses many points of resemblance to the Welch bacillus. The cultures studied differ from the Welch bacillus in their nonability to ferment visibly glycerol or starch; also, the action on saccharose is distinctly less than that on the other carbohydrates studied, or is absent.

These characteristics, taken in connection with the relatively slow fermentation of lactose in milk cultures, appear to be distinct points of difference between the two organisms.

It would appear that the saccharose fermenting and nonsaccharose fermenting strains comprise two distinct types, parallel in significance to the four types of Welch bacillus defined by Simonds [7] and so accepted by Henry.[4]

BACILLUS FALLAX

STUDY XLVI

Bacillus fallax is a rather small anaerobic bacillus, occurring singly or in pairs, which was first isolated from infected wounds and described by Weinberg and Séguin.[1] The organism has occasionally been recovered from the blood stream of the patient during the earlier days of the infection. The organism is distinctly more slender than most of the gunshot wound microbes, and the larger axis is frequently distinctly curved, when observed in stained preparations derived from actively growing cultures. These observations have received confirmation in the studies of Henry[2] and others.[3]

A majority of investigators have directed attention to the comparative infrequency with which spores are observed in culture mediums. This is in distinct contrast to the readiness with whch other anaerobic organisms sporulate under parallel conditions. Generally speaking, anaerobic bacteria, or indeed any bacteria, rarely produce spores in the tissues of animals or of man; also, anaerobes with the possible exception of the vigorous proteolytic microbes, such as B. sporogenes, fail to form spores in mediums containing utilizable carbohydrates.

B. fallax appears to be somewhat more exacting in regard to the environmental conditions governing sporulation than other organisms of the anaerobic group thus far studied, but it may be said that the cultures studied in the series reported in the following, and identified as B. fallax, formed spores consistently but not abundantly in mediums containing protein, such as gelatin or blood serum, in which the reaction remains at or near the neutral point. Spores were never observed in mediums containing utilizable carbohydrates, irrespective of the protein constituents of the medium.

The pathologic and cultural characteristics of B. fallax have been studied by Weinberg and Séguin,[4] and by Henry.[2] The most significant feature of the cultural complex is the apparent inability of the organism to utilize lactose. The organisms of the series reported herein are not in accord in this respect with those of Henry. A slow

[1] Compt. rend. Soc. biol., 1915, 78, p. 686; 1916, 79, p. 581.
[2] Jour. Path. & Bacteriol., 1916, 21, p. 344.
[3] Medical Research Committee, Report 39, 1919.
[4] La Gangrène Gazeuse, 1917.

evolution of gas in milk (utilization of lactose) with no concurrent evidence of proteolysis is in harmony with this view.

The production of gas in starch mediums is also an important cultural and diagnostic feature. The cultural complex suggests strongly that B. fallax is culturally similar to the gas bacillus (Welch bacillus) in that the hexoses and the better known bioses (lactose and saccharose) are fermented, while the alcohols of the hexose series, especially mannitol, are unattacked. The intensity of fermentation, both with respect to rate and amount, is decidedly less vigorous than that of the Welch bacillus, however. The organism is carbohydrophilic. Its action on protein is minimal.

Four cultures are studied in this series. They were obtained from the following sources:

Culture A—National Research Council, from an infected war wound.

Culture B—From the National Research Council, labeled "Gas Bacillus, from an infected wound."

Culture C—From the intestinal contents of a man suffering from an acute diarrhea.

Culture D—From intestinal contents.

The method of purification by the modified Barber single cell method and the general procedure followed in the study of the metabolism of these cultures is that described previously.[5]

RESULTS

Nitrogenous Changes.—The extremely small amounts of ammonia formed during the growth of B. fallax in cultural mediums show conclusively that the action of the organism on protein is minimal. It is not proteophilic. Even after 2 weeks' growth the ammonia has not increased to the extent of 15 mg. in 100 c c of culture medium in gelatin or in plain nutrient bouillon in which no utilizable carbohydrate is present, and in which, consequently, the greatest evidence of proteolysis might confidently be looked for. The change in amino-nitrogen, similarly, is equally insignificant.

The addition of glucose, saccharose, or starch results in a decided increase of activity, which is manifested by a moderate evolution of gas, principally CO_2 and H_2, and the gradual accumulation of titratable acid. The increase of acidity is greatest during the first 24 hours of growth. Lactose is less rapidly decomposed, and the total amount of gas is distinctly less than that of the other carbohydrates mentioned.

[5] Kendall, Ryan and Cook: Jour. Infect. Dis., 1921, 29, p. 227. Kendall, Day and Walker: Studies in Bacterial Metabolism, XLIV, XLV, ibid., 1922, 30, pp. 141 and 155.

TABLE 1

BACILLUS FALLAX

	Day	Plain: Reaction	Plain: Ammonia Nitrogen	Plain: Amino Nitrogen	Plain: Percentage Ammonia to Total Nitrogen	Gelatin: Reaction	Gelatin: Ammonia Nitrogen	Gelatin: Amino Nitrogen	Gelatin: Percentage Ammonia to Total Nitrogen	Glucose: Reaction	Glucose: Ammonia Nitrogen	Glucose: Amino Nitrogen	Glucose: Percentage Ammonia to Total Nitrogen
Control......	..	—0.50	3.5	23.1	2.08	—0.50	5.6	35.7	0.62	—0.20	3.5	21.7	2.08
Culture A....	1	—0.50	4.2	23.8	2.50	—0.40	5.6	36.4	0.62	+3.00	3.5	21.7	2.08
	3	—0.50	4.2	23.8	2.50	—0.30	5.6	36.4	0.62	+3.10	3.5	21.7	2.08
	6	—0.55	4.2	26.6	2.50	—0.20	5.6	37.8	0.62	+3.10	4.2	21.7	2.50
	13	—0.55	4.2	26.6	2.50	—0.30	5.6	40.6	0.62	+2.80	4.2	22.4	2.50
	21	—0.60	4.2	26.6	2.50	—0.30	5.6	40.6	0.62	+2.80	4.2	22.4	2.50
Control......	..	—0.45	3.5	23.1	1.85	—0.80	4.9	44.1	0.54	—0.20	3.5	21.7	1.85
Culture B....	1	—0.50	3.5	22.4	1.85	—0.80	7.0	46.2	0.77	+2.40	4.2	21.7	2.22
	3	—0.50	4.2	23.1	2.22	—0.70	7.7	46.9	0.85	+2.80	4.2	21.7	2.22
	6	—0.50	4.2	23.8	2.22	—0.50	7.7	46.9	0.85	+2.70	4.2	22.4	2.22
	13	—0.50	4.9	25.9	2.59	—0.40	7.7	47.6	0.85	+2.60	4.9	22.4	2.59
	21	—0.50	5.6	27.3	2.96	—0.40	8.4	47.6	0.93	+2.70	4.9	23.1	2.59
Control......	..	—0.40	2.1	21.7	1.25	—0.40	3.5	41.3	0.39	—0.20	2.8	19.6	1.66
Culture C....	1	—0.50	2.8	22.4	1.66	—0.60	3.5	41.3	0.39	+2.60	2.1	21.0	1.25
	3	—0.50	2.8	22.4	1.66	—0.60	4.2	41.3	0.46	+2.80	2.1	21.0	1.25
	6	—0.50	2.8	22.4	1.66	—0.60	4.2	41.3	0.46	+3.00	2.8	21.0	1.66
	12	—0.55	4.2	23.8	2.50	—0.50	4.9	42.0	0.54	+3.10	3.5	19.6	2.08
Control......	..	—0.40	2.1	21.7	1.25	—0.40	3.5	41.3	0.39	—0.10	2.8	19.6	1.66
Culture D....	1	—0.40	2.8	23.1	1.66	—0.40	2.8	41.3	0.31	+1.10	2.8	19.6	1.66
	3	—0.50	3.5	22.4	2.08	—0.50	4.9	39.2	0.54	+1.10	2.8	19.6	1.66
	6	—0.50	4.9	21.0	2.91	—0.50	5.6	40.6	0.62	+1.30	3.5	21.0	2.08
	12	—0.55	5.6	21.0	3.33	—0.50	4.9	40.6	0.54	+1.30	3.5	20.3	2.08

	Day	Mannitol: Reaction	Mannitol: Ammonia Nitrogen	Mannitol: Amino Nitrogen	Mannitol: Percentage Ammonia to Total Nitrogen	Glycerol: Reaction	Glycerol: Ammonia Nitrogen	Glycerol: Amino Nitrogen	Glycerol: Percentage Ammonia to Total Nitrogen	Lactose: Reaction	Lactose: Ammonia Nitrogen	Lactose: Amino Nitrogen	Lactose: Percentage Ammonia to Total Nitrogen
Control......	..	—0.50	3.5	23.1	2.08	—0.50	3.5	23.1	2.08	—0.50	3.5	23.1	2.08
Culture A....	1	—0.40	4.2	22.4	2.50	+2.20	4.2	23.1	2.50	+0.90	4.2	22.4	2.50
	3	—0.40	4.2	22.4	2.50	+2.30	4.2	23.1	2.50	+2.50	4.2	22.4	2.50
	6	—0.40	4.2	22.4	2.50	+2.30	4.2	23.1	2.50	+2.80	4.2	22.4	2.50
	13	—0.30	4.2	22.4	2.50	+2.20	4.2	23.1	2.50	+2.50	4.2	23.1	2.50
	21	—0.40	4.2	22.4	2.50	+2.20	4.9	23.1	2.92	+2.50	4.2	23.1	2.50
Control......	..	—0.40	3.5	23.1	1.85	—0.40	3.5	23.1	1.85	—0.40	3.5	23.1	1.85
Culture B....	1	—0.30	4.2	25.2	2.22	+0.60	3.5	22.4	1.85	+2.60	3.5	24.5	1.85
	3	—0.40	4.2	25.9	2.22	+0.70	2.8	22.4	1.48	+2.80	4.2	23.8	2.22
	6	—0.40	4.9	24.5	2.59	+0.70	3.5	23.1	1.85	+2.90	4.2	24.5	2.22
	13	—0.40	4.9	25.2	2.59	+0.80	4.2	23.8	2.22	+2.40	4.2	24.5	2.22
	21	—0.40	4.9	25.2	2.59	+0.80	4.2	23.8	2.22	+2.40	4.2	24.5	2.22
Control......	..	—0.40	2.1	23.1	1.25	—0.40	2.8	21.7	1.66	—0.40	2.8	20.3	1.66
Culture C....	1	—0.50	4.2	22.4	2.50	+2.10	2.1	20.3	1.25	+2.60	2.8	20.3	1.66
	3	—0.45	3.5	22.4	2.08	+2.00	2.1	20.3	1.25	+2.60	2.1	22.4	1.25
	6	—0.45	3.5	23.8	2.08	+2.10	2.8	20.3	1.66	+2.70	2.8	22.4	1.66
	12	—0.50	3.5	23.8	2.08	+2.10	2.8	20.3	1.66	+2.70	3.5	21.7	2.08
Control......	..	—0.40	2.1	23.1	1.25	—0.40	2.8	21.7	1.66	—0.40	2.1	20.3	1.25
Culture D....	1	—0.50	2.8	21.7	1.66	—0.40	3.5	21.7	2.08	+0.80	2.1	21.0	1.25
	3	—0.40	2.8	23.1	1.66	—0.40	4.2	20.3	2.50	+1.30	2.1	21.0	1.25
	6	—0.35	3.5	23.8	2.08	—0.30	3.5	20.3	2.08	+1.60	2.1	21.7	1.25
	12	—0.35	3.5	23.8	2.08	—0.20	4.9	21.7	2.91	+1.50	2.8	22.4	1.66

	Day	Saccharose: Reaction	Saccharose: Ammonia Nitrogen	Saccharose: Amino Nitrogen	Saccharose: Percentage Ammonia to Total Nitrogen	Starch: Reaction	Starch: Ammonia Nitrogen	Starch: Amino Nitrogen	Starch: Percentage Ammonia to Total Nitrogen	Milk: Reaction	Milk: Ammonia Nitrogen	Milk: Amino Nitrogen	Milk: Percentage Ammonia to Total Nitrogen
Control......	..	—0.40	3.5	23.1	2.08	—0.40	3.5	21.7	2.08	+1.10	4.2	22.4	0.88
Culture A....	1	+2.40	4.2	22.4	2.50	+2.50	4.2	21.0	2.50	+2.40	5.6	23.1	1.17
	3	+2.40	4.2	22.4	2.50	+2.90	4.2	21.0	2.50	+3.10	4.9	23.1	1.03
	6	+2.80	4.2	22.4	2.50	+3.10	4.2	21.0	2.50	+3.70	4.9	23.8	1.03
	13	+2.90	5.6	23.1	3.33	+3.00	4.2	21.0	2.50	+3.50	4.9	23.8	1.03
	21	+2.60	4.9	23.1	2.92	+2.80	4.2	21.0	2.50	+3.40	5.6	23.8	1.17
Control......	..	—0.50	3.5	23.1	1.85	—0.40	3.5	23.1	1.85	+1.40	7.7	23.1	1.47
Culture B....	1	+2.90	4.2	22.4	2.22	+2.80	3.5	23.1	1.85	+1.50	7.7	23.1	1.47
	3	+3.10	4.2	23.1	2.22	+3.00	4.2	23.8	2.22	+2.40	8.4	24.5	1.60
	6	+2.90	3.5	23.8	1.85	+3.10	4.2	23.8	2.22	+2.60	8.4	24.5	1.60
	13	+2.70	4.9	24.5	2.59	+3.00	4.9	23.8	2.59	+2.80	9.1	23.8	1.74
	21	+2.80	4.9	24.5	2.59	+3.00	5.6	24.5	2.96	+3.00	9.1	24.5	1.74
Control......	..	—0.40	2.1	20.3	1.25	—0.40	3.5	20.3	2.08	+3.20	2.8	21.0	0.56
Culture C....	1	+3.00	2.1	20.3	1.25	+2.80	2.8	21.0	1.66	+1.70	2.1	22.4	0.45
	3	+3.10	2.8	20.3	1.66	+2.90	2.8	21.0	1.66	+2.60	2.1	22.4	0.45
	6	+3.20	2.1	21.0	1.25	+3.10	2.8	21.0	1.66	+3.10	2.8	21.0	0.56
	12	+3.10	2.8	21.0	1.66	+3.10	3.5	21.0	2.08	+3.20	2.8	21.0	0.56
Control......	..	—0.40	2.1	20.3	1.25	—0.40	3.5	20.3	2.08	+1.30	2.8	25.2	0.56
Culture D....	1	+1.00	2.8	21.0	1.66	+1.40	2.8	21.7	1.66	+1.50	2.8	22.4	0.56
	3	+1.20	2.8	21.0	1.66	+1.30	3.5	21.7	2.08	+1.90	4.2	23.1	0.89
	6	+1.40	2.8	21.7	1.66	+1.40	4.2	22.4	2.50	+2.40	3.5	25.2	0.74
	12	+1.30	3.5	21.7	2.08	+1.30	4.2	22.4	2.50	+2.50	3.5	25.9	0.74

Reaction: — = alkaline to neutral red; + = acid to neutral red; c c normal acid or alkali per 100 c c of medium.
Ammonia and amino nitrogen expressed in milligrams per 100 c c of culture medium.
Control indicates initial composition of medium. Net results may be obtained by subtracting the control from the day's analysis.
Amino nitrogen is corrected in each instance for ammonia.

In milk, as well as lactose broth, however, there is a slow evolution of gas, and this factor, in association with the distinct and rapid development of an acid reaction, would appear to afford conclusive evidence that B. fallax is to be regarded as a lactose fermenter.

Cultures A and B fermented glycerol with moderate intensity. Cultures B and D failed to produce gas, but the reaction became somewhat acid, greater than the acidity developed in corresponding mediums containing no utilizable, non-nitrogenous source of carbon. Available evidence fails to furnish an adequate explanation for this phenomenon. It cannot be stated at this time whether Culture B is a nonglycerol fermenting variant of B. fallax, or whether a slight and unrecognized impurity in the glycerol furnished a small amount of substance utilizable for energy in place of the nitrogenous constituents, giving rise to this slight increase in acid above that characteristic of nonsaccharine mediums. The indifferent nitrogenous changes which characterize the proteolytic activities of the bacillus are insufficient to distinguish between these possibilities. Attempts to demonstrate a soluble, proteoclastic enzyme were wholly unsuccessful. As the gelatin medium failed to soften even after two weeks' incubation, however, this negative result is to be expected.

SUMMARY

B. fallax is a carbohydrophilic organism, whose general cultural properties are reminiscent in a moderate degree of those characteristic of B. welchii.

The fermentation of starch with the production of gas and acid appears to be a mark of resemblance to the Welch bacillus, and a point of differentiation from the other anaerobic bacteria which comprise the flora of infected wounds of warfare.

The relatively gradual evolution of gas, both in milk and in mediums containing utilizable carbohydrates, contrasts markedly with the rapid generation of gas in cultures of the Welch bacillus.

Lactose is decomposed more slowly than the other carbohydrates which are utilizable as sources of energy by Bacillus fallax. This appears to be a feature of considerable diagnostic importance.

The coagulum formed gradually in milk as a result of the slowly increasing acidity attributable to the fermentation of the lactose is quite unlike that characteristic of B. welchii and Vibrion septique. It lacks the ragged, torn appearance characteristic of the former, and it fails to exhibit the reddish coloration of the latter.

BACILLUS TERTIUS

STUDY XLVII

Bacillus tertius was isolated from infected war wounds and described by Henry.[1] It received its name because it was encountered third in point of frequency of occurrence among the anaerobic bacteria of wounds by Henry. The morphology, especially of young, rapidly growing cultures, is fairly distinctive. Spores are formed readily in protein mediums, which are always of the plectridial type, and oval in outline when fully mature. Immature spores, which may be stained by Gram's method, appear first as small, deeply staining enlargements on one end of the bacillary rods. As the spore matures, it becomes longer, larger, and tends to lose its ability to stain with ordinary dyes. Eventually the mature spore is nearly twice the diameter of the parent rod, distinctly longer, and stainable only by intensified methods of coloration, as for example, steaming with carbol fuchsin. Once stained, however, the mature spore retains the color tenaciously; in this respect, it resembles spores of other organisms. The peculiarity is the frequence with which immature polar spores may be detected in actively growing cultures in the earlier stages of incubation.

The organism has been identified by Miss Robertson[2] as indistinguishable from Bacillus III of Rodella[3] and as Bacillus IX of von Hibler.[4] It may be closely related to the organism described by Fleming as Bacillus Y,[5] but this is doubtful because the latter is said to decompose protein slowly. Published descriptions by Henry[1] and others are in accord in ascribing carbohydrophilic, but not proteolytic properties to B. tertius.

An important cultural diagnostic feature is the fermentation of mannitol by the organism. In general, the alcohol derivatives of the hexoses do not appear to be utilizable as sources of energy by the saccharolytic anaerobic organisms; mannitol, however, is fermented by B. tertius, but dulcitol is unattacked. The organisms identified as B. tertius in the series presented in the following agree in this detail with the organism originally described.

[1] Brit. Med. Jour., 1917, 1, p. 806; Jour. Path. & Bacteriol., 1916, 21, p. 344.
[2] Ibid., 1915, 20, p. 327.
[3] Ztschr. f. Hyg., 1902, 39, p. 201.
[4] Untersuchungen über die pathogenen Anaëroben, u. s. w., 1908.
[5] Lancet, 1915, 2, p. 376.

TABLE 1

Bacillus Tertius

	Day	Plain				Gelatin				Glucose			
		Reaction	Ammonia Nitrogen	Amino Nitrogen	Percentage Ammonia to Total Nitrogen	Reaction	Ammonia Nitrogen	Amino Nitrogen	Percentage Ammonia to Total Nitrogen	Reaction	Ammonia Nitrogen	Amino Nitrogen	Percentage Ammonia to Total Nitrogen
Control......	..	−0.40	2.1	21.7	1.25	−0.40	3.5	41.3	0.39	−0.10	2.8	19.6	1.66
Culture A....	1	−0.50	2.8	22.4	1.66	−0.60	4.9	42.7	0.54	+0.90	2.8	19.6	1.66
	3	−0.50	2.8	22.4	1.66	−0.50	4.9	42.7	0.54	+1.10	2.8	19.6	1.66
	6	−0.50	2.8	22.4	1.66	−0.50	4.9	42.7	0.54	+1.30	2.8	19.6	1.66
	12	−0.50	2.8	23.1	1.66	−0.40	4.9	42.7	0.54	+1.30	2.8	19.6	1.66
Control......	..	−0.50	3.5	23.1	2.00	−0.50	4.2	42.0	0.47	−0.10	3.5	21.7	2.00
Culture B....	1	−0.60	4.2	22.4	2.40	−0.60	4.2	42.0	0.47	+1.40	3.5	21.7	2.00
	3	−0.60	4.2	22.4	2.40	−0.60	4.9	42.0	0.55	+1.70	3.5	21.7	2.00
	6	−0.60	4.2	24.5	2.40	−0.60	4.9	42.7	0.55	+1.70	3.5	21.7	2.00
	13	−0.60	4.2	23.8	2.40	−0.60	5.6	44.1	0.63	+1.60	3.5	23.1	2.00
	21	−0.60	4.2	23.8	2.40	−0.60	5.6	44.1	0.63	+1.70	3.5	23.1	2.00

	Day	Mannitol				Glycerol				Lactose			
		Reaction	Ammonia Nitrogen	Amino Nitrogen	Percentage Ammonia to Total Nitrogen	Reaction	Ammonia Nitrogen	Amino Nitrogen	Percentage Ammonia to Total Nitrogen	Reaction	Ammonia Nitrogen	Amino Nitrogen	Percentage Ammonia to Total Nitrogen
Control......	..	−0.40	2.1	23.1	1.25	−0.40	2.8	21.7	1.66	−0.40	2.1	20.3	1.25
Culture A....	1	+1.50	2.8	21.7	1.66	−0.40	2.8	21.0	1.66	−0.40	2.1	21.7	1.25
	3	+1.60	2.8	21.0	1.66	−0.40	2.8	21.0	1.66	+1.40	2.8	23.1	1.66
	6	+1.60	2.8	19.6	1.66	−0.40	3.5	21.7	2.08	+1.70	2.8	23.1	1.66
	12	+1.80	2.8	21.0	1.66	−0.60	3.5	23.1	2.08	+1.80	2.8	22.4	1.66
Control......	..	−0.60	3.5	23.1	2.00	−0.60	3.5	23.1	2.00	−0.60	3.5	23.1	2.00
Culture B....	1	+0.90	3.5	22.4	2.00	−0.50	3.5	21.7	2.00	−0.40	3.5	21.7	2.00
	3	+1.60	4.2	22.4	2.40	−0.60	3.5	21.7	2.00	+1.80	4.2	21.7	2.40
	6	+1.60	4.2	23.8	2.40	−0.60	3.5	21.7	2.00	+1.90	4.2	23.1	2.40
	13	+1.60	4.2	23.8	2.40	−0.60	4.2	22.4	2.40	+1.90	4.2	23.1	2.40
	21	+1.70	4.2	23.8	2.40	−0.80	4.2	23.1	2.40	+1.80	4.9	24.5	2.80

	Day	Saccharose				Starch				Milk			
		Reaction	Ammonia Nitrogen	Amino Nitrogen	Percentage Ammonia to Total Nitrogen	Reaction	Ammonia Nitrogen	Amino Nitrogen	Percentage Ammonia to Total Nitrogen	Reaction	Ammonia Nitrogen	Amino Nitrogen	Percentage Ammonia to Total Nitrogen
Control......	..	−0.40	2.1	20.3	1.25	−0.40	3.5	20.3	2.08	+1.30	2.8	25.2	0.59
Culture A....	1	+0.60	2.8	19.6	1.66	−0.40	2.1	22.4	1.25	+1.50	3.5	21.7	0.69
	3	+1.70	2.8	22.4	1.66	−0.40	2.8	21.7	1.66	+1.70	4.2	21.0	0.89
	6	+1.80	2.1	21.7	1.25	−0.40	3.5	19.6	2.08	+1.90	4.2	21.0	0.89
	12	+1.70	2.8	22.4	1.66	−0.40	4.2	21.0	2.50	+1.80	4.2	24.5	0.89
Control......	..	−0.60	3.5	23.1	2.00	−0.60	3.5	23.1	2.00	+1.20	7.0	21.0	1.41
Culture B....	1	−0.40	3.5	22.4	2.00	−0.60	4.2	21.7	2.40	+1.60	7.0	22.4	1.41
	3	+1.00	3.5	22.4	2.00	−0.60	4.2	21.7	2.40	+2.20	7.0	21.0	1.41
	6	+1.20	4.2	23.1	2.40	−0.50	4.2	21.7	2.40	+2.10	7.0	21.7	1.41
	13	+1.50	4.2	23.8	2.40	−0.40	4.2	21.7	2.40	+2.20	6.3	21.7	1.27
	21	+1.60	4.2	24.5	2.40	−0.40	4.2	23.1	2.40	+2.10	6.3	21.7	1.27

Reaction: — = alkaline to neutral red; + = acid to neutral red; c c normal acid or alkali per 100 c c of medium.
Ammonia and amino nitrogen expressed in milligrams per 100 c c of culture medium.
Control indicates initial composition of medium. Net results may be obtained by subtracting the control from the day's analysis.
Amino nitrogen is corrected in each instance for ammonia.

Origin of Cultures.—B. tertius, Culture A, was obtained from Dr. Holman, who brought it from Paris.

B. tertius, Culture B, was isolated from the fecal contents of a man exhibiting an overgrowth of Welch bacilli in the alimentary canal.

DISCUSSION

Chemically, B. tertius is one of the more inert varieties of anaerobic bacilli. The nitrogenous changes induced by the organism are quantitatively very similar to those of B. fallax.[6] In mediums containing no utilizable carbohydrate, the nitrogenous changes even on prolonged incubation are minimal. Neither the ammonia nor the amino nitrogen exhibits a deviation from the uninoculated controls which is in excess of the probable error of the method, namely, about 2 mg. above or below the controls. The nitrogenous changes in plain broth, glycerol, and starch mediums (which have the same nitrogenous content) are almost identical, as might confidently be expected, as the glycerol and starch are not utilizable as sources of energy. In gelatin also the nitrogenous changes are practically negligible. Attempts to demonstrate a soluble, proteolytic enzyme in gelatin cultures of Bacillus tertius were uniformly negative. The gelatin remained firm even after three weeks' incubation. Glucose, lactose, saccharose and mannitol are fermented with the production of some gas, and a moderate but distinct increase in titratable acidity. The decomposition of the carbohydrates is slow, the evolution of gas is very moderate, and the accumulation of acid products of fermentation is very deliberate.

Culture B differed from culture A in that its action on milk was very slow. After a few weeks only a few cubic centimeters of gas were formed, and the direct examination of the milk cultures by the method of Gram staining revealed only a few bacilli. It would appear that this particular organism failed to develop with even moderate luxuriance in the milk medium.

SUMMARY

B. tertius is an anaerobic bacillus, characterized morphologically by the stainable properties of immature spores. The mature spores are terminal, and distinctly oval. This is a point of differentiation from Bacillus tetani, with which the organism might be confused on purely morphologic grounds.

[6] Kendall, Day and Walker: Jour. Infect. Dis., Study XLVI, 1922, p. 163.

Culturally, the organism is relatively inert. Its action on protein (or protein derivatives) is minimal, in which respect it suggests B. fallax strongly.

In mediums containing utilizable carbohydrates there is a very moderate evolution of gas, chiefly H_2 and CO_2, and a coincident increase in titratable acidity. Acid and gas are produced from glucose, lactose, saccharose, and the hexose alcohol, mannitol. In the latter respect, that is, the gaseous fermentation of mannitol, B. tertius is quite distinctive among the members of the carbohydrophilic anaerobic group, to which it belongs.

The inability of B. tertius to utilize either glycerol or starch for energy, together with its ability to ferment mannitol, would appear to be distinguishing features, definitely differentiating it culturally from B. welchii, Vibrion septique or B. fallax. Its negative effect on nitrogenous substances is an additional distinguishing characteristic.

BACILLUS TETANI

STUDY XLVIII

B. tetani is the most widely known of the anaerobic bacilli. Indeed, since Carle and Rattoni [1] inoculated a rabbit with pus from a human case of the disease and reproduced the essential clinical features of the disease in 1884, the occasional case of tetanus has been widely heralded even in the public press. The dread of the wound inflicted with a "rusty nail" has become a public heritage which perhaps has its origin in the experiments of Nicolaier,[2] who induced lesions in laboratory animals by the subcutaneous injection of garden soil. Kitasato's [3] great discovery of the toxin of the tetanus bacillus and the preparation of a specific antitoxin on a practical scale completed the really significant available information of the growth of the organism and the nature of its products up to the Great War.

The mechanism of the production of tetanus toxin is of no concern in the present discussion. An additional discovery of importance, produced as a result of the intensive study of tetanus bacilli derived from wounds of warfare is that of Tulloch,[4] who described four types of

[1] Gior. d. r. Accad. di med. di Torino, 1884, No. 3.
[2] Deutsch. med. Wchnschr., 1884, 10, p. 842.
[3] Deutsch. med. Wchnschr., 1889, 15, p. 635; Ztschr. f. Hyg., u. Infektionskr., 1889, 7, p. 225.
[4] Jour. Hygiene, 1919, 18, p. 103.

tetanus bacilli, each of which appears to be a serological entity. In this respect the tetanus bacillus is reminiscent of the four serological types of the meningococcus and the pneumococcus. Tetanus antitoxin, however, unlike the meningococcus immune serums, is qualitatively, and for practical purposes quantitatively, a specific neutralizing agent for the toxin of any of the four types.[4]

As the principal cultural substance formed by the tetanus bacillus as a result of its growth is the soluble, and tremendously potent toxin, it is not unnatural that the identification of the organism in the past has been restricted practically to the determination of this point. The cultural identification has been largely overlooked, or at best imperfectly scrutinized. The toxin, furthermore, is said not to be materially reduced in potency when it is developed by cultures of tetanus bacilli contaminated with alien organisms. For this reason, as the usual interest surrounding B. tetani is the production of toxin for purposes of immunization, few attempts at the cultural study of the organism, with adequate methods, are on record.

The commonly accepted characteristics of B. tetani suggest strongly a proteolytic aspect, and endowed with fermentative powers as well. Indeed, the directions for cultivating tetanus bacilli for toxin production stress the formation of considerable gas during the earlier stages of the process, and the gradual development of a foul odor later, when toxin begins to accumulate.

Achalme[5] appears to have been the first, or at least one of the earliest, investigators to call attention to the fact that the tetanus bacillus fermented no carbohydrates. This view apparently is accepted by the Medical Research Committee.[6] The latter, however, state that gelatin is liquefied, while coagulated serum exhibits little or no liquefaction, suggesting at least mild proteolytic powers. In this respect the Medical Research Committee would apparently place the Welch bacillus and Vibrion septique in a group exhibiting both saccharolytic and proteolytic activities, the former predominating. Undoubtedly, the fluidification of gelatin, exhibited by both the Welch organism and Vibrion septique, would be a determining factor in such a classification. Chemical analyses of gelatin cultures of the organisms inciting gas gangrene[7, 8] have shown that the quantitative nitrogenous changes in

[5] Ann. Inst. Past., 1902, 16, p. 633.

[6] Report on Anaerobic Infections of Wounds, 1919.

[7] Wolf: Jour. Path. & Bacteriol., 1917, 21, p. 386; ibid., 1918, 22, p. 115.

[8] Kendall, Day and Walker: Jour. Infect. Dis., Studies XLIV and XLV, 1922, 30, pp. 141 and 155.

TABLE 1

BACILLUS TETANI

	Day	Plain: Reaction	Plain: Ammonia Nitrogen	Plain: Amino Nitrogen	Plain: Percentage Ammonia to Total Nitrogen	Gelatin: Reaction	Gelatin: Ammonia Nitrogen	Gelatin: Amino Nitrogen	Gelatin: Percentage Ammonia to Total Nitrogen	Glucose: Reaction	Glucose: Ammonia Nitrogen	Glucose: Amino Nitrogen	Glucose: Percentage Ammonia to Total Nitrogen
Control......	..	—1.00	14.7	32.9	5.00	—0.40	24.5	39.9	3.21	—0.60	14.0	31.5	4.76
Culture A....	1	—0.80	16.8	25.9	5.72	—0.30	29.4	35.0	3.87	—0.40	15.4	20.3	5.22
	3	—0.80	20.3	26.6	6.90	—0.30	32.2	35.7	4.22	—0.20	18.2	21.7	6.19
	6	—0.70	25.2	28.7	8.57	—0.20	30.8	39.2	4.04	—0.10	20.3	22.4	6.90
	13	—0.60	28.0	32.9	9.53	—0.10	39.9	38.5	5.23	+0.10	21.7	23.8	7.38
	21	—0.60	28.0	31.5	9.53	—0.10	42.7	37.1	5.60	+0.20	22.4	27.3	7.62
Control......	..	—0.60	3.5	24.5	1.84	—0.70	4.2	46.2	0.44	—0.10	4.2	21.0	2.22
Culture B....	1	—0.40	7.7	19.6	4.07	—0.60	7.0	39.2	0.73	+0.20	4.9	16.1	2.59
	3	—0.30	12.6	21.7	6.66	—0.40	9.8	42.0	1.03	+0.30	9.8	16.1	5.18
	6	—0.20	14.7	24.5	7.78	—0.30	14.7	46.2	1.54	+0.50	10.5	18.2	5.56
	13	—0.20	18.2	24.5	9.63	—0.40	21.7	44.1	2.28	+0.50	11.9	17.5	6.30
	21	......	....	....	....	—0.30	23.8	42.0	2.50	+0.60	13.3	17.5	7.03
Control......	..	—0.70	2.8	26.6	1.43	—1.00	4.2	42.0	0.45	—0.10	2.8	22.4	1.43
Culture C....	1	—0.70	4.9	24.5	2.50	—0.80	6.3	32.9	0.68	+0.10	4.9	23.1	2.50
	3	—0.50	7.0	18.2	3.63	—0.70	10.5	32.9	1.13	+0.20	6.3	24.5	3.21
	6	—0.40	9.1	17.5	4.64	—0.70	16.1	32.9	1.74	+0.40	7.0	24.5	3.63
	13	—0.40	12.6	16.1	6.42	—0.60	19.6	32.9	2.12	+0.40	9.8	21.0	5.00

	Day	Mannitol: Reaction	Mannitol: Ammonia Nitrogen	Mannitol: Amino Nitrogen	Mannitol: Percentage Ammonia to Total Nitrogen	Glycerol: Reaction	Glycerol: Ammonia Nitrogen	Glycerol: Amino Nitrogen	Glycerol: Percentage Ammonia to Total Nitrogen	Lactose: Reaction	Lactose: Ammonia Nitrogen	Lactose: Amino Nitrogen	Lactose: Percentage Ammonia to Total Nitrogen
Control......	..	—0.90	14.7	32.2	5.00	—0.90	14.7	28.7	5.00	—0.80	14.0	30.8	4.76
Culture A....	1	—0.70	15.4	26.6	5.22	—0.70	14.7	25.2	5.00	—0.60	15.4	23.8	5.22
	3	—0.60	20.3	23.1	6.90	—0.20	18.2	26.7	6.19	—0.50	21.7	20.3	7.38
	6	—0.60	23.8	23.8	8.10	—0.10	20.3	25.2	6.90	—0.50	22.4	23.8	7.62
	13	—0.40	25.2	25.2	8.57	+0.10	23.8	25.9	8.10	—0.30	28.7	28.7	9.76
	21	—0.50	28.0	30.8	9.53	+0.20	27.3	30.8	9.30	—0.40	29.4	28.0	10.0
Control......	..	—0.60	3.5	24.5	1.84	—0.60	3.5	24.5	1.84	—0.50	3.5	24.5	1.84
Culture B....	1	—0.40	7.7	19.6	4.07	—0.30	4.2	18.2	2.22	—0.20	7.7	19.6	4.07
	3	—0.30	10.5	21.7	5.56	—0.40	10.5	19.6	5.56	—0.20	10.5	21.0	5.56
	6	—0.30	11.9	25.2	6.30	—0.30	11.2	23.1	5.93	—0.10	14.7	26.6	7.78
	13	—0.20	14.7	28.7	7.78	—0.30	16.1	26.6	8.52	—0.10	15.4	25.9	8.15
	21	—0.20	17.5	28.0	9.26	—0.20	16.1	26.6	8.52	.....	....	....	....
Control......	..	—0.70	3.5	25.9	1.78	—0.70	2.8	26.6	1.43	—0.60	3.5	25.9	1.78
Culture C....	1	—0.50	7.0	18.9	3.63	—0.40	4.9	26.6	2.50	—0.60	6.3	23.1	3.21
	3	—0.50	9.8	17.5	5.00	—0.30	9.1	22.4	4.64	—0.50	8.4	20.3	4.28
	6	—0.30	11.2	23.8	5.72	—0.20	12.6	21.7	6.42	—0.40	9.8	17.5	5.00
	13	—0.10	13.3	23.8	6.78	—0.20	13.3	22.4	6.78	—0.30	11.2	19.6	5.72

	Day	Saccharose: Reaction	Saccharose: Ammonia Nitrogen	Saccharose: Amino Nitrogen	Saccharose: Percentage Ammonia to Total Nitrogen	Starch: Reaction	Starch: Ammonia Nitrogen	Starch: Amino Nitrogen	Starch: Percentage Ammonia to Total Nitrogen	Milk: Reaction	Milk: Ammonia Nitrogen	Milk: Amino Nitrogen	Milk: Percentage Ammonia to Total Nitrogen
Control......	..	—1.00	14.0	32.2	4.76	—0.90	14.0	32.9	4.76	+1.70	5.6	21.0	1.14
Culture A....	1	—0.80	15.4	25.2	5.22	—0.60	15.4	25.9	5.22	+1.70	7.7	18.9	1.57
	3	—0.70	20.3	23.1	6.90	—0.60	23.1	22.4	7.86	+1.80	8.4	18.2	1.71
	6	—0.70	25.2	26.6	8.57	—0.60	26.6	27.3	9.06	+1.80	8.4	18.2	1.71
	13	—0.50	26.6	28.0	9.03	—0.50	30.8	28.7	10.4	+1.80	9.8	19.6	2.00
	21	—0.60	30.1	31.5	10.2	—0.60	32.2	35.7	10.9	+1.90	11.9	21.7	2.43
Control......	..	—0.60	3.5	24.5	1.84	—0.60	3.5	24.5	1.84	+1.40	7.0	21.0	1.43
Culture B....	1	—0.30	6.3	20.3	3.33	—0.30	7.7	19.6	4.07	+1.40	9.1	18.9	1.86
	3	—0.40	9.8	21.0	5.18	—0.40	11.2	21.7	5.93	+1.40	9.1	18.9	1.86
	6	—0.20	12.6	23.8	6.66	—0.20	13.3	25.9	7.03	+1.40	9.8	20.3	2.00
	13	—0.20	15.4	25.9	8.15	—0.20	14.0	27.3	7.40	+1.50	9.8	21.0	2.00
	21	—0.10	16.1	26.6	8.52	—0.30	15.4	28.0	8.15	+1.50	10.5	21.0	2.14
Control......	..	—0.70	3.5	25.9	1.78	—0.70	3.5	25.9	1.78	+1.00	5.6	22.4	1.12
Culture C....	1	—0.50	9.1	18.2	4.64	—0.50	5.6	18.2	2.85	+1.20	6.3	18.2	1.26
	3	—0.50	11.4	18.9	5.72	—0.50	9.8	18.9	5.00	+1.40	7.7	21.7	1.55
	6	—0.50	12.6	19.6	6.42	—0.40	12.6	19.6	6.42	+1.50	10.5	22.4	2.11
	13	—0.30	14.7	22.4	7.50	—0.20	15.4	21.7	7.86	+1.70	11.9	23.1	2.39

Reaction: — = alkaline to neutral red; + = acid to neutral red; c c normal acid or alkali per 100 c c of medium.
Ammonia and amino nitrogen expressed in milligrams per 100 c c of culture medium.
Control indicates initial composition of medium. Net results may be obtained by subtracting the control from the day's analysis.
Amino nitrogen is corrected in each instance for ammonia.

gelatin mediums are of very small magnitude, and wholly different from those characteristic of bacteria which cause deep-seated, true liquefactions in these mediums.[9]

It should be stated that those bacteria which produce powerful, soluble toxins incidentally to the utilization of protein for energy, as the diphtheria bacillus, are characterized by their slight action on protein, as shown by a study of the nitrogenous metabolism of such cultures.[10] So far as available information indicates, true toxin formation appears to be incompatible with marked proteolysis.

Origin of Cultures.—B. tetani A—A strain used extensively in the United States to produce tetanus toxin.

B. tetani B—An old culture obtained from Dr. Theobald Smith.

B. tetani C—Isolated from garden soil.

DISCUSSION

The nitrogenous changes are somewhat more marked than those characteristic of the carbohydrophilic organisms studied previously—B. welchii, B. fallax, and Vibrion septique. In each strain there is a moderate production of ammonia, amounting to approximately 20-30 mg. for each 100 c c of medium. These figures are of the same order of magnitude as those characteristic for the diphtheria bacillus for an equal period of incubation. The amino nitrogen shows a small but definite decrease in each instance. This suggests, but of course does not prove, that the tetanus bacillus utilizes that portion of the nitrogenous constituents of the various mediums which contain NH_2 groups capable of uniting with formaldehyde for at least a part of their energy. It will be remembered that Buchner[11] claimed to have demonstrated toxin formation to a limited extent in a modified Uschinsky medium, which contains no protein whatsoever. Asparagin was the only organized source of nitrogen available for the organism in his experiments. It should be stated that Brieger[12] failed to confirm Buchner's observations.

Some gas was formed in all the mediums studied. The amount was small and the rate of accumulation was small. The gas formed was not analyzed. It was as great in amount in plain, nutrient broth as

[9] Kendall and Walker: Ibid., 1915, 17, p. 442.

[10] Kendall and Farmer: Jour. Biol. Chem., 1912, 12, p. 13. Kendall, Day and Walker: Jour. Am. Chem. Soc., 1913, 35, p. 1201.

[11] München. med. Wchnschr., 1893, 40, 449.

[12] Ztschr. f. Hyg. u. Infektionskr., 1895, 19, p. 101.

in gelatin, glucose broth or any of the mediums studied. Coincidently, there was a slow rise in the titratable acidity of the mediums.

Gelatin was not softened, even after an incubation of nearly three weeks, and the nitrogenous changes induced by the organisms are quantitatively small and not suggestive of proteolytic tendencies.

The addition of the ordinary carbohydrates—glucose, lactose, saccharose, mannitol, or starch—failed to increase materially either the luxuriance of growth or to augment in a noteworthy manner the rate or amount of gas production. The changes observed in titratable acidity in carbohydrate mediums above those of corresponding nonsaccharine mediums, furthermore, with respect to titratable acidity or otherwise, were quantitatively undetectable.

SUMMARY

The strains of tetanus bacillus discussed herein produced a soluble toxin, a very small amount of which, amounting to 0.05 c c, would kill white mice. No attempt was made to determine the minimal lethal dose, however. The sole purpose of the mouse inoculation was to establish the presence of a soluble toxin which would induce qualitatively a typical fatal effect on the animal.

Morphologically the organisms were perfectly typical. Chemically they were relatively inert.

The changes induced in the nitrogenous constituents of the ordinary cultural mediums were limited. There was a small, but definite and gradual, accumulation of ammonia, which was quantitatively the same, irrespective of the non-nitrogenous constituents. Simultaneously, and at nearly the same rate, there was a diminution in the amount of "amino-nitrogen," as shown by the method of formol titration.[13]

Gelatin was not softened, and there was no visible change in the appearance of milk. A gradual increase in titratable acidity was demonstrated in each medium, and coincidently a slow and limited evolution of gas occurred. Presumably the gas was derived from some of the protein constituents of the mediums.

Carbohydrates were not decomposed in a measurable degree.

The cultures identified and studied as Bacillus tetani are not carbohydrophilic. They are feebly proteolytic. Chemically, the organisms are characterized by their relative inertness.

[13] Sörensen: Ztschr. physiol. Chem., 1910, 64, p. 120.

BACILLUS PSEUDOTETANI

STUDY XLIX

The organism discussed here as pseudotetanus appears to be identical with B. tetanomorphus of the Medical Research Committee.[1] They in turn establish identity with the B. pseudotetani of McIntosh and Feldes.[2] The organism described in 1898 by Tavel [3] as a pseudotetanus bacillus is very probably the earliest description which is in reasonable agreement with the organism under discussion. It is possible that Debono's organism, B. anaerobicus-alcaligenes,[4] Fleming's bacillus,[5] and the bacillus of Adamson and Cutler [6] may be identical or at least closely related forms.

The microbe, as the name suggests, exhibits the morphology of Bacillus tetani. It differs from B. tetani, however, in that no soluble toxin is demonstrable in cultures in any medium. Aside from the resemblance of B. pseudotetani to the true toxin producing B. tetani, it has no distinctive characteristics. The strain studied as B. pseudotetani was obtained by Dr. Holman in England.

It exhibits the characteristics described and agrees with the generally accepted description of the organism which it is supposed to represent in being practically without action on gelatin or other protein, and in inducing a gaseous fermentation in glucose. In addition a few gas bubbles evolve in a plain, cooked meat medium, which becomes somewhat red in color. A small amount of gas is evolved in all mediums. The volume, however, except in glucose cultures, is detectable but insignificant as indicating a true saccharine fermentation.

The nitrogenous changes induced in the ordinary mediums by B. pseudotetani are of moderate intensity. There is a slight, steady increase in the ammonia content of the mediums, amounting finally, after 2 weeks' incubation, to about 30 mg. per 100 c c of culture medium above that of the controls. Like B. tetani,[7] the amino-nitrogen decreases in amount as the ammonia increases. This is especially the case during the earlier days of incubation when the birth-rate of the organisms is very high. Later, when the products of metabolism slow

1 Report 39, 1919.
2 Report 12, 1917.
3 Centralbl. f. Bakteriol., 1898, 23, p. 538.
4 Centralbl. f. Bakteriol., I, O., 1912, 62, p. 229.
5 Lancet, 1915, 2, p. 376.
6 Lancet, 1917, 1, p. 688.
7 Kendall, Day and Walker: Study XLVIII, Jour. Infect. Dis., 1922, 30, p. 170.

TABLE 1

BACILLUS PSEUDOTETANI

	Day	Plain				Gelatin				Glucose			
		Reaction	Ammonia Nitrogen	Amino Nitrogen	Percentage Ammonia to Total Nitrogen	Reaction	Ammonia Nitrogen	Amino Nitrogen	Percentage Ammonia to Total Nitrogen	Reaction	Ammonia Nitrogen	Amino Nitrogen	Percentage Ammonia to Total Nitrogen
Control......	..	—0.90	14.7	35.0	5.53	—0.60	16.1	35.7	2.53	—0.50	14.0	32.2	5.26
Culture A....	1	+0.20	16.8	25.2	6.32	+0.10	14.7	36.4	2.31	+2.50	14.0	23.8	5.26
	3	+0.60	23.1	27.3	8.68	+0.20	15.4	37.1	2.42	+3.30	14.0	23.8	5.26
	6	+0.70	25.2	29.4	9.48	+0.40	19.6	35.7	3.07	+3.90	14.0	26.6	5.26
	13	+0.70	28.0	33.6	10.5	+0.50	21.0	37.1	3.29	+3.10	16.1	25.9	6.06
	21	+0.70	31.5	32.9	11.8	+0.60	21.7	40.6	3.41	+2.70	17.5	34.3	6.58

	Day	Mannitol				Glycerol				Lactose			
		Reaction	Ammonia Nitrogen	Amino Nitrogen	Percentage Ammonia to Total Nitrogen	Reaction	Ammonia Nitrogen	Amino Nitrogen	Percentage Ammonia to Total Nitrogen	Reaction	Ammonia Nitrogen	Amino Nitrogen	Percentage Ammonia to Total Nitrogen
Control......	..	—0.90	14.0	33.6	5.26	—0.90	14.0	35.0	5.26	—0.90	14.0	33.6	5.26
Culture A....	1	+0.50	14.7	27.3	5.53	+0.30	16.8	22.4	6.32	+0.60	16.1	23.1	6.06
	3	+0.60	16.1	25.9	6.06	+1.80	18.2	23.8	6.84	+0.70	21.7	20.3	8.16
	6	+0.70	22.4	28.0	8.43	+2.60	21.0	28.0	7.90	+0.70	23.1	25.9	8.68
	13	+0.60	26.6	29.4	10.0	+2.40	24.5	28.7	9.22	+0.80	26.6	32.2	10.0
	21	+0.60	23.8	32.2	8.96	+2.00	25.2	36.4	9.48	+0.90	26.6	32.2	10.0

	Day	Saccharose				Starch				Milk			
		Reaction	Ammonia Nitrogen	Amino Nitrogen	Percentage Ammonia to Total Nitrogen	Reaction	Ammonia Nitrogen	Amino Nitrogen	Percentage Ammonia to Total Nitrogen	Reaction	Ammonia Nitrogen	Amino Nitrogen	Percentage Ammonia to Total Nitrogen
Control......	..	—0.90	14.0	34.3	5.23	—0.90	14.7	35.0	5.53	+1.50	6.3	18.9	1.36
Culture A....	1	+0.30	16.8	23.1	6.32	+0.50	16.8	26.6	6.32	+1.60	6.3	18.9	1.36
	3	+0.60	20.3	23.8	7.63	+0.70	22.4	25.2	8.42	+1.90	7.7	18.9	1.63
	6	+0.70	23.1	23.8	8.68	+0.70	23.1	28.7	8.68	+1.80	7.7	20.3	1.66
	13	+0.60	25.9	28.0	9.74	+0.60	26.6	29.4	10.0	+2.00	7.7	21.7	1.66
	21	+0.80	30.1	33.6	11.3	+0.90	28.7	31.5	10.7	+2.20	8.4	23.1	1.81

Reaction: — = alkaline to neutral red; + = acid to neutral red; c c normal acid or alkali per 100 c c of medium.
Ammonia and amino nitrogen expressed in milligrams per 100 c c of culture medium.
Control indicates initial composition of medium. Net results may be obtained by subtracting the control from the day's analysis.
Amino nitrogen is corrected in each instance for ammonia.

up the reproductive process, the amino-nitrogen tends to increase somewhat, approaching finally in amount that of the uninoculated controls.

The total nitrogenous change, however, is so slight in comparison to the total nitrogenous content of the mediums that the pseudotetanus bacillus can hardly be classed as one of the proteophilic group.

Gelatin is not softened, even after prolonged incubation, and the nitrogenous changes in this medium are scarcely greater than those of plain, nutrient broth in which the amount of protein nitrogen is scarcely 20% as great. No evidences of a soluble, proteolytic enzyme were obtained. The only carbohydrate that was fermented was glucose. The analytic table shows the sharp rise in titratable acidity associated with the fermentation of this hexose sugar. A decided increase in acidity with an evolution of some gas was observed in glycerol. Glycerol, however, did not stimulate the rate or volume of gas formation in a marked degree, as did glucose. Indeed, the amount of gas observed in glycerol cultures was not greatly in excess of that formed in the other mediums not containing glucose.

B. pseudotetani, therefore, appears to be an anaerobic bacillus, exhibiting the morphology of B. tetani, but devoid of toxicogenic powers. The organism is culturally quite inert. It is without noteworthy proteolytic powers, and it is nearly devoid of fermentative powers, as well. Glucose (and maltose) appear to be the only carbohydrates which B. pseudotetani can utilize for energy. The principal significance of the microbe lies in its remarkable resemblance to B. tetani, and its possibility of occurrence in associations in which B. tetani would be sought for as a matter of routine.

BACILLUS BOTULINUS

STUDY L

Bacillus botulinus does not appear to have been isolated from infected wounds of warfare; as a majority of strains grow rather poorly at body temperature, it is not improbable that the microbe may be disregarded as an incitant of gunshot wound infections. The organism is a formidable toxin producer, although leading apparently a saprophytic existence; therefore it is to be regarded as one of the dangerous anaerobic bacteria. B. botulinus, as von Ermengem, its discoverer, showed many years ago,[1] forms a soluble toxin under appropriate con-

[1] Centralbl. f. Bakteriol., 1896, 19, p. 442; Ztschr. f. Hyg. u. Infektionskr., 1897, 26, p. 1.

TABLE 1

BACILLUS BOTULINUS

	Day	Plain: Reaction	Plain: Ammonia Nitrogen	Plain: Amino Nitrogen	Plain: Percentage Ammonia to Total Nitrogen	Gelatin: Reaction	Gelatin: Ammonia Nitrogen	Gelatin: Amino Nitrogen	Gelatin: Percentage Ammonia to Total Nitrogen	Glucose: Reaction	Glucose: Ammonia Nitrogen	Glucose: Amino Nitrogen	Glucose: Percentage Ammonia to Total Nitrogen
Control......	..	−0.60	5.6	19.6	3.33	−0.60	7.0	44.1	0.77	−0.30	5.6	16.8	3.33
Culture A....	1	−0.60	5.6	22.4	3.33	−0.30	5.6	38.5	0.62	+0.80	7.0	24.5	4.16
	3	−0.40	21.0	14.7	12.5	−0.10	15.4	42.0	1.69	+1.50	10.5	25.9	6.25
	6	−0.30	28.0	25.9	16.6	+0.20	33.6	45.5	3.69	+1.90	12.6	28.7	7.50
	13	−0.20	32.9	27.3	19.5	+0.60	38.5	59.5	4.23	+2.10	14.7	28.7	8.75
	21	−0.20	33.6	25.9	20.0	+0.70	37.1	56.0	4.08	+2.00	14.0	26.6	8.33
Control......	..	−0.60	5.6	19.6	3.33	−0.60	7.0	44.1	0.77	−0.30	5.6	16.8	3.33
Culture B....	1	−0.60	5.6	19.6	3.33	−0.50	6.3	36.4	0.69	+0.60	3.5	17.5	2.08
	3	−0.50	6.3	21.0	3.75	−0.30	15.4	42.0	1.69	+1.40	8.4	20.3	5.00
	6	−0.20	20.3	30.1	12.0	−0.10	28.0	49.7	3.07	+1.90	11.2	22.4	6.66
	13	−0.10	27.3	31.2	16.2	+0.20	34.5	56.0	3.77	+2.20	13.3	24.5	7.92
	20	−0.10	35.0	25.9	20.8	+0.40	39.2	56.7	3.21	+2.30	14.7	25.2	8.75
Control......	..	−0.60	3.5	18.9	1.92	−0.50	4.2	39.2	0.47	−0.10	3.5	17.5	1.92
Culture C....	1	−0.40	9.1	15.4	5.00	−0.30	4.9	33.6	0.55	+0.30	4.2	18.2	2.30
	3	−0.30	8.4	17.5	4.63	+0.10	16.1	39.9	1.81	+1.10	7.7	21.7	4.23
	6	−0.10	18.2	23.1	10.0	+0.10	25.2	47.6	2.83	+1.60	14.0	25.2	7.69
	12	+0.10	24.5	26.6	13.4	+0.20	31.5	49.7	3.54	+2.10	16.1	28.0	8.85
Control......	..	−0.60	5.6	19.6	3.33	−0.60	7.0	44.1	0.77	−0.30	5.6	16.8	3.33
Culture D....	1	−0.50	7.7	17.5	4.58	−0.50	11.2	34.3	1.23	+1.10	4.9	24.5	2.91
	3	−0.40	15.4	21.7	9.16	−0.40	20.3	44.1	2.23	+1.40	9.8	19.6	5.81
	6	−0.10	25.2	23.1	19.1	−0.10	26.6	56.0	2.92	+1.80	9.8	19.6	5.81
	13	−0.20	33.6	23.8	20.0	+0.10	34.3	59.5	3.77	+2.20	16.1	17.5	9.05
	20	−0.10	35.0	23.8	20.8	+0.20	38.5	57.4	4.23	+2.00	16.8	16.8	10.0
Control......	..	−0.70	11.2	21.0	5.16	−0.70	11.2	36.4	1.63	−0.80	17.5	27.3	8.06
Culture E....	1	−0.50	14.0	19.6	6.45	−0.60	14.0	36.4	2.04	+1.80	18.9	24.5	8.72
	3	−0.40	18.9	18.9	8.72	−0.10	17.5	41.3	2.50	+2.00	19.6	28.0	9.03
	6	−0.20	23.1	22.4	10.6	+0.20	21.7	42.7	3.16	+2.30	21.7	26.6	10.0
	9	+0.10	29.4	29.4	13.5	+0.30	35.7	44.1	5.20	+2.50	22.3	26.6	10.3
	14	+0.20	29.4	32.2	13.5	+0.30	41.3	50.4	6.02	+2.40	21.7	26.6	10.0
Control......	..	−0.70	16.8	26.6	7.74	−0.70	14.0	42.0	1.92	−0.40	16.1	24.5	7.42
Culture F....	1	−0.50	19.6	25.9	9.03	−0.50	19.6	37.1	2.62	+1.80	11.9	26.6	5.48
	3	−0.20	27.3	28.7	12.5	−0.10	21.0	41.3	2.84	+2.20	17.5	30.8	8.06
	6	−0.00	29.4	26.6	13.5	+0.10	27.3	46.2	3.75	+2.40	18.2	32.9	8.39
	9	+0.20	32.2	28.7	14.8	+0.30	29.4	48.3	4.04	+2.50	18.9	27.3	8.72
	14	+0.20	35.0	30.8	16.1	+0.40	39.2	48.3	5.38	+2.70	19.6	28.0	9.03

	Day	Mannitol: Reaction	Mannitol: Ammonia Nitrogen	Mannitol: Amino Nitrogen	Mannitol: Percentage Ammonia to Total Nitrogen	Glycerol: Reaction	Glycerol: Ammonia Nitrogen	Glycerol: Amino Nitrogen	Glycerol: Percentage Ammonia to Total Nitrogen	Lactose: Reaction	Lactose: Ammonia Nitrogen	Lactose: Amino Nitrogen	Lactose: Percentage Ammonia to Total Nitrogen
Control......	..	−0.60	5.6	19.6	3.33	−0.50	5.6	19.6	3.33	−0.60	5.6	19.6	3.33
Culture A....	1	−0.50	7.7	21.0	4.58	−0.10	5.6	19.6	3.33	−0.60	9.1	20.3	5.41
	3	−0.30	18.2	16.8	10.8	+0.60	9.1	17 5	5.41	−0.40	21.0	13.3	12.5
	6	−0.20	27.3	21.0	16.2	+1.10	14.0	20.3	8.33	−0.30	25.2	23.8	15.0
	13	−0.10	35.0	22.4	20.8	+1.30	15.4	21.7	9.16	−0.10	32.9	24.5	19.5
	21	−0.20	37.1	24.5	22.1	+1.30	12.6	23.1	7.50	−0.10	37.1	23.8	22.1
Control......	..	−0.60	5.6	19.6	3.33	−0.50	5.6	19.6	3.33	−0.60	5.6	19.6	3.33
Culture B....	1	−0.60	7.7	20.3	4.58	−0.50	7.0	19.6	4.16	−0.50	4.2	19.6	2.50
	3	−0.30	17.5	17.5	10.4	+1.10	6.3	20.3	3.75	−0.40	16.8	21.7	10.0
	6	−0.10	31.5	21.0	18.7	+1.20	9.1	19.6	5.41	−0.10	23.5	20.3	24.0
	13	−0.10	35.7	21.7	21.2	+1.50	12.6	21.0	7.50	−0.00	33.6	21.7	20.0
	20	+0.10	37.1	21.7	22.1	+1.60	13.3	22.4	7.92	+0.10	35.0	20.3	20.8
Control......	..	−0.60	3.5	18.9	1.92	−0.60	3.5	18.9	1.92	−0.50	3.5	18.9	1.92
Culture C....	1	−0.50	6.3	14.0	3.46	−0.10	3.5	22.4	1.92	−0.40	8.4	21.7	4.63
	3	−0.30	12.6	19.6	6.92	+1.10	9.1	21.7	5.00	−0.10	15.4	20.3	8.46
	6	−0.10	29.4	20.3	16.1	+1.60	11.2	23.1	6.16	+0.10	24.5	24.5	13.4
	12	+0.20	35.7	23.1	19.6	+1.70	15.4	25.2	8.46	+0.10	31.5	29.4	17.3
Control......	..	−0.60	5.6	19.6	3.33	−0.50	5.6	19.6	3.33	−0.60	5.6	19.6	3.33
Culture D....	1	−0.50	8.4	19.6	5.00	−0.40	7.0	15.4	4.16	−0.40	10.5	12.6	6.25
	3	−0.30	17.5	17.5	10.4	+0.10	8.4	11.2	5.00	−0.30	16.8	19.6	10.0
	6	−0.10	24.5	18.2	14.5	+1.00	10.5	21.7	6.25	−0.10	22.4	23.8	13.3
	13	−0.10	35.0	22.4	20.8	+1.30	15.4	23.1	9.16	−0.10	28.7	21.7	17.0
	20	+0.10	37.1	24.5	23.4	+1.70	15.4	23.1	9.16	+0.20	30.8	23.8	18.3
Control......	..	−0.90	17.5	21.0	8.05	−0.60	17.5	24.5	8.05	−0.80	17.5	27.3	8.05
Culture E....	1	−0.80	17.5	18.9	8.05	−0.10	16.8	30.8	7.74	−0.50	15.4	17.5	7.10
	3	−0.50	22.4	19.6	10.3	+1.60	17.5	30.8	8.05	−0.40	23.1	16.8	10.6
	6	−0.30	27.3	21.0	12.5	+1.70	18.2	32.9	8.39	−0.30	25.2	16.8	11.6
	9	−0.20	32.2	22.4	14.8	+1.90	18.9	33.6	8.72	−0.20	29.4	21.0	13.5
	14	+0.10	31.5	24.5	14.5	+2.10	19.6	33.6	9.03	−0.20	30.8	27.3	14.2
Control......	..	−0.60	16.8	16.8	7.74	−0.60	16.8	25.2	7.74	−0.50	16.8	25.2	7.74
Culture F....	1	−0.40	19.6	14.0	9.03	+1.20	14.7	28.0	6.76	−0.30	16.1	21.7	7.42
	3	−0.30	20.3	15.4	9.35	+1.70	14.7	29.4	6.76	−0.20	21.0	21.7	9.68
	6	−0.30	25.2	17.5	11.6	+1.90	19.6	31.5	9.03	−0.10	25.2	22.4	11.6
	9	−0.30	29.4	19.6	13.5	+2.10	19.6	31.5	9.03	0.00	28.7	24.5	13.2
	14	−0.20	32.2	21.0	14.8	+2.20	21.7	31.5	10.0	+0.20	31.5	25.9	14.5

	Day	Saccharose: Reaction	Saccharose: Ammonia Nitrogen	Saccharose: Amino Nitrogen	Saccharose: Percentage Ammonia to Total Nitrogen	Starch: Reaction	Starch: Ammonia Nitrogen	Starch: Amino Nitrogen	Starch: Percentage Ammonia to Total Nitrogen	Milk: Reaction	Milk: Ammonia Nitrogen	Milk: Amino Nitrogen	Milk: Percentage Ammonia to Total Nitrogen
Control......	..	−0.60	5.6	19.6	3.33	−0.60	5.6	19.6	3.33	+1.40	8.4	16.8	1.66
Culture A....	1	−0.60	6.3	22.4	3.75	−0.60	5.6	19.6	3.33	+1.40	9.1	19.6	1.80
	3	−0.30	18.2	18.9	10.8	−0.40	18.2	18.9	10.8	+1.50	22.4	18.9	4.45
	6	−0.20	30.1	20.3	17.7	−0.20	19.6	19.6	11.6	+1.90	29.4	25.2	5.83
	13	−0.10	35.0	23.8	20.8	−0.20	31.5	23.8	18.2	+2.00	31.5	27.3	6.25
	21	−0.20	34.3	22.4	20.4	−0.10	32.2	25.2	19.1	+2.10	30.8	26.6	6.11
Control......	..	−0.60	5.6	19.6	3.33	−0.60	5.6	19.6	3.33	+1.40	8.4	16.8	1.66
Culture B....	1	−0.60	7.0	19.6	4.16	−0.60	5.6	19.6	3.33	+1.40	4.2	17.5	0.83
	3	−0.40	14.0	21.7	8.33	−0.40	12.6	18.9	7.50	+1.70	17.5	21.7	3.45
	6	−0.30	21.7	20.3	12.9	−0.20	19.6	23.1	5.41	+1.90	24.5	23.1	4.86
	13	−0.00	24.5	23.1	14.5	−0.10	22.4	27.3	13.3	+2.10	26.1	26.1	5.18
	20	−0.20	29.6	25.2	17.6	0.00	24.5	26.6	14.5	+2.00	28.7	28.7	5.69
Control......	..	−0.60	3.5	18.9	1.92	−0.60	3.5	18.9	1.92	+1.50	5.6	20.3	1.19
Culture C....	1	−0.50	5.6	18.9	3.07	−0.50	7.7	20.3	4.23	+1.60	7.7	22.4	1.64
	3	−0.20	17.5	21.7	9.62	−0.10	18.2	22.4	10.0	+1.60	16.8	27.3	3.58
	6	−0.00	25.2	26.6	13.8	+0.10	22.4	25.2	12.3	......	....	....	.....
	12	+0.10	30.8	27.3	16.9	+0.10	26.6	28.0	14.6	+1.90	27.3	29.4	5.82
Control......	..	−0.60	5.6	16.8	3.33	−0.60	5.6	19.6	3.33	+1.40	8.4	16.8	1.66
Culture D....	1	−0.30	9.1	18.2	5.42	−0.40	9.4	13.3	5.00	+1.20	8.4	18.2	1.66
	3	−0.10	13.3	16.8	7.92	−0.30	16.1	16.1	9.05	+1.50	11.2	16.8	2.22
	6	+0.10	19.6	21.7	11.6	−0.10	16.8	22.4	10.0	+1.80	11.2	21.7	2.22
	13	+0.20	25.2	22.4	15.0	+0.10	20.3	22.4	12.0	+1.90	16.8	22.4	3.33
	20	+0.20	28.7	23.8	17.0	+0.10	24.5	25.2	14.5	+2.20	20.2	27.3	4.03
Control......	..	−0.70	17.5	27.3	8.05	−0.60	17.5	27.3	8.05	+1.60	5.6	18.2	1.23
Culture E....	1	+1.20	18.2	25.9	8.39	−0.50	16.1	22.4	7.42	+1.80	6.3	18.9	1.38
	3	+1.60	19.6	25.9	9.03	−0.30	15.4	26.6	7.10	+2.10	18.2	20.3	4.00
	6	+1.90	22.4	34.3	10.3	−0.10	19.3	35.7	9.03	+2.10	19.6	21.0	4.31
	9	+2.20	21.0	34.3	9.68	+0.20	22.4	38.5	10.3	+2.40	21.0	23.1	4.61
	14	+2.30	21.0	34.3	9.68	+0.30	25.2	38.5	11.6	+2.30	21.7	26.6	4.55
Control......	..	−0.60	16.8	25.2	7.74	−0.60	16.8	25.2	7.74	+1.70	4.2	21.0	0.88
Culture F....	1	+1.80	16.1	26.6	7.42	−0.40	16.3	21.0	7.74	+1.70	4.2	21.0	0.88
	3	+2.00	16.1	27.3	7.42	−0.00	27.3	22.4	12.5	+1.80	4.9	20.3	1.02
	6	+2.10	20.3	27.3	9.36	0.00	29.4	26.6	13.5	+2.00	5.6	21.0	1.17
	9	+2.40	21.7	27.3	10.0	+0.10	33.6	27.3	15.5	+2.30	8.4	18.2	1.76
	14	+2.40	20.3	28.7	9.36	+0.10	33.6	28.0	15.5	+2.40	11.2	23.1	2.35

Reaction: — = alkaline to neutral red; + = acid to neutral red; c c normal acid or alkali per 100 c c of medium.
Ammonia and amino nitrogen expressed in milligrams per 100 c c of culture medium.
Control indicates initial composition of medium. Net results may be obtained by subtracting the control from the day's analysis.
Amino nitrogen is corrected in each instance for ammonia.

ditions which possesses the unique and deadly property of passing the gastro-intestinal tract of man and of animals unharmed. The ingestion of various foods, therefore, has from time to time given rise to single or multiple cases of botulism. As the toxin and not the bacillus is the causative agent of the poisoning, the organism must be sought for, if it is to be recovered, in infected food.[2]

As the organisms described as B. botulinus are recognized and identified chiefly through the ability to produce the soluble toxin which resists gastro-intestinal digestion, it is not surprising to find that the published descriptions are somewhat meager and varied. The original description [1] attributed proteolytic properties to B. botulinus, and these observations are concurred in up to the present time by many, if not a majority, of observers. Liquefaction of gelatin is described as one of the essential characteristics by the British Medical Committee.[3]

Cultures have been obtained, exhibiting the property of forming a digestion-resistant, soluble toxin, which are without marked proteolytic action on gelatin or other protein. Such cultures may frequently be isolated from supposedly pure strains of B. botulinus that induce liquefaction in gelatin after several days' incubation. In such cases the contaminating organism, present at the start in small numbers, gradually becomes prominent and induces a true liquefaction of the medium through the agency of soluble proteolytic enzyme.

Six cultures are studied here. All were purified as described in preceding studies.[4]

B. botulinus A was obtained from the Bureau of Animal Industry.
Culture B, from the same source.
Culture C, from a can of pimentoes.
Culture D, from Miss Nevin.
Culture E, from Dr. Karl Meyer.
Culture F, from Dr. Karl Meyer.

DISCUSSION

The nitrogenous changes observed in the metabolism of the 6 strains of B. botulinus [5] were approximately the same, quantitatively speaking, as those characteristic for cultures of B. tetani [6] in so far as

[2] Dickson: Monograph 8, Rockefeller Institute, 1918, contains references to literature to that date.
[3] Report 39, London, 1919.
[4] Kendall, Cook and Ryan: Jour. Infect. Dis., 1921, 29, p. 227.
[5] Toxin that kills guinea-pigs and is resistant to gastro-intestinal digestion was determined in each instance by soaking a crumb of bread in a 10-day culture and feeding it to the animal. The time required to kill varied from approximately 20 to 48 hours.
[6] Kendall, Day and Walker: Study XLVIII, Jour. Infect. Dis., 30, p. 170.

ammonia formation is concerned. The increases observed amount to about 30 or 40 mg. per 100 c c of medium, in those instances in which utilizable carbohydrate is not available as a source of energy. In other words, the strains of B. botulinus considered in this series are not proteophilic. Their action for energy on protein or protein derivatives is comparatively slight. This observation is in harmony with the rather general tendency of bacteria to incite moderate changes in protein, even though the observations are carried out for considerable periods of time.

The addition of utilizable carbohydrate to protein mediums reduces materially the amount of ammonia produced. This reduction amounts to 50% in most instances, or even more. Coincidently, a somewhat greater amount of titratable acidity is noticed. In all mediums, however, there is a moderate but definite increase in titratable acidity, and a slow, slight, but readily detectable evolution of gas takes place. This evolution of gas is more rapid and greater in amount in mediums containing utilizable carbohydrate.

The fermentation reactions of B. botulinus are very much in doubt. Some observers claim no carbohydrates are fermented, while others attribute considerable versatility to B. botulinus with respect to its ability to utilize carbohydrate for energy. It seems to be generally conceded that glucose is fermented, and polymers of glucose—maltose and starch—also seem to be available sources of non-nitrogenous energy. Glycerol also is said by many observers to be fermented.

The Medical Research Committee [7] states that lactose but not saccharose is fermentable. While information on this point that is wholly satisfactory is not at present available, it may be stated as a somewhat general observation that bacteria which are not parasitic on man or animals frequently fail to utilize lactose, which, it will be remembered, is an animal sugar.

The cultures studied here fermented glucose, maltose and glycerol consistently, although the evolution of gas was rather slow and the general process was relatively sluggish. Starch was slowly decomposed by cultures B and F. Lactose was not visibly attacked. Saccharose was slowly decomposed by cultures F and G. The toxicity of these strains was materially less than that of cultures A, B, C, and D.

The amino-nitrogen changes differed somewhat in type from those observed in cultures of B. tetani. The initial decrease of amino

[7] Report 39, 1919.

nitrogen, common to both organisms, was followed by a decided tendency toward an increase above that of the uninoculated controls in the botulinus cultures, as incubation proceeded. The actual change was never great, amounting to less than 40 mg. in 100 c c of medium. This change was less marked in mediums containing utilizable carbohydrate than in purely protein mediums. The significance to be attached to this slight quantitative difference between B. botulinus and B. tetani cannot be determined in such a limited series of cultures. In this respect, however, the entire field of anaerobic metabolism is yet to be developed.

The nitrogenous changes observed in gelatin and in milk were of the same order of magnitude as those occurring in the simpler protein mediums, such as plain nutrient bouillon. Gelatin was softened after prolonged incubation to a point where it would no longer solidify when placed for several hours at the temperature of the icebox (40 C.), but there was no evidence of a soluble proteolytic enzyme in gelatin cultures, and it appears probable that the action of the organism on protein is relatively limited. It will be remembered that the same phenomenon of softening in gelatin cultures was observed in cultures of the Welch bacillus,[8] and the same explanation is offered for the phenomenon exhibited by B. botulinus as that advanced for the corresponding change induced by the Welch bacillus.

SUMMARY

The strains of B. botulinus studied in this series formed varying amounts of toxin which are resistant to gastro-intestinal digestion.

The fermentation reactions were somewhat variable. Generally speaking, glucose and the polymers of glucose—maltose and starch—appear to be rather more acceptable sources of non-nitrogenous energy than lactose. Saccharose was slowly fermented by two strains. Glycerol was fermented slowly by all.

Some gas was produced even in protein mediums, and the quantitative difference in gas production and gas volume between purely protein and protein-carbohydrate mediums is not great. Considerable caution is required, therefore, in the interpretation of fermentation reactions (gas production) in cultures of B. botulinus.

The nitrogenous changes induced by B. botulinus in protein mediums are relatively insignificant. The organism cannot be classed as a proteophilic anaerobe. Culturally B. botulinus is chemically relatively inert.

[8] Kendall, Day and Walker: Study XLIV, Jour. Infect. Dis., 1922, 30, p. 141.

BACILLUS BIFERMENTANS

STUDY LI

Bacillus bifermentans (Bacillus bifermentans-sporogenes) was described originally by Tissier and Martelly [1] as an anaerobic bacillus exhibiting both carbohydrophilic and proteophilic properties. The organism has been cultured from infected wounds of warfare by Tissier [2] and by Hemple.[3]

The organism fails to exhibit any striking or noteworthy morphologic, serologic or toxicologic features; the changes it induces in culture mediums are quite sharply defined, but not vigorous. One rather definite cultural characteristic is the gradual accumulation of a mucinous deposit in cultures containing utilizable carbohydrate. Small amounts of gas bubbles are slowly evolved from all ordinary cultural mediums. The rate of formation of this gas, and the volume, however, are small. This ability to produce a small amount of gas from cultural mediums, even those containing no carbohydrates, is a rather general one exhibited by nearly all anaerobic bacilli. The origin of the gas, its composition, and its significance, are yet to be determined. The phenomenon is of real importance in connection with gas production from utilizable carbohydrates by anaerobes, however, because the question of fermentability of non-nitrogenous compounds with the liberation of gas is a cultural procedure of diagnostic importance in this group. Elaborate controls must be made to distinguish between the small volume of fundamental gas common to all mediums from the additional evolution of gas from utilizable carbohydrates. Usually the phenomenon is most confusing when determinations are made in small volumes, such as "shake cultures" or Smith fermentation tubes. When larger volumes of mediums—100 c c or more—are studied, the fundamental gas volume becomes less difficult of evaluation because of the larger proportionate accumulation of gaseous products from the decomposition of significant amounts of sugars or their derivatives.

The fermentation reactions accredited to B. bifermentans comprise the gaseous fermentation of glucose, levulose, and maltose.[4] From these acid is produced, and gas is slowly evolved. Tissier and Martelly [1]

[1] Ann. Inst. Past., 1902, 16, p. 865.
[2] Ibid., 1916, 30, p. 681.
[3] Jour. Hygiene, 1918, 17, p. 13 (Organism No. 2).
[4] Weinberg and Séguin, La Gangrène Gazeuse, 1917.

speak of a fermentation of glycerol as well, acid alone being produced. Gelatin and other enriched protein mediums are rather deeply decomposed.

Two cultures are studied in this series:

B. bifermentans A, from Miss Hemple.

B. bifermentans B, from Miss Hemple.

They were typical morphologically, and they induced a slow, but definite gaseous fermentation in glucose, maltose and glycerol. The volume of gas was smaller in glycerol than that observed in the sugar mediums. Gelatin was liquefied, and a soluble proteolytic enzyme was obtained from filtrates of the gelatin cultures which would induce liquefaction in a solution of gelatin in 0.5% phenol solution. In such a medium the bacteria of course could not grow. Consequently, there was no increase in ammonia. The amino-nitrogen content of the medium, however, increased somewhat, indicating a gradual breaking of the protein tie in the gelatin molecule with a coincident liberation of free NH_2 groups as mono-amino acids, and as polypeptids of varying degrees of complexity. As the amino-acid content of gelatin cultures decreased during bacterial growth while it increased in the carbol gelatin containing the soluble enzyme of the organism but no live bacteria, it would appear that the amino acids and polypeptids formed as a result of the cleavage of the protein molecule were utilized as sources of energy by the microbes. It will be noticed in the analytic table that the amino nitrogen of cultures containing no utilizable carbohydrate shows a moderate but definite decrease as a result of bacterial development with a concomitant formation of ammonia. In mediums containing utilizable carbohydrate—glycerol and glucose—on the contrary, the amino nitrogen does not undergo a diminution, and the concomitant ammonia formation is proportionately lessened.

This phenomenon is another manifestation of the sparing action of utilizable carbohydrate for protein as a source of energy for bacteria. In milk, in spite of the fact that the lactose is not apparently utilizable for the microbes, there is an increase in titratable acidity and a moderate increase in amino nitrogen formation. It would seem probable that a part of this carbohydrate type of reaction is due to the small but definite amount of glucose in the milk. Available evidence suggests also that B. bifermentans is able to effect a cleavage of fats, and the subsequent fermentation of glycerol resulting therefrom is possibly a factor in the accumulation of acid.

TABLE 1

BACILLUS BIFERMENTANS

	Day	Plain				Gelatin				Glucose			
		Reaction	Ammonia Nitrogen	Amino Nitrogen	Percentage Ammonia to Total Nitrogen	Reaction	Ammonia Nitrogen	Amino Nitrogen	Percentage Ammonia to Total Nitrogen	Reaction	Ammonia Nitrogen	Amino Nitrogen	Percentage Ammonia to Total Nitrogen
Control......	..	—0.60	10.5	27.5	3.95	—0.40	7.0	30.8	1.19	0.00	10.5	27.3	3.95
Culture A....	1	+0.40	39.2	20.3	14.7	+0.50	22.4	25.2	3.52	+2.00	14.0	31.5	5.26
	3	+0.90	65.1	19.6	24.4	+0.80	36.4	24.5	5.70	+2.40	18.2	29.4	6.84
	6	+1.10	66.5	19.6	25.0	+1.00	53.2	23.1	8.35	+2.50	18.9	31.5	7.10
	13	+1.10	75.1	20.3	28.2	+1.40	76.3	25.9	11.9	+3.00	19.6	31.5	7.37
	20	+0.90	71.4	21.7	26.8	+1.20	56.7	26.6	8.91	+2.80	21.7	32.9	8.16
Control......	..	—0.70	11.9	27.3	4.25	—0.80	7.7	28.7	1.14	—0.20	11.9	23.1	4.25
Culture 2.....	1	+0.30	35.7	19.6	12.7	—0.80	8.4	29.4	1.25	+1.80	11.9	30.8	4.25
	3	+0.50	50.4	18.9	18.0	+0.10	36.4	25.9	5.42	+2.20	16.1	28.7	5.75
	6	+0.90	58.1	19.6	20.7	+0.70	59.2	25.9	8.53	+2.70	16.8	29.4	6.00
	13	+0.90	58.1	19.6	20.7	+0.80	95.2	24.5	14.1	+2.80	14.0	30.1	5.00
	20	+0.90	65.1	20.3	23.2	+0.70	94.5	23.1	14.0	+2.70	18.9	29.4	6.75

	Day	Mannitol				Glycerol				Lactose			
		Reaction	Ammonia Nitrogen	Amino Nitrogen	Percentage Ammonia to Total Nitrogen	Reaction	Ammonia Nitrogen	Amino Nitrogen	Percentage Ammonia to Total Nitrogen	Reaction	Ammonia Nitrogen	Amino Nitrogen	Percentage Ammonia to Total Nitrogen
Control......	..	—0.60	10.5	27.3	3.95	—0.60	10.5	27.3	3.95	—0.60	10.5	27.3	3.95
Culture A....	1	+0.70	35.0	21.0	13.1	+2.50	16.8	31.5	6.32	+0.40	31.5	23.8	11.8
	3	+0.90	58.1	19.6	21.8	+3.10	18.2	32.9	6.84	+1.00	56.0	19.6	21.0
	6	+1.10	67.2	18.9	25.2	+3.20	18.2	34.3	6.84	+1.20	65.8	18.9	24.7
	13	+1.10	67.9	19.6	25.5	+3.10	18.2	31.5	6.84	+1.20	70.7	20.3	26.5
	20	+1.00	68.6	20.3	25.7	+2.90	18.9	31.5	7.10	+1.00	63.0	19.6	23.7
Control......	..	—0.70	11.9	27.3	4.25	—0.70	11.9	27.3	4.25	—0.70	11.9	25.9	4.25
Culture 2.....	1	—0.30	35.0	18.9	12.5	+1.50	9.8	31.5	3.50	+0.40	28.7	18.9	10.2
	3	0.00	57.4	20.3	20.5	+2.10	14.7	36.4	5.25	+0.70	42.0	19.6	15.0
	6	+0.50	57.4	21.7	20.5	+2.60	14.7	36.4	5.25	+0.90	52.5	21.0	18.7
	13	+1.20	63.7	22.4	22.7	+2.60	16.1	35.0	5.75	+1.10	61.6	19.6	22.0
	20	+1.20	65.8	23.1	23.5	+2.70	21.7	34.3	7.75	+1.10	64.4	21.7	23.0

	Day	Saccharose				Starch				Milk			
		Reaction	Ammonia Nitrogen	Amino Nitrogen	Percentage Ammonia to Total Nitrogen	Reaction	Ammonia Nitrogen	Amino Nitrogen	Percentage Ammonia to Total Nitrogen	Reaction	Ammonia Nitrogen	Amino Nitrogen	Percentage Ammonia to Total Nitrogen
Control......	..	—0.60	10.5	27.3	3.95	—0.60	10.5	27.3	3.95	+1.60	7.0	22.4	1.53
Culture A....	1	+0.40	39.2	19.6	14.7	+0.80	51.1	14.0	19.2	+1.60	7.0	22.4	1.53
	3	+1.10	58.1	18.9	21.8	+1.10	67.2	16.1	25.2	+2.60	80.5	39.9	17.6
	6	+1.10	59.5	20.3	22.3	+1.30	71.4	16.1	26.8	+2.70	114.1	53.9	25.0
	13	+1.10	66.5	21.0	25.0	+1.20	79.8	18.9	30.0	+2.50	126.0	56.0	27.7
	20	+1.10	71.4	21.7	26.8	+1.00	71.9	19.6	27.0	+2.60	141.4	58.8	31.0
Control......	..	—0.70	11.9	27.3	4.25	—0.70	11.9	27.3	4.25	+1.20	4.9	21.7	1.03
Culture 2.....	1	+0.40	37.8	20.3	13.5	+0.50	31.5	20.3	11.2	+2.00	18.9	28.0	3.97
	3	+0.70	49.7	21.0	17.7	+0.80	56.7	19.6	20.2	+2.30	113.4	51.8	23.8
	6	+0.90	59.5	22.4	21.2	+1.40	63.7	17.5	22.7	+2.50	133.0	43.4	27.9
	13	+1.30	65.1	22.4	23.2	+1.10	66.5	21.0	23.7	+2.70	143.5	39.9	30.1
	20	+1.20	70.0	23.1	25.0	+1.10	70.7	21.7	25.5	+2.80	152.6	38.3	32.0

Reaction: — = alkaline to neutral red; + = acid to neutral red; c c normal acid or alkali per 100 c c of medium.
Ammonia and amino nitrogen expressed in milligrams per 100 c c of culture medium.
Control indicates initial composition of medium. Net results may be obtained by subtracting the control from the day's analysis
Amino nitrogen is corrected in each instance for ammonia.

The titratable acidity of all mediums increases, and some gas is evolved. The increase in titratable acidity in glucose and glycerol mediums, which are fermentable by B. bifermentans, are, however, marked and unmistakable.

SUMMARY

B. bifermentans is an anaerobic bacillus exhibiting, as its name suggests, both carbohydrophilic and proteophilic characteristics.

The former are indicated by a gaseous fermentation of glucose and glycerol with the concomitant development of acid and the production of a mucinous substance which accumulates in these cultures.

The proteophilic properties are manifested by the formation of a soluble gelatin-liquefying enzyme which possesses the property of cleaving the gelatin molecule with the gradual liberation of NH_2 groups, which are detectable and measurable by the method of formol titration.

BACILLUS OEDEMATIENS

STUDY LII

Bacillus oedematiens was isolated from several cases of gas gangrene by Weinberg and Séguin [1] early in the war. It was soon discovered that the organism produces a soluble poison, formed during the first 2 days of growth, which will kill guinea-pigs within 48 hours, as a rule. This soluble poison, like that of the Welch bacillus and Vibrion septique, loses its potency on prolonged incubation. It would appear, therefore, that the poison is a substance formed incidental to the growth of the organism rather than a toxin produced as a result of the utilization of protein for energy by the organism.[2]

B. oedematiens appears to be very similar to, or identical with Novy's B. oedematis maligni II.[3] Weinberg and Séguin [4] also suggest a possible identity of their organism with Costa and Troisier's "Bacillus Neigeux," [5] and with Aschoff's "Gas oedema bacillus." [6] The organism has been isolated by a number of investigators from the bacterial flora of infected wounds, and as it has been recovered from the soil, it is

1 Compt. rend. Soc. biol., 1915, 78, p. 274, p. 507.
2 Kendall, Day and Walker: Study XLIV, Jour. Infect. Dis., 1922, 30, p. 141.
3 Ztschr. f. Hyg. u. Infektionskr., 1894, 17, p. 209.
4 La Gangrène Gazeuse, 1917.
5 Compt. rend. Soc. biol., 1915, 78, p. 352.
6 Veröffentl. a. d. Geb. d. Mil. Sanitätswesens, 1918, 68, p. 1.

not surprising to find Bacillus oedematiens among the microbes of infected gunshot wounds.

Morphologically, B. oedematiens resembles the Welch bacillus rather closely. On the whole, it is longer and the ends are usually more rounded, however. The shorter individuals observed in rapidly growing cultures, when segmentation is taking place rapidly, may, however, appear more nearly oblong. The ends of such organisms are more nearly square cut, and at this stage of development it would be difficult indeed to distinguish the microbe from the gas bacillus (Bacillus welchii). The spores of B. oedematiens occur at one end of a bacillary rod, or, more accurately, the residual bacillary substances project from one pole of the spore, which is oval and greater in diameter than the parent cell. The mature spore with its adherent parental cell resembles a tennis racquet quite closely. The Welch bacillus spore, although somewhat greater in diameter than the parent cell, is usually central or subterminal. The spore bacillary rod complex in this instance consists of a fragment of bacillary substance at each end of the oval, distended spore. B. oedematiens sporulates much more readily than Bacillus welchii. Weinberg and Séguin[4] state that the former will produce mature spores even in glucose-containing mediums. The cultures identified and discussed as B. oedematiens in this study failed to form spores in mediums containing utilizable sugars; at least, spores were not observed under these conditions, although search was made for them.

Culturally, B. oedematiens is not very distinctive. Weinberg and Séguin[4] state that gas and acid are produced in mediums containing glucose, levulose and maltose. Henry[7] states that starch and xylose are also fermented. The cultures described in the following failed to ferment starch. Xylose was not investigated.

Wolf[8] has studied the metabolism of B. oedematiens in peptone solution, glucose peptone solution, milk, and the cooked meat medium. His experiments show that the organism produces considerably less nitrogenous change in a simple peptone medium than in the cooked meat medium, containing much more highly complex protein. This is indicated both by the greater amount of ammonia formed, and by the accumulation of amino nitrogen. The addition of glucose to peptone solution clearly spares the protein constituents of the medium, shown both by a lessened ammonia formation and amino nitrogen content.

[7] Jour. Path. & Bacteriol., 1916, 21, p. 344.
[8] Ibid., 1919, 23, p. 254.

	Day	Plain: Reaction	Plain: Ammonia Nitrogen	Plain: Amino Nitrogen	Plain: Percentage Ammonia to Total Nitrogen	Gelatin: Reaction	Gelatin: Ammonia Nitrogen	Gelatin: Amino Nitrogen	Gelatin: Percentage Ammonia to Total Nitrogen	Glucose: Reaction	Glucose: Ammonia Nitrogen	Glucose: Amino Nitrogen	Glucose: Percentage Ammonia to Total Nitrogen
Control......	..	-0.60	3.5	23.1	1.78	-0.50	3.5	39.9	0.39	-0.20	3.5	18.9	1.78
Culture A....	1	+0.20	6.3	18.9	3.21	+0.50	12.6	43.4	1.41	+1.40	5.6	22.4	2.85
	3	+0.20	23.1	24.5	11.7	+0.80	37.8	56.7	4.50	+1.40	9.1	23.1	4.64
	6	+0.40	26.8	25.2	13.6	+1.20	46.2	63.0	5.20	+1.70	11.9	23.1	6.07
	13	+0.50	42.0	25.2	21.4	+1.50	54.6	61.6	6.11	+1.40	12.6	21.7	6.42
Control......	..	-0.50	3.5	23.1	2.08	-0.70	4.2	46.2	0.44	-0.20	3.5	21.7	2.08
Culture B....	1	+0.10	8.4	16.1	5.00	+0.70	14.7	41.3	1.54	+1.10	8.4	25.2	5.00
	3	+0.20	27.3	21.0	16.2	+1.00	30.8	63.0	3.23	+1.60	10.5	26.6	6.22
	6	+0.40	31.5	22.4	18.7	+1.30	44.8	68.6	4.71	+1.50	12.6	25.2	7.50
	13	+0.30	38.5	27.3	21.9	+1.60	56.0	65.8	5.88	+1.50	15.4	25.2	9.17
	21	.....	....	....	.....	+1.50	55.3	64.4	5.79	+1.30	16.8	23.8	10.0
Control......	..	-0.60	3.5	23.1	1.78	-0.50	3.5	39.9	0.39	-0.20	3.5	18.9	1.78
Culture C....	1	+0.10	6.3	22.4	3.21	+0.30	16.8	35.0	0.89	+0.80	9.8	23.1	5.00
	3	+0.30	28.7	21.0	14.6	+1.20	39.2	49.0	4.41	+1.20	11.2	24.5	5.77
	6	+0.30	34.3	23.1	17.4	+1.80	47.6	63.7	5.35	+1.60	12.6	24.5	6.42
	13	+0.30	45.5	23.8	23.2	+1.60	57.4	64.4	6.46	+1.70	17.5	28.0	8.93
	20	+0.30	46.2	25.2	23.5	+1.70	59.5	62.3	6.59	+1.50	18.9	22.4	9.63
Control......	..	-0.50	3.5	23.1	1.85	-0.80	4.9	44.1	0.54	-0.20	3.5	21.7	1.85
Culture D....	1	-0.10	14.7	22.4	7.82	+1.10	10.5	37.8	1.16	+1.20	10.5	22.4	5.56
	3	+0.20	28.0	16.8	14.8	+1.00	41.3	56.0	4.57	+1.60	12.6	23.1	6.67
	6	+0.30	34.3	25.9	18.1	+1.80	45.5	53.2	5.04	+1.40	14.0	27.3	7.41
	13	+0.20	41.3	27.3	21.8	+1.80	58.8	67.9	6.51	+1.20	16.8	22.4	8.90
	21	+0.20	43.4	26.6	22.9	+2.00	61.6	66.5	6.80	+1.20	16.1	22.4	8.52
Control......	..	-0.50	3.5	23.1	1.85	-0.80	4.9	44.1	0.54	-0.20	3.5	21.7	1.85
Culture E....	1	+0.10	16.1	19.6	8.53	+0.10	10.5	43.4	1.16	+1.00	6.3	21.0	3.33
	3	+0.20	39.2	18.9	20.7	+1.30	39.2	56.0	4.24	+1.60	7.7	23.8	4.07
	6	+0.30	42.0	23.1	22.2	+1.70	45.5	59.5	5.04	+1.40	13.3	23.8	7.04
	13	+0.30	43.4	22.4	22.9	+1.90	63.0	64.4	6.47	+1.40	18.9	22.4	10.0
	21	+0.20	44.1	23.1	23.3	+1.90	66.5	66.5	7.36	+1.00	20.3	21.0	10.7
Control......	..	-0.50	3.5	23.1	1.85	-0.80	4.9	44.1	0.54	-0.20	3.5	21.7	1.85
Culture F....	1	0.00	15.4	19.6	8.15	+0.70	14.7	34.3	1.63	+1.00	5.6	25.2	2.96
	3	+0.30	23.8	25.2	12.5	+1.40	29.4	54.6	3.26	+1.00	7.7	23.1	4.07
	6	+0.40	35.0	28.0	18.5	+1.60	54.6	68.6	6.04	+1.20	9.8	22.4	5.18
	13	+0.40	45.5	28.0	24.0	+2.00	61.6	71.3	6.82	+1.30	10.5	23.1	5.56
	21	+0.40	46.9	29.4	24.8	+2.00	63.0	68.6	6.47	+1.20	12.6	24.5	6.67

	Day	Mannitol: Reaction	Mannitol: Ammonia Nitrogen	Mannitol: Amino Nitrogen	Mannitol: Percentage Ammonia to Total Nitrogen	Glycerol: Reaction	Glycerol: Ammonia Nitrogen	Glycerol: Amino Nitrogen	Glycerol: Percentage Ammonia to Total Nitrogen	Lactose: Reaction	Lactose: Ammonia Nitrogen	Lactose: Amino Nitrogen	Lactose: Percentage Ammonia to Total Nitrogen
Control......	..	-0.60	3.5	21.7	1.78	-0.40	2.8	22.4	1.42	-0.50	3.5	21.7	1.78
Culture A....	1	+0.20	5.6	18.2	2.85	+1.00	10.5	24.5	5.34	+0.20	8.4	19.6	4.28
	3	+0.20	16.8	20.3	8.58	+1.00	14.7	25.2	7.50	+0.20	12.6	20.3	6.42
	6	+0.30	25.2	21.7	12.8	+1.20	15.4	29.4	7.86	+0.40	31.5	21.0	16.0
	13	+0.30	34.3	23.8	17.5	+1.20	16.8	28.7	8.57	+0.40	39.9	23.8	20.3
Control......	..	-0.50	3.5	23.1	2.08	-0.50	3.5	23.1	2.08	-0.50	3.5	23.1	2.08
Culture B....	1	+0.10	7.7	18.9	4.57	+0.10	7.7	16.8	4.57	+0.20	8.4	17.5	5.00
	3	+0.20	23.8	23.8	14.1	+0.40	24.5	23.8	14.5	+0.20	23.1	18.2	13.7
	6	+0.40	35.0	22.4	20.8	+0.90	27.3	26.6	16.2	+0.40	28.7	20.3	17.0
	13	+0.20	37.8	28.7	22.5	+1.10	33.6	82.9	20.0	+0.30	36.4	23.8	21.6
	21	+0.20	41.3	29.4	24.5	+1.00	36.4	35.0	21.6	+0.20	39.9	24.5	23.7
Control......	..	-0.60	3.5	21.7	1.78	-0.40	2.8	22.4	1.42	-0.50	3.5	21.7	1.78
Culture C....	1	-0.60	9.1	18.9	4.64	+0.10	5.6	16.8	2.85	+0.10	16.8	16.1	8.58
	3	+0.10	19.6	20.3	10.0	+0.90	5.6	22.4	2.85	+0.10	22.4	19.6	11.4
	6	+0.30	26.6	25.2	13.5	+0.90	13.3	22.4	6.79	+0.20	33.6	16.8	17.1
	13	+0.30	35.7	25.2	18.2	+0.90	14.7	22.4	7.50	+0.20	32.2	18.9	16.4
	20	+0.20	37.8	25.9	19.2	+0.90	15.4	29.4	7.75	+0.10	32.2	23.8	16.4
Control......	..	-0.40	3.5	23.1	1.78	-0.40	3.5	23.1	1.85	-0.40	3.5	23.1	1.85
Culture D....	1	-0.10	6.3	22.4	4.64	+0.80	12.6	24.5	6.67	+0.40	14.7	18.2	7.82
	3	+0.20	18.2	19.6	10.0	+1.40	14.7	26.6	7.82	+0.30	24.5	15.4	12.9
	6	+0.20	22.4	25.9	13.5	+1.20	17.2	28.0	9.10	+0.40	27.3	20.3	14.4
	13	+0.20	30.8	21.7	18.2	+1.00	21.7	27.3	11.4	+0.20	31.5	21.7	16.6
	21	+0.10	34.3	23.1	19.2	+1.20	21.0	29.4	11.1	+0.20	33.6	26.6	17.7
Control......	..	-0.40	3.5	23.1	1.85	-0.40	3.5	23.1	1.85	-0.40	3.5	23.1	1.85
Culture E....	1	-0.40	8.4	23.1	4.44	+0.90	11.9	25.2	6.29	+0.50	27.3	16.1	14.4
	3	+0.20	39.9	21.0	21.1	+1.00	14.7	28.7	7.77	+0.20	14.7	19.6	7.77
	6	+0.40	41.3	28.0	21.8	+1.00	16.8	32.2	8.89	+0.60	36.4	21.0	19.2
	13	+0.40	46.8	25.9	24.7	+1.10	22.4	28.7	11.8	+0.60	38.5	27.3	20.3
	21	+0.40	47.5	27.3	25.1	+1.10	23.1	27.3	12.2	+0.50	39.2	29.4	20.7
Control......	..	-0.40	3.5	23.1	1.85	-0.40	3.5	23.1	1.85	-0.40	3.5	23.1	1.85
Culture F....	1	+0.10	19.6	19.6	10.3	+1.00	11.9	26.6	6.30	+0.30	22.4	16.8	11.8
	3	+0.40	25.9	23.1	13.7	+1.20	10.5	24.5	5.56	+0.10	11.2	18.9	5.92
	6	+0.40	34.3	25.2	18.1	+1.40	11.9	22.4	6.30	+0.40	37.1	21.0	19.6
	13	+0.50	42.0	24.5	22.2	+1.70	11.9	22.4	6.30	+0.30	45.5	21.7	24.0
	21	.....	....	....	.....	+1.60	11.9	23.8	6.30	+0.40	43.4	28.0	23.1

	Day	Saccharose: Reaction	Saccharose: Ammonia Nitrogen	Saccharose: Amino Nitrogen	Saccharose: Percentage Ammonia to Total Nitrogen	Starch: Reaction	Starch: Ammonia Nitrogen	Starch: Amino Nitrogen	Starch: Percentage Ammonia to Total Nitrogen	Milk: Reaction	Milk: Ammonia Nitrogen	Milk: Amino Nitrogen	Milk: Percentage Ammonia to Total Nitrogen
Control......	..	-0.60	3.5	21.7	1.78	-0.60	3.5	21.7	1.78	+1.20	4.9	22.4	1.06
Culture A....	1	+0.20	5.6	17.5	2.85	+0.20	7.7	23.1	3.93	+1.70	14.0	24.5	3.03
	3	+0.20	20.3	16.1	10.3	+0.30	18.9	26.6	9.63	+2.30	29.4	28.0	6.33
	6	+0.20	27.3	20.3	13.9	+0.30	23.8	29.4	12.1	+2.00	33.6	31.5	7.23
	13	+0.30	35.0	21.7	17.8	+0.20	31.5	26.6	16.0	+1.90	42.0	42.0	9.09
Control......	..	-0.40	3.5	23.1	2.08	-0.40	3.5	21.7	2.08	+1.10	4.2	22.4	0.88
Culture B....	1	+0.10	10.5	16.1	6.22	+0.20	11.2	17.5	6.67	+1.80	9.8	21.0	2.05
	3	+0.20	21.7	18.9	12.3	+0.30	28.0	19.6	16.6	+2.40	31.5	26.6	6.62
	6	+0.40	32.2	23.8	19.1	+0.60	35.7	20.3	21.2	+2.50	36.4	28.7	7.65
	13	+0.30	36.4	25.2	21.6	+0.40	38.5	24.5	21.9	+2.30	45.5	35.0	9.35
	21	+0.50	37.8	25.2	22.5	+0.30	41.3	27.3	24.5	+2.00	48.3	39.2	10.1
Control......	..	-0.60	3.5	21.7	1.78	-0.60	3.5	21.7	1.78	+1.20	4.9	22.4	1.06
Culture C....	1	+0.10	14.7	18.9	7.50	+0.10	16.1	16.8	8.21	+1.50	7.0	20.3	1.51
	3	+0.10	21.7	18.9	11.0	+0.10	24.5	22.4	12.5	+2.60	37.8	28.0	8.18
	6	+0.30	33.6	16.1	17.1	+0.30	33.6	18.9	17.1	+2.70	42.0	26.6	9.09
	13	+0.30	35.7	20.3	18.2	+0.30	35.7	20.3	18.2	+2.60	45.5	32.2	9.85
	20	+0.40	35.7	23.8	18.2	+0.30	36.4	19.6	18.5	+2.60	46.2	34.3	10.0
Control......	..	-0.50	3.5	23.1	1.85	-0.40	3.5	23.1	1.85	+1.40	7.7	23.1	1.46
Culture D....	1	+0.10	14.7	21.0	7.82	-0.40	8.4	24.6	4.44	+1.60	14.7	21.7	2.80
	3	+0.30	26.6	21.7	14.0	+0.20	18.9	17.5	10.0	+2.40	27.3	26.6	5.20
	6	+0.50	31.5	25.2	16.6	+0.40	30.8	20.3	16.3	+2.60	35.7	28.0	6.80
	13	+0.40	39.9	23.1	21.1	+0.30	33.6	22.4	17.7	+2.60	42.7	33.6	8.13
	21	+0.40	39.9	25.2	21.1	+0.30	37.8	25.2	19.9	+2.60	45.5	41.3	8.67
Control......	..	-0.50	3.5	23.1	1.85	-0.40	3.5	23.1	1.85	+1.40	7.7	23.1	1.46
Culture E....	1	+0.50	25.2	22.4	13.3	+0.10	16.8	17.5	8.89	+1.80	9.8	23.8	1.86
	3	+0.20	12.6	20.3	6.67	+0.50	28.0	23.8	14.8	+1.90	13.3	26.6	2.53
	6	+0.70	34.3	24.5	18.1	+0.60	31.5	22.4	16.6	+2.10	41.3	31.6	7.87
	13	+0.50	38.5	21.7	20.3	+0.60	35.0	23.8	18.5	+2.10	45.5	35.7	8.67
	21	+0.50	37.8	24.5	20.0	+0.70	35.7	28.7	18.8	+2.30	49.0	42.7	9.34
Control......	..	-0.50	3.5	23.1	1.85	-0.40	3.5	23.1	1.85	+1.40	7.7	23.1	1.46
Culture F....	1	+0.30	25.9	23.1	13.7	+0.10	15.4	18.2	8.15	+1.50	14.0	21.7	2.66
	3	+0.10	13.3	18.2	7.04	+0.20	21.7	21.7	11.3	+2.40	21.7	28.7	4.13
	6	+0.30	34.3	25.2	18.1	+0.40	30.1	22.4	15.9	+2.60	37.8	36.4	7.20
	13	+0.30	44.1	23.8	23.3	+0.40	40.6	21.7	21.4	+2.40	43.4	43.4	8.27
	21	+0.20	46.2	27.3	24.4	.....	....	....	.....	+2.20	39.2	43.4	7.47

Reaction: — = alkaline to neutral red; + = acid to neutral red; c c normal acid or alkali per 100 c c of medium.
Ammonia and amino nitrogen expressed in milligrams per 100 c c of culture medium.
Control indicates initial composition of medium. Net results may be obtained by subtracting the control from the day's analysis.
Amino nitrogen is corrected in each instance for ammonia.

Milk was fermented, according to Wolf's observations. His conclusions are that B. oedematiens exhibits both saccharolytic and proteolytic characteristics, the former greatly predominating. He notes, however, that "large quantities of gas are produced in cooked meat mediums containing no free carbohydrates. Notable quantities of amino acids and ammonia may be formed."

ORIGIN OF CULTURES

B. oedematiens A—From intestinal contents.

B. oedematiens B—From National Research Council.

B. oedematiens C—Culture incorrectly named Bacillus chauvœi.

B. oedematiens D—Culture incorrectly named Bacillus welchii.

B. oedematiens E—Culture incorrectly named Bacillus of Malignant oedema.

B. oedematiens F—Culture from National Research Council.

DISCUSSION

Milk is slowly changed by the growth of B. oedematiens. The reaction becomes acid, more rapidly with some strains, distinctly less rapidly with others. There is a tendency for the acid reaction to recede during the later days of incubation, although the reaction never reaches the initial titer. The casein is usually precipitated slowly, but the evidence of digestion of the clot is usually wanting. The reaction in reaction (see analytic table) appears to be associated with a gradual increase in the amount of ammonia formed as a result of the intracellular utilization of the protein constituents of the milk. There is some evidence of a parallelism between the development of acid in milk and in glycerol mediums. In both instances, the reaction becomes somewhat greater than in corresponding mediums not containing utilizable carbohydrate. Also, the amount of amino nitrogen detectable in cultures of the organism in milk and glycerol is greater than that found in other mediums, except gelatin. The suggestion is made that glycerol is slowly utilized as a source of energy with the liberation of acid substances which in turn give rise to the somewhat greater titratable acidity of these mediums. There appears to be justification for it in light of the quantitative differences in amino nitrogen and titratable acidity observed in these cultures. They do not seem to be accidental. This explanation is not without objections, however, and it is to be regarded as purely tentative.

The ammonia, except in glucose broth, is produced in moderate amounts which increase from day to day. The total accumulation is not very large, even on prolonged incubation, however. It is distinctly greater in mediums rich in complex nitrogenous substances, such as gelatin or milk, lesser in mediums containing protein derivatives of the order of peptones and polypeptids. It is perhaps to be expected that the evidences of intense, intracellular decomposition of protein would be lacking in cultures of B. oedematiens because the organism forms a soluble poison early in the growth of the culture. Intense proteolytic powers and toxin production appear to be incompatible.

In glucose broth, the amount of ammonia formed is distinctly less than in other corresponding mediums which do not contain a utilizable, non-nitrogenous source of energy. This is indicative of the sparing action of utilizable carbohydrate for protein.

The amino nitrogen detectable in the various mediums is moderate in amount, particularly with respect to those nutritive solutions whose nitrogenous constituents are peptones and polypeptids. A greater amino acid content is found in gelatin and milk cultures. The increase is suggestive of the greater suitability of complex protein for the energy requirements of the organisms. The greater amino-nitrogen content of glycerol and milk mediums has been discussed. In gelatin a considerable amount of amino nitrogen is characteristic of each of the six strains studied. The ammonia content of the medium is also greater than that of the others. Gelatin appears to be a suitable medium for the growth of B. oedematiens.

Acid is produced in all mediums irrespective of the nonprotein constituents; it is greater in peptone mediums containing glucose than in any other of the series studied. This is presumably due to the acid products arising from the utilization of the glucose for energy. The sparing action of the sugar for the protein is shown by the decrease in amino nitrogen in this medium in contrast to that of the mediums of the same nitrogenous composition but containing no utilizable non-nitrogenous source of energy. A similar but somewhat less intense action is observed in glycerol mediums, especially in cultures A, D, and F. Cultures B and C do not appear to be active fermenters of glycerol.

The chemical identification of B. oedematiens appears to be less precise than that of the purely fermentative or carbohydrophilic anaerobes. The organism exhibits moderate fermentative activities both with reference to its ability to utilize the commonly used sugars, and with respect to the intensity of the reaction induced in these carbohydrates. Also, its proteophilic qualities are moderate. There is no evidence of a rapid deep-seated degradation of protein, although gelatin and the proteins of milk are progressively decomposed with the formation of gradually increasing amounts of ammonia and a corresponding increase of amino nitrogen.

The recognition of B. oedematiens would appear to rest largely on its morphology and ability to produce a soluble poison. For confirmation, the rather negative chemistry of the organism in contrast to B. welchii and Vibrion septique, would be a feature of importance. The differentiation from Bacillus botulinus would hinge directly on the labile nature of the poison of Bacillus oedematiens in contrast to the cumulative development of soluble toxin in cultures of B. botulinus, as well as the resistance of the latter to gastro-intestinal digestion.

BACILLUS AEROFOETIDUS

STUDY LIII

Bacillus aerofoetidus was first described by Weinberg and Séguin [1] as Bacillus D. Later they conferred the name "aerofoetidus" on it. Henry [2] confirmed the occurrence of B. aerofoetidus in infected wounds of warfare, and redetermined and extended the fermentation reactions of the organism, previously made by McIntosh and Feldes,[3] that glucose, maltrose, and lactose were fermented with the production of considerable gas and acid by adding levulose and salicin to the list of non-nitrogenous sources of energy.

Weinberg and Séguin failed to detect spores in cultures of aerofoetidus, but Henry, and McIntosh and Feldes, found occasional spores which were subterminal, oval and apparently slightly greater in diameter than the parent bacterial cell. The cultures identified as B. aerofoetidus in the series reported in the following sporulated sparsely in mediums not containing utilizable carbohydrates.

The organism resembles B. fallax in its morphology, but it differs culturally in several particulars. The foul odor of protein cultures of B. aerofoetidus seems to have been one of the prominent qualitative features characteristic of the microbe, and it is to this factor that Weinberg and Séguin were led to formulate the specific name of the organism.

[1] Compt. rend. Soc. biol., 1916, 79, p. 116; La Gangrène Gazeuse, 1917.
[2] Henry: Jour. Path. & Bacteriol., 1916, 21, p. 367.
[3] Med. Res. Committee, Special Report Series 19, 1917.

TABLE 1

Bacillus Aerofoetidus

	Day	Plain: Reaction	Plain: Ammonia Nitrogen	Plain: Amino Nitrogen	Plain: Percentage Ammonia to Total Nitrogen	Gelatin: Reaction	Gelatin: Ammonia Nitrogen	Gelatin: Amino Nitrogen	Gelatin: Percentage Ammonia to Total Nitrogen	Glucose: Reaction	Glucose: Ammonia Nitrogen	Glucose: Amino Nitrogen	Glucose: Percentage Ammonia to Total Nitrogen
Control......	..	−0.70	13.3	25.9	5.59	−0.60	9.8	39.2	1.21	−0.40	12.6	25.2	5.30
Culture A....	1	+0.20	22.4	15.6	9.43	+0.20	27.3	25.2	3.39	+1.80	14.0	27.3	5.89
	3	+0.40	62.3	22.4	26.1	+1.50	97.3	31.5	12.1	+2.50	17.5	35.7	7.35
	6	+0.40	61.6	23.8	25.9	+1.80	145.6	32.9	18.1	+2.70	18.2	37.9	7.65
	13	+0.60	77.7	26.6	32.6	+2.00	219.6	39.9	27.3	+3.10	19.6	37.2	8.23
	20	+0.70	79.8	28.7	33.5	+1.90	224.7	44.8	27.9	+3.30	19.6	39.5	8.23
Control......	..	−0.20	13.3	25.9	5.59	−0.60	9.8	39.2	1.21	−0.80	12.6	25.2	5.30
Culture B....	1	+0.30	21.7	15.4	9.12	+0.10	22.4	31.5	2.78	+2.10	13.3	27.3	5.59
	3	+0.70	53.2	18.2	22.3	+1.60	78.4	36.4	9.75	+2.40	14.7	28.0	6.18
	7	+0.60	50.4	19.6	21.1	+2.00	117.6	42.7	14.6	+2.70	19.6	31.5	8.23
	13	+0.60	63.0	25.2	26.4	+2.20	218.4	44.8	27.1	+2.90	19.6	36.4	8.23
	20	+0.50	65.1	27.8	27.3	+2.10	226.1	47.6	28.1	+3.10	21.7	36.4	9.12

	Day	Mannitol: Reaction	Mannitol: Ammonia Nitrogen	Mannitol: Amino Nitrogen	Mannitol: Percentage Ammonia to Total Nitrogen	Glycerol: Reaction	Glycerol: Ammonia Nitrogen	Glycerol: Amino Nitrogen	Glycerol: Percentage Ammonia to Total Nitrogen	Lactose: Reaction	Lactose: Ammonia Nitrogen	Lactose: Amino Nitrogen	Lactose: Percentage Ammonia to Total Nitrogen
Control......	..	−0.70	11.9	25.9	5.00	−0.70	11.9	25.9	5.00	−0.60	11.2	25.2	4.71
Culture A....	1	+0.10	11.9	18.2	5.00	+0.50	13.3	23.8	5.59	+0.40	20.3	19.6	8.53
	3	+0.40	43.4	13.3	18.2	+1.40	40.6	23.1	17.0	+0.70	18.2	23.8	7.65
	6	+0.70	78.6	23.8	33.0	+1.40	51.8	20.3	21.7	+0.60	24.5	27.3	10.3
	13	+0.80	80.5	26.8	33.8	+1.80	68.6	20.3	28.7	+0.40	35.0	26.6	14.7
	20	+0.90	79.9	28.0	33.5	+1.90	67.2	21.7	28.2	+0.50	42.7	24.5	17.9
Control......	..	−0.70	11.9	25.9	5.00	−0.70	11.9	25.9	5.00	−0.60	11.2	25.2	4.71
Culture B....	1	−0.70	8.4	23.8	3.52	+0.10	21.0	17.5	8.83	+0.70	18.9	20.3	7.94
	3	−0.20	37.8	16.1	15.8	+0.80	37.8	25.9	15.8	+0.70	19.6	25.9	8.23
	7	+0.30	51.1	19.6	21.4	+1.40	50.4	23.1	21.1	+0.90	31.5	27.3	13.2
	13	+0.80	72.8	24.5	30.5	+1.40	60.2	23.8	25.2	+0.90	42.0	28.0	17.6
	20	+0.80	77.7	26.6	32.6	+1.80	69.3	30.8	29.1	+0.70	42.0	26.6	17.6

	Day	Saccharose: Reaction	Saccharose: Ammonia Nitrogen	Saccharose: Amino Nitrogen	Saccharose: Percentage Ammonia to Total Nitrogen	Starch: Reaction	Starch: Ammonia Nitrogen	Starch: Amino Nitrogen	Starch: Percentage Ammonia to Total Nitrogen	Milk: Reaction	Milk: Ammonia Nitrogen	Milk: Amino Nitrogen	Milk: Percentage Ammonia to Total Nitrogen
Control......	..	−0.70	11.9	25.9	5.00	−0.70	11.9	25.9	5.00	+1.10	3.5	21.7	0.75
Culture A....	1	+0.40	27.3	14.7	11.4	+0.40	21.0	16.8	8.83	+2.00	5.6	19.6	1.21
	3	+0.30	59.5	16.8	24.9	+0.70	53.9	18.9	22.6	+2.40	18.9	20.3	4.09
	6	+0.50	65.1	19.6	27.3	+0.80	79.1	22.4	33.2	+2.80	56.7	28.7	12.2
	13	+0.60	85.4	21.7	35.8	+0.90	81.9	24.5	34.4	+2.90	64.4	31.5	13.9
	20	+0.50	85.4	26.6	35.8	+0.70	84.0	27.5	35.2	+3.10	68.5	35.7	14.8
Control......	..	−0.70	11.9	25.9	5.00	−0.70	11.9	25.9	5.00	+1.10	3.5	21.7	0.75
Culture B....	1	+0.50	23.1	14.7	9.72	+0.10	20.3	15.4	8.53	+1.80	6.3	21.0	1.36
	3	+0.50	46.2	16.8	19.4	+0.50	44.8	18.2	18.8	+2.10	25.9	23.1	5.60
	7	+0.40	49.0	20.3	20.5	+0.90	55.3	21.0	23.2	+2.80	54.6	30.1	11.8
	13	+0.70	72.8	22.4	30.5	+0.70	65.8	25.2	17.6	+2.90	65.8	35.7	14.2
	20	+0.80	70.0	27.3	29.4	+0.60	64.4	27.3	17.0	+2.90	67.9	34.3	14.7

Reaction: − = alkaline to neutral red; + = acid to neutral red; c c normal acid or alkali per 100 c c of medium.
Ammonia and amino nitrogen expressed in milligrams per 100 c c of culture medium.
Control indicates initial composition of medium. Net results may be obtained by subtracting the control from the day's analysis.
Amino nitrogen is corrected in each instance for ammonia.

Culturally, B. aerofoetidus is of the saccharo-proteolytic type—it ferments some of the more commonly used carbohydrates with the production of considerable acid and gas, and it is a moderately proteoclastic organism as well, producing a soluble proteolytic enzyme which will effect the liquefaction of gelatin in the absence of the microbes.

Origin of Cultures.—Culture B. aerofoetidus "A" was obtained from Dr. Holman. It came originally from Paris.

Culture B. aerofoetidus "B" was obtained from the National Research Council. It is said to have been isolated from an infected wound.

DISCUSSION

The nitrogenous changes induced by B. aerofoetidus in mediums containing peptone and meat extractives as the source of nitrogen are characterized by a considerable liberation of ammonia. The addition of utilizable carbohydrate (glucose) effects a decided reduction in the amount of this substance formed, suggesting a sparing action of the non-nitrogenous source of energy for the protein. At the same time the fermentative activities of B. aerofoetidus do not appear to be as marked in mediums containing utilizable protein as those corresponding for B. welchii and the Vibrion septique, which are carbohydrophilic rather than proteolytic in their activities. It appears to be a rather general characteristic of bacteria which produce soluble proteolytic enzymes to effect a deeper cleavage of the protein molecule even in the presence of utilizable carbohydrate than occurs with the less actively proteolytic types.

B. proteus, for example, forms relatively more ammonia (greater deamination) when it utilizes protein for energy than does B. coli under similar circumstances, and B. coli in turn forms more ammonia under like conditions than B. diphtheriae. It will be remembered that B. proteus is more proteophilic than B. coli; and B. coli in turn effects a deeper degradation of protein than B. diphtheriae. Vigorous decomposition of protein is incompatible, apparently, with toxicogenesis. B. aerofoetidus partakes of the proteophilic type. In gelatin the amount of ammonia formed is relatively large, amounting to a material proportion of the total nitrogen of the medium. Culture A is rather more active in this respect than culture B.[4]

[4] Slight variations in the intensity of proteolysis even in the same kind of microbe are common. Cultures of B. proteus are noteworthy in this regard. The older division of proteus bacilli into B. proteus-vulgaris, micrabilis, zenkeri and zopfii in a descending scale of proteolytic activity was based on the qualitative proteolytic powers of current strains of the proteus bacillus. It is now surmised that the four "species" are naturally occurring variants of the same organism, which tends to lose its exuberant proteolytic powers on prolonged cultivation in cultural mediums.

Cultures of B. aerofoetidus exhibit a decided reduction in the amount of amino nitrogen in mediums containing no utilizable carbohydrate during the first days of growth. Even in gelatin, in which ammonia formation (deamination) proceeds with relatively great rapidity, this phenomenon is clearly discernible. In mediums containing utilizable carbohydrate, on the contrary, such as glucose and lactose broths and in milk (which of course contains lactose) the amino nitrogen increases during incubation. That this phenomenon is associated with the sparing action of carbohydrate for protein would appear to be almost certain.

The reaction (titratable acidity) becomes progressively acid even in nonsaccharine mediums, but in mediums containing utilizable carbohydrates the acidity increases more rapidly and reaches a greater concentration than is the case in corresponding mediums containing no utilizable sugars.

B. aerofoetidus, to summarize, appears to be an organism whose primary action is proteolytic. Certain carbohydrates—such as glucose and lactose—can be utilized by it for energy, thereby reducing noticeably the attack on protein. The organism would appear to be best classified as being of the proteophilic anaerobic bacilli.

BACILLUS SPOROGENES

STUDY LIV

Bacillus sporogenes, or that group of organisms which resembles this type of proteophilic microbe very closely, was first isolated from the intestinal contents and described by Metchnikoff.[1] In reality, Metchnikoff described two organisms, differing somewhat in morphology and in colony formation. One of these, which he called type A, was pictured as a rather slender rod, sometimes occurring in short chains, with subterminal spores. The other, called type B, was said to be stouter with centrally placed spores. The bacilli were studied chemically by Berthelot.[2] It was stated that both type A and B fermented glucose, galactose, maltose, lactose, and the alcohol mannitol; saccharose and starch were unfermented. McIntosh and Feldes[3] also described two anaerobic bacilli, one of which (No. XI) was identified

[1] Ann. Inst. Past., 1908, 22, p. 929.
[2] Ibid., 1909, 23, p. 85.
[3] Med. Res. Committee, Special Report 12, 1917.

by them as B. sporogenes. A second, unidentified bacillus with central spores (No. XII) exhibited quantitative rather than qualitative differences from their No. XI. They state, however, that the two are serologically unlike. Donaldson's "Reading bacillus" [4] (used by him to remove necrotic tissue from infected wounds, due to its soluble proteoclastic enzyme) is also in all probability a member of the B. sporogenes group.[5] The great problem confronting investigators of anaerobic bacteria is not that of obtaining cultures of B. sporogenes, however; it is to keep this organism out of cultural mediums and stock cultures of other anaerobes. The microbe is widely disseminated in nature, it forms resistant spores, and the most disagreeable and characteristic feature of all is its ability to grow in association with almost all other anaerobes as an unrecognized contaminant. Such "pure mixed cultures" containing unrecognized B. sporogenes in strains of B. welchii, Vibrion septique, B. chauvœi, B. tetani,[6] that organism called "Bacillus putrificus," B. botulinus and B. fallax, are fruitful sources of controversy. Of these cultures of the fermentative type of anaerobic bacilli, those first named are more commonly infected with B. sporogenes as an impurity. From the standpoint of the metabolism of anaerobic bacilli, it may be stated dogmatically that any culture containing living bacteria which shows little proteolysis for a week or 10 days followed by a sudden and noteworthy jump in the chemical evidences of proteolysis is contaminated with B. sporogenes, or somewhat less commonly, another of the proteophilic anaerobic bacilli.

In addition to the chemical observations of Berthelot,[2] Wolf and Harris [5, 7] have studied the metabolism of a strain of B. sporogenes, obtained from Henry.[8] Observations were made in various mediums, including milk and peptone broth. In milk they found a moderate and deliberate evolution of gas, gradually increasing in volume for 5 days At the end of that period the amount of gas evolved was equal in amount to a third, or even a half, the original volume of milk. The gas was mainly CO_2 and H_2 in the proportion of about $\frac{CO_2}{H_2} = 2/1$. A striking feature of the reaction was a progressive increase in titratable acidity, as the incubation was protracted. The previous statements of reaction in milk were almost unanimously indicative of an alkaline

[4] Jour. Path. & Bacteriol., 1918, 22, p. 129.

[5] Harris: Jour. Path. & Bacteriol., 1919, 23, p. 30.

[6] Donaldson (footnote 4) states that B. sporogenes destroys, or at least reduces, the potency of tetanus toxin as a result of its growth in mediums containing the toxin.

[7] Jour. Path. & Bacteriol., 1916, 21, p. 386.

[8] Ibid., p. 359.

change. The cultures studied in the following series are in accord with this increase in titratable acidity.

Wolf and Harris found also that the ammonia production was considerable; in this respect, B. sporogenes stands in marked contrast to the fermentative type of organisms, as for example, B. welchii.

The amino nitrogen also was found to be greatly increased; it amounted, according to the figures presented, to more than twice that of the ammonia increase. In plain peptone mediums, on the contrary, a distinct loss of amino nitrogen occurred. Wolf and Harris,[5, 7] in discussing the formation of gas in milk, make the statement that "Bacillus sporogenes possesses a ferment which hydrolyzes this sugar (lactose) to glucose and galactose." As the fermentation of glucose and lactose solutions (glucose and lactose bouillon) were apparently not tried out in the experiments recorded, the evidence for this statement is based exclusively on a slight increase in reducing power of the milk cultures after incubation, as shown by the Fehling test. Approximately the same volume of gas was obtained by them from alkaline casein solution; therefore, it would not seem necessary to bring in a cleavage of lactose to explain the evolution of gas in milk or protein solutions. As a matter of fact, B. sporogenes seems to possess the ability to generate gas in any protein solution, provided a sufficient amount of the cultural medium is inoculated to detect the gas. Amounts less than 100 c c are unsuited for this purpose.

The salient features of Wolf and Harris' study of B. sporogenes indicate that the organism is an energetic deaminizer of protein (or protein derivatives) and that in mediums relatively rich in protein, such as milk or alkaline casein, a considerable increase in amino nitrogen takes place. In mediums containing less highly organized nitrogen, such as peptone solution, an actual deficit in amino nitrogen occurs. Berthelot [2] called attention to the deep-seated changes B. sporogenes induces in protein, and Donaldson [4] demonstrated the presence of a soluble proteolytic enzyme. Wolf and Harris state: Ammonia was formed in such large quantity that it more than balanced the original amino-acids present in the medium. There is therefore a very vigorous deamination taking place, with an effort to keep the concentration of amino-acids up to the original level. Only one other explanation would be possible, namely, that bacteria attacked higher complexes and degraded them directly to ammonia, a type of reaction for which we have no analogy in higher metabolism." It appears reasonable to explain the relationship between ammonia formation and amino-nitro-

TABLE 1

BACILLUS SPOROGENES

	Day	Plain: Reaction	Plain: Ammonia Nitrogen	Plain: Amino Nitrogen	Plain: Percentage Ammonia to Total Nitrogen	Gelatin: Reaction	Gelatin: Ammonia Nitrogen	Gelatin: Amino Nitrogen	Gelatin: Percentage Ammonia to Total Nitrogen	Glucose: Reaction	Glucose: Ammonia Nitrogen	Glucose: Amino Nitrogen	Glucose: Percentage Ammonia to Total Nitrogen
Control	..	-0.60	22.4	29.4	6.28	-0.40	22.4	32.2	3.09	-0.20	22.4	28.0	6.28
Culture A	1	+1.00	36.0	20.3	15.6	+1.70	47.6	26.6	7.82	+3.00	18.2	28.0	5.10
	3	+2.00	110.6	21.0	30.9	+2.60	119.0	26.6	19.5	+4.50	37.1	21.7	10.4
	6	+2.30	128.8	25.2	36.0	+3.00	151.9	28.7	24.9	+3.90	56.0	35.0	15.6
	13	+2.40	147.0	33.6	41.1	+3.70	174.3	45.5	28.1	+3.50	70.7	35.7	19.7
	20	+2.20	147.7	38.5	41.3	+3.20	196.0	43.4	32.1	+3.40	78.4	36.4	21.9
Control	..	-0.90	29.4	35.0	10.5	-0.60	16.1	35.7	2.52	-0.50	29.4	32.2	10.5
Culture B	1	+1.70	60.9	38.5	21.7	+2.50	78.4	29.4	12.3	+3.10	32.2	30.8	11.5
	3	+2.10	95.9	28.7	34.2	+3.80	149.1	30.8	23.4	+3.70	32.9	30.1	11.7
	6	+2.50	109.9	27.3	39.2	+4.60	182.0	33.6	28.5	+3.60	54.6	37.8	19.5
	13	+2.30	113.4	30.8	40.5	+4.20	258.3	42.0	41.1	+3.50	72.8	49.7	26.0
	20	+2.20	117.6	33.6	42.0	+3.90	309.4	42.7	48.6	+3.60	73.5	53.2	26.2

	Day	Mannitol: Reaction	Mannitol: Ammonia Nitrogen	Mannitol: Amino Nitrogen	Mannitol: Percentage Ammonia to Total Nitrogen	Glycerol: Reaction	Glycerol: Ammonia Nitrogen	Glycerol: Amino Nitrogen	Glycerol: Percentage Ammonia to Total Nitrogen	Lactose: Reaction	Lactose: Ammonia Nitrogen	Lactose: Amino Nitrogen	Lactose: Percentage Ammonia to Total Nitrogen
Control	..	-0.50	22.4	29.4	6.28	-0.50	22.4	29.4	6.28	-0.50	22.4	28.0	6.28
Culture A	1	+1.10	56.0	19.6	15.6	+3.00	19.6	25.2	5.48	+1.10	49.0	21.7	13.7
	3	+1.70	111.3	20.3	31.1	+3.60	22.4	29.4	6.28	+1.90	101.5	23.1	28.4
	6	+2.00	122.5	24.5	34.3	+3.90	32.2	35.0	9.0	+1.90	123.9	21.7	34.7
	13	+2.30	142.1	25.9	39.8	+2.70	35.0	34.3	9.82	+2.20	135.1	25.2	37.8
	20	+2.30	142.1	31.5	39.8	+2.40	50.4	32.2	14.1	+1.80	135.8	30.8	38.0
Control	..	-0.90	30.8	33.6	11.0	-0.90	29.4	35.0	10.5	-0.90	28.0	33.6	10.0
Culture B	1	+1.70	55.3	39.9	29.7	+2.90	27.3	31.5	9.75	+1.80	64.4	30.1	23.0
	3	+2.30	91.0	36.4	32.5	+3.60	30.8	32.2	11.0	+2.10	91.0	32.2	32.5
	6	+2.30	106.4	37.8	38.0	+3.80	40.6	35.7	14.5	+2.40	105.7	35.0	37.7
	13	+2.30	121.4	39.2	43.2	+3.40	41.3	37.8	14.7	+2.10	113.4	35.7	40.5
	20	+2.30	119.0	34.3	42.5	+3.30	39.2	38.5	14.0	+2.20	119.7	38.5	42.7

	Day	Saccharose: Reaction	Saccharose: Ammonia Nitrogen	Saccharose: Amino Nitrogen	Saccharose: Percentage Ammonia to Total Nitrogen	Starch: Reaction	Starch: Ammonia Nitrogen	Starch: Amino Nitrogen	Starch: Percentage Ammonia to Total Nitrogen	Milk: Reaction	Milk: Ammonia Nitrogen	Milk: Amino Nitrogen	Milk: Percentage Ammonia to Total Nitrogen
Control	..	-0.50	22.4	29.4	6.28	-0.50	22.4	29.4	6.28	+1.50	7.0	19.6	1.51
Culture A	1	+1.00	57.4	21.0	16.0	+0.80	35.0	18.2	9.82	+1.80	14.0	22.4	3.03
	3	+2.10	98.7	21.0	27.6	+2.00	105.7	18.9	29.6	+3.20	101.5	27.3	21.9
	6	+2.30	118.7	23.1	33.2	+1.90	122.5	19.6	34.3	+3.40	131.6	30.8	28.4
	13	+2.70	128.1	24.5	35.8	+2.20	145.6	24.5	40.8	+3.40	149.1	41.3	32.2
	20	+2.80	192.5	29.4	53.9	+2.00	145.6	30.8	40.8	+3.40	158.2	46.2	34.2
Control	..	-0.90	30.1	28.0	10.7	-0.90	29.4	35.0	10.5	+1.50	6.3	18.9	1.36
Culture B	1	+2.10	71.4	25.2	25.5	+2.10	75.6	26.6	27.0	+1.60	9.1	18.9	1.96
	3	+2.40	105.7	37.1	37.7	+2.10	88.2	39.2	31.5	+2.50	116.9	28.7	25.3
	6	+2.70	114.8	41.3	41.0	+2.40	107.8	38.5	38.5	+3.20	135.8	39.2	29.4
	13	+2.70	112.0	40.6	40.0	+2.40	122.5	42.7	43.7	+3.40	150.5	45.5	32.5
	20	+2.70	119.7	39.2	42.7	+2.10	133.0	43.4	47.5	+3.40	160.5	46.9	34.7

Reaction: — = alkaline to neutral red; + = acid to neutral red; c c normal acid or alkali per 100 c c of medium.
Ammonia and amino nitrogen expressed in milligrams per 100 c c of culture medium.
Control indicates initial composition of medium. Net results may be obtained by subtracting the control from the day's analysis.
Amino nitrogen is corrected in each instance for ammonia.

gen content of the mediums, on the probable effect of the proteoclastic enzyme of B. sporogenes. This cleaves the protein molecule to amino-acids, or polypeptids, thus continually renewing, as it were, the supply of amino-acids utilizable for energy. This supply of amino-acids is continuously deaminized (but at an unknown rate), and the results would be those obtained by Wolf and Harris in mediums rich in protein. In protein-poor mediums, such as peptone water, the supply of cleavable protein is much less, and consequently the deaminizing power is presumably greater in proportion, and an actual deficit in amino-acids below that of the uninoculated controls results.

Origin of Cultures.—Two cultures were studied in this series, A and B. Culture A was isolated from feces. Culture B was a contaminant obtained from an impure strain of the organism of symptomatic anthrax (B. chauvœi). Both cultures fermented glucose and maltose with the production of gas. Lactose, saccharose, starch and mannitol were not fermented with the formation of gas above that of nonsaccharine mediums.

It should be stated that a slow, gradual evolution of gas was observed in plain peptone bouillon, a somewhat greater liberation in mediums rich in protein, such as gelatin and milk. The reaction in glycerol became strongly acid, and although the gaseous evolution was not materially greater than that observed in plain broth, nevertheless the impression gained was that the organisms utilized glycerol as a non-nitrogenous source of energy. Organisms of the general type of B. sporogenes are difficult to classify with respect to their fermentation reactions, because the liberation of gas and development of progressive titratable acidity occur with moderate intensity in nonfermentation mediums. The excess of gas and acid in true fermentation mediums is measurable only by rigid comparison.

Both cultures contained a soluble, proteolytic enzyme which effected a fairly rapid cleavage of gelatin (carbol gelatin) in the absence of bacteria. This soluble enzyme is probably the most distinctive chemical characteristic of the organism. It appears early in the incubation of the medium, and it acts with considerable rapidity.

DISCUSSION

The analytic statistics of the metabolism of the two cultures of B. sporogenes exhibit a feature of proteophilic bacteria which deserves passing comment. Culture A is distinctly more active in all its manifestations than Culture B, although the differences are quantitative rather than qualitative.[9]

In milk, the nitrogenous changes are on the whole quite similar in type to those observed by Wolf and Harris—a marked deamination, indicated by the steady increase in ammonia and the decided increase in amino nitrogen. The former—ammonia formation—indicates the intracellular utilization of nitrogenous protein derivatives by the microbes, and the latter suggests strongly the action of the soluble proteolytic enzyme, mentioned previously. The action of this enzyme affords a relatively simple explanation for the simultaneous development of the bacteria, the rapid formation of ammonia, and the ascending tendency of the amino-acid content of the medium in spite of the probable utilization of amino acids or amino acid complexes by the bacteria for their combined structural and energy requirements. The reaction, in terms of titratable acidity, becomes progressively acid. This is true qualitatively in all mediums, however. The reactions in gelatin are much the same.

In mediums containing peptone and meat extractives as sources of nitrogen the reactions were less intense. The amino acid residuum was smaller from day to day in mediums not containing glucose or glycerol than those in the corresponding uninoculated controls. In other words, the organisms reduced the content of amino acids in mediums not containing highly organized nitrogen, such as gelatin or milk. It will be remembered that Wolf and Harris found the same phenomenon in peptone water cultures.

In mediums containing glucose or glycerol, on the contrary, the amino nitrogen content was nearly stationary, or even a little above the uninoculated controls. At the same time, the rate and amount of ammonia formation was distinctly less than that found in corresponding mediums containing no utilizable carbohydrate. This is suggestive of a sparing action of the carbohydrate for protein.

SUMMARY

B. sporogenes is a striking example of the group of the proteophilic anaerobic bacilli. It forms a potent, soluble proteolytic enzyme, which effects a relatively rapid cleavage of proteins, and it utilizes protein for energy with the liberation of considerable amounts of ammonia. In

[9] Harris (footnote 5) has also found this same phenomenon in his careful studies of the "Reading bacillus" and B. sporogenes.

mediums rich in protein—gelatin and milk—the amino acid content increases materially in spite of the utilization of the products of protein cleavage for both the structural and energy requirements of the organisms. In mediums containing protein of the peptone type, however, the amino-nitrogen content diminishes incidentally to the growth of the organisms; the ammonia formation, however, is of about the same rate and intensity in either type of medium. The addition of utilizable, non-nitrogenous sources of energy, such as glucose or glycerol, reduces noticeably both the formation of ammonia and the utilization of amino acids for energy.

BACILLUS HISTOLYTICUS

STUDY LV

Bacillus histolyticus is a member of the plectridial group of anaerobic bacilli. It was isolated and its most characteristic property described by Weinberg and Séguin [1] in 1915. B. histolyticus derives its name from the remarkable proteolytic ability it possesses of liquefying injured or necrotic tissue.[2] Legros and Vaucher [3] have observed this digestive action in the tissues surrounding wounds of warfare, and Nicolas [4] has made similar observations in horses. Unlike B. sporogenes,[5] however, which dissolves injured tissue without serious results to the patient, the presence of B. histolyticus in infected wounds leads frequently to serious signs and symptoms of toxemia, which may result fatally. The pathogenicity of strains, however, varies considerably. The more virulent strains cause a progressive necrosis which may eventually become widespread. Weinberg and Séguin [6] have found a soluble poison which appears in cultures of the organism during the earlier hours of incubation in its greatest potency. In this respect the soluble poison resembles that of B. welchii and Vibrion septique, rather than the soluble toxins of B. tetani, B. botulinus, and the diphtheria bacillus, which are cumulative and apparently formed as a result of the utilization of protein derivatives for energy.

The cultural identification of B. histolyticus appears to be a subject of controversy. Apparently the tissue-liquefying properties of the

[1] Compt. rend. Soc. biol., 1915, 78, p. 274.
[2] Ibid., 1917, 80, p. 157.
[3] La Gangrène Gazeuse, 1917, p. 318.
[4] Ibid., p. 319.
[5] Donaldson: Jour. Path. & Bacteriol., 1918, 22, p. 129. Donaldson and Joyce. Lancet, 1917, 2, p. 445.
[6] La Gangrène Gazeuse, p. 171.

TABLE 1

BACILLUS HISTOLYTICUS

	Day	Plain				Gelatin				Glucose				Lactose				Saccharose				Milk			
		Reaction	Ammonia Nitrogen	Amino Nitrogen	Percentage Ammonia to Total Nitrogen	Reaction	Ammonia Nitrogen	Amino Nitrogen	Percentage Ammonia to Total Nitrogen	Reaction	Ammonia Nitrogen	Amino Nitrogen	Percentage Ammonia to Total Nitrogen	Reaction	Ammonia Nitrogen	Amino Nitrogen	Percentage Ammonia to Total Nitrogen	Reaction	Ammonia Nitrogen	Amino Nitrogen	Percentage Ammonia to Total Nitrogen	Reaction	Ammonia Nitrogen	Amino Nitrogen	Percentage Ammonia to Total Nitrogen
Control	..	—0.70	11.9	27.3	4.72	—0.50	7.0	36.4	0.96	—0.40	11.9	25.9	4.72	—0.60	11.9	25.9	4.72	—0.70	11.9	27.3	4.42	+1.40	5.6	19.6	0.89
Culture A	1	+0.20	54.9	35.0	21.8	+1.50	161.7	78.4	23.1	+0.20	49.7	28.0	19.7	+0.20	50.4	30.1	20.0	+0.20	53.9	33.6	21.3	+1.40	7.0	21.0	1.12
	3	+0.10	67.2	34.3	26.6	+1.70	250.6	57.0	34.4	+0.10	58.1	32.2	23.0	+0.10	61.6	32.9	24.4	+0.10	65.8	31.5	26.1	+2.70	51.1	55.3	8.20
	6	+0.20	67.2	35.0	26.6	+1.70	269.5	54.6	37.0	+0.10	61.6	32.9	24.4	+0.10	61.6	32.9	24.4	+0.20	67.9	33.6	26.9	+2.80	90.3	80.5	14.5
	13	+0.10	70.7	37.8	28.2	+1.50	270.9	70.7	37.2	—0.10	62.3	35.0	24.7	0.00	65.8	33.4	26.1	+0.10	70.0	35.7	27.7	+2.80	100.1	83.3	16.2
	20	+0.20	72.8	39.9	28.8	+.120	276.5	80.5	38.0	—0.20	63.7	35.0	25.2	—0.30	66.5	35.0	26.4	+0.20	72.1	35.0	28.5	+2.90	100.1	86.1	16.2
Control	..	—1.00	18.9	30.1	6.75	—0.70	11.9	37.1	1.54	—0.70	18.9	25.9	6.75	—0.90	16.1	27.3	5.72	—1.00	18.9	27.3	6.72	+1.20	3.5	21.7	0.80
Culture B	1	+0.40	51.8	34.3	18.4	+0.30	175.7	51.8	22.8	+0.50	45.5	29.4	16.2	+0.70	49.0	27.3	17.5	+0.70	49.7	32.9	17.7	+1.50	6.3	21.7	1.45
	3	+0.70	55.3	39.2	19.7	+0.50	249.2	94.1	32.4	+0.60	51.1	32.2	18.2	+0.70	53.9	33.6	19.2	+0.60	56.0	37.1	20.0	+1.80	46.2	35.0	10.6
	6	+0.70	59.5	39.2	21.2	+0.40	290.5	93.8	37.7	+0.50	54.6	37.1	19.5	+0.70	56.0	35.7	20.0	+0.50	58.8	35.7	21.0	+2.10	90.3	46.9	20.8
	13	+0.30	64.4	41.3	23.0	+0.20	298.6	119.0	38.2	+0.30	56.7	38.5	20.2	+0.30	56.0	35.7	20.0	+0.20	60.2	39.9	21.5	+2.40	100.8	79.1	23.2
	20	+0.10	65.8	45.5	23.5	+0.20	301.7	126.7	39.2	+0.30	58.7	42.7	20.9	+0.10	56.7	40.6	20.2	—0.10	63.7	44.8	22.7	+2.70	100.1	84.0	23.0
Control	..	—0.80	10.5	23.1	4.55	—0.90	11.2	42.0	1.33	—0.70	10.5	23.1	4.55	—0.70	10.5	23.1	4.55	—0.70	10.5	23.1	4.55	+1.30	3.5	20.3	0.74
Culture C	1	+0.20	48.3	27.3	21.0	+0.10	185.5	86.1	22.2	+0.20	47.6	20.6	20.6	......	....	....	.....	......	....	....	.....	+1.90	8.4	19.6	1.79
	3	+0.40	56.0	32.9	24.2	+1.40	272.3	86.1	32.4	+0.10	53.2	23.1	23.0	+0.20	51.1	22.4	22.1	+0.30	53.9	....	23.3	+2 00	33.6	44.8	7.16
	7	+0.80	60.9	30.8	26.3	+1.90	290.5	77.7	34 6	+0.60	56.0	24.5	24.2	......	....	....	.....	......	....	....	.....	+2.20	57.4	56.0	12.2
	10	+0.80	59.5	33.6	25.9	+1.80	350.3	81.9	35.7	+0.70	56.0	24.5	24.2	......	....	....	.....	......	....	....	.....	+2.20	72.1	62.3	15.3
	14	+0.60	60.9	37.8	26.3	+1.70	308.0	77.7	36.6	+0.50	57.4	25.2	24.8	+0.40	57.4	24.5	24.8	+0.40	57.4	24.5	24.8	+2.00	90.3	70.7	19.2
Control	..	—0.80	10.5	23.1	4.55	—0.90	11.2	42.0	1.33	—0.70	10.5	23.1	4.55	—0.70	10.5	23.1	4.55	—0.70	10.5	23.1	4.55	+1.30	3.5	20.3	0.74
Culture D	1	+0.50	51.1	24.5	22.1	+0.40	210.7	84.7	25.8	+0.50	51.7	22.4	22.1	......	....	....	.....	......	....	....	.....	+1.80	11.2	16.8	2.38
	3	+0.60	56.7	25.2	24.5	+1.50	273.7	69.3	32.1	+0.50	55.3	23.8	23.9	+0.50	54.6	25.2	23.6	+0.60	54.6	23.6	23.6	+1.70	14.0	32.2	2.98
	7	+0.50	57.4	28.7	24.8	+1.90	282.1	84.7	33.6	+0.50	56.7	24.5	24.5	......	....	....	.....	......	....	....	.....	+2.00	37.8	49.0	8.06
	10	+0.40	57.4	30.8	24.8	+2.20	307.3	76.3	36.5	+0.30	57.4	25.2	24.8	......	....	....	.....	......	....	....	.....	+2.30	72.8	50.4	15.5
	14	+0.40	58.1	32.9	25.1	+2.10	322.0	70.0	38.3	+0.40	57.4	28.0	24.8	+0.30	58.1	29.4	25.1	+0.70	55.3	27.3	23.9	+2.10	80.5	49.7	17.1
Control	..	—0.80	10.5	23.1	4.55	—0.90	11.2	42.0	1.33	—0.70	10.5	23.1	4.55	—0.70	10.5	23.1	4.55	—0.70	10.5	23.1	4.55	+1.30	3.5	20.3	0.74
Culture E	1	+0.50	51.1	22.1	22.1	+1.80	198.8	91.7	23.6	+0.50	49.7	21.5	21.5	......	....	....	.....	......	....	....	.....	+1.90	7.7	15.4	1.64
	3	+0.30	56.0	24.5	24.2	+1.80	296.8	98.0	35.3	+0.40	55.3	23.8	23.9	+0.30	53.9	23.8	23.3	+0.40	53.9	24.5	23.3	+2.10	9.8	29.4	2.08
	7	+0.30	58.1	25.2	25.1	+2.10	272.3	91.7	32.4	+0.30	57.4	24.5	24.8	......	....	....	.....	......	....	....	.....	+1.90	30.1	47.6	6.32
	10	+0.20	58.1	25.2	25.1	+2.20	312.9	77.7	37.2	+0.10	58.1	25.2	25.1	......	....	....	.....	......	....	....	.....	+1.30	50.4	56.0	10.7
	14	+0.10	58.1	25.2	25.1	+1.90	333.9	77.7	39.7	+0.10	58.8	25.9	25.4	+0.10	55.3	26.6	23.9	+0.10	56.0	25.2	24.2	+1.50	80.5	69.3	17.1
Control	..	—0.80	10.5	23.1	4.55	—0.90	11.2	42.0	1.33	—0.70	10.5	23.1	4.55	—0.70	10.5	23.1	4.55	—0.70	10.5	23.1	4.55	+1.50	3.5	20.3	0.74
Culture F	1	+0.20	52.5	22.4	22.7	+1.70	220.5	68.6	26.2	+0.90	51.8	21.0	22.4	......	....	....	.....	......	....	....	.....	+1.80	8.4	14.7	1.79
	3	+0.40	62.3	26.6	26.9	+1.70	310.8	70.0	37.0	+0.80	59.5	25.2	25.7	+0.40	60.2	26.6	26.0	+0.20	60.9	25.9	26.3	+1.80	10.5	26.6	2.23
	7	+0.30	63.7	27.3	27.5	+1.90	315.7	67.9	37.5	+0.90	60.2	28.7	26.0	......	....	....	.....	......	....	....	.....	+2.20	65.1	44.1	13.8
	10	+0.20	63.7	27.3	27.5	+2.00	318.5	70.7	37.9	+0.60	61.6	25.9	26.6	......	....	....	.....	......	....	....	.....	+2.30	70.7	46.6	15.0
	15	+0.10	62.3	26.6	26.9	+1.80	324.1	77.7	38.5	+0.50	62.3	25.2	26.9	+0.10	59.5	25.9	25.7	—0.10	60.2	26.6	26.0	+2.10	70.0	57.4	14.9

Reaction: — = alkaline to neutral red; + = acid to neutral red; c c normal acid or alkali per 100 c c of medium
Ammonia and amino nitrogen expressed in milligrams per 100 c c of culture medium.
Control indicates initial composition of medium. Net results may be obtained by subtracting the control from the day's analysis.
Amino nitrogen is corrected in each instance for ammonia.

microbe rather than cultural peculiarities have been the basis for identification.

The fermentation reactions are variously reported by different observers. Henry[7] states that glucose, levulose and maltose are fermented. Weinberg and Séguin[1] have found that the fermentative powers, if indeed any are demonstrable, proceed very slowly. They were unable to discover an evolution of gas or the formation of acid in any mediums. McIntosh and Feldes[8] state that the acid production is weak, but after seven days it is distinct in glucose, maltose and starch.

Bundles of gray-white crystals, which are acicular, form in the meat medium after several days' incubation. These crystals have been regarded as impure tyrosin.[9] They do not give the reactions of tyrosin, however. Their composition is still in doubt.

Six strains of B. histolyticus were studied in the series reported below. They were obtained from the following sources:

Culture, B. histolyticus A, from Dr. Holman.
Culture, B. histolyticus B, from Dr. Holman.
Culture, B. histolyticus C, from the National Research Council.
Culture, B. histolyticus D, from the National Research Council.
Culture, B. histolyticus E, from Dr. Meyer.
Culture, B. histolyticus F, from Dr. Meyer.

DISCUSSION

The biochemistry of B. histolyticus was studied by Wolf and Harris.[10] In a peptone water medium they found a measurable evolution of gas, amounting to about 70 c c in 4 days. There was also a considerable formation of ammonia, amounting to 24 mg. in the same time, and an equal increase in the amount of amino nitrogen. The reaction in terms of hydrogen-ion concentration remained practically the same during the entire period of incubation. In milk the gas formation was materially greater, amounting to about 300 c c for each liter of medium. It should be stated, however, that the time of incubation in the latter medium was 12 days. The formation of ammonia was decidedly greater in the milk medium which contained a greater total amount of protein, and of course a very material amount of highly

[7] Jour. Path. & Bacteriol., 1916, 21, p. 344.
[8] Med. Res. Committee, Special Report 12, 1917.
[9] Med. Res. Committee, Special Report 39, 1919.
[10] Jour. Path. & Bacteriol., 1918, 22, p. 1.

organized protein. In milk the ammonia production rose to the relatively considerable amount of 82 mg. per 100 c c of medium. The amino nitrogen content increased during the same incubation interval to 178 mg. per c c. It appears probable from these analytic figures that histolyticus forms a soluble proteolytic enzyme which cleaves the milk proteins to amino acids and polypeptids greater in amount than the bacillus can utilize.

The strains of the organism identified as B. histolyticus in the series reported herein agree in salient metabolic features with the ones studied by Wolf and Harris.

In plain, glucose, lactose, saccharose, glycerol, starch and mannitol broths the nitrogenous changes, indicated by ammonia production and amino nitrogen accumulation, were quantitatively the same, suggesting that the presence of the non-nitrogenous sources of energy exercised no sparing action on the nitrogenous constituents of the medium. Furthermore, the cultures mentioned became slowly, but progressively acid, during the first few days of incubation. Later the titratable acidity decreased, suggesting that the gradual accumulation of basic products, typified by ammonia, exceeded in amount the acidic products which accumulated in the earlier days of growth, when the numbers of bacilli were increasing rather rapidly. At the same time there was a slow, indolent production of gas. Wolf and Harris [10] found this gas to consist chiefly of carbon dioxide (70 to 78%). The amino nitrogen formation is not large, proportionate to the ammonia formation in mediums containing peptone and meat extractives as the sole sources of nitrogen. It is not improbable that this may be explained in part by the relatively simple state of aggregation of the amino-acid complex which comprises the peptone molecule. The proteolytic enzyme of B. histolyticus might confidently be expected to have a less favorable field of activity in such relatively simple nitrogenous compounds. In opposition to this proportionately small accumulation of amino acid in the peptone mediums, the rapid and large amount of amino acids in mediums containing complex protein—gelatin and milk—stands in marked contrast. Here the amino acid accumulation (except in culture E, which failed to develop typically in milk) is strikingly characteristic. The bacilli are quite unable to utilize enough of the amino acids formed by the action of the proteolytic enzyme to reduce significantly the rapid accumulation of these substances, and the analytic figures show clearly how quickly the protein cleavage takes place.

The evolution of ammonia in milk is proportionately less than in gelatin. The action of B. histolyticus on the milk proteins is quantitatively different from that on gelatin. In both mediums, with the exception noted in the foregoing, the amino acid formation proceeds briskly, but in milk—for some reason for which an adequate explanation fails to present itself—the ammonia formation proceeds decidedly more slowly, and fails to approach that observed in the gelatin medium. It is a fact that the total nitrogen content of the gelatin medium used in these studies is about twice on the average that of the milk medium, but this explanation fails to account for the relatively exuberant formation in the former medium, because the amino-nitrogen content of both mediums during the entire course of the growth of the organism runs quantitatively nearly parallel.

SUMMARY

The strains of the anaerobic bacillus identified herein as B. histolyticus do not appear to be fermentative; the analytic tables fail to show any quantitative differences in mediums containing exactly the same nitrogenous constituents but differing in their carbohydrate content. In all mediums there is a progressive increase in titratable acidity for the first few days, followed by a slight recession of acidity as the basic products accumulate. There is coincidently a slow, indolent evolution of gas, produced in approximately equal amounts in mediums containing peptone and meat extractives, irrespective of the carbohydrate content. In gelatin and milk, the gas production was quantitatively greater. The gaseous metabolism suggests that the origin of the gaseous products of growth is from the protein, and not influenced by the presence of any of the commoner carbohydrates. Glycerol also appears to exert no appreciable influence on the growth of the organism. This feature appears to be rather characteristic of B. histolyticus. Many anaerobes utilize glycerol.

On the other hand, the organism is actively proteolytic. The nitrogenous changes appear to be related quantitatively to the complexity of the nitrogenous constituents of the medium, at least in so far as gelatin and milk are concerned. The influence of other proteins was not tested.

The analytic tables indicate clearly that the organism described herein as B. histolyticus must be classed as of the obligately proteolytic group.

BACILLUS PUTRIFICUS

STUDY LVI

That group of anaerobic bacilli which is characterized morphologically by the formation of terminal spores greater in diameter than the parent rod has been a subject of controversy for several years. The isolation from infected wounds of warfare of several apparently distinct varieties or species exhibiting somewhat striking characteristics has redirected attention to them.

The first member of the group to be studied appears to have been Bacillus putrificus, described by Bienstock [1] in 1884. It was obtained from intestinal contents. It will be remembered that Escherich [2] described, but failed to isolate, his "Köpfchen bacillus" in the dejecta of young infants.

In the next two decades Klein,[3] Passini,[4] Rodella [5] and others obtained anaerobic bacilli of morphology similar to B. putrificus from feces, laboratory dust, soil and putrifying mixtures. These microbes were so similar in size, shape and sporulation, but so unlike in cultural characteristics that a somewhat acrimonious controversy arose among various observers regarding their identity. It seemed to be quite clear that at least two rather distinct varieties were obtained, differing in their apparent fermentative capacities, and Bienstock [6] published a description of a new organism exhibiting the morphology of B. putrificus, but apparently endowed with distinctly greater fermentative powers. The latter organism has been less thoroughly discussed than the preceding group.

The significance of B. putrificus to the bacteriologist resides rather in its theoretical relationship to that form of protein decomposition known as "putrefaction" than in its participation in human activities as an incitant of specific infection. In other words, B. putrificus seems to possess a chemical, rather than a pathogenic interest to the bacteriologist.

For many years the microbe was regarded as the type organism which induces that type of bacterial activity which Bienstock and,

[1] Ztschr. f. klin. Med., 1884, 8, p. 1; Arch. f. Hyg., 1889, 36, p. 335; 1901, 39, p. 390.
[2] Darmbakterien des Säuglings, 1886.
[3] Centralbl. f. Bakteriol., 1899, 25, p. 278; 1901, 29, p. 991.
[4] Ztschr. f. Hyg. u. Infektionskr., 1905, 49, p. 135.
[5] Ann. Inst. Past., 1905, 19, p. 804.
[6] Ann. Inst. Past., 1906, 20, p. 497.

somewhat later, Rettger [7] termed "putrefaction." Two other anaerobic bacilli were regarded by Rettger as belonging to the group of true "putrefactive" bacteria, namely, B. oedematis (Bacillus oedematis maligni, or, as it is now termed, Vibrion septique), and B. chauvœi (the Rauschbrand bacillus, or B. anthracis symptomatici).[8]

The subsequent history of the conception of putrefaction, and the bacteria which are or were supposed to be the active incitants is interwoven with the gradual recognition of the difficulties attending the isolation and cultivation of cultures of anaerobic bacteria of unquestioned purity. Thus, Rettger's first studies on putrefaction [7] were recognized by him to have been vitiated by the presence of unrecognized contaminants in his cultural mediums.[8, 9] Even in 1912, however, before intensive studies of the bacilli of malignant edema and symptomatic anthrax were made with cultures of undoubted purity, Rettger still maintained that these two organisms were examples of the "putrefactive" type.[10]

More recent studies by Meyer,[11] and the striking work of Miss Robertson,[12] the Medical Research Committee,[13] and Weinberg and Séguin [14] have shown beyond reasonable doubt that the bacillus of malignant edema and the organism of symptomatic anthrax are practically devoid of proteolytic powers. In this respect they resemble the strongly fermentative anaerobic bacteria, such as the Welch bacillus.

Achalme [15] and others have studied cultures identified as B. putrificus with varied results, and comparatively recently Sturges and Rettger [16] have reopened the question of the identity of B. putrificus with observations apparently at variance with all previous work. They say: "All the strains of B. putrificus isolated by us exhibit a peculiar reluctance in undergoing development and in attacking the egg-meat medium in pure culture. The putrefaction is very much delayed and does not begin as a rule until twenty to thirty days after the beginning of incubation under anaerobic conditions. When once begun, however, the putrefaction is rapid and typical. This is in striking contrast with the other well-known putrefyers (B. oedematis and B. chauvœi) which usually begin to decompose the protein within a period of three to

[7] Am. Jour. Physiol., 1903, 8, p. 284.
[8] Rettger: Jour. Biol. Chem., 1906, 2, p. 85.
[9] Ibid., 1908, 4, p. 45.
[10] Ibid., 1912, 13, p. 341.
[11] Jour. Infect. Dis., 1915, 17, p. 458.
[12] Brit. Med. Jour., 1918, 1, p. 583.
[13] Special Report Series 39, 1919.
[14] La Gangrène Gazeuse, 1917.
[15] Ann. Inst. Past., 1902, 16, p. 633.
[16] Jour. Bacteriol., 1919, 4, p. 171.

four days. This delayed putrefaction of B. putrificus occurs only in pure cultures."

It is unusual for pure cultures of known anaerobic bacilli to exhibit a latent period of from two to three weeks in cultural mediums (where the gradual entrance of air would tend to create progressively unfavorable conditions for growth), followed by an apparently abrupt entrance into the vegetative state associated with rather intense chemical activity. Quantitative studies of the metabolism of such bacilli might throw some light on the nature of the process taking place, and possibly explain the cause or causes for the delayed growth. Whatever the explanation for this phenomenon may be, it is clear that the identity of B. putrificus, and even of the entire anaerobic plectridial group, with the exception of B. tetani, is still a matter of some doubt.

The important members of the plectridial group of anaerobes thus far described, comprise the following: B. tetani, B. tertius,[17] B. tetanomorphus,[18] (B. pseudotetani?), B. cochlearius,[19] B. histolyticus,[20] B. putrificus, and B. paraputrificus. It is not improbable that other members of this group, characterized morphologically by plectridial spores, may be isolated in the future.

The salient characteristics of those members of the group which appear to be sufficiently distinctive to identify a microbic entity, excluding B. tetani, B. tertius, B. pseudotetani and B. histolyticus (discussed in earlier communications of this series of studies), are inserted for purposes of orientation. In making this table, it is specically understood that the final description of B. putrificus is yet to be elucidated. For historical reasons B. putrificus is specifically designated a proteolytic anaerobic bacillus, notwithstanding the fact that some observers have recently ascribed to the organism characteristics which would definitely remove it from the proteophilic group. It appears probable that the descriptions of these tabulated organisms, excluding B. putrificus and B. paraputrificus, are sufficiently well established to warrant at least their temporary acceptance as well defined microbic entities.[18] This would leave B. putrificus indeterminate but exhibiting historical characteristics not in opposition to those of two strains of anaerobic plectridial bacilli which have been isolated in this laboratory. One was obtained from feces (culture A), the other from a culture sent for diagnosis

[17] Henry: Jour. Path. & Bacteriol., 1916, 21, p. 344.

[18] McIntosh and Feldes: Bacillus tetanomorphi, Med. Res. Committee, Special Report Series 12, 1917.

[19] Type 3 C, McIntosh and Feldes, footnote 18.

[20] Weinberg and Séguin: Compt. rend. Soc. de biol., 1915, 78, p. 274; 1917, 80, p. 157.

from an unknown source (culture B). These two strains exhibit in common the ability to induce a gaseous fermentation in glucose and a rather noteworthy ability to produce evidence of proteolysis in mediums containing gelatin or milk proteins.

It should be emphasized that the proteolytic changes are decidedly less marked than those characteristic of B. histolyticus or of B. sporogenes, as evidenced by amino nitrogen formation. It is also wholly distinct from B. tertius,[17] both in its fermentative properties and in its ability to induce visible changes in milk and gelatin. It also differs from B. pseudotetani [18] in its biochemical properties.

TABLE A

PLECTRIDIAL ANAEROBES

	B. cochlearius	B. pseudotetani	B. putrificus (?)	B. paraputrificus
Morphology.	Slender rod	Slender rod	Slender rod	Slender rod
Size..........	Same as tetanus	Same as tetanus	0.6–0.8× 5–6 μ	Same as putrificus
Motility......	Active	Active	Acitve	Active
Grouping....	Singly, pairs	Singly, pairs	Singly, pairs, rarely short chains	Same as putrificus
Capsule......	Not demonstrated	Not demonstrated	Not demonstrated	Not demonstrated
Spore........	Terminal, oval or spherical	Terminal, spherical	Terminal, oval or spherical	Terminal, oval or spherical
Stain.........	Gram + readily becomes Gram —	Gram + may become Gram —	Gram +*	Gram +*
Meat medium	Very little change	Pink color, some gas	Meat slowly digested	Gas, then digested
Gelatin.......	No softening	No softening	Liquefied	Liquefied
Milk..........	No visible change	No visible change	Peptonized	Gas and acid clot
Fermentation	None	Glucose and maltose	Glucose, maltose, glycerol, acid, some gas	Glucose, lactose, possibly other sugars

* Old cultures may become irregularly gram-negative.

The relations of the cultural characteristics of the two strains under discussion to B. cochlearius, B. pseudotetani, and to the imperfectly described B. paraputrificus, are indicated in the tabulation (Table A). It is expressly understood that the designation "Bacillus putrificus" is to be construed as suggestive, rather than final. The organism agrees in essential details with that described as B. putrificus by the British Medical Research Committee.[13]

TABLE 1

BACILLUS PUTRIFICUS

	Day	Plain				Gelatin				Glucose				Lactose				Saccharose				Milk			
		Reaction	Ammonia Nitrogen	Amino Nitrogen	Percentage Ammonia to Total Nitrogen	Reaction	Ammonia Nitrogen	Amino Nitrogen	Percentage Ammonia to Total Nitrogen	Reaction	Ammonia Nitrogen	Amino Nitrogen	Percentage Ammonia to Total Nitrogen	Reaction	Ammonia Nitrogen	Amino Nitrogen	Percentage Ammonia to Total Nitrogen	Reaction	Ammonia Nitrogen	Amino Nitrogen	Percentage Ammonia to Total Nitrogen	Reaction	Ammonia Nitrogen	Amino Nitrogen	Percentage Ammonia to Total Nitrogen
Control	..	−0.80	12.6	21.0	5.61	−0.70	9.1	34.3	1,27	−0.60	12.6	21.0	5.61	−0.60	12.6	21.0	5.61	−0.80	12.6	21.0	5.61	+1.50	7.0	19.6	1.51
Culture A	1	+0.50	31.5	14.0	14.0	+0.90	32.9	23.8	4.61	+2.70	15.4	23.8	6.86	.....	....	....	.....	......	....	....	.....	+2.50	9.1	17.5	1.96
	3	+1.00	54.6	24.5	24.3	+2.10	85.4	27.3	11.9	+3.20	17.5	25.9	7.80	+1.20	66.5	29.7	29.6	+1.10	51.8	19.6	23.1	+2.80	30.8	18.2	6.67
	6	+1.40	69.3	30.8	30.9	+2.40	121.8	29.4	17.0	+3.60	14.0	28.7	6.25	.....	....	....	.....	......	....	....	.....	+3.00	77.7	30.8	16.8
	10	+1.50	77.7	34.3	34.6	+2.70	147.7	35.7	20.7	+3.30	9.8	30.8	4.37	.....	....	....	.....	......	....	....	.....	+2.80	141.4	31.5	30.6
	14	+1.60	70.7	31.5	31.5	+3.00	157.5	37.8	22.0	+3.20	14.7	32.2	6.56	+1.40	78.4	35.0	34.9	+1.80	62.3	28.7	27.8	+2.90	140.0	31.5	30.3
Control	..	−0.80	12.6	22.4	5.61	−0.70	9.1	34.3	1.27	−0.60	12.6	21.0	5.61	−0.60	12.6	21.0	5.61	−0.80	12.6	21.0	5.61	+1.50	7.0	19.6	1.51
Culture B	1	+0.20	15.4	18.2	6.86	+0.10	16.8	28.0	2.35	+1.60	11.2	24.5	5.00	.....	....	....	.....	......	....	....	.....	+2.60	22.4	22.4	5.07
	3	+0.90	56.0	16.8	24.9	+1.30	60.2	26.6	8.43	+3.30	11.9	24.5	5.30	+0.50	39.9	17.8	17.8	+1.70	44.8	20.3	20.0	+2.90	74.9	36.4	16.2
	6	+1.20	71.4	25.2	31.9	+2.90	142.1	36.4	19.9	+3.60	13.3	29.9	5.94	.....	....	....	.....	......	....	....	.....	+3.10	137.9	34.3	29.8
	10	+1.30	70.7	28.7	31.5	+2.90	165.9	39.2	23.2	+3.60	14.0	31.5	6.25	.....	....	....	.....	......	....	....	.....	+3.10	143.5	31.5	31.0
	14	+1.30	75.6	33.6	33.3	+2.90	182.0	42.7	25.5	+3.40	16.8	32.2	7.50	+1.00	72.1	32.2	32.1	+2.00	60.2	26.6	26.8	+3.20	143.5	34.5	31.0

Reaction: − = alkaline to neutral red; + = acid to neutral red; c c normal acid or alkali per 100 c c of medium.
Ammonia and amino nitrogen expressed in milligrams per 100 c c of culture medium.
Control indicates initial composition of medium. Net results may be obtained by subtracting the control from the day's analysis.
Amino nitrogen is corrected in each instance for ammonia.

DISCUSSION

The nitrogenous changes induced by the anaerobic plectridial bacilli, tentatively designated B. putrificus, are quite different from those described for other members of the terminal spore group, previously studied.[21] In plain, lactose, and saccharose mediums, there is a moderate formation of ammonia, and a relatively small accumulation of amino nitrogen which succeeds an initial decrease in these substances, containing NH_2 groups which can be removed by the addition of liquor formaldehydi. The amount of nitrogenous change in these mediums, taken by themselves, would unquestionably place these organisms in a group characterized by moderate changes in protein mediums. Even after prolonged cultivation the amount of ammonia fails to exhibit an increase which would suggest a tendency toward marked proteolysis. The change in titratable acidity becomes slowly, but distinctly, acid, without however a marked departure from uninoculated controls. The

[21] See Kendall, Day and Walker: Studies XLVII, XLVIII, XLIX, and L, Jour. Infect. Dis., 1922, 30, pp. 167-177.

addition of glucose to the plain broth medium causes a distinct rise in titratable acidity; at the same time, an evolution of gas takes place which contrasts in amount and in the rate of formation with the indolent collection of bubbles of gas in the medium containing the same protein constituents, but not glucose. Also, the amino nitrogen fails to exhibit the decrease observed in the peptone mediums not containing this carbohydrate. The ammonia formation is distinctly less. The addition of glucose to peptone mediums, therefore, appears to exhibit that series of nitrogenous changes which are indicative of a sparing action of this carbohydrate for the protein constituents.

In gelatin and milk, the nitrogenous changes are distinctly greater, although they do not rise to the amounts formed by some of the active proteolytic anaerobic bacteria. In gelatin, the amount of ammonia formed is more than twice that produced in peptone mediums, and greater on the whole than that observed in milk. The amino nitrogen also falls below that of uninoculated controls during the earlier days of growth, but rises as the culture becomes older. Unlike B. histolyticus, the amino nitrogen content is less in gelatin than in milk, suggesting perhaps that the milk proteins are on the whole somewhat more utilizable for energy than the gelatin protein. The action of B. putrificus, judging from these results, is comparatively slight on peptones and meat extractives; this is in harmony with the more recent observations of a number of observers who have stated that B. putrificus is not a strongly proteolytic organism when grown in nutrient broth mediums. The action on gelatin also, while distinct, is on the whole not marked. Here again the contention that the organism is not of the marked proteolytic type would appear to be substantiated. In milk, the action on protein is distinctly more pronounced than on the other mediums studied. It is worthy of note that the initial decrease of amino acid and the formation of ammonia follows that characteristic of glucose broth rather than that observed in gelatin or peptone meat extractive mediums not containing a utilizable source of carbohydrate. After the first day or two, however, the increase in titratable acidity, the formation of ammonia and the accumulation of amino nitrogen is more in accord with the corresponding changes induced in mediums not containing a utilizable source of non-nitrogenous energy.[22] As milk contains about 0.1% of a substance appar-

[22] The tenth day flask of culture B in milk shows clearly that development has failed to take place at the normal rate. The value of the use of separate flasks for each day's analysis is shown by this culture, which is exceptional. As a rule, the flasks show a uniform "curve of growth" which is a valuable check on the purity of the culture.

ently glucose, the similarity of the growth curve for the first day in milk cultures is plausibly explained. After that time, or at least before the third day of growth was reached, the sugar of the medium was exhausted, and attack of the organisms was of necessity on the protein constituents of the medium.

SUMMARY

The organisms identified as B. putrificus are plectridial anaerobic bacilli of fairly definite proteolytic properties. On peptone-meat extractive mediums the nitrogenous transformations are moderate. There is a considerable formation of ammonia, an initial deficit in amino nitrogen, followed later by a progressive increase in amino nitrogen which usually exceeds by a small amount that of uninoculated controls. In peptone mediums the organism is not an active transformer of nitrogenous energy. The addition of glucose to these mediums reduces materially the formation of ammonia, and protects the amino nitrogen to a degree from bacterial transformation. In gelatin mediums the evidences of proteolytic activity are decidedly but not markedly greater. Gelatin is softened so that it will no longer solidify on cooling to the temperature of the icebox. The formation of ammonia is decidedly greater than in peptone medium, and there is a final concentration of amino nitrogen greater than in peptone mediums.

Milk proteins are somewhat more energetically attacked than gelatin in peptone proteins. Somewhat less ammonia, proportionately, is formed, and relatively more amino nitrogen is produced. The early hours of incubation in milk give rise to more acid, less ammonia, and a reduced diminution in amino nitrogen, suggesting an initial attack of the bacteria on the small amount of glucose in the milk. After this is used, the characteristic nitrogenous changes appear, suggestive of a greater cleavage of milk protein than gelatin protein, as evidenced by the greater amino acid accumulation.

B. putrificus appears to be an organism possessed of relatively limited but perfectly distinct proteolytic powers. Its fermentative properties are limited. The impression derived from a consideration of the respective proteolytic activities in peptone mediums, gelatin, and milk, in the order named, form a gradual progression in nitrogenous activity which would be misleading if each were considered by itself. It would appear that the milk proteins are most adapted to the nitrogenous requirements of B. putrificus in so far as these metabolic studies permit of comparison.

THE SIGNIFICANCE AND QUANTITATIVE MEASUREMENT OF THE NITROGENOUS METABOLISM OF BACTERIA

STUDIES IN BACTERIAL METABOLISM. LVII

Arthur Isaac Kendall

From The Patten Research Foundation and the Department of Bacteriology, Northwestern University Medical School, Chicago, Ill.

One of the significant indications of a transition in the biologics from the condition of an art to the status of a science is the development within them of suitable quantitative methods. This follows because qualitative observations, frequently more striking than quantitative measurements, require the application of methods of precision for their elucidation. Thus, the phenomena of growth and repair in health and disease have been explored through the rise of the science of nutrition and metabolism. The development of the science of pharmacology followed logically the perfection of methods for recording accurately the physiologic effects of drugs and chemicals. The physiologic assay of the potency of bacterial toxins has progressed along lines previously employed in pharmacology. Similarly, the rise of the youngest of the biologic sciences, immunology, has been dependent on the acquisition of procedures sufficiently accurate to estimate the nature and extent of those complex relationships which exist between microbe and host, in infection and in resistance to infection. Furthermore, the determination of the potency of lysins, agglutinins and precipitins has assumed practical significance in medicine since their numerical relations to infection and resistance have been established.

The application of quantitative chemical methods to the study of bacterial metabolism is in its infancy. This might confidently be expected because qualitative observations involving phenomena of bacterial metabolism are few in number, inconspicuous in their relations to medicine, in whose domain they have largely been associated, and difficult of recognition. Nevertheless, some results have been recorded which not only shed light on the mode of action of bacteria, but also indicate lines of approach to underlying and fundamental principles of cellular behavior in general.

Received for publication Oct. 12, 1921.

Among the available indications of the possible results that may flow from the study of bacterial chemistry, the observations of Theobald Smith [1] that glucose in cultures of the diphtheria bacillus prevents the formation of diphtheria toxin, may be cited. This phenomenon is an example of a great group of related reactions which seem to depend on the physiologic dictum that "carbohydrate spares protein from utilization for energy." [2] Stated differently, the specificity of action of a majority of pathogenic bacteria depends on their utilization of protein for energy.[3] Simonds'[4] study of the relation of the composition of mediums to the immunologic reactions of bacteria developed therein is an important contribution to the same field. The effects of cultural sources of energy on the development of soluble enzymes [5] is still another indication of the relationship that exists between the nature of the nutrition of bacteria and the character of their activities. The ever-increasing developments along chemical lines in those industries in which bacteria play a part is a suggestion of the capitalization of utilitarian bacterial transformations in processes of economic importance. Even in the domain of therapeutics there is evidence that a knowledge of bacterial metabolism may prove to be the starting point for dietary procedures of importance in the treatment of bacillary dysentery, [3, 6] typhoid fever,[7] and other excrementitious diseases.

THE NATURE OF BACTERIAL METABOLISM

The life history of a bacterium, like that of any living entity, may be divided into two distinct phases, the structural phase and the energy phase. The structural phase comprises those phenomena which result in the transformation of suitable nutrient substances, together with water and salts, into the mature bacterial cell. The structural phase is complete, aside from losses incidental to the formation of enzymes and other nitrogenous substances necessary for the maintenance of the organism, when the phenomenon of fission from the mother cell is complete. The amount of substance required to build a bacterial cell is little indeed; an average sized typhoid bacillus weighs about 0.000,000,002 of a milligram, its volume being very nearly one two-thousand-millionth of a cubic millimeter.[8] In other words, two million

[1] Jour. Exper. Med., 1899, 4, p. 373.
[2] Kendall: Chem. and Metall. Jour., 1921, 24, p. 56.
[3] Kendall: Am. Jour. Med. Sc., 1918, 156, p. 157.
[4] Jour. Infect. Dis., 1915, 17, p. 500.
[5] Auerbach: Arch. f. Hyg., 1897, 31, p. 311. Kendall and Walker: Jour. Infect. Dis., 1915, 17, p. 442.
[6] Kendall: Boston Med. & Surg. Jour., 1911, 154, p. 288.
[7] Torrey: Jour. Med. Res., 1919, 39, p. 415.
[8] Kendall: Med. Rec., 1913, 84, p. 151.

million typhoid bacilli would be required to balance a gram weight. About 87% of this is water. The amount of organic substance is comparatively small.

The energy requirements of bacterial cells are as disproportionately extensive as the structural requirements are inconspicuous. The surface area of the typhoid bacillus mentioned in the foregoing, whose weight is one two-thousand-millionth of a milligram, is one hundred-thousandth of a square millimeter. Expressed numerically, the surface area of the microbe to its weight is as 0.000,01 is to 0.000,000,002.[9] As the energy requirements of living things vary with the surface area rather than with the volume, the well-known ability of bacteria to effect transformations of nutritive material far in excess of the amount their extremely minute size would apparently permit, receives some explanation. The rapid development of bacteria in favorable mediums, in which successive generations may appear at intervals as frequent as every 15 or 20 minutes in the early hours of growth in a fresh environment furnishes the factor of enormous numbers of microbes which is necessary to complete the background for those rapid chemical transformations, which bacteria are capable of.

Nitrogen is the corner stone of the structural requirement of living things, and bacteria are of course no exception. Nitrogen in available form is absolutely essential for the growth of bacteria. The significant element in the energy phase of bacterial metabolism, however, is carbon; nitrogen not only is not a source of energy for most bacteria, but it also is useless for this purpose. This is equally true, so far as available information indicates, in the animal kingdom. The well-known utilization of available carbohydrates (which possess the requisite stereo-configuration to fit the bacterial cytoplasm) for energy in mediums containing both protein derivatives and sugars is illustrative of this fact. There is no nitrogenous residuum in carbohydrate, and the partially oxidized carbon of the sugar molecule possessing the requisite stereo-configuration appears to be a peculiarly readily utilized source of energy. If, however, the carbohydrate is withdrawn from the medium, leaving the protein derivatives alone for both the structural (nitrogenous) and energy (carbonaceous) requirements, the nitrogen of the amino acids and polypeptids is eliminated quantitatively as ammonia (deamination prior to the utilization of the non-nitrogenous residium for energy). In this instance, the amount of ammonia

[9] For purposes of comparison, a man 200 centimeters tall, weighing 100 kg. has a surface area of almost exactly 2.36 square meters.

accumulating as a result of deamination is a very exact measure of the intracellular utilization of amino acids or their complexes for bacterial energy.[10]

It is a well attested fact that the amount of urea excreted from the animal body increases with the increase of protein in the diet above that minimum necessary to establish nitrogen equilibrium; therefore, a purely protein diet is associated with much urea excretion. The substance antecedent to urea is of course ammonia, which results from the deamination of amino acids or their complexes. In this sense, urea excreted in the urine of mammals and ammonia excreted in cultures of bacteria have an almost parallel significance.

Unfortunately, no methods are available for directly measuring the amount of carbon utilized for energy either in animals or bacterial cultures. It is possible, however, to follow the change in the nitrogenous constituents of bacterial cultures utilized for structure, and for structural repair, as they are liberated through recessive and autolytic changes, and as they are liberated from proteins or protein derivatives incidental to their intracellular utilization for energy (deamination).

Folin has devised two important methods for the measurement of nitrogenous substances, one for the determination of ammonia by the air current method, the other for nonprotein nitrogen, which in connection with the Sörensen formol titration method or the Van Slyke amino nitrogen method, and the Kjeldahl method for total nitrogen, make it possible to divide the nitrogenous constituents of culture mediums into several fractions, as follows: Knowing the total nitrogen and the total nonprotein nitrogen, it follows that their difference may be designated appropriately "protein nitrogen." Also, the nonprotein nitrogen may be fractionated into ammonia nitrogen, amino nitrogen (corrected of course for ammonia) and residual nonprotein nitrogen. In ordinary cultural mediums the nonprotein residual nitrogen may consist—in addition to polypeptids, the most important constituents—of creatin or creatinin, urea, uric acid (the latter two in traces at most), purin bases and possibly also pyrimidin bases. Mediums containing meat extract as a basis are richer in creatinin and purin bases than mediums compounded from "meat juice." In any event, no great error is introduced if the term "polypeptid nitrogen" be substituted for residual nonprotein nitrogen, and the term will be so used in this and subsequent communications.

[10] Kendall and Walker: Jour. Infect. Dis., 1915, 17, p. 442.

As an example of the fractionation of nitrogen on this basis, the composition of three samples of gelatin are appended:

TABLE 1

COMPOSITION OF THREE SAMPLES OF GELATIN

Milligrams per 100 c c Sample	Sample A	Sample B	Sample C
Total nitrogen	0.672	1.001	1.064
Protein nitrogen	0.542	0.721	0.762
Nonprotein nitrogen	0.130	0.280	0.302
Polypeptid nitrogen	0.102	0.209	0.213
Amino nitrogen	0.020	0.039	0.032
Ammonia nitrogen	0.008	0.032	0.057

A, 5 % gelatin in water, no peptone or meat extractives.
B, plain nutrient gelatin (5% gelatin, 1% peptone, 0.3% meat extract).
C, another lot of plain, nutrient gelatin prepared as under B.

It will be seen that the combined amino nitrogen and ammonia nitrogen comprise less than 10% of the total nitrogen.

It is highly important, as will be indicated in succeeding studies, to determine changes in nitrogen distribution during experiments in bacterial metabolism. The intermediary metabolism, especially experiments in bacterial metabolism between the protein and polypeptid nitrogen fractions, furnishes much information concerning the nature of bacterial attack on the nitrogenous constituents under various conditions.

It should be mentioned in passing that the creatinin fraction of the "polypeptid" nitrogen section may be determined by the colorimetric method of Folin.[11] Some bacteria [12] act on creatinin. Also, the purin and pyrimidin bases may be estimated separately, if desired.

METHODS

Total Nitrogen.—Total nitrogen is determined either by the Folin-Farmer micro method,[13] making duplicate determinations, or by the Gunning modification of the Kjeldahl procedure. If nonprotein nitrogen determinations are to be made on the same sample, the latter is somewhat less time-consuming. The procedure is as follows:

To 10 c c of the sample to be analyzed, discharged into a 300 c c pyrex Kjeldahl flask, add 5 gm. of C. P. potassium sulphate, 5 drops of a 10% copper sulphate solution, and 15 c c of nitrogen-free sulphuric acid. Digestion is practiced until the residual solution is clear, but bluish-green in color. The digestion mixture is cooled to the point of commencing viscosity; then about

[11] Jour. Biol. Chem., 1914, 17, p. 463.
[12] Popoff: Centralbl. f. Bakteriol., 1890, 7, p. 585. Antonoff: Ibid., I, O., 1907, 43, 209. Burri and Andrejew: Ibid., 1910, 56, p. 217.
[13] Jour. Biol. Chem., 1912, 11, p. 493.

50 c c of distilled water are added, and the contents poured carefully into a 100 c c graduated pyrex flask. After cooling, enough water is added to the flask in small amounts to bring the entire volume of washings to exactly 100 c c. Duplicate portions of 2 c c each are placed in 8x1 inch pyrex test tubes, enough NaOH added to make the solution strongly alkaline,[14] and the free ammonia is blown out into 250 c c flasks, each containing exactly 10 c c of N/50 HCl., a drop of alizarin, and enough water to make a total volume of about 75 c c, using the apparatus and procedure described in the following, under the Folin air current method for ammonia. It will be seen that the only departure from the classical process is the dilution of the digestion mixture, and the subsequent "blowing out" of the ammonia from an aliquot part, in duplicate or in triplicate, in place of the ordinary steam distillation of the entire amount.

As the duplicates agree, with ordinary care, within 0.10 c c of N/50 alkali, it is clear that the advantage of this method of "blowing out" the ammonia in duplicate aliquot parts is to afford a check on the entire process.

It is customary in this laboratory to run duplicate samples, both in the digestion itself, and on the subsequent determination of ammonia, from each digestate. This procedure controls both the uniformity of digestion and the accuracy of the determination of the ammonia. The satisfaction which flows from the checking of duplicate determinations on duplicate samples far outweighs the slight additional expenditure of time required to effect this procedure.

There is no criterion for the computation of the total nitrogen content of organic compounds such as cultural mediums. It is quite probable that certain combinations of carbon and nitrogen may exist, or be formed during the digestion process, which fail to be broken up by the combination of sulphuric acid and temperature of digestion. These cyanogen compounds, if they exist, are in all probability small in amount, and as the total nitrogen determination holds only for one particular lot of medium, and is repeated for each succeeding lot made from essentially the same ingredients put together in substantially the same way, the error is relatively constant, and therefore relatively insignificant. Of greater consequence is the concentration of nitrogenous substances in cultural mediums due to the loss of water by evaporation, as incubation proceeds. The practice of weighing all cultural mediums in their containers at the start of an experiment, and of restoring the loss due to evaporation before making analyses, has much to commend it.

Nonprotein Nitrogen.—The method devised by Folin and Wu[15] for the determination of "nonprotein nitrogen" in the blood has been found to be very satisfactory for the estimation of the nonprotein

[14] A drop of alizarin is added as an indicator.
[15] Jour. Biol. Chem., 1919, 38, p. 81.

nitrogen of bacterial cultures. The method in essence consists of two stages: first, the precipitation of molecules of nitrogenous substance of a rather definite but of course unknown size from solution; and, second, the determination of the nitrogen in the filtrate (which contains "nonprotein nitrogen") after the larger sized molecules are removed by filtration.

The academic question of the nature or size of nitrogenous molecules in solution in cultural mediums which are precipitated by the Folin reagent is left to others for elucidation. The remarkable fact that a quantitative separation of the constituents of a gelatin medium, containing approximately 5% of gelatin, 1% of peptone, and 0.3% of meat extractives may be made in duplicate, with astonishingly exact results, is shown in table 2, in which are shown the results when seven samples of gelatin, containing the same nitrogenous ingredients but with ascending amounts of glucose were digested in duplicate, and the nitrogen of each digestion determined in duplicate, according to the procedure outlined.

TABLE 2

GELATIN

Sample		Plain	0.1 Glucose	0.2 Glucose	0.3 Glucose	0.4 Glucose	0.5 Glucose	0.75 Glucose	
Titration	a	8.40	8.45	8.55	8.50	8.50	8.55	8.50	Digestion A
		8.45	8.45	8.40	8.50	8.45	8.40	8.40	
	b	8.40	8.40	8.40	8.40	8.50	8.50	8.40	Digestion B
		8.50	8.40	8.50	8.45	8.50	8.50	8.55	
Average milligrams nonprotein nitrogen per 100 c c of medium		8.45	8.40+	8.45	8.45+	8.50	8.50	8.45	
		0.347	0.358	0.347	0.347	0.347	0.336	0.347	

The figures represent the number of cubic centimeters of N/50 alkali required to neutralize 10 c c of N/50 HCl., into which there has been blown the ammonia resulting from the digestion of the various samples (by the Folin air current method), in accordance with the analytic procedure soon to be described.

The analysis of many samples of gelatin has given results which are consistent, and there appears to be no doubt that the Folin nonprotein method, if followed with reasonable care, will furnish results which have a definite value in the quantitative study of the nitrogenous metabolism of bacterial cultures. Of course the "nonprotein nitrogen" fraction will decrease somewhat and the "protein nitrogen" fraction will increase somewhat as bacterial multiplication results in the formation of bacterial protein. Also, the bacterial formation of mucin or mucin-like substances may add to the "protein nitrogen" fraction.

The filtration or centrifugalization of such cultures will separate the "bacterial protein nitrogen" from the soluble "protein nitrogen," should such a procedure be desirable. It is also clear that autolytic or recessive processes in old bacterial cultures will probably result in a decrease in protein nitrogen during the later stages of incubation. Such recessive changes may be expected after seven or eight days' continual development at body temperature.

Procedure: Ten c c of culture are diluted with exactly 70 c c of distilled water, and thoroughly mixed. Exactly 10 c c of a 10% aqueous solution of sodium tungstate are added with constant agitation, and then exactly 10 c c of ⅔ normal sulphuric acid. The resulting solution (100 c c) should be faintly acid to congo red paper. Continuous agitation is practiced for several minutes. The turbid solution containing a tenacious precipitate is filtered through a moderately coarse filter paper. The filtrate is usually clear at first, but soon becomes milky, due apparently to the formation of an oxidization product of tungsten. Such a filtrate containing glucose frequently becomes blue on standing in the sunlight.

Digestion:[16] 25 c c duplicate samples of the filtrate are placed in 300 c c pyrex digestion flasks. To each is added about 15 c c nitrogen-free sulphuric acid, about 5 gm. potassium sulphate, and 5 drops of a 10% solution of copper sulphate. Digestion is carried out in precisely the same manner as that for the determination of total nitrogen.

When digestion is complete and the contents of the flasks have cooled somewhat, the digestion mixture is made up to a volume of exactly 100 c c (at room temperature). Two portions of 5 c c each are removed to 8 x 1 inch pyrex test tubes. The contents are made strongly alkaline with NaOH, and the free ammonia is blown out into flasks, containing exactly 10 c c of N/50 HCl., about 70 c c of water, and a drop of alizarin. The entire amount of nitrogen as ammonia is removed by this air current method in less than 30 minutes. Back titration of the contents of each flask with N/50 NaOH completes the process. Duplicate determinations of duplicate digestion on the same sample may be confidently expected to agree within 0.10 c c N/50 NaOH. Much time is conserved in calculation by the use of tables, which are readily prepared to show at a glance the back titration in terms of N/50 NaOH, and the corresponding number of milligrams of nonprotein nitrogen per 100 c c of culture medium.

Experience indicates that no precautions other than reasonable care in measurements and ordinary skill in Kjeldahl determinations are necessary to insure the precision of results indicated in the foregoing. The titration method

[16] The Folin phosphoric-sulphuric acid digestion mixture has been found to be somewhat less suitable for culture mediums than the Kjeldahl-Gunning digestion mixture. Undoubtedly the nitrogenous constituents of cultural mediums are more difficult to break up than those of the blood for which the Folin mixture is excellent.

offers some advantages over the Nesslerization of the digestion mixture as carried out by Folin. When large numbers of determinations are made (the writer has frequently carried out 50 unaided in a morning), the cost of the Nessler reagent becomes a potent factor.

It is clear that the difference between the "nonprotein nitrogen" and the total nitrogen represents nitrogenous substances of molecular aggregation precipitable by the tungsten. This fraction is advantageously termed "protein nitrogen."

Amino Nitrogen.—Henriques,[17] and Henriques and Sörenson,[18] have taken advantage of the reaction between formaldehyde and free NH_2 groups in proteins and protein derivatives to produce methylated nitrogenous groups, thus destroying the basicity of the NH_2 group, in their method of "formol titration." The reaction is as follows:

$$R. CH_2. CHNH_2. COOH + HCOH = R. CH_2. CHN : CH_2. COOH + H_2O.$$

The basicity of the amino group being eliminated, the full acidity of the carboxyl group becomes titratable, and it may be measured quantitatively by titration with standard caustic soda solution, using phenolphthalein as an indicator. It is clear that free ammonia that may be present in solution also reacts with formaldehyde—in this case, however, to form hexamethylene tetra amine. A correction should be made for the free ammonia in the determination.[19]

It should be remembered that the only free NH_2 groups are thus determinable; the remaining amino groups of a polypeptid are united chemically to the carboxyl groups, forming the well-known "protein or 'peptid' tie." In a dipeptid, only one free amino group is ordinarily present, and, generally speaking, it is very probable that polypeptids possess for the most part only one free amino group and one free carboxyl group.[20] The remaining amino and carboxyl groups are united in order to link together the amino acids which collectively comprise the

[17] Ztschr. f. physiol. Chem., 1909, 60, p. 1.

[18] Ibid., 1910, 54, p. 120.

[19] It appears probable that much of the ammonia, even in plain gelatin mediums is in combination with CO_2 as ammonium carbonate. The change of the ammonia to hexamethylene tetra-amine by the addition of neutral formaldehyde, therefore, would remove the basicity of the ammonia. Also, the neutralization of basic digestion mixtures of bacterial causation will result in the union of ammonia with the acid (HCl) up to the neutral point of the indicator used. The addition of formaldehyde and the subsequent neutralization of the acidity of the mixture containing free carboxyl groups will probably go to a point where sodium will replace ammonium in ammonium chloride; the slowly liberated ammonia will tend to unite with formaldehyde to form hexamethylene tetra-amine, and in proportion to the ammonia present. If, however, this supposition of the influence of ammonia is incorrect, the net effect on the calculation of the distribution of nitrogen is after all quite small, because the amino nitrogen fraction changes relatively little during the period of incubation.

[20] Of course the dicarboxylic acids, aspartic and glutamic, are specifically exceptions to this $NH_2 — COOH$ ratio.

polypeptid. It is not surprising, therefore, to find that proteins, or even peptones, possess comparatively few free NH_2 groups. Their formol titrations are relatively small. For example, alanin and alanyl-alanin have the same theoretical formol titration. Thus:

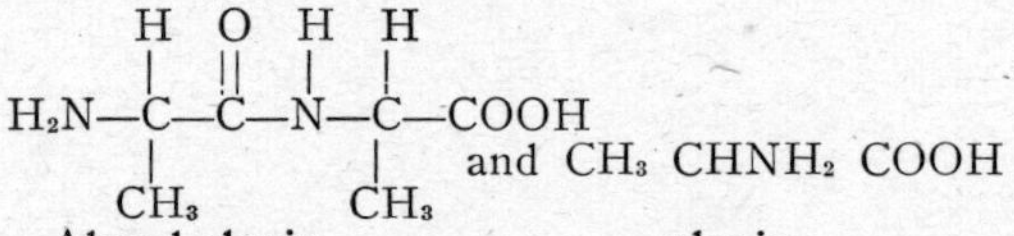

Alanyl-alanin alanin

have each one free NH_2 group. Hence, their formol titrations would be the same. A determination of the formol titration, and of the "non-protein nitrogen" (correcting both solutions for ammonia), would offer a theoretical means of determining the respective amounts of each in a culture medium. It is very evident that the usual cultural mediums will contain much more "polypeptid" nitrogen than "amino" nitrogen.

Procedure: Ten c c of culture medium are introduced into a beaker, together with about 40 c c of neutral, distilled water. The reaction is brought to the neutral point of phenolphthalein (P_H 8.3) by the cautious addition of N/10 HCl or N/10 NaOH, as may be required. Five c c of formaldehyde, exactly neutral to phenolphthalein, are added to the solution, which immediately becomes acid due to the reduction in basicity through the removal of the NH_2 groups, as outlined in the foregoing.

A second titration to neutrality will measure the acidity of the carboxyl group. As one free COOH occurs for one free NH_2 group in most amino acids and polpeptids,[20] the equivalent amount of standard ammonia corresponding to the amount of standard alkali in the titration after the addition of the neutral formaldehyde solution will be a measure of the "amino nitrogen" of the solution. Duplicate determinations will check with 0.10 c c N/10 NaOH without any difficulty. The precision of this reaction is about that of the nonprotein nitrogen and the total nitrogen determinations, if it is carried out with reasonable care. Rarely solutions are so highly colored that the end point is obscured somewhat.

An alternative procedure, much more time-consuming and presumably somewhat more exact, is the Van Slyke [21] method for the determination of amino nitrogen. The correction to be applied for free ammonia is somewhat more difficult to evaluate, since ammonia reacts relatively slowly with nitrous acid, which is the reagent used in the Van Slyke procedure. Generally speaking, the precision of the Sörensen titration wherever it can be used in the study of the nitrogenous metabolism of bacterial cultures is commensurate with the accuracy attending the parallel development of bacterial growths.

[21] Jour. Biol. Chem., 1912, 12, p. 275.

The amino nitrogen changes in bacterial cultures, as might be expected, are less marked and less significant than the concomitant changes in total nonprotein nitrogen and the gradual accumulation of free ammonia.

Free Ammonia.—Available evidence indicates that the accumulation of free ammonia in cultures of bacteria (probably present in no inconsiderable degree as ammonium carbonate) is very largely, if not practically exclusively, the result of the intracellular utilization of protein or protein derivatives for structural requirements (including the formation of enzymes and other structural replacements) and more particularly for energy. The extrusion of ammonia from the amino acid complex prior to the oxidation of the carbon is known as deamination. It is a measure of the intracellular utilization of amino acids for energy.

The difference in the amount of ammonia formation in protein and protein-carbohydrate mediums, respectively, is an indication of the sparing action of utilizable carbohydrate for protein as a source of energy. The analogy of the sparing action of carbohydrate for protein for bacterial cultures has its analogy in the sparing action of carbohydrate for protein in the human and animal body. Urea in the urine and ammonia in cultures of ordinary bacteria have approximately analogous significance.

Determination of Free Ammonia.—The determination of free ammonia in cultures of bacteria is readily accomplished with the Folin-MacCallum [22] modification of the Folin [23] air current method.

PROCEDURE

Two c c of culture medium are measured accurately with an Oswald pipet into an 8x1 inch pyrex test tube. One c c of an aqueous solution saturated both with sodium carbonate and sodium oxalate is added to the tube, and 1 c c of kerosene [24] to prevent foaming. The tube is closed with a two-hole tightly fitting rubber stopper. Air freed from ammonia by passage through a wash bottle containing 25% H_2SO_4 is led to the bottom of the tube, and bubbled through the solution. The air, containing ammonia, is passed through glass and rubber tubing to a glass tube terminating in a small bulb containing a crown of small openings. This tube reaches to the bottom of a 250 c c Erlenmeyer flask containing exactly 10 c c (or a multiple of 10 c c when necessary) of N/50 HCl, about 65 c c of water (neutral to alizarin), and a drop of aqueous alizarin solution (0.5%). It will be seen that this is a closed system through

[22] Jour. Biol. Chem., 1912, 11, p. 363.

[23] Ztschr. physiol. Chem., 1902, 37, p. 161.

[24] Old kerosene is better than fresh, because some of the more volatile constituents disappear on standing.

which ammonia-free air is forced through an alkaline solution of culture medium containing ammonia. The air current in its passage through the culture medium forces the ammonia (which is in the free state) quantitatively out of the medium, and carries it to the acid in the flask where it is quantitatively absorbed. After 15 minutes, with a fairly brisk air current, the entire amount of ammonia is gathered in the acid flask. The difference in titration between the original amount of N/50 HCl and that remaining free after the absorption of the ammonia as NH_4Cl, gives an accurate measure of the latter. The results of duplicate determinations check readily within 0.1 c c of N/50 alkali on back titration.

A number of details add to the rapidity with which the process may be carried out.

The most satisfactory air pump is the Westinghouse automatic type, driven by steam. A reservoir of 50 to 100 gallons to draw from is a necessity. The air pump will maintain a very nearly uniform pressure in such a tank without any human interference.

The delivery of air is readily accomplished through a long pipe set at 6-inch intervals with two opposite lateral openings. Each opening is controlled with a pet cock, or, better, with a gate valve. From each individual valve the air passes through a 2 liter bottle ⅛ filled with 25% of H_2SO_4. The air is forced through the acid (which frees it from ammonia), and from the bottle it passes to a tube which can be connected with one of the two delivery tubes in the pyrex test tube, as indicated in the foregoing. A battery of 20 pairs of independent air openings, each with its control valve, can be set up on a table less than 14 feet long and 3 feet wide.

For convenience the test tubes containing the solutions to be freed from ammonia can be supported in the double clamp so commonly used for burettes in chemical analyses. The occurrence of the tubes in pairs adds greatly to the convenience of keeping track of duplicate determinations. A pipe ¾ inch in diameter with ½ inch lateral openings, carrying 30 pounds' air pressure, is ample to carry 20 pairs of apparatus at one time. A drain cock should be placed at the distal end of the pipe to permit of the removal of condensation water which usually collects in the system.

The Oswald pipet should deliver exactly 2 c c. Such pipets may be purchased at any reputable chemical supply house. They should be tested for delivery, however. The dispensing of many flasks, each containing exactly 10 c c of N/50 HCl is best accomplished by the use of an automatic 10 c c pipet connected with the reservoir of acid. Such pipets are purchasable, but they must be tested for accurate delivery. Once a perfect pipet is obtained, it saves many times its cost in economy of time.

The N/50 alkali must be prepared, using alizarin as an indicator. Solutions that are the equivalent of N/1 HCl and N/1 NaOH, using phenolphthalein as an indicator, will not be exactly equivalent when they are diluted to N/50 strength. About 39.38 c c of N/1 NaOH will make exactly 2 liters of N/50 NaOH that will agree with N/50 HCl diluted in the proportion of 40 c c N/1 HCl to 1,960 c c of water.

The distilled water must be neutral to alizarin. Not all stills will deliver water of this reaction.

When the ammonia is removed from the culture solution, and the air is turned off, the delivery tube in the flask containing acid must be washed down with distilled water before the solution is titrated, otherwise some acid adheres to the tube and is lost.

Ammonia determinations performed in this manner check with the greatest ease to 0.10 c c of N/50 solution. This degree of precision should be adhered to in the methods described for total nitrogen, nonprotein nitrogen, and ammonia. All of these determinations, it will be remembered, are made with the air current method for removing the ammonia from solution and combining it with N/50 HCl. One c c of N/50 standard alkali corresponds to 0.00028 gm. ammonia nitrogen. Therefore, duplicate determinations check within 0.000,028 gm. nitrogen as ammonia, plus or minus. This is a relatively small error.

SUMMARY

The determination of total nitrogen, "nonprotein nitrogen," amino nitrogen and ammonia nitrogen, as outlined, permits a fractioning or division of the nitrogen in cultural mediums as follows:

1. Total Nitrogen.
2. Protein Nitrogen: Obtained as the difference between total nitrogen and nonprotein nitrogen.
3. Nonprotein Nitrogen.
4. "Polypeptid Nitrogen:" Obtained as the difference between the nonprotein nitrogen and the sum of the amino and ammonia nitrogen.
5. Amino Nitrogen: Obtained from the formol titration after subtraction of the free ammonia.
6. Free Ammonia: Obtained by the air current method as outlined. The relations of the several fractions are indicated briefly in the following examples:

TABLE 3

RELATIONS OF THE SEVERAL FRACTIONS

	A	B	C
Total nitrogen	1.064	1.064	1.064
Protein nitrogen	0.762	0.863[25]	0.885[25]
Nonprotein nitrogen	0.302	0.201	0.179
"Polypeptid nitrogen"	0.213	0.092	0.092
Amino nitrogen	0.032	0.030	0.037
Ammonia nitrogen	0.057	0.079	0.050
Reaction	+0.60	—1.70	+5.80
PH	7.0	8.1	4.9

A, control, uninoculated medium.
B, plain, sugar-free nutrient broth.
C, plain, sugar-free nutrient broth: (A), containing in addition 1% glucose; (B and C), parallel 7-day cultures of Bacillus coli.

The changes are readily explainable and need no comment. The least significant change appears to be that induced in the amino nitrogen fraction.

[25] Increase due chiefly to protein in the bacterial cells.

More energetic proteolytic bacteria, such as B. proteus, induce far greater changes, thus:

TABLE 4

CHANGES PRODUCED BY B. PROTEUS

	Control	A, Plain Gelatin	B, 1.5% Glucose Gelatin
Total nitrogen	1.001	1.001	1.001
Protein nitrogen	0.721	0.038	0.732
Nonprotein nitrogen	0.280	0.963	0.269
Polypeptid nitrogen	0.209	0.696	0.186
Amino nitrogen	0.039	0.036	0.044
Ammonia nitrogen	0.032	0.204	0.039

7-day incubation.

Here again the amino nitrogen fraction changes but little, although the free ammonia in the plain gelatin (deamination) increases very much indeed. In glucose gelatin the deamination is minimal.

That the increase in free ammonia is due to the intracellular utilization of the protein for energy is shown by the following experiments, in which 5 c c of culture A and of culture B, respectively, were placed in 95 c c of 10% carbol gelatin. No bacterial development took place of course. Incubation was practiced for 3 days to allow the enzyme in "A" to act.

TABLE 5

SEVEN-DAY CULTURE IN CARBOL GELATIN

	Control	A	B
Total nitrogen	1.330	1.330	1.330
Protein nitrogen	1.061	0.332	1.051
Nonprotein nitrogen	0.269	1.008	0.279
Polypeptid nitrogen	0.211	0.916	0.222
Amino nitrogen	0.040	0.073	0.040
Ammonia nitrogen	0.018	0.019	0.017

Here, as might be confidently expected, the deamination failed to take place. This shows strikingly what the sparing action of utilizable carbohydrate for protein really means in the nitrogen spectrum of a bacterial culture. The action of the enzyme in "A" is very clearly indicated.

THE NITROGENOUS METABOLISM OF B. DYSENTERIAE (SHIGA), BACILLUS TYPHOSUS, B. PARATYPHOSUS ALPHA AND B. PARATYPHOSUS BETA

STUDIES IN BACTERIAL METABOLISM LVIII-LXI

Arthur Isaac Kendall and Reba Cordelia Haner

Department of Bacteriology, Northwestern University Medical School, Chicago, Ill.

The discovery of the newer and more complete methods for the measurement of nitrogenous substances which possess significance in the metabolism of the human body, by Folin,[1] has opened new avenues of approach to the problem of intermediary nitrogenous metabolism in bacterial cultures. Slight changes in the technic of Folin's method for the determination of nonprotein nitrogen,[2] which do not affect the principle involved but do add somewhat to their applicability to bacterial mediums, have made it possible to fractionate the nitrogenous constitutents of bacterial cultures and to follow the quantitative distribution of these fractions under varying conditions. The precision of measurement attainable by these methods is of such a degree that even the finer and less conspicuous phases of bacterial growth may be definitely evaluated; the simplicity of the chemical manipulation requisite for close duplication of results places the entire process within the reach of the average student.

Hitherto the changes in nitrogenous constituents of cultural mediums during bacterial growth have been restricted almost entirely to the measurement of the amino nitrogen and ammonia nitrogen, and their respective ratios to the total nitrogen of the medium. Ammonia formation, resulting from deamination incidental to the intracellular utilization of protein or protein derivatives, is of much greater significance than the variation in amino nitrogen.[3] Indeed, the determination of the so-called "amino nitrogen" is limited to those NH_2 groups of protein, of the various products of protein cleavage by hydrolysis or otherwise, of polypeptids and free amino acids which are free and not chemically combined with carboxyl groups of other amino acids to form the "protein tie." It will be remembered that a dipeptid and a single amino acid would give exactly the same theoretical "amino" nitrogen

Received for publication Oct. 12, 1921.

[1] Jour. Biol. Chem., 1919, 38, p. 81.

[2] Kendall: Jour. Infect. Dis., Study LVII, 1922, 30, p. 211.

[3] Kendall and Walker: Ibid., 1915, 17, p. 442.

titer if they were examined molecule for molecule. Thus, alanin, and alanylalanin (the latter composed of two molecules of alanin minus hydrogen and oxygen in the proportions to form water), would each possess one free NH_2 group. Folin's nonprotein nitrogen method permits a much more extensive survey of the nitrogenous constituents than has hitherto been possible. The fractions that may be measured comprise the following: total nitrogen, protein nitrogen, nonprotein nitrogen, ammonia nitrogen, and that portion of nitrogen which is obtained by the difference between the total nonprotein nitrogen and the sum of the ammonia and amino nitrogen. This fraction in ordinary cultural mediums is undoubtedly made up of creatin and creatinin,[4] purin and pyramidin bases, and polypeptids from which the nitrogen of the "protein tie" is liberated by the digestion with acid in the process of determination of nonprotein nitrogen. For convenience, this residual nonprotein nitrogen will be designated "polypeptid" nitrogen,[2] it being expressly understood that the term as used is symbolical rather than definitive.

It is clear that any method which opens up possibilities of quantitative measurement is of material importance in the biologic sciences. A series of studies on important pathogenic bacteria indicates that considerable light may be thrown on the mechanism of their metabolism through the application of the new Folin procedures.

BACILLUS DYSENTERIAE

STUDY LVIII

One of the important pathogenic bacterial groups is that of the dysentery bacilli. During the Great War the members of this group were much studied because of their formidable effects on troops in the warmer areas fought over. The Shiga bacillus is the most formidable of the group, both on account of its great toxicity and because of the residual incapacity for work which Shiga bacillus carriers exhibit after recovery from the acute stage of the infection.[5]

In previous communications,[6] a peculiarity of Shiga cultures was pointed out, namely, the parallelism in ammonia formation in plain and glucose broth cultures during the earlier days of incubation. This stands in distinct contrast to the other members of the dysentery group,[7]

[4] It would be perfectly possible to determine the creatinin fraction of the polypeptid nitrogen by the method of Folin. Jour. Biol. Chem., 1914, 17, p. 475.

[5] Med. Res. Committee, Special Report 29, 1919.

[6] Kendall and Farmer: Jour. Biol. Chem., 1912, 12, p. 13.

[7] Except the Schmitz bacillus, which will be discussed later.

which attack from the start the protein constituents of plain broth, forming therefrom progressive amounts of ammonia, and generating coincidently a constantly increasing alkalinity. The same phenomenon is observed in cultures of staphylococci, and the explanation advanced tentatively is that the so-called carbohydrate fraction of the protein

TABLE 1

BACILLUS DYSENTERIAE SHIGA

Mg. per 100 C c	Control	Day	Plain Broth	Glucose Broth
Total nitrogen	1.064	1	1.064	1.064
Protein nitrogen	0.762		0.762	0.762
Nonprotein nitrogen	0.302		0.302	0.302
Polypeptid nitrogen	0.213		0.213	0.206
Amino nitrogen	0.032		0.032	0.029
Ammonia nitrogen	0.057		0.055	0.057
Reaction	+0.60		+0.60	+1.30
PH	7.0		.....	.....
Total nitrogen	1.064	3	1.064	1.064
Protein nitrogen	0.762		0.806	0.818
Nonprotein nitrogen	0.302		0.258	0.246
Polypeptid nitrogen	0.213		0.178	0.165
Amino nitrogen	0.032		0.029	0.027
Ammonia nitrogen	0.057		0.051	0.054
Reaction	+0.60		+1.00	+2.10
PH	7.0		7.1	5.5
Total nitrogen	1.064	6	1.064	1.064
Protein nitrogen	0.762		0.829	0.896
Nonprotein nitrogen	0.302		0.235	0.168
Polypeptid nitrogen	0.213		0.137	0.079
Amino nitrogen	0.032		0.045	0.040
Ammonia nitrogen	0.057		0.053	0.049
Reaction	+0.60		+1.20	+4.00
PH	7.0		7.2	5.9
Total nitrogen	1.064	10	1.064	1.064
Protein nitrogen	0.762		0.806	0.840
Nonprotein nitrogen	0.302		0.258	0.224
Polypeptid nitrogen	0.213		0.158	0.135
Amino nitrogen	0.032		0.045	0.040
Ammonia nitrogen	0.057		0.055	0.049
Reaction	+0.60		+0.70	+3.90
PH	7.0		.....	.....
Total nitrogen	1.064	15	1.064	1.064
Protein nitrogen	0.762		0.818	0.818
Nonprotein nitrogen	0.302		0.246	0.246
Polypeptid nitrogen	0.213		0.144	0.159
Amino nitrogen	0.032		0.047	0.044
Ammonia nitrogen	0.057		0.055	0.043
Reaction	+0.60		+0.30	+4.00
PH	7.0		7.9	5.8

molecule is peculiarly vulnerable to the action of the Shiga bacillus and the staphylococcus. These microbes utilize the carbohydrate moiety, producing therefrom the acid, and also sparing the nitrogenous constituents from attack until the carbohydrate is exhausted. In the staphylococcus cultures which were studied, the attack on the nitrogenous constituents of plain broth for energy, usually after five days' incubation, was indicated by a sudden increase in ammonia formation, the abrupt decrease in the initial acid reaction and the disappearance of the Molisch test, which is supposed to depend on the presence of a carbohydrate in the protein molecule.[8]

A study of the metabolism of the Shiga bacillus in 5% nutrient gelatin, both with and without the addition of 1% of glucose, has substantiated the observations made previously, and has shown in addition some of the more intimate details of its action on the nitrogenous constituents of the mediums.

Reaction: The change in titratable acidity, both in plain and glucose gelatin, during the first week of incubation is toward the acid side, although much less in the plain than in the glucose medium. An attempt was made to follow the change in hydrogen-ion concentration, using phenol sulphonephthalein (phenol red) for values above 6.8 and below 8.3, and dibromo ortho cresol sulphonephthalein (brom cresol purple) for ranges below 6.8 and above 5.4.[9] The observations were made in comparitor tubes, practically as suggested in Clark's monograph. The results were disappointing, chiefly because the "protein error," due to the gelatin not only diminishes the brilliancy of the dye, but it also, in some way not clearly understood, alters the quality of the color so that the comparisons with standard solutions are difficult and uncertain. The gas chain method of measuring the electrical potential would undoubtedly have been satisfactory, but the amount of information elicited in this particular series of studies would have been disproportionately small to the time required to obtain it.

NITROGENOUS CHANGES

Although the Shiga bacillus is one of the more inert bacteria, chemically speaking, the changes in the nitrogenous constitutents of the mediums are clear cut. Whatever attack the microbe may make on the protein nitrogen of the medium is more than compensated for by the increase in protein nitrogen of the culture attributable to the growth of the bacilli. This formation of bacterial protein, furthermore, is at the expense of the residual nonprotein nitrogen after the subtraction therefrom of the amino and ammonia nitrogen. Neither the amino nitrogen nor the ammonia nitrogen show noteworthy changes, even during the late days of incubation (10 days) when the recessive changes and

[8] Kendall and Farmer: Jour. Biol. Chem., 1912, 12, p. 215.
[9] Clark: Determination of Hydrogen Ions, 1920.

autolytic processes seem to redissolve and restore to the nonprotein fraction some of the substance that was built up into the bacterial bodies in the earlier days of growth.

It would appear that in these gelatin mediums the Shiga bacillus found the best structural nitrogenous compounds in the residual, nonprotein nitrogen moiety, which contains, as explained in the foregoing, polypeptids, together with smaller and unknown amounts of purin and pyramidin bases and creatinin. It is not surprising to find that the bacilli grow more rapidly in the medium containing glucose. This is shown by the more rapid and greater accumulation of "protein nitrogen" in the glucose medium. Also, as might be expected perhaps, the rate and extent of autolysis is somewhat less in the glucose medium. As soon as the evidences of carbohydrate in the gelatin-peptone molecules are gone (approximately 10 days), the evidences of proteolysis become somewhat more apparent, although at that late stage the process cannot presumably go very far. It would appear that the addition of gelatin to cultural mediums intended for the growth of B. dysenteriae would not materially enrich them; there is practically no evidence that the bacilli produce any significant alteration in that portion of the total nitrogen fraction which would obviously belong to the true gelatin-protein moiety.

BACILLUS TYPHOSUS

STUDY LIX

The belief is fairly widespread that cultures of pathogenic bacteria kept on artificial mediums for long periods of time tend to lose some of those qualities which are collectively spoken of as "virulence." In some instances this loss is manifested by a decreased ability to incite lesions or cause death in experimental animals. In other cases there may be a distinct loss or even complete disappearance of toxin-producing power. On the other hand, it is a matter of common observation that the initial growths of pathogenic bacteria outside the body are difficult to obtain, and also that successive transfers of such organisms on artificial mediums are more and more readily produced. It might be confidently expected that there may be some relationship expressible in chemical terms which would be parallel to this phenomenon, as increased ability to grow under the conditions imposed by cultural conditions would suggest an adaptability to the chemical nutrients of artificial pabula. In one definite instance, a quantitative but not qualitative difference between a virulent and a nonvirulent strain was detected, namely, in two cultures of hog cholera bacilli, obtained from Dr. Theobald Smith several years ago.[1] The virulent strain was noticeably less proteolytic than the avirulent one. There was no evidence available at that time to indicate whether this difference was due wholly to incomplete adaptation of the virulent strain of the hog cholera bacillus to

TABLE 1

BACILLUS TYPHOSUS, 1

Mg. per 100 C c	Control	Day	Plain Broth	Glucose Broth
Total nitrogen	1.080	1	1.080	1.080
Protein nitrogen	0.778		0.800	0.790
Nonprotein nitrogen	0.302		0.280	0.290
Polypeptid nitrogen	0.210		0.175	0.196
Amino nitrogen	0.042		0.048	0.045
Ammonia nitrogen	0.050		0.057	0.049
Reaction	+0.80		+1.30	+5.10
PH	7.2		7.3	5.0
Total nitrogen	1.080	4	1.080	1.080
Protein nitrogen	0.778		0.811	0.801
Nonprotein nitrogen	0.302		0.269	0.279
Polypeptid nitrogen	0.210		0.167	0.181
Amino nitrogen	0.042		0.044	0.051
Ammonia nitrogen	0.050		0.058	0.047
Reaction	+0.80		—0.80	+5.40
PH	7.2		7.8	5.0
Total nitrogen	1.080	7	1.080	1.080
Protein nitrogen	0.778		0.923	0.913
Nonprotein nitrogen	0.302		0.157	0.167
Polypeptid nitrogen	0.210		0.044	0.067
Amino nitrogen	0.042		0.043	0.052
Ammonia nitrogen	0.050		0.070	0.048
Reaction	+0.80		—1.40	+5.80
PH	7.2		8.4	5.0
Total nitrogen	1.080	10	1.080	1.080
Protein nitrogen	0.778		0.868	0.890
Nonprotein nitrogen	0.302		0.212	0.190
Polypeptid nitrogen	0.210		0.097	0.102
Amino nitrogen	0.042		0.038	0.040
Ammonia nitrogen	0.050		0.077	0.048
Reaction	+0.80		—2.10	+4.20
PH	7.2		8.7	5.3

artificial conditions (it grew somewhat less luxuriantly, but not decidedly so, than the avirulent strain), or whether other and wholly unsuspected or unknown factors played a prominent part in this definite phenomenon.

An opportunity presented itself to study two strains of typhoid bacilli, 1 and 2, under nearly parallel conditions. Culture 1 has been kept as a stock laboratory culture with monthly transfers, for a period

[1] For analytical details, see Kendall and Farmer, Jour. Biol. Chem., 1912, 12, p. 19.

of at least 12 years. Culture 2 is said to have been isolated within a recent period, less than a month. The nitrogenous metabolism of these 2 cultures was studied, using methods previously described,[2] and extending over a period of 10 days for the older strain and 15 days for the newer strain, respectively.

DISCUSSION

Certain quantitative differences in the intensity of the reactions induced by the two strains are clearly discernible, but it is quite evident that the significance to be attached to them is not great. It is quite probable that the variations in the amount of growth, suggested by the increases in protein nitrogen, are potent factors in evaluating these changes. Culture 1 at the end of the seventh day, for example, in plain nutrient gelatin had increased the protein nitrogen fraction 14.5%, while culture 2 had increased the corresponding fraction less than 8%. A more distinctive change is that of the accumulation of free ammonia. Here the deamination in culture 1 was equal to 2.7% of the total nitrogen of the culture medium, while that of culture 2 was almost exactly 1%. The tendency, on the whole, is for culture 1 to be somewhat more active in deamination than culture 2, a phenomenon which had its counterpart in the avirulent and virulent hog cholera bacilli, referred to previously. The tables show quite clearly that the increase in protein nitrogen, due presumably to the actual increase in bacterial protein is largely at the expense of the residual nonprotein nitrogen, the "polypeptid nitrogen," after deduction of the amino nitrogen and ammonia nitrogen. The autolytic changes in both cultures after the seventh day of incubation are quite clearly indicated by the decrease in protein nitrogen at that time. This change is materially greater in culture 1 than in culture 2.

The sparing action of glucose for the protein constituents of the mediums utilizable for energy is shown by the differences in deamination in plain and glucose cultures, respectively. The total amount of bacterial protein, evidenced by the increase of protein nitrogen as incubation proceeds, is roughly parallel in each culture, and in each medium. The amino nitrogen undergoes little change, although whatever difference there may be favors an increase in the glucose gelatin and a reduction in the plain gelatin. In the former medium, however, there is a slight but actual diminution in the amount of ammonia (no

[2] Kendall: Jour. Infect. Dis., Study LVII, 1922, 30, p. 211.

increase in deamination), whereas in the plain gelatin the tendency is toward an increase. This is in harmony with many previous investigations on this subject. Final evidence of the effects of carbohydrate on the energy requirements of bacteria will be obtained when adequate methods for measuring accurately the carbon metabolism of bacteria

TABLE 2

BACILLUS TYPHOSUS, 2

Mg. per 100 C c	Control	Day	Plain Broth	Glucose Broth
Total nitrogen	1.064	1	1.064	1.064
Protein nitrogen	0.762		0.762	0.762
Nonprotein nitrogen	0.302		0.302	0.302
Polypeptid nitrogen	0.213		0.213	0.210
Amino nitrogen	0.032		0.032	0.038
Ammonia nitrogen	0.057		0.057	0.054
Reaction	+0.60		+0.30	+3.00
PH	7.0		.....	.....
Total nitrogen	1.064	3	1.064	1.064
Protein nitrogen	0.762		0.829	0.840
Nonprotein nitrogen	0.302		0.235	0.224
Polypeptid nitrogen	0.213		0.156	0.143
Amino nitrogen	0.032		0.026	0.035
Ammonia nitrogen	0.057		0.053	0.046
Reaction	+0.60		—0.60	+4.70
PH	7.0		7.8	5.5
Total nitrogen	1.064	6	1.064	1.064
Protein nitrogen	0.762		0.840	0.874
Nonprotein nitrogen	0.302		0.224	0.190
Polypeptid nitrogen	0.213		0.127	0.102
Amino nitrogen	0.032		0.037	0.042
Ammonia nitrogen	0.057		0.060	0.046
Reaction	+0.60		—1.40	+4.60
PH	7.0		7.9	5.9
Total nitrogen	1.064	10	1.064	1.064
Protein nitrogen	0.762		0.795	0.829
Nonprotein nitrogen	0.302		0.269	0.235
Polypeptid nitrogen	0.213		0.169	0.147
Amino nitrogen	0.032		0.033	0.041
Ammonia nitrogen	0.057		0.067	0.047
Reaction	+0.60		—1.60	+4.90
PH	7.0		.....	.....
Total nitrogen	1.064	15	1.064	1.064
Protein nitrogen	0.762		0.739	0.806
Nonprotein nitrogen	0.302		0.325	0.258
Polypeptid nitrogen	0.213		0.220	0.158
Amino nitrogen	0.032		0.041	0.052
Ammonia nitrogen	0.057		0.064	0.048
Reaction	+0.60		—1.90	+5.20
PH	7.0		8.6	5.8

are available. It should be stated, however, that the decided change in reaction exhibited by the cultures in glucose gelatin, as evidenced by change in titratable acidity and hydrogen-ion concentration, point unmistakably to a vigorous action on carbohydrate in the glucose mediums.

The alterations in reaction in purely nitrogenous mediums under otherwise parallel conditions are distinct, but quantitatively much less. The basicity of the protein reaction is, in proportion to the increase of protein nitrogen, rather at the relative expense of the residual or polypeptid nitrogen in the plain gelatin cultures, however.

It appears to be quite clear that the addition of gelatin to cultures of typhoid bacilli, containing the usual peptone and meat extractives, is of no material benefit in so far as the purely nutritional value of the nitrogenous constituents of the gelatin is concerned. Whether the colloidal conditions of the solution are improved for bacterial growth by the addition of gelatin is not answered by these experiments.

BACILLUS PARATYPHOSUS ALPHA

STUDY LX

Bacillus paratyphosus alpha is a member of the intermediate, or paratyphoid group of bacilli, which, it will be remembered, usually incite infections in man similar to but usually less severe than typhoid fever. The alpha type is somewhat less commonly encountered in human infections in the United States than the beta type, judging from available statistics. Also, the type of infection induced is said to be more nearly typhoidal both in course and severity. Chemically, the alpha organism approaches quite closely in its general reactions the more commonly encountered typhoid strain; that one which induces a persistent acid reaction in milk. Milk cultures of both the typhoid bacillus type just mentioned and B. typhosus alpha may exhibit somewhat lessened acidity after several days' incubation, but this tendency is by no means as marked as that characteristic of milk cultures of B. typhosus beta. Milk cultures of the beta type exhibit an initial acidity in milk under normal conditions which soon (three days on the average) turns toward the alkaline side. The older cultures not infrequently assume a semitranslucent appearance, due chiefly to a slow degradation of the milk proteins. This digestion is rather of the peptic than the tryptic type, so far as chemical analyses indicate, because the change in the amino nitrogen fraction is relatively slight and quite unlike that of actively proteolytic bacteria, as, for example, typical strains of B. proteus.

A study of the nitrogenous metabolism of a typical strain of B. paratyphosus alpha, using the newer procedure which furnishes several distinct fractions of nitrogenous nutritive substances,[1] has thrown some light on the character of the intermediary changes in the gelatin-peptone-meat extractive medium during the growth of the organism, and also the effect of adding glucose to the protein constituents as an additional source of energy.

BACILLUS PARATYPHOSUS ALPHA

Mg. per 100 C c	Control	Day	Plain Broth	Glucose Broth
Total nitrogen	1.080	1	1.080	1.080
Protein nitrogen	0.778		0.789	0.790
Nonprotein nitrogen	0.302		0.291	0.290
Polypeptid nitrogen	0.210		0.184	0.199
Amino nitrogen	0.042		0.049	0.039
Ammonia nitrogen	0.050		0.056	0.052
Reaction	+0.80		+1.90	+3.90
PH	7.2		7.1	5.9
Total nitrogen	1.080	4	1.080	1.080
Protein nitrogen	0.778		0.811	0.801
Nonprotein nitrogen	0.302		0.269	0.279
Polypeptid nitrogen	0.210		0.167	0.188
Amino nitrogen	0.042		0.041	0.043
Ammonia nitrogen	0.050		0.061	0.048
Reaction	+0.80		—0.60	+4.90
PH	7.2		7.7	5.0
Total nitrogen	1.080	7	1.080	1.080
Protein nitrogen	0.778		0.923	0.879
Nonprotein nitrogen	0.302		0.157	0.201
Polypeptid nitrogen	0.210		0.055	0.104
Amino nitrogen	0.042		0.038	0.049
Ammonia nitrogen	0.050		0.064	0.048
Reaction	+0.80		—1.00	+5.20
PH	7.2		8.4	5.3
Total nitrogen	1.080	10	1.080	1.080
Protein nitrogen	0.778		0.890	0.890
Nonprotein nitrogen	0.302		0.190	0.190
Polypeptid nitrogen	0.210		0.085	0.103
Amino nitrogen	0.042		0.025	0.040
Ammonia nitrogen	0.050		0.080	0.047
Reaction	+0.80		—1.10	+5.30
PH	7.2		8.7	5.3

DISCUSSION

The growth of the organism in both the plain and the glucose gelatin was luxuriant, judging from the increase in the protein nitrogen fraction, and the corresponding decrease in the nonprotein constituents. At the end of the seventh day, when the change was greatest, and before autolytic changes had brought about a partial resolution of the bacterial substance, there was an increase in protein nitrogen of 145 mg. in each 100 c c of culture medium (plain gelatin). This amounts almost exactly to 14.5% increase in the protein nitrogen fraction. The

[1] Kendall: Jour. Infect. Dis., Study LVII, 1922, 30, p. 211.

ammonia increased somewhat during this time, but there was no proportionate variation in the amino-nitrogen fraction. Indeed, this remained practically constant; the small fluctuation, amounting to 0.04 of 1% (4 mg.) at the height of the protein nitrogen increase, is almost within the limits of error of the method.

The great and significant change corresponding to the increase in protein nitrogen (protein of the bacterial substance itself) is that observed in the residual nonprotein nitrogen after correction for the amino and ammonia-nitrogen fractions, respectively. This corresponds to the polypeptid nitrogen discussed in an earlier communication.[1]

In glucose gelatin the same relative increase in protein nitrogen is observed, although the maximum is not as great in this medium as in plain gelatin. In actual figures, it amounts to slightly more than 11% in glucose gelatin compared with 14.5% in plain gelatin. The amino-nitrogen fraction undergoes practically no change in the glucose gelatin, as was the case in the plain gelatin cultures.

The evidences of deamination, shown by the free ammonia fraction, are absent in glucose gelatin; the extreme variation in this fraction is 3 mg. from the uninoculated controls. Three milligrams' variation in 100 c c of medium corresponds in this instance to 0.3 of 1% of the total nitrogen. On the contrary, the deamination in the plain gelatin cultures, in which the organisms obtain their energy from protein derivatives (polypeptids chiefly), amounts progressively from 0.6 of 1% in the 24-hour cultures to 3% in the 10-day cultures. As deamination is a measure of the intracellular utilization of protein derivatives for energy, this result might have been confidently expected in plain broth cultures.

The glucose gelatin cultures contain a readily utilizable non-nitrogenous source of energy as well as the nitrogenous polypeptid fraction in common with the plain gelatin medium. The absence of evidence of deamination in the glucose gelatin, therefore, points clearly to the sparing action of glucose for the protein derivatives in glucose gelatin cultures of this organism. It will be remembered that B. paratyphosus alpha produces gas (CO_2 and H_2) and acid in glucose mediums; a basic reaction, no gas and no acid in plain nutrient broth. Here again the sparing action of the glucose for the protein constituents of the medium as a source of energy is manifested. This is expressed in determinative or diagnostic bacteriology by stating that B. paratyphosus alpha "ferments glucose."

BACILLUS PARATYPHOSUS BETA

STUDY LXI

The appended analytic tables illustrative of the nitrogenous metabolism of a culture of B. paratyphosus beta are confirmatory of the general phenomena observed in cultures of B. typhosus and of B. paratyphosus alpha.[1] The growth of the beta strain herein described was somewhat less luxuriant than is the case with many current strains, but the general character of the results is unmistakable. The increase in protein nitrogen is, as before, indicative of the luxuriance of the development of the bacteria.

BACILLUS PARATYPHOSUS BETA

Mg. per 100 C c	Control	Day	Plain Gelatin	Glucose Gelatin
Total nitrogen	1.064	1	1.064	1.064
Protein nitrogen	0.762		0.762	0.762
Nonprotein nitrogen	0.302		0.302	0.302
Polypeptid nitrogen	0.213		0.207	0.210
Amino nitrogen	0.032		0.035	0.035
Ammonia nitrogen	0.057		0.060	0.057
Reaction	+0.60		+0.60	+2.60
PH	7.0		.....	.....
Total nitrogen	1.064	3	1.064	1.064
Protein nitrogen	0.762		0.829	0.863
Nonprotein nitrogen	0.302		0.235	0.201
Polypeptid nitrogen	0.213		0.152	0.117
Amino nitrogen	0.032		0.023	0.029
Ammonia nitrogen	0.057		0.060	0.054
Reaction	+0.60		—0.60	+4.80
PH	7.0		7.8	5.5
Total nitrogen	1.064	6	1.064	1.064
Protein nitrogen	0.762		0.829	0.863
Nonprotein nitrogen	0.302		0.235	0.201
Polypeptid nitrogen	0.213		0.135	0.112
Amino nitrogen	0.032		0.031	0.038
Ammonia nitrogen	0.057		0.069	0.051
Reaction	+0.60		—1.60	+6.20
PH	7.0		7.9	5.9
Total nitrogen	1.064	10	1.064	1.064
Protein nitrogen	0.762		0.806	0.840
Nonprotein nitrogen	0.302		0.258	0.224
Polypeptid nitrogen	0.213		0.155	0.137
Amino nitrogen	0.032		0.024	0.039
Ammonia nitrogen	0.057		0.079	0.048
Reaction	+0.60		—1.90	+5.70
PH	7.0		.....	.....
Total nitrogen	1.064	15	1.064	1.064
Protein nitrogen	0.762		0.762	0.818
Nonprotein nitrogen	0.302		0.302	0.246
Polypeptid nitrogen	0.213		0.201	0.161
Amino nitrogen	0.032		0.034	0.038
Ammonia nitrogen	0.057		0.067	0.047
Reaction	+0.60		—2.10	+6.30
PH	7.0		8.8	5.8

[1] Kendall and Haner: Studies LVIII and LIX, Jour. Infect. Dis., 1922, 30, pp. 226, 229.

In the series under consideration, the growth in the glucose gelatin culture was somewhat more vigorous than that in the plain gelatin culture. The sparing action of the glucose for the protein constituents of the medium, manifested by the uniform absence of an increase in ammonia, is clear cut. Although there was an undoubted disparity of growth in the plain and glucose mediums in favor of the latter, the evidence of deamination (ammonia increase) is exhibited only in the plain gelatin cultures.

The maximum development in both plain and glucose cultures is reached on or about the seventh day of incubation. By the tenth day recessive changes, associated with a partial resolution of the protein locked up in the bodies of the bacteria (autolysis) are clearly discernible. The gelatin protein, as before noted,[1] plays a minor and negligible part in providing nitrogenous nutriment for the bacilli, even in plain gelatin. The conclusion that gelatin protein is not as favorable a source of nitrogenous energy as the polypeptid fraction of the medium for B. paratyphosus beta seems to be clearly demonstrated through the fact that the increase in protein nitrogen is paralleled by a corresponding decrease in the residual nonprotein fraction of the nitrogenous constituents of the medium after correction for the amino-nitrogen and ammonia-nitrogen portions.

The influence of glucose on the utilization of protein derivatives for energy is clearly shown not only by the difference in deamination, previously mentioned, but also by a comparison of the increase in protein nitrogen, due to the transformation of nonprotein nitrogen into actual bacterial substance with the corresponding change in residual nonprotein nitrogen after allowance for deamination.

The increase in protein nitrogen in the plain gelatin culture is (10 days) 44 mg.; in glucose broth, in which the development was more luxuriant, 78 mg. Twenty-two mg. of ammonia were produced by the simultaneous deamination of nitrogenous substances in the plain gelatin, whereas there was a slight deficit in ammonia in the glucose gelatin incidental to the production of 78 mg. of protein nitrogen (bacterial protein). Corresponding to the increase of 78 mg. of protein nitrogen in the glucose-gelatin culture, there was a decrease of 76 mg. of residual nonprotein nitrogen after correction for the amino nitrogen and free ammonia. In contrast to this close relationship between polypeptid decrease and protein nitrogen increase, the plain broth nitrogenous changes appear significant.

The protein nitrogen increase in the plain gelatin amounted to 44 mg. (10-day culture), and the corresponding polypeptid nitrogen decrease was 48 mg., or nearly 25% more. This disproportion between bacterial protein increase and polypeptid nitrogen decrease in the two mediums is again an indication of the sparing action of utilizable carbohydrate for energy by many bacteria. In other words, B. paratyphosus beta appears to multiply in a glucose gelatin medium to a greater extent with a smaller concomitant expenditure of nitrogenous substance than is the case in plain gelatin, in which both the structural and energy requirements for the entire metabolic process must be derived from the nitrogenous constituents of the medium.

THE NITROGENOUS METABOLISM OF BACILLUS COLI

STUDIES IN BACTERIAL METABOLISM. LXII

Arthur Isaac Kendall and Robert S. Bly

Department of Bacteriology, Northwestern University Medical School, Chicago, Ill.

Bacillus coli is normally the most abundant organism of the lower intestinal contents in adolescence and adult life. Observations are not wanting which would suggest that it is equally commonly found in the feces of domestic animals. Even in severe infections of the intestinal tract by exogenous bacteria, such as typhoid or dysentery bacilli, the colon bacillus persists in variable but relatively considerable numbers, and protracted starvation fails to eliminate the microbe.[1] It appears to possess characteristics which meet those of the intestinal environment without apparent discomfort to the host.

Chemically and culturally, B. coli is distinctly more active than those exogenous intestinal invaders which incite specific disease, such as B. typhosus and members of the dysentery bacillus group. The colon bacillus is less active chemically than the cholera group, however. In general, it may be stated that intense chemical and cultural activity is incompatible with etiologic participation in progressively pathogenic disease. Cholera is apparently a striking exception to this statement, however.

Previous studies of the nitrogenous metabolism of certain members of the pathogenic intestinal group of bacilli[2] have shown that the changes in the nitrogenous constituents of ordinary mediums (containing no utilizable carbohydrate) which are utilized for energy are chiefly centered in that portion of the nitrogen spectrum designated, for purposes of discussion, "polypeptid" nitrogen.[3] This fraction consists of the polypeptids, creatin and creatinin, purin and pyrimidin bases chiefly. The diminution of this polypeptid fraction as growth proceeds, aside from a small increase in free ammonia indicating the utilization of some amino acid for the requisite energy of the microbes, is closely

Received for publication Oct. 12, 1921.

[1] Kendall: Observations on the Bacterial Intestinal Flora of a Starving Man. Publication 203, Carnegie Institute, Washington, 1915, p. 232.

[2] Studies LVII-LXI, inclusive, Jour. Infect. Dis., 1922, 30, pp. 211-238.

[3] Kendall: Study LVII, ibid., 1922, 30, p. 211.

paralleled by a corresponding increase in the protein-nitrogen fraction of the nitrogen content. The most direct explanation for this apparent transformation of nonprotein nitrogen is that an actual production of bacterial protein has taken place. In other words, this is a measure of the growth of bacteria in the medium.

It should be stated that centrifugalization of such a culture will throw out an amount of nitrogen almost exactly equal to the increase of bacterial nitrogen as growth proceeds. A microscopic examination of the sediment will reveal the fact that it is essentially made up of the bodies of bacteria. Within the limits of precision of available methods, therefore, pathogenic bacteria of the typhoid-dysentery-paratyphoid group appear to build their bodies from the "polypeptid" fraction of ordinary nutrient gelatin mediums, rather than from the gelatin protein which is also present. The absence of certain aromatic amino acids from gelatin, such as tyrosin, may be of some significance in this connection, although the evidence is on the whole against it.

If utilizable carbohydrate is present in the gelatin medium, the requisite energy of the microbes is obtained from it; the increment in the protein nitrogen occurs without appreciable change in the free ammonia. If, on the contrary, protein and protein derivatives alone are present, the protein fraction increases with a concomitant augmentation in free ammonia, suggesting the utilization of a certain amount of nitrogen-containing substance for energy.

As B. coli is more reactive than the pathogenic intestinal bacteria referred to in the foregoing, it is a matter of some theoretical importance to determine the effects of its growth on nitrogenous constituents of cultural mediums. Nutrient gelatin, both with and without the addition of glucose, was selected because the protein fraction is much greater in this enriched medium than would be the case in the peptone mediums usually employed for cultural observations.

The same series of observations as those reported in previous studies were made in cultures of B. coli.[2] In addition, an effort was made to determine whether a soluble proteolytic enzyme was present, which might cause cleavage of some of the gelatin or peptone protein. The method used to detect such an enzyme has been described previously.[4] It consists essentially in adding 5 c c of a growing culture of the organism at stated intervals to 95 c c of a 5% solution of gelatin in water to which is added 0.5% phenol. The phenol prevents the

[4] Kendall and Walker: Jour. Infect. Dis., 1915, 17, p. 442.

growth of the bacteria, and experience has shown that the soluble enzyme of organisms, such as B. proteus, is not prevented from acting in such a medium. It is necessary to make careful controls each time a culture is examined for enzyme activity. One control is examined immediately after the culture is added. Incubation of the culture—carbol gelatin mixture is practiced 3 days to afford time for the enzyme to act.

TABLE 1

BACILLUS COLI

Mg. per 100 C c	Control	Day	Plain Broth	Glucose Broth
Total nitrogen	1.064	1	1.064	1.064
Protein nitrogen	0.762		0.773	0.773
Nonprotein nitrogen	0.302		0.291	0.291
Polypeptid nitrogen	0.213		0.202	0.203
Amino nitrogen	0.032		0.022	0.032
Ammonia nitrogen	0.057		0.067	0.056
Reaction	+0.60		+0.20	+3.80
PH	7.0		.....	.....
Total nitrogen	1.064	3	1.064	1.064
Protein nitrogen	0.762		0.840	0.840
Nonprotein nitrogen	0.302		0.224	0.244
Polypeptid nitrogen	0.213		0.137	0.144
Amino nitrogen	0.032		0.014	0.030
Ammonia nitrogen	0.057		0.073	0.050
Reaction	+0.60		—1.40	+5.50
PH	7.0		7.8	5.0
Total nitrogen	1.064	6	1.064	1.064
Protein nitrogen	0.762		0.863	0.885
Nonprotein nitrogen	0.302		0.201	0.179
Polypeptid nitrogen	0.213		0.092	0.092
Amino nitrogen	0.032		0.028	0.037
Ammonia nitrogen	0.057		0.081	0.050
Reaction	+0.60		—1.70	+5.80
PH	7.0		8.1	4.9
Total nitrogen	1.064	10	1.064	1.064
Protein nitrogen	0.762		0.840	0.852
Nonprotein nitrogen	0.302		0.224	0.212
Polypeptid nitrogen	0.213		0.113	0.124
Amino nitrogen	0.032		0.027	0.039
Ammonia nitrogen	0.057		0.084	0.049
Reaction	+0.60		—2.10	+4.30
PH	7.0		.....	5.8
Total nitrogen	1.064	15	1.064	1.064
Protein nitrogen	0.762		0.717	0.750
Nonprotein nitrogen	0.302		0.347	0.314
Polypeptid nitrogen	0.213		0.239	0.219
Amino nitrogen	0.032		0.031	0.041
Ammonia nitrogen	0.057		0.078	0.054
Reaction	+0.60		—3.10	+4.70
PH	7.0		8.9	5.8

DISCUSSION

In general, the nitrogenous changes produced by B. coli are qualitatively similar to those found for B. typhosus, B. dysenteriae and B. paratyphosus.[2] Quantitatively, the increase in protein nitrogen, indicative of the growth of the organisms with the transformation of some of the nonprotein constituents of the medium into the actual bacterial substance, is not very different from that observed in cultures of the pathogenic members of the intestinal group. In other words, the rate of growth of all the microbes studied in this series is relatively about the same. The development in glucose gelatin appears to be more rapid and somewhat more extensive than in the plain gelatin. This is indicated by the slightly greater increase in protein nitrogen in the former medium. There is not much change in the amino nitrogen, but the tendency is toward a reduction in the plain gelatin, whereas the glucose gelatin change in this fraction of the cultural nitrogen is, within the limits of error of the method, practically negligible.

The changes in free ammonia, on the contrary, are unmistakable. In the glucose gelatin, in spite of an apparently more luxuriant growth of the bacteria, the amount of this substance not only fails to increase —on the contrary, there is a slight diminution. This contrasts sharply with the unmistakable increase in the plain, glucose-free gelatin up to the period of maximal development of the culture, namely, the tenth day. At this time, the increase in free ammonia above that of the uninoculated control is very nearly 3%. As this increase is the quantitative measure of the intracellular utilization of protein for energy by the bacteria, the significance becomes apparent. Expressed differently, it may be stated that the increase in protein nitrogen (bacterial protein) in plain gelatin, amounting in terms of nitrogen to 10% of the total nitrogen of the medium, was accomplished at the expense of nearly 3% of nitrogen liberated as free ammonia. In glucose gelatin, on the contrary, approximately 12% of the total nitrogen of the medium was transformed into bacterial substance (protein nitrogen) without the slightest discernible increase in free ammonia. In the former instance (sugar-free gelatin), the requisite energy of the bacteria appears to have been obtained by the combustion of nonprotein nitrogenous constituents, whereas in glucose gelatin the energy was derived in such a manner as to leave the nonprotein constituents relatively intact. This is shown, on the one hand, by the constancy of the amino and ammonia nitrogen fractions, and, on the other hand, by the almost direct parallelism between polypeptid decrease and protein nitrogen increase. This would appear to lend additional weight to the theory that utilizable carbohydrate protects or spares cultural protein from utilization of bacteria for energy.[5] The change in reaction, progressively more

[5] Kendall: Bacteriology, General, Pathological and Intestinal, Ed. 2, 1921, Chapter IV, for literature.

alkaline in the sugar-free medium and progressively more acid in the glucose medium, is indicative of the same phenomenon. It is well known that the products derived from the putrefaction of protein by bacteria are basic, whereas those of the fermentation of carbohydrate are acidic in character and reaction.

It must be admitted that the analytic figures, striking as they are, fail theoretically to eliminate the possibility that the increase in the protein fraction, due to the accumulation of bacteria in the culture, may not be a resultant between an unrecognized breaking down of some of the protein nitrogen of the original medium which is overshadowed and therefore masked by the relatively rapid growth of the bacteria. As the increase in the protein fraction amounts to 10% or more of the total nitrogen of the medium, this possibility clearly exists.

To obtain some evidence on this point, an attempt was made to detect enzymic changes in gelatin which might be caused by the activities of an hitherto undetected proteolytic enzmye produced by B. coli. It must be admitted that all previous evidence is against this view because the organism, by universal consent, is stated not to liquefy gelatin.

The method employed is one familiar to bacteriologists. It consists essentially in adding a small, definite amount of culture to a larger definite amount of 5% gelatin, containing 0.5% phenol to prevent growth. After two or three days' incubation of such cultures of organisms as B. proteus, which excrete soluble enzymes, such sterile mediums will become liquefied without the slightest evidence of growth.[4]

Table 2 shows the results of two experiments, respectively, in which 3 and 6 day cultures of B. coli in plain and glucose gelatin were added to carbol gelatin in the proportions of 5 c c of culture to 95 c c of the carbol gelatin. The results are wholly negative with respect to the demonstration of a soluble proteolytic enzmye. The variations between control and inoculated carbol gelatin mixtures are within the limits of error of the method employed. Under similar conditions, those bacteria which excrete soluble proteolytic enzymes would show physical and chemical signs of activity.

It cannot be claimed of course that this observation absolutely excludes the possibility of the existence of a soluble proteolytic enzyme, but it does make the probability of the occurrence of an enzyme in an active state unlikely. Considering all the factors in the metabolism of

B. coli, as exhibited in tables 1 and 2, it may be stated that the gelatin protein is of little or no value to the organism as a source of nitrogenous energy. The somewhat greater nitrogenous waste attending the growth and activity of B. coli in plain gelatin in comparison with the dysentery and typhoid cultures stands in relation to the fact that

TABLE 2

ENZYME STUDY; CARBOL GELATIN. BACILLUS COLI

	Plain Culture		Glucose Culture	
	Control	Three Days' Incubation	Control	Three Days' Incubation
Total nitrogen	0.675	0.675	0.675	0.675
Protein nitrogen	0.541	0.529	0.541	0.552
Nonprotein nitrogen	0.134	0.146	0.134	0.123
Polypeptid nitrogen	0.096	0.109	0.098	0.087
Amino nitrogen	0.028	0.028	0.028	0.028
Ammonia nitrogen	0.010	0.009	0.008	0.008
Reaction	+0.60	+0.70	+0.90	+0.90
PH	6.3	6.3	5.9	5.9
Total nitrogen*	0.675	0.675	0.675	0.675
Protein nitrogen	0.552	0.563	0.541	0.541
Nonprotein nitrogen	0.123	0.112	0.134	0.134
Polypeptid nitrogen	0.085	0.084	0.098	0.098
Amino nitrogen	0.028	0.028	0.028	0 028
Ammonia nitrogen	0.010	0.011	0.008	0.008
Reaction	+0.20	+0.20	+1.10	+1.20
PH	6.6	6.8	5.6	5.6

* 6 days incubation.

progressively pathogenic bacteria produce less deep seated changes, generally speaking, in protein mediums than the parasitic and saprophytic types. The presence of indol in cultures of B. coli and the practical absence of this substance in cultures of B. typhosus, is suggestive but not conclusive evidence on this point.

THE NITROGENOUS METABOLISM OF THE SCHMITZ BACILLUS

STUDIES IN BACTERIAL METABOLISM. LXIII

Arthur Isaac Kendall; Reba Cordelia Haner, and Robert S. Bly

Department of Bacteriology, Northwestern University Medical School, Chicago, Ill.

The Schmitz bacillus, so called because it was first isolated and described by an observer by that name,[1] was found on the Roumanian and Salonika fronts in the feces of patients exhibiting the general symptoms of bacillary dysentery. It also appears to have been rather widely disseminated among the British troops in Macedonia. Serologically, the Schmitz bacillus appears to be an entity definitely distinguishable from the Shiga bacillus and the members of the Flexner group of dysentery bacilli. Culturally, it resembles the Shiga bacillus closely, both chemically and morphologically. A point of differentiation between the two appears to be indol formation. The Schmitz bacillus practically always changes tryptophan to indol, whereas the Shiga bacillus has never been reported as inducing noteworthy decomposition of this amino acid. It is quite clear from the meager literature on the Schmitz bacillus that comparatively little is known about it other than the circumstantial evidence surrounding its occurrence in the feces of patients exhibiting a syndrome similar to, or indistinguishable from, mild to severe bacillary dysentery.

Two cultures were available for study, one from the Army Medical School, the other from the laboratory of Dr. Andrewes in England. As they agreed culturally and chemically, the details of only one are herewith presented.

A cultural difference between the Shiga bacillus [2] and the Schmitz bacillus is at once discernible. The Shiga bacillus produces a moderate but distinct increase in reaction up to and including the first week of growth, during which time the amount of deamination (ammonia formation) is minimal, and the evidence points to the availability of a nonnitrogenous source of energy during this period. Then the reac-

Received for publication Oct. 12, 1921.

[1] Schmitz: München. med. Wchnschr., 1917, 64, p. 1571.

[2] Kendall and Haner: Jour. Infect. Dis., Study LVII, 1922, 30, p. 226.

tion becomes alkaline and the deamination begins. This was tentatively explained as an indication of the utilization of the so-called carbohydrate fraction of the protein molecule for which the Shiga bacillus and the staphylococcus seem to possess a predilection. On the exhaustion of this moiety of the protein constituents of the medium, the attack on the residual nitrogenous portion begins.

The Schmitz bacillus fails to exhibit signs indicative of this utilization of the carbohydrate portion of the protein molecule. Indeed, the

TABLE 1

BACILLUS OF SCHMITZ

Mg. per 100 C c	Control	Day	Plain Broth	Glucose Broth
Total nitrogen	1.080	1	1.080	1.080
Protein nitrogen	0.778		0.811	0.790
Nonprotein nitrogen	0.302		0.269	0.290
Polypeptid nitrogen	0.210		0.170	0.198
Amino nitrogen	0.042		0.044	0.042
Ammonia nitrogen	0.050		0.055	0.050
Reaction	+0.80		+1.40	+3.80
P_H	7.2		6.9	5.8
Total nitrogen	1.080	4	1.080	1.080
Protein nitrogen	0.778		0.822	0.812
Nonprotein nitrogen	0.302		0.258	0.268
Polypeptid nitrogen	0.210		0.156	0.166
Amino nitrogen	0.042		0.044	0.052
Ammonia nitrogen	0.050		0.058	0.050
Reaction	+0.80		+0.80	+5.10
P_H	7.2		7.1	5.3
Total nitrogen	1.080	7	1.080	1.080
Protein nitrogen	0.778		0.879	0.890
Nonprotein nitrogen	0.302		0.201	0.190
Polypeptid nitrogen	0.210		0.088	0.098
Amino nitrogen	0.042		0.051	0.042
Ammonia nitrogen	0.050		0.062	0.050
Reaction	+0.80		−0.80	+5.00
P_H	7.2		7.8	5.0
Total nitrogen	1.080	10	1.080	1.080
Protein nitrogen	0.778		0.856	0.857
Nonprotein nitrogen	0.302		0.224	0.223
Polypeptid nitrogen	0.210		0.121	0.135
Amino nitrogen	0.042		0.037	0.040
Ammonia nitrogen	0.050		0.066	0.048
Reaction	+0.80		−1.50	+4.80
P_H	7.2		8.5	5.3

growth suggests strongly that of the typhoid bacillus in intensity of action on the protein constituents of plain gelatin. In glucose gelatin the sparing action of utilizable carbohydrate for protein is clearly indicated through the practical absence of deamination. These observations on the nitrogenous changes in plain gelatin cultures of the Schmitz bacillus are in accord with the known facts, namely, that the organism is clearly distinguishable from the Shiga bacillus, both serologically and because the former induces deeper seated changes in specific constituents of the nitrogenous cultural medium.

With respect to indol formation, the Schmitz bacillus resembles more closely the members of the dysentery group of the Flexner type than the Shiga type. On the other hand, the inability of the Schmitz bacillus to ferment mannitol separates it sharply from the Flexner types and places it with the Shiga type in so far as the relationship between the cytoplasm of the microbes and the stereo-configuration of the carbohydrates utilizable for energy is concerned. The available evidence suggests that the Schmitz bacillus is a distinct member of the dysentery group but not a variant of the Shiga bacillus.

THE NITROGENOUS METABOLISM OF BACILLUS ALKALESCENS

STUDIES IN BACTERIAL METABOLISM. LXIV

ARTHUR ISAAC KENDALL AND ALEXANDER ALFRED DAY

Department of Bacteriology, Northwestern University Medical School, Chicago, Ill.

Bacillus alkalescens is an organism of somewhat obscure origin and significance which was isolated from diarrheal feces by English observers during investigations of bacillary dysentery. Like the Schmitz bacillus, described previously,[1] the position of B. alkalescens in the group of intestinal bacteria is somewhat indeterminate, although there is on the whole less evidence that B. alkalescens is of material significance in the etiology of a dysenteric syndrome than is the case with the Schmitz bacillus. Culturally, B. alkalescens, as its name would suggest, is characterized by the production of basic substances as the result of its action on proteins. In this respect, it differs quantitatively from B. alkaligenes, however. The latter ferments no known carbohydrates, and in general its nitrogenous activity is similar to that of B. typhosus in so far as available quantitative methods indicate.[2] The nitrogenous metabolism of B. alkalescens in sugar-free mediums resembles more closely that of the Bacillus of Morgan.[3] The carbohydrate fermentation, however, is different in that the Morgan bacillus produces gas (H_2 and CO_2) as well as acid from the fermentation of glucose, whereas B. alkalescens produces acid only under parallel conditions. The organism, furthermore, ferments mannitol. The Morgan bacillus does not.

DISCUSSION

B. alkalescens, in conformity with its name, brings about a rather vigorous change in reaction toward the alkaline side of neutrality in plain, sugar-free gelatin. Not only is there a considerable deamination (ammonia formation) and a distinct reduction in amino nitrogen in the cultures after several days' incubation, but the reaction becomes decidedly alkaline as well. The increase in protein nitrogen, indicative

Received for publication Oct. 12, 1921.

[1] Kendall, Haner and Bly: Study LXIII, Jour. Infect. Dis., 1922, 30, p. 245.
[2] Kendall, Day & Walker: Jour. Am. Chem. Soc., 1913, 35, p. 1213.
[3] Ibid., p. 1225.

of the incorporation of the nitrogenous constituents of the medium into the bodies of the bacteria, is even more energetic in the glucose medium than the sugar-free medium. In the former, 10% of the nitrogen is thus converted; in the latter, about 13%. The same sparing action of utilizable carbohydrate for protein is clearly shown by a comparison of the respective changes in protein nitrogen and ammonia nitrogen in the plain and glucose mediums. In the former, nearly 4% of the nitrogen of the medium is liberated as free ammonia (intracellular deamina-

TABLE 1

BACILLUS ALKALESCENS

Mg. per 100 C c	Control	Day	Plain Broth	Glucose Broth
Total nitrogen	1.080	1	1.080	1.080
Protein nitrogen	0.778		0.822	0.778
Nonprotein nitrogen	0.302		0.258	0.302
Polypeptid nitrogen	0.210		0.161	0.211
Amino nitrogen	0.042		0.038	0.041
Ammonia nitrogen	0.050		0.059	0.050
Reaction	+0.80		+1.30	+3.90
PH	7.2		7.0	5.3
Total nitrogen	1.080	4	1.080	1.080
Protein nitrogen	0.778		0.811	0.790
Nonprotein nitrogen	0.302		0.269	0.290
Polypeptid nitrogen	0.210		0.172	0.195
Amino nitrogen	0.042		0.035	0.048
Ammonia nitrogen	0.050		0.062	0.047
Reaction	+0.80		+0.80	+5.10
PH	7.2		7.1	5.3
Total nitrogen	1.080	7	1.080	1.080
Protein nitrogen	0.778		0.879	0.913
Nonprotein nitrogen	0.302		0.201	0.167
Polypeptid nitrogen	0.210		0.098	0.070
Amino nitrogen	0.042		0.022	0.048
Ammonia nitrogen	0.050		0.081	0.049
Reaction	+0.80		—0.60	+5.30
PH	7.2		8.5	5.0
Total nitrogen	1.080	10	1.080	1.080
Protein nitrogen	0.778		0.856	0.890
Nonprotein nitrogen	0.302		0.224	0.190
Polypeptid nitrogen	0.210		0.116	0.101
Amino nitrogen	0.042		0.020	0.041
Ammonia nitrogen	0.050		0.088	0.048
Reaction	+0.80		—2.40	+5.20
PH	7.2		8.7	5.3

tion) during the period when 10% of the total nitrogen is added to the protein fraction. This is interpreted as profound utilization of protein for energy by the bacteria during the first week of the incubation of the culture. On the contrary, in a medium of exactly the same composition, containing 1% of glucose in addition to the nitrogenous ingredients, the protein nitrogen fraction increases 13%, suggesting, if not proving, a larger proliferation of bacteria with no apparent change in the ammonia content of the medium. The substitution of a carbohydrate source of energy for the protein source of energy results in more luxuriant growth, with a great saving of the protein constituents of the culture.

The changes in reaction in glucose gelatin are as great, or even greater proportionately than those in the plain gelatin cultures, although of opposite sign. The general behavior of the organism known as B. alkalescens, therefore, is that of a parasite rather than that of a pathogenic microbe, in so far as the magnitude of the changes in the utilizable constituents of the mediums in which it may be grown can determine this point. This agrees in essence with the general consensus of opinion relative to its importance in the etiology of dysenteric infection. In this respect it would appear to stand in rather close resemblance to the Morgan bacillus.

THE NITROGENOUS METABOLISM OF BACILLUS PROTEUS

STUDIES IN BACTERIAL METABOLISM. LXV

ARTHUR ISAAC KENDALL; HAROLD C. CHEETHAM, AND CLIFF S. HAMILTON

Department of Bacteriology, Northwestern University Medical School, Chicago, Ill.

One of the most conspicuous, versatile and puzzling groups of bacteria commonly encountered is that one on which Hauser [1] conferred the very appropriate appellation "Proteus." Originally, the term "Proteus" seems to have referred to four varieties or members of a peculiar morphologic type of bacillus which differed quantitatively in their respective abilities to induce liquefaction in gelatin mediums. Later and more intensive studies have revealed other peculiarities which emphasize especially the apparent heterogenicity of the immunologic armamentarium of at least certain strains of the type organism. Thus Frost [2] has isolated a strain of B. proteus which is agglutinated in high dilution with a specific typhoid serum. Felix and Weil [3] have shown that at least two strains of B. proteus [4] (X_2 and X_{19}) will agglutinate with serums from a majority of typhus fever patients. It is significant that the latter strains are distinctly less active proteolytically than the ordinary, freshly isolated varieties of the Hauser type, designated by him Proteus vulgaris.

Many observers have failed to recognize the striking proteolytic activity of typical strains of the vulgaris type. Berman and Rettger,[5] criticising Kendall and Walker's [6] work on the influence of utilizable carbohydrate on the appearance of an active, soluble proteolytic enzyme of B. proteus, say: "A bacterial proteolytic enzyme, as a rule, is not produced within the first twenty-four hours, but requires a longer period before it makes its appearance in detectable quantities."

It is quite evident that Berman and Rettger were not familiar with the more typical and active strains of B. proteus, as will be shown

Received for publication Oct. 12, 1921.

[1] Weber: Fäulnisbakterien und deren Beziehungen zur Septikäme, 1885.
[2] Public Health and Marine Hospital Laboratory, Bull. 66, 1910, Washington, D. C.
[3] Wien. klin. Wchnschr., 1916, 29, pp. 873, 974.
[4] Bengston: Public Health Reports, 1919, 34, p. 2446.
[5] Jour. Bacteriol., 1918, 3, p. 389.
[6] Jour. Infect. Dis., 1915, 17, p. 442.

later. Wolf [7] also states that cultures of B. proteus do not induce that rapid liquefaction of gelatin mediums which have been ascribed to them. It seems not improbable from a perusal of this article that Wolf was working with one of the two cultures of B. proteus, X_2 or X_{19}, which agglutinate with typhus serums. These strains, as Miss Bengston [4] has shown, are rather indolent in their gelatin liquefying powers.

The question naturally presents itself: What is Bacillus proteus? Flügge [8] classifies the members of the group primarily on their respective abilities to liquefy gelatin—Proteus vulgaris being the most active, Proteus mirabilis less so, and Proteus zenkeri quite without liquefying powers. In this connection, it will be remembered that the ability of strains of B. proteus (Proteus vulgaris) to induce liquefaction in gelatin is frequently decreased or lost through prolonged development in artificial mediums. Also, the saccharose-fermenting power may be lost on prolonged cultivation. A strain that has lost its gelatin-liquefying and saccharose-fermenting powers assumes superficially many of the cultural characteristics of the Morgan bacillus.[9] Theobald Smith [10] made the highly important observation that Proteus vulgaris ferments glucose and saccharose with the production of gas and acid, lactose being unattacked. It is now known that mannitol also is unfermented. A point of some importance also is the inability of a majority, if indeed not of all, of the true members of the Proteus vulgaris type to ferment mannose.

A typical strain of B. proteus (Proteus vulgaris), therefore, induces a rapid liquefaction of gelatin by means of a soluble, or exo-enzyme. It ferments glucose and saccharose with the formation of gas and acid, but fails to ferment lactose, mannose or mannitol. A restriction or loss of gelatin-liquefying power and the loss of saccharose-fermenting power are rather common modifications of cultural and chemical properties of the typical organism. The association of Proteus vulgaris with human lesions is accompanied frequently by one or more of these modifications.

The study of the nitrogenous metabolism of B. proteus reported in the following was undertaken to determine the changes induced in nitrogenous constituents of a gelatin-peptone-meat juice medium by an active culture of the organism after various periods of incubation. The

[7] Jour. Path. & Bacteriol., 1919, 22, p. 284.
[8] Die Mikroorganismen, 1896, 2, p. 272.
[9] Morgan: British Med. Jour., 1906, 1, p. 908.
[10] The Fermentation Tube, Wilder Quarter Century Book, 1893, p. 213.

medium contained the usual ingredients, including 5% of gelatin and 1% of peptone, made up in meat infusion. The reaction at the start was slightly alkaline—P_H 7.3 to be exact. The cultures were studied at various intervals, and, also, an effort was made to measure the activity

TABLE 1

B. PROTEUS

Proteus No. 1 June 28, 1921 Cultures	Day	Control	Plain	Percentage of Glucose						
				0.1	0.2	0.3	0.4	0.5	0.75	1.5
Total nitrogen	1	1.001	1.001	1.001	1.001	1.001	1.001	1.001	1.001	
Protein nitrogen		0.721	0.531	0.564	0.598	0.609	0.665	0.676	0.721	
Nonprotein nitrogen		0.280	0.470	0.437	0.403	0.392	0.336	0.325	0.280	
Polypeptid nitrogen		0.209	0.389	0.361	0.330	0.319	0.265	0.253	0.213	
Amino nitrogen		0.039	0.032	0.028	0.028	0.029	0.030	0.032	0.029	
Ammonia nitrogen		0.032	0.049	0.048	0.045	0.044	0.041	0.040	0.038	
Total nitrogen	2	1.001	1.001	1.001	1.001	1.001	1.001	1.001	1.001	1.001
Protein nitrogen		0.721	0.262	0.195	0.385	0.419	0.453	0.497	0.497	0.743
Nonprotein nitrogen		0.280	0.739	0.806	0.616	0.582	0.548	0.504	0.504	0.258
Polypeptid nitrogen		0.209	0.638	0.709	0.527	0.415	0.475	0.429	0.434	0.191
Amino nitrogen		0.039	0.032	0.030	0.029	0.029	0.028	0.027	0.026	0.030
Ammonia nitrogen		0.032	0.069	0.067	0.060	0.048	0.045	0.048	0.044	0.037
Total nitrogen	3	1.001	1.001	1.001	1.001	1.001	1.001	1.001	1.001	
Protein nitrogen		0.721	0.239	0.239	0.284	0.352	0.430	0.453	0.531	
Nonprotein nitrogen		0.280	0.762	0.762	0.717	0.649	0.571	0.548	0.470	
Polypeptid nitrogen		0.209	0.647	0.647	0.608	0.536	0.473	0.469	0.400	
Amino nitrogen		0.039	0.036	0.036	0.032	0.030	0.047	0.030	0.028	
Ammonia nitrogen		0.032	0.089	0.089	0.077	0.056	0.051	0.049	0.042	
Total nitrogen	4	1.001	1.001	1.001	1.001	1.001	1.001	1.001	1.001	
Protein nitrogen		0.721	0.060	0.073	0.139	0.228	0.262	0.307	0.351	
Nonprotein nitrogen		0.280	0.941	0.928	0.862	0.773	0.739	0.694	0.650	
Polypeptid nitrogen		0.209	0.796	0.777	0.709	0.696	0.654	0.613	0.571	
Amino nitrogen		0.039	0.028	0.035	0.035	0.018	0.035	0.032	0.030	
Ammonia nitrogen		0.032	0.117	0.116	0.118	0.059	0.050	0.049	0.049	
Total nitrogen	5	1.001	1.001	1.001	1.001	1.001	1.001	1.001	1.001	1.001
Protein nitrogen		0.721	0.161	0.127	0.161	0.206	0.206	0.239	0.340	0.822
Nonprotein nitrogen		0.280	0.840	0.847	0.840	0.795	0.795	0.762	0.661	0.179
Polypeptid nitrogen		0.209	0.663	0.694	0.679	0.654	0.667	0.648	0.567	0.103
Amino nitrogen		0.039	0.033	0.031	0.032	0.024	0.025	0.035	0.030	0.039
Ammonia nitrogen		0.032	0.144	0.149	0.129	0.117	0.103	0.079	0.064	0.037
Total nitrogen	7	1.001	1.001	1.001	1.001	1.001	1.001	1.001	1.001	1.001
Protein nitrogen		0.721	0.038	0.094	0.071	0.060	0.083	0.094	0.105	0.732
Nonprotein nitrogen		0.280	0.963	0.907	0.930	0.941	0.918	0.907	0.896	0.269
Polypeptid nitrogen		0.209	0.696	0.687	0.703	0.757	0.750	0.730	0.722	0.185
Amino nitrogen		0.039	0.036	0.025	0.032	0.035	0.042	0.040	0.033	0.044
Ammonia nitrogen		0.033	0.204	0.195	0.195	0.149	0.126	0.137	0.141	0.039
Total nitrogen	14	1.001	1.001	1.001	1.001	1.001	1.001	1.001	1.001	
Protein nitrogen		0.721	0.162	0.151	0.140	0.218	0.151	0.106	0.106	
Nonprotein nitrogen		0.280	0.839	0.850	0.861	0.783	0.850	0.895	0.895	
Polypeptid nitrogen		0.209	0.587	0.577	0.566	0.511	0.580	0.600	0.624	
Amino nitrogen		0.039	0.039	0.026	0.030	0.059	0.057	0.079	0.050	
Ammonia nitrogen		0.033	0.213	0.247	0.265	0.213	0.213	0.216	0.221	

of the soluble proteolytic enzyme at the same periods. The methods have been described previously.[6,11,12] The results are shown in the tables.

[11] Kendall: Study LVII, Jour. Infect. Dis., 1922, 30, p. 211.
[12] Kendall and Bly: Ibid., Study LXII.

DISCUSSION ON TABLE 1

Cultures: The salient features of the changes in the nitrogenous constituents of the various gelatin-glucose-mediums are indicated clearly by the analytic figures, which express the results of duplicate determinations in terms of milligrams of nitrogen per 100 c c of culture. The most striking change is that of the protein nitrogen fraction, which even within 24 hours of incubation has diminished from 72% (that of the uninoculated control) to 53% in the glucose-free gelatin. It must be remembered that this remarkable decrease in protein nitrogen, due to the activity of the soluble enzyme of the organism, is somewhat greater than the figures indicate because there is produced simultaneously some increase in this fraction due to the formation of bacterial protein.[13]

There is coincidently a not inconsiderable increase in ammonia nitrogen, greater in the glucose-free and 0.1% glucose gelatin, less in the mediums containing larger proportions of sugar. The increase in ammonia from the first day of incubation, when it amounts to less than 2%, to the second week of incubation when it reaches almost 20%, is an indication of the deaminizing activity of the microbe. It is a striking fact that the amino-nitrogen fraction shows little increase during this time. Apparently the significant change is a degradation of the original protein nitrogen directly to the nonprotein-nitrogen fraction, and specifically to that residual nonprotein nitrogen fraction which for convenience of discussion is termed "polypeptid" nitrogen.[11] This change amounts to an increase of "polypeptid" nitrogen from about 20% in the uninoculated control to over 70% in the 7-day culture in plain and low percentage glucose mediums, as is clearly shown in the tables.

In concentrations of glucose exceeding 0.3%, the protein-nitrogen fraction, even after several days' incubation, fails to reach quite as low a level as in the plain gelatin cultures and those containing lesser amounts of glucose. The suggestion is made, which has considerable evidence in its favor, that the amount of bacterial protein is somewhat greater in the higher glucose concentrations; in other words, bacterial development has proceeded further. Filtration of the bacteria from one such culture reduced the protein nitrogen of the filtrate from 10% to

[13] Compare Bacillus dysenteriae (Study LVIII), typhosus (Study LVII), and Studies LX to LXIV, inclusive, for quantitative measurements of the increase in protein nitrogen due to the growth of nonliquefying bacteria.

6% of the original protein nitrogen.[14] The addition of 1.5% glucose to the gelatin medium effectively prevented evidences of proteolysis. The organisms apparently failed to ferment all the glucose, presumably because the accumulation of acid products of fermentation prevented the growth of the bacteria after a few days' incubation. With the progressive increase in glucose content the delay in ammonia formation is clearly outlined.

Berman and Rettger,[5] criticising Kendall and Walker's study on the influence of glucose on the metabolism of B. proteus, state: "The present investigation has shown conclusively that fermentable sugars in moderate amounts do not affect the nitrogen metabolism of bacteria—under conditions of favorable environment." Their contention is based on the study of cultures of B. proteus and other bacteria using the method of formol titration of Sörensen and the biuret test of Vernon as measures of nitrogenous change. Their tests were made in two kinds of mediums, one containing 0.5% peptone, 0.25% beef extract, 0.5% NaCl, and 0.2 and 0.4% glucose, respectively, and the same mediums containing in addition 0.5% K_2HPO_4. This is a large amount of phosphoric acid in proportion to the other constituents of the medium. Their results are puzzling.

In the control medium, containing 0.2% glucose and 0.5% K_2HPO_4, they record sugar as absent; in each culture of B. proteus in this medium, however, sugar is invariably recorded as "present." It is very significant, as Jones[15] has pointed out, that in the 0.2% glucose medium without the K_2HPO_4, sugar is reported "absent" after 24 hours' incubation. It would appear from their own tables that Berman and Rettger's conclusions relative to the influence of small amounts of utilizable sugar on the metabolism of B. proteus are incorrect; unless their tables contain unrecognized typographical errors. Perhaps the most striking instance of such incompatibility is the reported absence of sugar in the control phosphate—0.2% glucose medium on page 397 of their article.

The nitrogenous metabolism of a culture of B. proteus in the gelatin-peptone-meat infusion medium described in the foregoing, with graded amounts of glucose from 0.1% to 1.5%, shows therefore several distinctive features: The sparing action of utilizable carbohydrate in sufficient amounts to provide more than the organism can completely utilize is shown clearly in the column in which the nitrogenous change in this medium is recorded. Smaller amounts of glucose in descending order retard the rate of deamination by the bacilli and, also, as the table shows clearly, retard in regular order, but do not ultimately prevent, the decrease in protein nitrogen and the corresponding increase in "polypeptid" nitrogen.

[14] This experiment was made on the 7-day culture in 0.75 glucose gelatin. Before filtration the protein nitrogen was 105 mg. per 100 c c culture medium. After filtration the protein nitrogen was only 61 mg. per 100 c c culture medium.

[15] Journal Infect. Diseases, 1920, 27, 169.

The question naturally arises: What proportion of the decrease in protein nitrogen, and therefore what proportion of the increase in the "polypeptid" nitrogen is due to the soluble enzyme of the bacteria, and what part is due to the intracellular nitrogenous metabolism of the bacteria, respectively?

TABLE 2

B. PROTEUS

Carbol Gelatin Enzyme	Day	Control	Plain	Percentage of Glucose						
				0.1	0.2	0.3	0.4	0.5	0.75	1.5
Total nitrogen	1	0.672	0.672	0.672	0.672	0.672	0.672	0.672	0.672	
Protein nitrogen		0 542	0.325	0.280	0.381	0.392	0.426	0.426	0.471	
Nonprotein nitrogen		0.130	0.347	0.392	0.291	0.280	0.246	0.246	0.201	
Polypeptid nitrogen		0.102	0.314	0.360	0.257	0.252	0.217	0.217	0.172	
Amino nitrogen		0.020	0.025	0.024	0.028	0.022	0.023	0.023	0.023	
Ammonia nitrogen		0.008	0.008	0.008	0.006	0.006	0.006	0.006	0.006	
Total nitrogen	2	0.672	0.672	0.672.	0.672	0.672	0.672	0.672	0.672	0.672
Protein nitrogen		0.542	0.235	0.246	0.314	0.403	0.414	0.358	0.370	0.515
Nonprotein nitrogen		0.130	0.437	0.426	0.358	0.269	0.258	0.314	0.302	0.157
Polypeptid nitrogen		0.098	0.384	0.379	0.314	0.235	0.227	0.285	0.273	0.125
Amino nitrogen		0.023	0.044	0.038	0.035	0.026	0.022	0.022	0.020	0.023
Ammonia nitrogen		0.009	0.009	0.009	0.008	0.008	0.009	0.007	0.009	0.009
Total nitrogen	3	0.672	0.672	0.672	0.672	0.672	0.672	0.672	0.672	
Protein nitrogen		0.542	0.078	0.112	0.146	0.202	0.258	0.291	0.347	
Nonprotein nitrogen		0.130	0.594	0.560	0.526	0.470	0.414	0.381	0.325	
Polypeptid nitrogen		0.097	0.534	0.498	0.475	0.430	0.368	0.344	0.294	
Amino nitrogen		0.023	0.048	0.052	0.042	0.031	0.038	0.029	0.023	
Ammonia nitrogen		0.010	0.012	0.010	0.009	0.009	0.008	0.008	0.008	
Total nitrogen	4	1.330	1.330	1.330	1.330	1.330	1.330	1.330	1.330	
Protein nitrogen		1.061	0.389	0.447	0.524	0.515	0.793	0.793	0.804	
Nonprotein nitrogen		0.269	0.941	0.883	0.806	0.815	0.537	0.537	0.526	
Polypeptid nitrogen		0.119	0.860	0.819	0.737	0.459	0.484	0.484	0.478	
Amino nitrogen		0.035	0.065	0.048	0.053	0.041	0.038	0.037	0.032	
Ammonia nitrogen		0.015	0.016	0.016	0.016	0.015	0.015	0.016	0.016	
Total nitrogen	5	1.330	1.330	1.330	1.330	1.330	1.330	1.330	1.330	1.330
Protein nitrogen		1.061	0.322	0.332	0.390	0.390	0.424	0.547	0.670	1.051
Nonprotein nitrogen		0.269	1.008	1.008	0.940	0.940	0.906	0.783	0.660	0.279
Polypeptid nitrogen		0.211	0.916	0.907	0.844	0.847	0.812	0.700	0.575	0.222
Amino nitrogen		0.040	0.073	0.083	0.078	0.075	0.077	0.066	0.067	0.040
Ammonia nitrogen		0.018	0.019	0.018	0.018	0.018	0.017	0.017	0.018	0.017
Total nitrogen	7	1.330	1.330	1.330	1.330	1.330	1.330	1.330	1.330	1.330
Protein nitrogen		1.061	0.367	0.390	0.333	0.547	0.524	0.524	0.524	0.983
Nonprotein nitrogen		0.269	0.963	0.940	0.997	0.883	0.806	0.806	0.806	0.347
Polypeptid nitrogen		0.205	0.861	0.832	0.884	0.778	0.706	0.706	0.708	0.279
Amino nitrogen		0.039	0.076	0.082	0.086	0.081	0.076	0.075	0.073	0.043
Ammonia nitrogen		0.025	0.026	0.026	0.027	0.024	0.024	0.025	0.025	0.025
Total nitrogen	14	1.330	1.330	1.330	1.330	1.330	1.330	1.330	1.330	1.330
Protein nitrogen		1.061	0.413	0.547	0.402	0.402	0.367	0.379	0.469	
Nonprotein nitrogen		0.269	0.917	0.883	0.928	0.928	0.963	0.951	0.861	
Polypeptid nitrogen		0.191	0.821	0.738	0.820	0.826	0.854	0.847	0.750	
Amino nitrogen		0.049	0.067	0.070	0.078	0.073	0.082	0.076	0.082	
Ammonia nitrogen		0.029	0.029	0.030	0.030	0.029	0.027	0.028	0.029	

An answer to this question was sought for, using the carbol-gelatin method previously described by Kendall and Walker.[6] Briefly, the method was to add 5 c c of culture of B. proteus at the intervals stated to 95 c c of a solution of gelatin in 0.5% phenol (carbolic acid) solution. Two samples were prepared simultaneously from each of the cultures of a particular date. One of these was analyzed at once in accordance with the nitrogenous constituents tabulated. This was the control. The other sample was incubated 72 hours at 37 C. to allow the enzyme to act. The same determinations were then made.[16]

DISCUSSION OF TABLE 2

Two distinctive features stand out clearly in carbol gelatin inoculated from the mediums containing the smaller amounts of glucose, namely, the rapid reduction in the protein-nitrogen fraction, indicating a cleavage of the gelatin protein molecule by a soluble enzyme, and also no appreciable change in the ammonia nitrogen. The former is a measure of the activity of the soluble proteolytic enzyme. The latter shows distinctly that the deaminizing process depends on the presence of living bacteria. This is in harmony with the theory advanced by Kendall and Walker [6] that deamination is a measure of the intracellular utilization of protein or protein derivatives for energy by bacteria.

Little change is noticed in the amino nitrogen fraction; the greatest change amounts to less than 4% of the total nitrogen of the medium.

The great change is between the protein nitrogen and the "polypeptid" nitrogen. The former is reduced from 54% to less than 8% in the first few days (plain gelatin culture; very little change is noted in the 1.5 glucose culture). During the first 24 hours of growth the change amounts to rather more than 20%.[17] On the other hand, the polypeptid nitrogen rises from less than 13% to more than 59% in the same time. In this respect the protein-nitrogen and polypeptid-nitrogen fractions of the carbol gelatin follow closely those observed in the cultures containing living bacteria. It would appear that the significant change, therefore, is due to the activity of the soluble enzyme. The absence of deamination in the carbol gelatin, on the contrary, is in striking contrast to the rapid deamination in the plain gelatin culture, and the mediums containing the lower percentages of glucose.

[16] The table (table 2) shows only one control for each day. A separate control for each sample was made, because the amounts of ammonia, protein nitrogen, and polypeptid nitrogen varied somewhat with the culture used. To save space, all controls are reduced to that of the plain gelatin culture, and the results of incubation reduced accordingly. It was found necessary on the fourth day to increase the gelatin to 10%. This explains the apparently abrupt change in total nitrogen and other nitrogenous constituents on this date in comparison with the preceding days.

[17] This unequivocal result would appear to controvert Berman and Rettger's unsupported surmise that "a bacterial proteolytic enzyme, as a rule, is not produced within twenty-four hours," etc.

It is quite clear that the methods employed [11] offer a much more complete study of the nitrogen spectrum, both of cultures and of enzymes, than those previously utilized by Berman and Rettger. These methods, furthermore, appear to be applicable to the study of the action of enzymes, such as pepsin and trypsin, as well as bacterial enzymes, on nitrogenous substrates.

CONCLUSIONS

These quantitative measurements of the nitrogenous metabolism of B. proteus in various mediums, and of the nature and extent of the soluble enzyme of B. proteus, confirm and extend the observations of Kendall and Walker, referred to in the foregoing, in the following particulars, which were specifically studied:

"Bacillus proteus forms a soluble proteolytic enzyme in plain gelatin. The mature enzyme may be obtained in an active state freed from bacteria."

"The enzyme appears to be a preparatory enzyme in the sense that it prepares protein for assimilation by the bacteria; it has no demonstrable rôle in the intracellular utilization of the protein by the bacteria."

"The liquefaction of gelatin by the bacteria-free enzyme is not accompanied by the liberation of ammonia; deamination is an independent phenomenon associated with the intracellular utilization of the products of proteolysis by the organisms themselves."

HYDROGEN-ION STUDIES

I. CHANGES IN THE REACTION OF THE BLOOD DURING ANAPHYLACTIC SHOCK *

Edwin F. Hirsch and J. Lisle Williams

From the Pathological Laboratory of St. Luke's Hospital, Chicago

There seems to be no mention in the literature of changes in the H-ion concentration of the blood during anaphylactic shock. Recently Eggstein [1] reported a lowering of the alkali reserve, apparently in proportion with the severity of the shock. Changes in the alkali reserve of the blood are said to occur without appreciable alteration of the H-ion concentration. A study of the reaction of the blood in anaphylactic shock by the gas chain method should demonstrate changes, and should there be any, these may be compared with parallel alkali reserve values. Such a study is reported here, including mention of certain changes observed in the concentration of the sugar of the blood.

Rabbits were sensitized by intraperitoneal injections of the proteins on three successive days. The H-ion concentration of the blood was determined by the gas chain method. These estimations were made with the Hg-HgCl-$\frac{N}{10}$-KCl | sat. KCl | PtH_2 system, a McClendon electrode being used to contain the blood. The electromotive force readings were made with a Leeds and Northrup type K potentiometer and were properly corrected for temperature in converting them to the equivalent P_H expressions. This system was checked against known standard solutions. The rabbits were bled from the ear veins into a clean glass tube containing a little neutral powdered potassium oxalate. When markedly prostrated, the rabbits were bled from the heart with a syringe. The electrometric readings were made immediately to avoid as much as possible the loss of carbon dioxide, or other changes which might alter the reaction of the blood. Whole blood was used in all the determinations. The carbon dioxide combining power of the blood was estimated according to Van Slyke and Cullen,[2] the sugar concentration by the Folin and Wu [3] method.

Received for publication Oct. 21, 1921.

* Aided by the Winfield Peck Memorial Fund.

[1] Jour. Lab. & Clin. Med., 1921, 6, p. 555.

[2] Jour. Biol. Chem., 1917, 30, p. 289.

[3] Ibid., 1919, 38, p. 81; ibid., Supplement 1, 1920, 41, p. 367.

In the chart are graphically represented the changes in the reaction and in the alkali reserve of the blood during anaphylactic shock and in the table are recorded the results of individual experiments. In all of these experiments there is a diminished alkalinity of the blood during anaphylactic shock, as well as a lowering of the alkali reserve as Eggstein has reported. When it is remembered that the entire

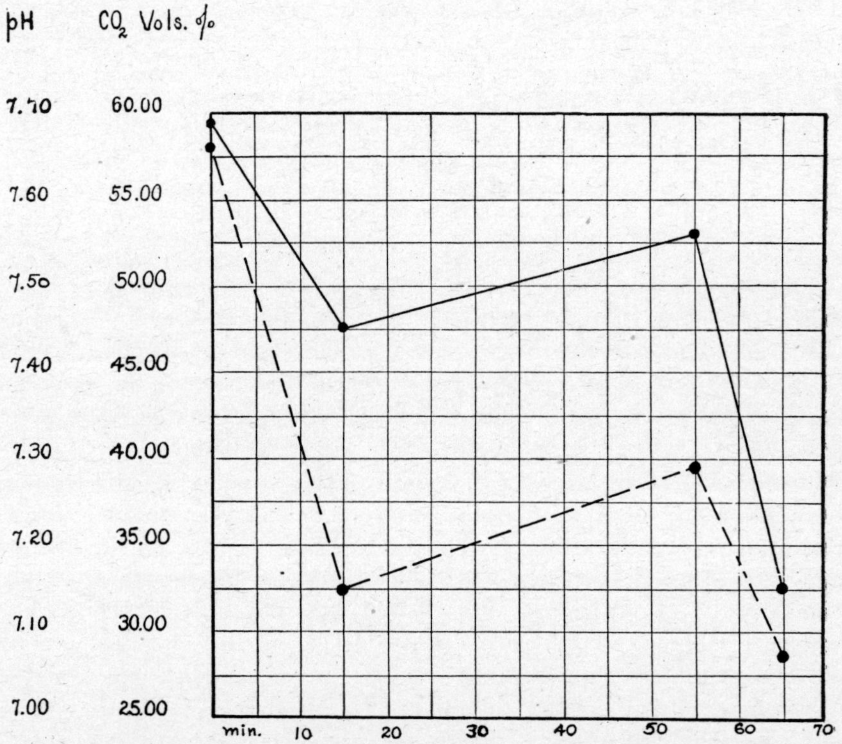

Chart 1.—Changes in the reaction and alkali reserve of the blood during anaphylactic shock. Death occurred in this experiment. The broken line indicates alkali reserve; the continuous line indicates the hydrogen-ion concentration.

range of reaction of the blood compatible with life lies between P_H 7.0 and 7.8 [4] the changes in the H-ion concentration of the blood mentioned are considerable. In only a few of the experiments is there an appreciable change in the concentration of the sugar of the blood. This absence of change in concentration may be due largely to the comparatively

[4] Van Slyke, D. D.: Jour. Biol. Chem., 1921, 48, p. 154.

short time in which the animal is in shock, for it is known generally that in acidosis there is a hyperglycemia.

When death occurs soon after the shock injection, the change in the reaction of the blood is not as great as when death follows prolonged prostration. This is similar to the change when death is produced suddenly by the intravenous injection of acid substances, and each probably is a condition in which acid and basic substances in the tissues and fluids of the body are not in a neutralized equilibrium. It may be that the maximum acidity occurs in tissue cells other than the blood, and that the changes in the reaction of the blood are secondary to those occurring in other tissues.

TABLE 1

RESULTS OF EXPERIMENTS WITH ANAPHYLACTIC SHOCK

Antigen	Before Anaphylactic Shock			During Anaphylactic Shock			Comment
	Alkali Reserve	P_H	Sugar, %	Alkali Reserve	P_H	Sugar, %	
Sheep serum	54.79	7.64	0.14	37.84	7.43	0.224	Lived
Sheep serum	64.62	7.56	0.095	50.21	7.39	Not determined	Died
Sheep serum	62.37	7.64	0.093	42.97	7.52	0.111	Lived
Human serum	60.92	7.79	0.13	50.26	7.49	0.182	Lived
Human serum	57.19	7.80	0.13	32.54	7.24	0.157	Lived
Human serum	57.28	7.69	0.084	28.54	7.15	0.084	Died
Human serum	67.02	7.72	0.127	54.40	7.70	0.113	Lived
Human serum	57.19	7.80	0.13	22.63	6.88	Not determined	Died
Human serum	57.71	7.61	0.088	42.97	7.46	0.116	Lived
Human serum	63.21	7.61	0.098	44.12	7.40	0.128	Lived
Sheep corpuscles	63.24	7.64	0.126	52.18	7.52	0.105	Lived
Egg white	69.03	7.68	0.104	48.93	7.45	0.082	Lived
Egg white	56.47	7.68	0.134	42.81	7.58	0.076	Lived

Changes in reaction during anaphylactic shock may account for some of the physical changes of the blood, such as diminished viscosity and coagulability that accompany this state. The H-ion concentration of the blood during anaphylactic shock may become so great as to make life incompatible and when such a change occurs it is, no doubt, important in explaining death.

Rapid changes in the alkali reserve of the blood, which when plotted in graphs make curves of similar contour, have been observed after intravenous injections of bacteria,[5] in protein [6] and in anaphylactic shock.[7] This similarity of change suggests that the H-ion concentration of the blood quite likely varies in each as it does in

[5] Jour. Am. Med. Assn., 1920, 75, p. 204; Jour. Infect. Dis., 1921, 28, p. 275.

[6] Jour. Lab. & Clin. Med., 1921, 6, p. 481.

[7] Ibid., 1921, 6, p. 555.

anaphylactic shock. These probably are important immune reaction changes. Such variations in the H-ion concentration of the blood are significant also in considering the pathologic changes observed in the organs with all of these abnormal conditions, for alterations in the reaction of the body fluids are likely the result of, or occur with, similar changes in the body tissues.

SUMMARY

There is a diminished alkalinity of the blood during anaphylactic shock, apparently in proportion with the severity of the symptoms. This change in reaction may become so great as to be incompatible with life. The altered reaction of the blood is accompanied by a roughly proportional lowering of the alkali reserve. Slight changes (usually an increase) in the concentration of the sugar of the blood occur in anaphylactic shock, but not to the degree observed in prolonged acidosis.

HYDROGEN-ION STUDIES

II. CHANGES IN THE REACTION OF SERUM ON THERMAL DESTRUCTION OF COMPLEMENT *

Edwin F. Hirsch and Ebba C. Peters

From the Pathological Laboratory of St. Luke's Hospital, Chicago

Numerous attempts have been made to determine the chemical nature of the thermolabile substance "complement" in normal blood serum. Its resemblance in certain respects to an enzyme has suggested that it is a lipase or a protease. Other properties suggest that it is a protein or lipin, or possibly a combination of soaps or lipins with serum proteins. Complement in serum is said to consist of two portions, an "end-piece" present in the albumin fraction and a "mid-piece" contained in the globulin portion. Bronfenbrenner and Noguchi [1] regard this so-called complement-splitting phenomenon merely an inactivation of the complement and not an actual cleavage. Brooks [2] recently expressed the opinion that the hemolytic action (complement) of serum is due primarily to a single substance which may be destroyed by ultraviolet rays according to a monomolecular reaction. There is considerable evidence, he says, that fatty acids are important in immune reactions and this taken with other facts known for complement suggests the presence of some fatty-acid compound acting as hemolysin in complement. He proposes that serum contains a hemolytic substance derived from a precursor (may resemble lecithin), and is constantly being formed and simultaneously being broken down.

Most of the methods for investigating complement have subjected normal serum to the action of chemicals. These modify to a great extent the menstruum in which complement exists and may even change the substance or substances constituting the complement. The extreme thermolability of complement makes a direct chemical examination very difficult. It seems possible with the precision of the gas-chain method to study the changes in the H-ion concentration of serum on heating to 56 C., and perhaps in this way to gain new information regarding the chemical behavior of complement.

Received for publication Oct. 21, 1921.

* Aided by the Winfield Peck Memorial Fund.

1 Jour. Exper. Med., 1912, 15, pp. 598 and 625.

2 Jour. Gen. Physiol., 1920-21, 3, p. 185.

Normal guinea-pig and rabbit serum was used in these experiments. The serum separating from coagulated blood kept in the icebox over night was thoroughly mixed in a large clean glass tube, and then distributed quickly into 4 c c glass test tubes, each one filled to within a short distance of the top and closed with a paraffined stopper. The tubes were heated in a water bath at 56 C. for periods of 1 minute to 2 hours, the length of time being measured from the moment the

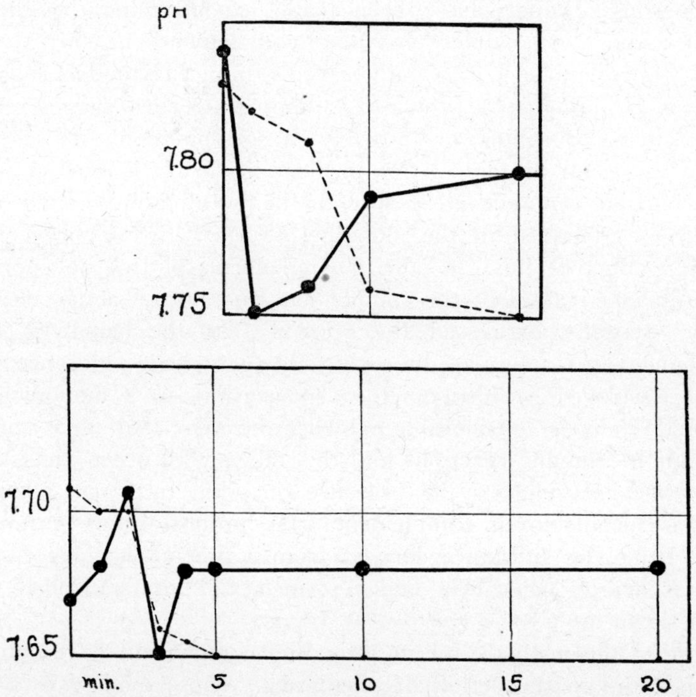

Chart 1.—Changes in the reaction of guinea-pig serum during thermal destruction of the complement. The continuous line represents the hydrogen-ion concentration; the broken line represents hemolysis.

tube was placed in the water bath until it was removed. This method, of course, in the short intervals disregards the lowering of the temperature of the water bath caused by introducing the tubes, as well as the time necessary to bring the serum and water in the bath to 56 C. On the other hand, the tendency by this method is to extend over longer periods of time any changes in the H-ion concentration brought about by heating the serum. Immediately after heating, the tubes were chilled in an ice bath, and kept there until the H-ion determinations were made. About 2 hours were required to complete a single experiment (9 H-ion determinations). Sealing the tubes and chilling them immediately after heating seemed to guard against reaction changes due to the escape of carbon dioxide, and those caused by autolysis; at least, such changes were reduced to a minimum. The H-ion concentration of unheated serum was determined with separate portions at the beginning and at the end of each experiment. These estimations were made with the Hg-HgCl-$\frac{N}{10}$-KCl | sat. KCl | PtH_2 system, a McClendon electrode being used to contain the serum. The electromotive force readings were made with a Leeds and Northrup type K potentiometer. This system was checked against known standard solutions, and all the estimations were made at room temperature (about 25 C.), there being little change in temperature during the period of each experiment. All the glass containers were washed with distilled water and dried, the McClendon electrode with water triple distilled in glass. The potentiometer readings were converted into the equivalent P_H expressions by the formula:

$$\frac{\text{E. M. F. (observed)} - \text{E (calomel electrode)}}{0.000\ 1983\ \text{T}} = \log. \frac{1}{(\text{H}+)} = P_H.$$

The complement activity of the serum was determined by the usual sheep red corpuscle, rabbit amboceptor system, the guinea-pig serum being diluted to 10%, the rabbit to 40%.

The results of these experiments are contained in the table, and those of two are graphically represented in the chart. On heating normal guinea-pig or rabbit serum, there is a prompt change in its reaction. In the experiments made, there seems to be a H-ion concentration of about P_H 7.74 to 7.76 which determines the direction of the initial change in reaction. When the P_H is greater, namely, 7.77, etc., the serum becomes less alkaline; when the P_H is smaller, namely, 7.73, etc., it becomes more alkaline. This initial change frequently reaches its maximum during the first minute of heating. When the initial change in reaction is an increased alkalinity there usually follows within 3 to 5 minutes a return to approximately the original reaction, and then again a change to a more alkaline reaction which remains fairly constant after the complement has been completely destroyed. When the initial change in reaction is a diminished alkalinity there is a subsequent return but not as great an alkalinity as that of the original unheated serum.

The reaction of the unheated serum kept in the ice water bath during the period of experiment (2 hours) changed in each experiment in the same direction and practically to the same degree as the initial change caused by heating the serum. A slight variation from this was observed once with guinea-pig serum (8) and once with rabbit serum (9).

TABLE 1

TABLE OF RESULTS OBTAINED WITH HEATING GUINEA-PIG AND RABBIT SERUM TO 56 C.

No.	Kind	Serum P_H. Heated 56 C. (Min.)										Unheated	
		1	2	3	4	5	10	20	30	60	120	0	120
1	Guinea-pig...........	7.75	....	7.76	....	7.79	7.80*	....	....	7.80	7.80	7.84	7.76
2	Guinea-pig...........	7.68	....	7.68	*	7.68	7.70	....	7.70	....	....	7.80	7.68
3	Guinea-pig...........	7.80	....	7.83	....	7.83	7.83*	....	7.82	7.82	7.82	7.85	7.80
4	Guinea-pig...........	7.79	....	7.80	....	7.75	7.79	....	7.76*	7.75	7.76	7.74	7.78
5	Guinea-pig...........	7.69	....	7.66	....	7.68	7.69	....	7.73*	....	7.72	7.76	7.68
6	Guinea-pig...........	7.75	7.74	7.78	7.76	7.75	7.75	7.76*	....	....	....	7.76	7.76
7	Guinea-pig...........	7.68	7.71	7.65	7.68	7.68*	....	7.68	....	....	....	7.67	7.71
8	Guinea-pig...........	7.47	....	7.49	7.49	7.51	7.47	7.51*	....	....	....	7.47	7.47
9	Rabbit...............	7.50	7.41	7.42	7.41*	7.41	7.41	7.41	....	....	....	7.40	7.42
10	Rabbit...............	7.46	7.49*	7.49	7.49	7.49	7.49	7.48	....	....	....	7.45	7.49
11	Rabbit...............	7.40	7.42	7.40	7.40	7.40†	....	7.40	....	....	....	7.38	7.43

* Complement destroyed completely.
† Slight hemolysis, serum not tested further.

DISCUSSION

An interpretation of the changes in the reaction of rabbit and guinea-pig serum when heated to 56 C. probably must be made on the basis of dissociation changes of a certain substance or substances (complement) in the serum. It seems that the dissociation of the complement substance occurs with the liberation of an acid radical, which spontaneously and with heating is volatilized or is removed by combining with some other substance. The H-ion concentration of serum seems to be the factor determining how much of this acid radical is present as such, above the P_H 7.74 very little, below this point more, so that when the serum is heated, in the former instance the complement substance rapidly dissociates, liberating its acid radical which then is removed by volatilization or chemical combination. In the latter instance its removal occurs first, and then dissociation and removal until the complement substance is completely destroyed.

The possibility that some volatile acid itself may be the complement suggested attempting to collect in inactivated serum (4 c c) the gases driven off from a larger amount (20 c c) of guinea-pig or rabbit serum during the heating at 56 C. for half an hour. These experiments demonstrated that such reactivation does not occur, and in order to be certain that a volatile acid substance was driven over, the H-ion concentration of inactivated serum was determined with a portion before, and with a portion after the gas had been forced through it. The reaction of the inactivated serum was changed by the substances volatilized (20 c c guinea-pig serum) from P_H 7.86 to 7.82, and from 7.81 to 7.76. That this change in reaction is not due entirely to carbon dioxide was demonstrated by testing inactivated serum before and after it had been exposed to pure carbon dioxide gas in amounts equal to the volume of gas driven off from heated serum. The reaction of each portion differed only to a slight degree. In order to satisfy the criticism that the glassware used contributed to the reaction changes, a set of tubes was thoroughly steamed under pressure in an auto clave, then placed in acid cleaning solution, thoroughly washed with water, finally with distilled water, and then dried. The results obtained with these tubes are similar to those obtained in the other experiments.

CONCLUSIONS

The destruction by heat (56 C.) of complement in normal guinea-pig and rabbit serum is accompanied by changes in the H-ion concentration. These probably are caused by dissociation of the complement substance or substances.

CULTIVATION OF THE GONOCOCCUS *

Mary J. Erickson and Henry Albert

From the Laboratories of the Department of Pathology and Bacteriology, University of Iowa, Iowa City, Iowa

The gonococcus was first cultivated by Bumm[1] on coagulated human placental serum in 1885, six years after its discovery by Neisser.[2] Wertheim[3] used a peptone agar with serum as a medium; the serum was inoculated with the infected material and added to the fluid agar in the proportion of two to one. Wassermann[4] used pig serum agar with glycerol and nutrose. Thalman[5] cultivated the gonococcus on plain agar, using a medium which in reaction was between the neutral points of litmus and phenolphthalein. He emphasized the importance of the reaction of the medium. Vannod[6] isolated and maintained several strains of gonococcus on plain agar. Gurd[7] suggested a medium of nutrient agar with a small quantity of defibrinated sterile human blood. Martin[8] published a review of methods of cultivating the gonococcus and of its differentiation from other gram-negative diplococci. He used beef infusion agar, the reaction of which was 0.6% acid to phenolphthalein, and moistened the surface with inactivated human serum. Hirshfelder[9] published a new formula using bullock testicular infusion agar. Warden[10] used a culture medium which contained ascitic or hydrocele fluid, blood or blood serum; later he used defibrinated rabbit blood with salt-free veal-peptone-agar, neutral to phenolphthalein, the medium being dried until the surface cracked. Vedder[11] described a starch agar, the reaction of which was 0.2 to 0.5% acid to phenolphthalein. Hall[12] made a testicular infusion agar. Thomson[13] used agar with human blood plasma. The more recent contributions on the cultivation of the gonococcus deal chiefly with the oxygen tension requirements and the importance of hydrogen-ion concentration. Nowak, in 1908, and Wherry and Oliver[14] reduced the oxygen tension for the cultivation of the gonococcus with a growth of B. subtilis. Chapin[15] suggested the cultivation of the gonococcus in an atmosphere of CO_2. Ruediger[16] felt that the exclusion of air was

Received for publication Oct. 3, 1921.

* This paper represents a part of the work done under a grant from the Interdepartmental Social Hygiene Board and the Graduate College of the University of Iowa. The main problem "A Selective Medium for the Cultivation of the Gonococcus," is still under investigation.

1 Deutsch. med. Wchnschr., 1885, 53, p. 910.
2 Centralbl. f. d. med. Wissensch., 1879, 17, p. 497.
3 Deutsch. med. Wchnschr., 1891, 17, p. 1351.
4 Berl. klin. Wchnschr., 1897, 34, p. 685.
5 Centralbl. f. Bakteriol., I, O., 1900, 27, p. 828.
6 Centralbl. f. Bakteriol., I, O., 1905, 40, p. 62.
7 Jour. Med. Research, 1908, 18, p. 291.
8 Jour. Path. & Bacteriol., 1910-11, 15, p. 76.
9 Jour. Am. Med. Assn., 1914, 62, p. 776.
10 Jour. Infect. Dis., 1913, 12, p. 93.
11 Jour. Infect. Dis., 1915, 16, p. 385.
12 Jour. Bacteriol., 1916, 1, p. 343.
13 Brit. Med. Jour., 1917, 1, p. 869.
14 Jour. Infect. Dis., 1916, 19, p. 288.
15 Ibid., 23, p. 342.
16 Ibid., 24, p. 376.

advantageous. Herrold[17] reduced the oxygen tension on plates in conjunction with B. subtilis. Swartz[18] described a simple method for reducing oxygen tension by heating inoculated tubes at the mouth by passing them over a flame to rarify the air within and then inserting a rubber stopper.

From this brief resume, it is evident that there is no uniformly satisfactory culture medium or method of cultivation of the gonococcus.

NOTES ON THE DIFFERENT KINDS OF CULTURE MEDIUMS

A comparison of various kinds of culture mediums that have been used for the isolation and cultivation of the gonococcus was made. The mediums tried were ascitic agar, blood agar, nutrient agar with blood serum, Vedder's[11] starch agar, Loeffler's blood serum, testicular agar, and Avery's[19] oleate-hemoglobin culture medium. Testicular infusion agar made according to Hall's[12] formula gave the most luxuriant growth of stock cultures. To this was added substances, such as blood or serum, which would favor the growth of gonococci from clinical cases. The addition of from 0.5 to 2.5% human blood to testicular agar produces a very good growth and is well adapted for isolation purposes. Defibrinated rabbit blood in proportions of 1 to 5% may be used. Blood, either human or rabbit, is added to agar at 40 C. Unheated or red blood agar produces a slightly better growth than chocolate or heated blood agar.

Human blood serum placed on the surface of testicular agar increases the growth materially. There was no difference in the growth of the organisms whether the serum was unheated or heated for one half hour at 56 C. The mixing of blood serum with the agar in proportions of one to three gives no better results than when the serum is simply smeared on the surface.

Martin[8] asserts that the value of blood serum and urine is not due to the addition of albuminous material but to substances such as phosphates, which act as buffers and equalize the reaction.

Vedder's starch agar, Avery's[19] oleate-hemoglobin medium, gelatin and nutrient agar cannot be relied on for isolation purposes since some strains of the organism refuse to grow on these mediums.

The importance and value of each supposedly essential ingredient of culture mediums, as well as the effect of the addition of other substances, such as bile, starch, etc., were studied.

[17] Jour. Am. Med. Assn., 1920, 74, p. 1716.
[18] Jour. Urology, 1920, 4, p. 325.
[19] Jour. Am. Med. Assn., 1918, 71, p. 2050.

The Effect of Glucose.—Ruediger [16] thinks that the addition of glucose is unfavorable. Cole [20] says that 1% glucose has no effect on initial growth, but shortens the viability of the cultures.

We have found that the presence of 0.5% glucose will cause certain strains to present visible colonies earlier, and also to show a more luxuriant growth than when no glucose was used. With other strains there seems to be no appreciable difference.

The Value of Peptone.—The importance of peptone was shown by experiments with 6 strains of the gonococcus. It was found that the growth is better on medium containing from 1.5 to 3% peptone than when lesser amounts are used.

The Effect of Salt.—Warden [10] states that physiologic salt solution and also distilled water favor autolysis. Martin [5] says that the organism loses its vitality in normal salt solution. We have confirmed these statements. Gonococci suspended in normal salt solution (0.7%) and transferred to tubes of culture medium failed to grow. Whenever we wished to use suspensions of the organisms we used a testicular infusion of P_H 7.4 which contained 0.3% monobasic sodium phosphate, 0.5% of glucose and 2% peptone. The gonococcus can also be grown in this broth.

We used monobasic sodium phosphate in from 0.2 to 0.3% in place of sodium chloride in the preparation of all culture mediums for gonococci. It is essential to use chemically pure salt since others seem to vary considerably in composition and ability to ionize. On several occasions we experienced considerable difficulty with the reaction of culture mediums. When using 0.3% of the phosphate (as recommended by Hall) the reaction changed from P_H 7.4 to P_H 6.5 by autoclaving, although the routine method of preparation was used and great care was taken not to autoclave longer than 20 minutes at 15 pounds of pressure. When the amount of monobasic sodium phosphate was reduced to 0.2%, the reaction adjusted to P_H 7.8 was found after autoclaving to be P_H 7.4. We consider the reaction of the medium to be of great importance as even stock cultures which show considerable adaptability to changes of medium, reaction, etc., show inhibition of growth when the reaction does not come within the optimum range.

Temperature Requirements.—One of the distinctive characteristics of the gonococcus is its failure to grow at room temperature. The

[20] Jour. Path. & Bacteriol., 1916-17, 21, p. 267.

maximum growth of the gonococcus occurs at 37.5 C. Jenkins[21] states that at a temperature of 35 C., in a moist atmosphere growth appears at the eighth to tenth hour, whereas in a dry atmosphere at 37.5 C. growth was not noticed until the sixteenth hour.

We have found that growths will occur at temperatures as low as 33 C., and as high as 39 C. The growths were, however, scanty and cultures kept at these temperatures lose their viability in a few days. A temperature of 42 C., maintained for several hours does not kill cultures—growth again taking place after the temperature is reduced to 37.5 C.

Herrold[17] emphasizes the necessity of warming the plates in the incubator for one-half hour before inoculation as a measure for inducing a good growth of the gonococcus. We have found this practice desirable and have adopted it for routine work.

The Reaction of Culture Mediums.—The optimum reaction for the growth of the gonococcus on artificial culture mediums is from P_H 7.4 to 7.6. This was determined by a series of tests with several strains, on mediums ranging in reaction from P_H 5.4 to 8.0. The results are shown in table 1.

TABLE 1

INFLUENCE OF HYDROGEN-ION CONCENTRATION ON GROWTH OF GONOCOCCUS

Gonococcus Strains	P_H 5.4	P_H 6.0	P_H 6.4	P_H 7.0	P_H 7.4	P_H 7.6	P_H 8.0
1	+	+	+	+	++	++	+
2	+	+	+	+	++	++	+
3	0	+	+	+	++	++	+
4	0	+	+	+	++	++	+
5	0	0	+	+	++	++	+
6	0	0	+	+	++	++	+

0 = no growth, + = slight growth, ++ = good growth.

As seen in table 1, certain strains failed to show any growth when the hydrogen-ion concentration was 6 or lower. All strains had been growing artificially for some time.

Cole[20] gives a P_H range for the gonococcus from 6.5 to 9.1 with the optimum at P_H 7.6. Swartz[18] found that growth occurred within a range of P_H 6.6 to 8.6; he states that the reaction of the culture mediums is not an important factor in the growth of the gonococcus. Martin[8] maintains that the reaction of culture mediums is of prime importance. He found that the best growths of the organism were obtained when the medium was 0.6% acid to phenolophthalein. He

[21] Ibid., 1921, 24, p. 160.

also states that "degrees of reaction beyond the limits of neutrality to an 0.8% acidity to phenolphthalein are distinctly unfavorable."

The Importance of Moisture in Culture Mediums.—It is of great importance to have the medium of the right moisture content. On too dry a medium the growth is scant or absent. We have found that the proper amount of moisture can be insured by using 2.5% granular agar. Shredded agar varies somewhat in moisture content and composition and culture mediums in which it is used accordingly are not uniform in consistency and constituents.

The tubes are stored in a moist chamber and slanted just before use. If tubes are slanted immediately after sterilization, the cotton plugs should be replaced by corks and dipped in paraffin. These tubes contain a moderate amount of water of condensation. With the exception of Warden,[10] all workers have seen the necessity of a moderately moist culture medium.

We have found it advantageous to keep a dish of water in the incubator at all times in order to insure proper moisture conditions.

Reduced Oxygen Tension.—It has been claimed by Wherry and Oliver,[14] Herrold,[17] Swartz,[18] and others, that reduced oxygen tension is essential if a good growth of the gonococcus is to be obtained.

Herrold reduced the oxygen tension by means of the B. subtilis; Swartz reduced it by passing the mouth of the inoculated tube through a flame several times and maintaining the diminished oxygen tension by corking the tube tightly with a rubber stopper. Reduction of the amount of oxygen has also been obtained by replacing a portion of the air with carbon dioxide.

We have tried the several methods suggested but have not been able to secure better results than when the organisms were grown in the presence of a normal oxygen tension. It is probable that the more satisfactory results attained by certain investigators is due, not to a reduced oxygen tension, but to the presence of an increased amount of moisture due to the technic used to exclude air.[22]

The Effect of Liver and Bile.—The addition of dry powdered liver to testicular agar did not improve the growth of the gonococcus. Culture mediums made from distilled water with 1 and 2% dry liver, peptone, glucose and monobasic sodium phosphate and the reaction adjusted to P_H 7.4, maintained the gonococcus for two subcultures. The third subcultures failed to grow.

[22] Kolaman, E. F.: J. Bacteriol., 1919, 4, p. 571.

Fresh ox-bile added to testicular agar in from 0.3 to 0.5% inhibited the growth of several strains of gonococci and slightly improved the growth of several others. Dry ox-gall added to testicular agar in from 0.5 to 1.0% inhibited the growth of gonococci slightly but did not inhibit the growth of the two strains of strephylococci and one of the colon bacillus on which such was tried. In a 0.2% preparation it also failed to influence the growth of the gonococcus. Bile salts in the form of sodium taurocholate and sodium glycocholate were added to testicular agar in proportions of 3 to 5%. The growth of five strains of gonococci was slightly inhibited by this. No effect was noticed on a culture of the colon bacillus, nor on two strains of staphylococci whereas one strain of the latter was slightly inhibited.

Fresh Tissue as Vitamines.—The addition of fresh tissue such as the liver and kidney of guinea-pigs to the testiculaı agar did not augment the growth of the gonococcus.

The Effect of Sodium Oleate.—Sodium oleate in the proportion of 1:1,000 was added to testicular agar for the purpose of reducing surface tension. Fairly good growths were obtained with 4 strains of the gonococcus but growth appeared later than in the controls. One strain showed no growth in 48 hours. The growth of 3 strains of staphylococci on this medium was as good as that on the control tubes.

The Effect of Starches.—A comparison was made of the growth of the gonococcus on agars containing the following starches: arrow-root, barley, bean, buckwheat, corn, ginger, pea, potato, rye, rice, sago and tapioca. Starch added to testicular agar does not improve the growth. Vedder [11] used cornstarch. We have found that the use of potato starch will in some instances result in better growths than when corn or other starches are used.

PHENOL RED AS AN INDICATOR IN FERMENTATION REACTIONS OF THE GONOCOCCUS

The gonococcus is very sensitive to the reaction of the medium. To get the best results in any test which depends on the growth of the organism, optimum conditions for growth should be provided. In most of the work on fermentation reactions of the gonococcus, litmus has been used as the indicator. The color change of litmus is approximately at P_H 6.8, while the maximum growth of the gonococcus is obtained at P_H 7.4. Phenolsulphonephthalein or "phenol red" is an indicator which has its range at the optimum reaction for the gonococcus. Enough indicator was added to the medium to give a decided rose-red color. Phenol red does not have any inhibitory action on the gonococcus when used in testicular agar in concentrations decidedly higher than necessary to show the changes in the reaction of the medium caused by the growth of the gonococcus.

In most of the previous work on the fermentation of sugars by the gonococcus, liquid mediums with a sugar concentration of 1% was used. Growth in liquid medium is always slower than on solid. We used solid culture mediums with 0.5% sugar. Dextrose was the only sugar in which acid production was observed. Lactose, saccharose and levulose in 1% concentration did not show acidity in 48 hours.

The results produced with 0.5% dextrose differed somewhat from those with 1.0% of the sugar. Acid is produced in both. When 0.5% dextrose was used, acidity was present in 9 hours. There was no apparent change in reaction of the medium after it had become acid until about the twenty-second hour; at this time 4 out of 5 strains began to show a change from acidity to alkalinity. The reaction gradually changed to complete alkalinity at about the fifty-seventh hour when the medium was strongly alkaline in all cases except one. When 1.0% dextrose was used no secondary alkalinity was observed. Fermentation of 0.5% dextrose in testicular agar is shown in table 2.

TABLE 2

FERMENTATION OF 0.5% DEXTROSE IN TESTICULAR AGAR WITH A REACTION OF PH 7.4, AND USING "PHENOL RED" AS AN INDICATOR

Strain	5 Hours	6 Hours	8 Hours	9 Hours	10 Hours	12 Hours	22 Hours	23 Hours	24 Hours	32 Hours	57 Hours	64 Hours
1	+	+	A	A	A	A	A+alk.	A+alk.	A+alk.	A+alk.	Alk.	Alk.
2	+	+	+	A	A	A	A	A	A	A	A+alk.	A+alk.
3	+	+	A	A	A	A	A+alk.	A+alk.	A+alk.	A+alk.	Alk.	Alk.
4	+	+	+	A	A	A	A+alk.	A+alk.	A+alk.	A+alk.	Alk.	Alk.
5	+	A	A	A	A	A	A+alk.	A+alk.	A+alk.	A+alk.	Alk.	Alk.

+ = Growth—no change in reaction of medium.
A = Acidity of medium.
A + alk. = Acid medium, showing begining secondary alkalinity.
Alk. = Secondary alkalinity complete.

The reason for this difference in acid and alkali formation probably lies in the fact that the 1% dextrose medium contains more dextrose than can be utilized by one culture of the organism, whereas in the 0.5% medium the dextrose is used up before the culture reaches the end of its growth. In all probability, if we could keep a given culture growing for a long period of time on a 1% dextrose medium, the same phenomenon of primary acidity and secondary alkalinity would be observed.

The Care of Stock Cultures.—Stock cultures of the gonococcus can be kept best by daily transfers on testicular agar: If transfers are made at less frequent intervals the growths are uncertain and less abundant.

A moist atmosphere, a temperature of 37.5 C., and the proper reaction of the mediums are necessary. A poorly growing culture, if changed to another favorable culture medium, begins to grow more abundantly. The addition of serum to the surface of an agar slant will also improve the growth.

The Addition of Dyes to Culture Mediums.—Studies of the effect of dyes on the growth of the gonococcus and contaminating organisms, have been made. The reaction of the medium and the quantity of nutrient substances, such as glucose and peptone, influence the effectiveness of dyes. We used testicular agar of P_H 7.4 and a 24-hour culture of gonococci and staphylococci.

TABLE 3

THE EFFECT OF VIOLET DYES ON THE GROWTH OF STAPHYLOCOCCI

Staphylococci Different Strains	Aniline Violet		Crystal Violet		Gentian Violet		Methyl Violet	
	Growth	No Growth	Growth	No Growth	Growth	No Growth	Growth	No Growth
Stock culture	1:25,000	1:10.000	1:25,000	1:10,000	1:50,000	1:40,000	1:40,000	1:25,000
Clinical 1	1:10,000	1:5,000	1:75,000	1:50,000	1:50.000	1:40,000	1:5,000	1:2,500
Clinical 2	1:40,000	1:25,000	1:75,000	1:50,000	1:10,000	1:5,000	1:10,000	1:5,000
Clinical 3	1:2.500	1:1,000	1:5,000	1:1,250	1:10,000	1:5,000	1:5,000	1:2.500
Clinical 4	1:50,000	1:40,000	1:10,000	1:5,000	1:75,000	1:50,000	1:40,000	1:25,000
Clinical 5	1:40,000	1:25,000	1:140,000	1:120,000	1:60,000	1:50,000	1:60,000	1:50,000
Clinical 6	1:60,000	1:50,000	1:140,000	1:120,000	1:60,000	1:50,000	1:60,000	1:50,000
Clinical 7	1:40,000	1:25,000	1:120,000	1:100,000	1:25,000	1:20,000	1:60,000	1:50,000
Clinical 8	1:50,000	1:40,000	1:180,000	1:160,000	1:100,000	1:75,000	1:75,000	1:60,000
Clinical 9	1:60,000	1:50,000	1:20,000	1:10,000	1:10,000	1:50,000	1:40,000	1:25,000
Clinical 10	1:60,000	1:50,000	1:20,000	1:10,000	1:10,000	1:5,000	1:40,000	1:25,000

Staphylococci and other gram-positive contaminants [23] can be inhibited to a marked degree by violet and green dyes. Staphylococci vary considerably in their ability to grow in the presence of violet dyes, as shown in table 3. There is also some difference in the bactericidal effect of a given dye made by different firms.[24] Aniline, crystal, gentian and methyl violet, and aniline, brilliant, malachite, methyl and solid green were used in our experiments. Methyl violet was found to be the most effective one for the isolation of the gonococcus in cases of mixed infection.

The comparative effect of violet dyes on gonococci and staphylococci is shown in table 4.

[23] Churchman, J. W., and Michael, W. H.: Jour. Exper. Med., 1912. 16, p. 822.

[24] Churchman, J. W., and Herz, L. F.: Ibid., 1913, 18, p. 579.

TABLE 4

THE COMPARATIVE EFFECT OF VIOLET DYES ON GONOCOCCI AND STAPHYLOCOCCI

No. of Cultures	Methyl Violet	Methyl Violet	Aniline Violet
Gonococcus................	1:100,000	1:500,000	1:100,000
Strain 1..................	+++	+++	++
Strain 2..................	+++	+++	++
Strain 3..................	++	+++	++
Strain 4..................	++	++	++
Saphylococcus			
Strain 1..................	+	+	++
Strain 2..................	+	+	++
Strain 3..................	+	+	++
Strain 4..................	++	+	++

+ = Slight growth. ++ = Fair growth. +++ = Good growth.

Combinations of green and violet dyes have also been tried; a concentration of 1:500,000 of each dye (as methyl green and methyl violet) is approximately as effective as a greater concentration—1:200,000—of a single dye.

The dye mediums are prepared by adding a sufficient quantity of a 1:1,000 stock solution of the dye to a measured amount of culture medium. The stock solution of dye is prepared by weighing the dye on tinfoil, and washing it into a sterile flask with sterile distilled water. Neutral glassware must be used and evaporation guarded against.

Victoria blue, janus green, hydroquinone, quinone, pyronine, magenta red, congo red and pyoktanin blue vary in their inhibitory action. None of them are of value in inhibiting contaminating organisms in a mixed culture. Hexamethylenamine was added to testicular agar of different reactions. It does not inhibit the growth of staphylococci or colon bacilli as much as that of the gonococcus. The practical importance of violet dyes, especially methyl in 1:200,000 to 1:500,000 concentration for isolation purposes was demonstrated in acute cases. In approximately 40% of acute cases we were able to obtain a growth of the gonococcus on methyl violet tubes, with marked inhibition of the staphylococcus, as indicated by comparison with tubes which contained no violet dyes. This is best demonstrated by the growth of transplants from the violet tubes on blood testicular agar. By this method the isolation of the gonococcus from acute and subacute cases of vaginitis of children was simplified. It is difficult to isolate the gonococcus from a chronic infection of the female genital tract. Nevertheless, because of the great practical importance of making a definite diagnosis, it is well worth while to attempt the isolation.

In transferring exudates[25] to plates or tubes, dry cotton swabs are not reliable; the swab should first be moistened in the water of condensation of a tube of culture medium or a platinum wire should be used.

SUMMARY AND CONCLUSIONS

Testicular blood agar with a reaction of P_H 7.4-7.8 is the most favorable medium for the isolation and subsequent cultivation of the gonococcus. The medium is prepared thus:

Beef testicle from which all connective tissue has been removed is put through a meat grinder, weighed and with twice its weight of distilled water added, is infused over night on ice. The following morning the mixture is heated in a double boiler to 50 C., allowed to stand for one hour and then brought to the boiling point. Let it stand for another hour to permit the solid particles to settle, after which the liquor is decanted off and used as the infusion for the preparation of culture mediums.

For the preparation of testicular infusion agar, 2% peptone, 0.5% glucose, 0.2 to 0.3% monobasic sodium phosphate and 2.5% granular agar are added. This is heated over a flame and stirred constantly until the agar is dissolved. The medium is titrated with phenol red as an indicator and the reaction adjusted to P_H 7.4 to 7.8; if phenolphthalein is used as an indicator, it should be adjusted to a 0.6 reaction. The medium is tubed and autoclaved for 20 minutes at 15 lbs. The titration is checked after sterilization. While the tubes are still liquid (just before the agar solidifies) human blood in the proportion of 0.5 to 2.5% is added. If human blood is not available, defibrinated rabbit's blood (1-5%) may be substituted.

The absence of sodium chloride, the proper reaction and moisture content are especially important.

Blood or blood serum mixed with the testicular agar or smeared on the surface of slanted tubes is necessary for the ready isolation of the gonococcus, but is not essential for the securing of growths of stock cultures.

Fermentation tests made with solid mediums containing 0.5% glucose and phenol red as an indicator results in a significant primary acidity and secondary alkalinity.

[25] Van Gieson, Ira: N. Y. Med. Rec., 1910, p. 1001.

Reduced oxygen tension is of no practical value for either the isolation or subsequent cultivation of the gonococcus.

Aniline dyes of the violet and green colors tend to inhibit the growth of staphylococci more than that of gonococci from cases of mixed infection. Methyl violet added to blood-testicular agar in a proportion of 1:200,000 to 500,000 appears to be of greatest value.

THE HEART RHYTHM IN DIPHTHERIA

CARL SCHWENSEN

From Blegdams-Hospital, Copenhagen

For the last 25 years of the past century clinicians have agreed on the serious significance of the symptoms of cardiac weakness during an attack of diphtheria, and numerous are the publications on this question. All authors hold that the chief features are: murmurs, dilatation and irregularities of the rhythm of the heart. Unfortunately, they have not been able to record the latter graphically, but several, such as Dubrisay,[1] and Huguenin,[2] describe this abnormal rhythm distinctly, in fact so distinctly that we are able to classify many of the disturbances. After the study of the rhythm of the heart gained ground in the ordinary clinical examinations, the following cases were published with sufficient graphic evidence.

Cases of acute heart-block by: Bøe,[3] Fleming and Kennedy,[4] Hecht,[5] Hume,[6] and Rohmer.[7] A most interesting case of acute heart-block combined with auricular fibrillation is reported by J. Parkinson.[8] His patient first developed complete heartblock; 4 days later auricular fibrillation set in. The fibrillation was, as shown by the electrocardiograph, still present 6 months after its onset. This is the only case of auricular fibrillation during diphtheria recorded with definite evidence. In a case recorded by Price and Ivy Mackenzie[9] the tracings are not convincing.

Cases of auricular flutter during diphtheria are reported by Hume,[6] who proposes that the tracings should be of "nodal-rhythm" with attacks of flutter.

A case of paroxysmal tachycardia is reported also by Hume.[6] The patient had had extrasystoles from the 15th day of his illness.

Records are published by Aviragnet, Lutembacher et le Soulier[10] and Aviragnet et Lutembacher[11] who declare them to be the result of extrasystoles and heart-block; but the tracings are not convincing.

Received for publication, August 29, 1921.

1 Union med., 1877, p. 288.
2 Rev. de med., 1888, pp. 790 and 995.
3 Med. Rec., 1913, 30, p. 73.
4 Heart, 1910, 2, p. 77.
5 Erg. d. inn. Med. u. Kinderh., 1913, 11, p. 324.
6 Heart, 1913, 5, p. 25.
7 Ztschr. f. exper. Path. u. Therap., 1912, 11, p. 426.
8 Heart, 1918, 6, p. 13.
9 Ibid., 1911, 3, p. 233.
10 Arch. d. mal. d. Coeur., 1918, 11, p. 41; 1920, 13, p. 1.
11 Jour. d. med. Fr., 1920.

METHODS OF INVESTIGATION

For about 4 years I have had the opportunity of following several thousands of patients with diphtheria during their stay in the hospital. As the toxicity of diphtheria vares in different epidemics I have thought it best to consider only patients seen during a limited space of time, and I have chosen patients who were discharged or who died between Jan. 1 and July 1, 1918. As cardiac disturbances usually occur only in patients with grave cases of diphtheria, I determined to follow these specially and to follow the lighter cases only when the patients had shown symptoms of cardiac trouble. By "grave" diphtheria is understool diphtheria with membrane on both the tonsils, more or less of the uvula and the soft palate. In several of the cases it even reached the gums. Furthermore, there was a more or less pronounced periadenitis of the glands of the neck.

In all, 568 patients suffering from diphtheria passed through the hospital during the period mentioned; 118 had cases of grave diphtheria. These patients were followed throughout their stay in hospital. From the day of admittance they were examined 2 or 3 times weekly. In the gravest cases, in which I could expect a quick development of the symptoms, I examined the patients daily, often several times daily. The pulse was taken morning and evening. The examinations have been: ordinary stethoscopic examination, graphic recording if signs of disordered action of the heart was found, and determination of the blood pressure.

Stethoscopic Findings.—Dilatation of the heart was found in 60 cases, in 42 patients the dilatation involved both the right and left half, in 11 only the right and in 7 only the left half.

We often saw systolic murmurs develop during the stay in hospital; they were usually soft, but might be very harsh; a general feature of the murmurs was that they often changed from day to day. Besides the murmurs, another change of the sounds was found: they became accentuated; then they were muffled and faint; at times they became quite inaudible. The last was a bad prognostic sign and was only found at the first sound in very serious cases. These alterations may vary much from day to day, even from hour to hour. Ordinary systolic murmurs were found in 88 cases; in 74 cases the murmurs were both apical and pulmonal; in 9 cases the murmur was only apical, and in 5 only pulmonal.

Disturbances in Rate and Rhythm.—The rate usually fell with the temperature and was low for a fortnight, whereafter it rose again.

Often it was constantly low in the beginning, morning and evening alike; later came a jumping of the rate, a difference of about 20 not being uncommon. The rate was then always highest in the evening. In several of these ordinary cases of bradycardia during convalescence injection of atropine gave a pronounced rise in the pulse rate.

During the daily work with the patients it soon became evident that 2 quite distinctly different types of irregularities occur besides the ordinary respiratory irregularity; the latter was often found even in patients who at the same time or later on in the course of the illness showed undeniable signs of impairment of the heart. I therefore find it quite impossible to consider this irregularity as a proof that the heart has escaped damage, as Mackenzie does.

The two types of disturbed rhythm were: (a) One which occurred early in the disease, usually before the membrane had entirely disappeared. These patients all died with symptoms of heart failure in the course of a few hours or days after the abnormal rhythm was found. Of the 118 grave cases, 5 were fatal in the acute stage of the disease; all died with symptoms of heart-failure; in 3 of these this abnormal ryhthm was found. (b) One which appeared late in the disease consisted of extrasystoles. In some cases they were found only at one examination, but usually they were present for several weeks until at last they disappeared. None of these patients died with symptoms of heart-failure.

When the abnormal rhythm started in the early stage of the illness (in my cases latest on the 11th day), it was always quite impossible to determine the type by simple comparison of the pulse and the auscultation; in these cases I have taken polygraphic tracings, as I unfortunately had no opportunity of using the electrocardiograph. I have also taken tracings from several of the patients with extrasystoles with the object of verifying the diagnosis, but all authors agree that it is possible to recognize this irregularity of the pulse by simultaneous comparison between the pulse and the auscultation, and these abnormal contractions often occurred with such long intervals that it would have been practically impossible to catch them. Furthermore, I found several times that they had disappeared during the application of the polygraph; as the children became anxious their pulse-rate rose, and it is well known that the premature contractions disappear when the rate of the normal irritations from the sinus is high enough to prevent the heterotope irritation from producing a contraction of the heart-muscle. For these reasons I ceased using the polygraph at this stage of the diphtheria.

A. THE "EARLY" TYPE

In the limited space of time between 1/1—1/7, 1918, I only had the opportunity of examining 3 cases displaying an early appearing irregularity, but as I later on have examined 8, I have in all examined 11 cases of this kind.

The age varied from 1¼ to 9½ years; 6 of the patients were boys, 5 girls. All 11 died. Death occurred at the earliest on the 7th day of illness, at the latest on the 13th day, on an average on the 10th day. The irregularity was earliest found on the 6th day, latest on the 11th, on an average on the 8th day of the diphtheria

The time that passed between the appearance of the irregularity and death was as follows: One patient died on the same day as the irregularity appeared; 5 patients died the day after; two died 2, one 3,

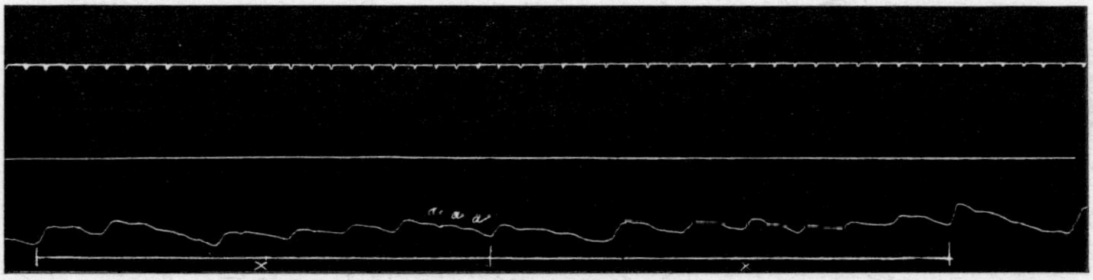

Chart 1, Case 1.—The tracings showed a regular pulse for 13 beats, then the rate of the radial pulse became as shown in the chart. There is pronounced spacing. These tracings were taken with a Jacquet's polygraph. The time-marking always corresponds to 1/5". The upper curve is always the jugular, the lower the radial.

one 4 and one 6 days after the irregularity had appeared. In 10 of the 11 cases I found, besides the irregularity, ordinary symptoms of heart-failure (dilatations, murmurs); in 1 case the irregularity was the sole symptom (case 11). As mentioned before, I took polygraphic tracings in all but one case in which the patient was 1¼ year old. None of the patients were under treatment with digitalis or similar drugs.

In 5 of the cases I made the atropine-test with negative results (cases 2, 5, 6, 7 and 9).

In 4 cases (Nos. 1, 2, 4 and 5) I examined the bundle of His-Tawara histologically according to Tawara.[12] I found it the seat of pathologic changes to the same degree as the myocardium surrounding it; most pronounced was a diffuse cellular infiltration. In none of the cases was an interruption of the bundle found.

[12] Reiszleitung-syst. d. Säugetiereherzen, 1906, p. 37.

I shall give a short summary of the cases with regard to the abnormalities in rate and rhythm, together with the tracings obtained.

SUMMARY OF CASES

CASE 1.—A 4 year old girl, admitted on the 4th day, died on the 12th day of illness. On the 11th day the pulse rate fell from about 100 to 62, it was alternately regular (fig. 1).

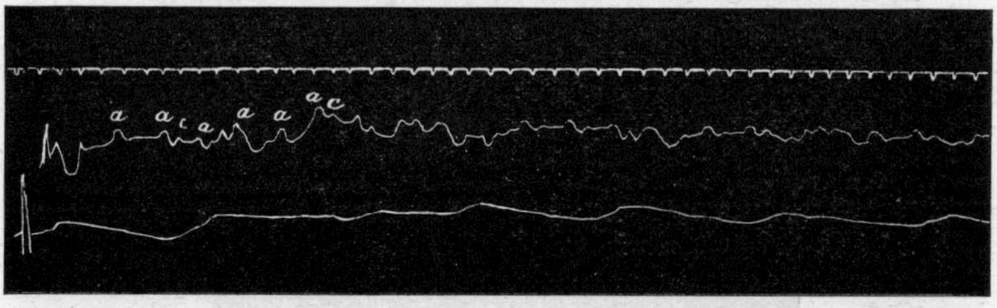

Chart 2, Case 2.—The tracings show partial heartblock. The auricular rate is about 120 per minute, the ventricular rate only about 50.

CASE 2.—A 3 year old boy, admitted on the 5th day, died on the 13th day of illness. The pulse rate fell during the night between the 9th and the 10th day from 120 to 68, and the pulse became irregular. Tracings (fig. 2) showed partial heartblock. The atropine test gave negative results. The tracings remained unaltered until death.

CASE 3.—An 8 year old girl, admitted on the 3rd day, died on the 12th day of illness. During the night between the 5th and 6th day the pulse rate fell from 100 to 48; the tracings showed partial heartblock (fig. 3). On the 7th

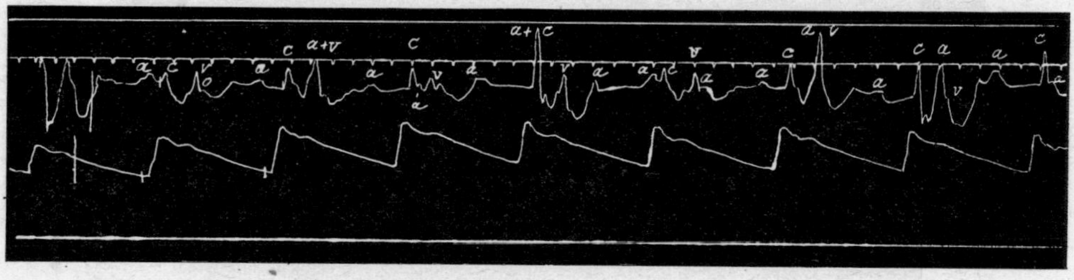

Chart 3, Case 3.—Typical partial heartblock. The a-c interval varies with great regularity.

and the 8th day the tracings still showed varying degrees of partial heartblock, but on the 9th day the pulse had become more irregular and changing. After I had obtained 3 tracings like fig. 4 the pulse suddenly changed and became fast and regular (120 per minute) as in fig. 5. During 20 minutes the pulse remained unaltered, but thereafter the tracings again became like those in fig. 4. The last days the patient lived the pulse showed features like those on the 9th day (figs. 6 and 7).

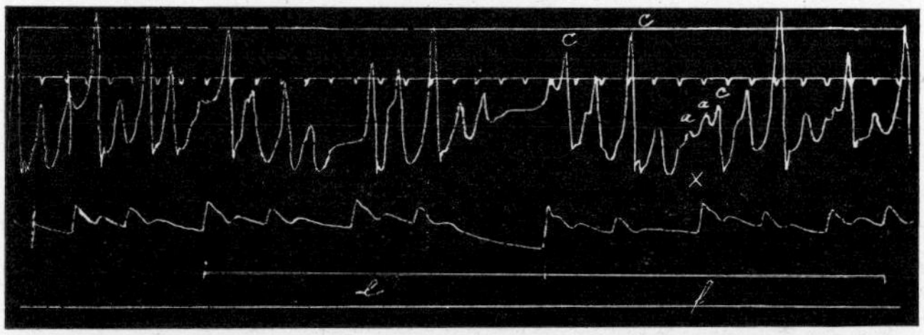

Chart 4, Case 3.—The radial curve is very irregular, but there is pronounced spacing. There are great, rather uniform waves in the jugular curve. At "x" small waves are seen marked "a," which may signify auricular contractions.

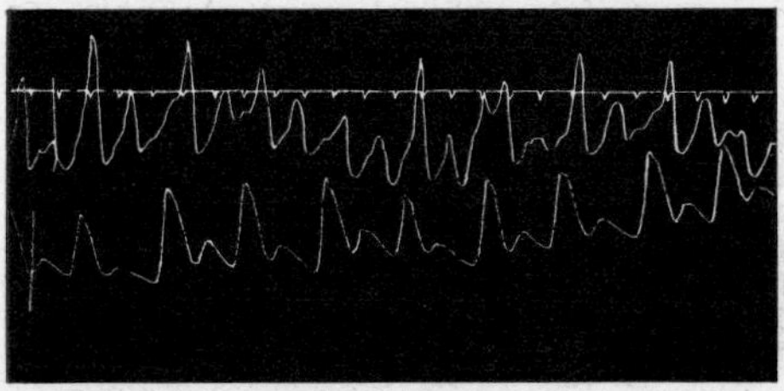

Chart 5, Case 3.—Tachycardia with a rate of about 120. The jugular curve is of the ventricular form.

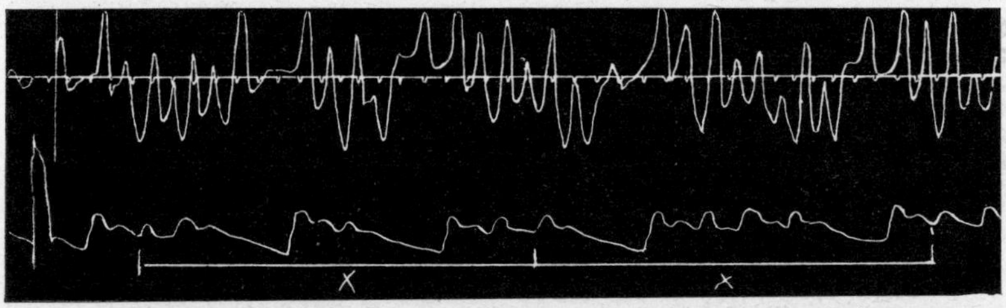

Chart 6, Case 3.—There are uniform big waves in the jugular curve. The radial curve shows pronounced spacing.

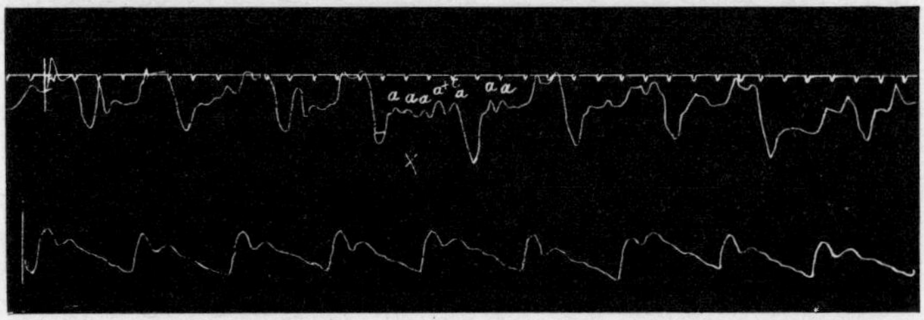

Chart 7, Case 3.—The radial curve is now regular. At "x" in the jugular tracing small waves marked "a" are seen.

CASE 4.—A 5 year old boy admitted on the 3rd day died on the 8th day of illness. On the 6th day the pulse became irregular (fig. 8) about 80. The same day as the patient died the pulse was about 180, regular.

CASE 5.—An 8 year old girl admitted on the 4th day died on the 9th day of illness. On the 6th day the tracings showed partial heartblock (fig. 9); the atropine-test gave negative results. On the 7th day consecutive tracings were like those of fig. 10 and 11, the pulse varying highly. On the 8th day tracings were like fig. 11.

CASE 6.—An 8 year old boy admitted on the 4th day died on the 13th day of illness. On the 12th day the pulse rate had fallen to between 40 and 50. Tracings showed partial heartblock (fig. 12). The atropine-test gave negative results. On the 13th day the pulse varied much in rate and rhythm, in the morning it was 40, in the forenoon 140. Later it was 72 and irregular, and while I observed it, it suddenly changed to 112, regular (fig. 13).

CASE 7.—An 8 year old boy admitted on the 3rd day, died on the 8th day of illness. On the 7th day the pulse became irregular but no tracings were obtained. On the 8th day the rate in the morning was 120, later it fell to

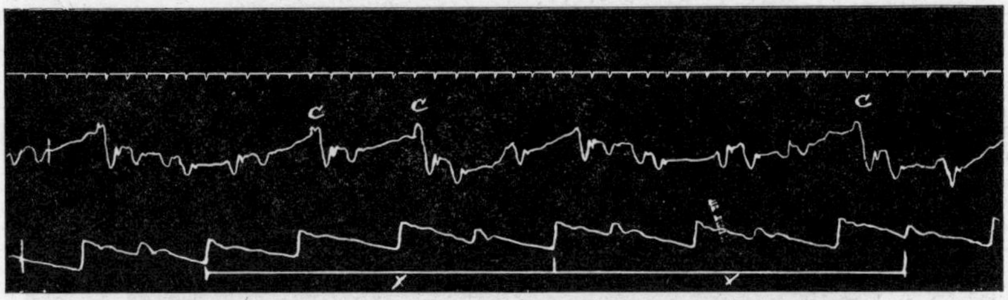

Chart 8, Case 4.—The radial curve is irregular but with spacing.

between 60 and 64, and the pulse was quite regular. At 8 o'clock in the evening a tracing was obtained which showed irregularity as in fig. 14. The atropine-test gave negative results; the tracings remained as before. Half an hour later he suddenly was seized by convulsions and died in a minute.

CASE 8.—A 9½ year old boy admitted on the 3rd day died on the 12th day of illness. The rate was about 60 on the 9th day, rose to 120 on the 11th day, and the pulse became irregular. Tracings obtained were like those in fig. 15. The tracings obtained on the following day were unaltered. He died during a fit of convulsions.

CASE 9.—A 2½ year old girl admitted on the 3rd day died on the 7th day of illness. In the course of the night between the 4th and the 5th day the pulse rate had fallen from 100 to 68, the rhythm was quite regular. On the 6th day the rate was 68, but the rhythm was now irregular (fig. 16). The atropine-test gave negative results. On the 7th day the pulse changed much in rhythm (sometimes it was slow, sometimes fast), the rate being about 96; later the rate increased to 132, and the rhythm was nearly regular, with only an occasional speeding up of the beat. She died in the course of the afternoon.

CASE 10.—A 7 year old boy admitted on the 5th day, died on the 11th day of illness. In the course of the 10th day the pulse rate fell from 112 in the morning to 66-68 in the middle of the day. Tracings showed features like those in fig. 17. After I had obtained one tracing the rhythm changed and the rate increased to 112-120. Tracings were like those in fig. 18. On the 11th day the pulse varied much in rate and rhythm; tracings were like those in figs. 17 and 18 except that occasionally there was a longer pause in the radial pulse.

CASE 11.—A 15 month old girl admitted on the 4th day died on the 7th day of illness. On the 7th day the pulse became irregular with dropped beats (determined by auscultation) and the child died in the evening. No tracings were obtained.

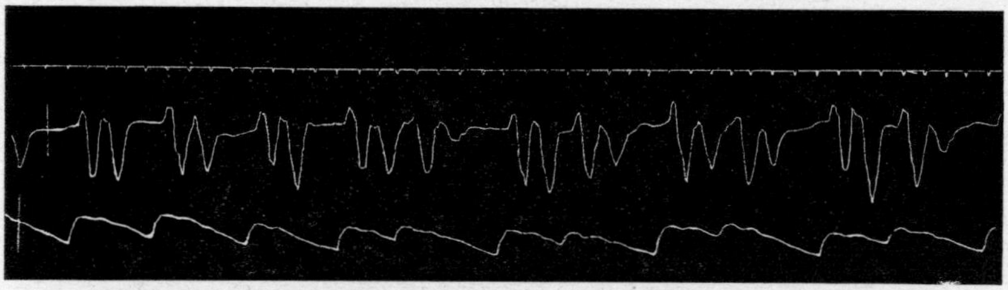

Chart 9, Case 5.—The tracings probably show partial heartblock. The atropine test gave negative results, the curves remaining unaltered.

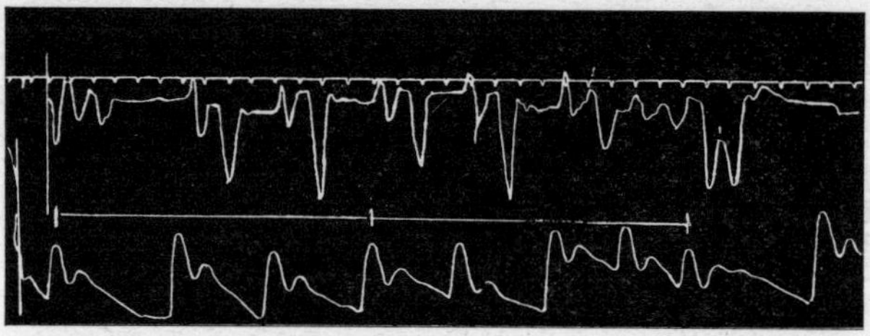

Chart 10, Case 5.—The radial pulse is irregular with pronounced spacing.

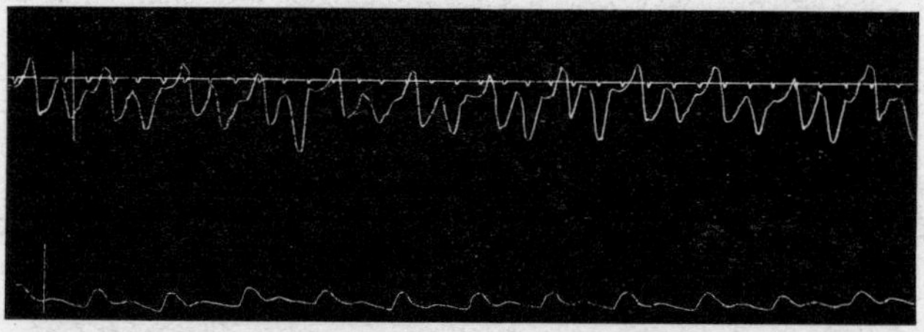

Chart 11, Case 5.—Regular tachycardia, the rate being about 90. The venous curve is of the ventricular form.

As mentioned, only the electrocardiograph would have determined definitely the type of irregularities found in these cases, but unfortunately I have not had the opportunity of using one. On this account I have not deemed it correct to take each tracing alone, but I have reached the following conclusions by considering both the tracings and the ordinary clinical symptoms and, last but not least, by comparing the findings from the different patients:

In the fatal cases of diphtheria, bradycardia often occurs at the end of the 1st or at the beginning of the 2nd week of illness. In some patients there was in a few hours a sudden drop in the pulse rate to about one half of the original rate.

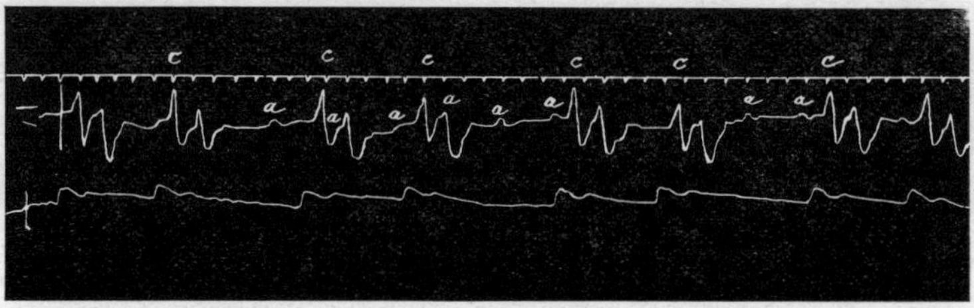

Chart 12, Case 6.—Typical partial heartblock.

The bradycardia was usually irregular, at times it was bigeminate; by auscultating, it was easy to distinguish between these bigeminate periods and extrasystoles.

In 4 of the 10 cases I obtained tracings in this period of bradycardia, and they all showed partial heartblock. In 3 of these cases the atropine-test gave negative results, the block, therefore, must have been caused by a direct affection of the bundle and could not have been due to vagal irritation.

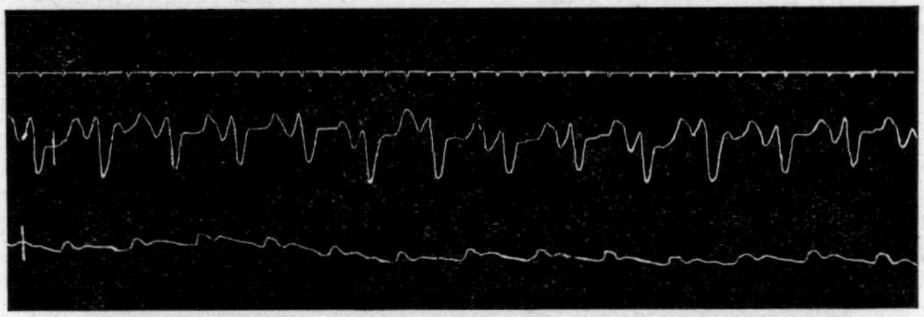

Chart 13, Case 6.—Regular tachycardia. The jugular curve is of the ventricular form.

In one of the cases the block persisted unaltered until death occurred on the 3rd day after the block had set in. In the 3 other cases the pulse later changed in rate and rhythm; at times the pulse rate was slow and regular, at others, bigeminate; occasionally there were series of quicker beats followed by a longer pause. Sometimes a regular tachycardia suddenly set in, followed by one of the other types. Auscultation showed that this varying irregularity did not in the least resemble extrasystoles. Soon the pulse rate became complex, and its most conspicuous character was the great instability of rhythm.

In the 6 cases in which I did not obtain tracings in the bradycardial period, the tracings obtained showed features just like those in tracings

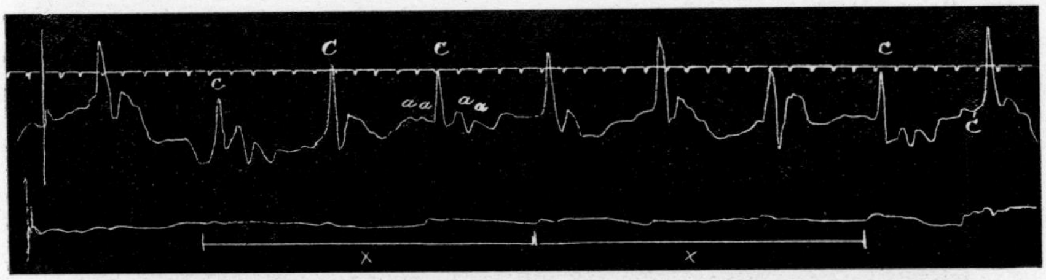

Chart 14, Case 7.—The radial tracing is irregular with spacing. In the jugular curve some small waves marked "a" are seen; probably they are due to very quick auricular contractions.

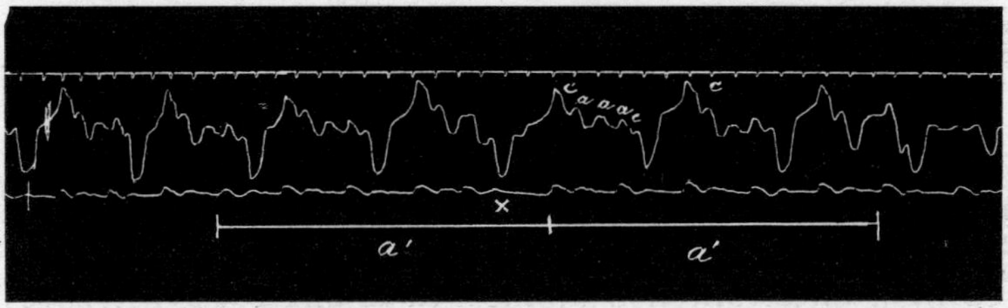

Chart 15, Case 8.—The radial curve shows spacing. The small waves marked "a" may correspond to auricular contractions.

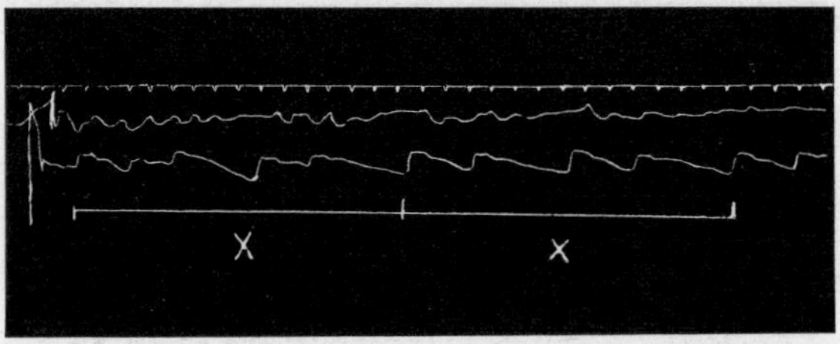

Chart 16, Case 9.—The radial tracing shows irregularity with spacing.

made during the complex period mentioned in the foregoing. In 2 of these cases the atropine test also gave a negative result.

With regard to the tracings from the complex period, I think it evident that they show the same type of irregularity in all of the 9 cases. Clinically there was no difference between these cases, and it was easy to recognize the irregularity by making the usual comparison between pulse and auscultation.

The most remarkable features of this disturbance of the rhythm are: (1) the instability of the rate and the rhythm, (2) the great waves which are found in several of the jugular tracings, (3) the pronounced "spacing" (Lewis [13]) shown by all these radial tracings, (4) smaller waves marked a in some of the jugular tracings may correspond to fast auricular contractions, and (5) the fact that the tracings are identical with tracings made in cases of flutter verified electrocardiographically (Lewis,[14] Ritchie [15]).

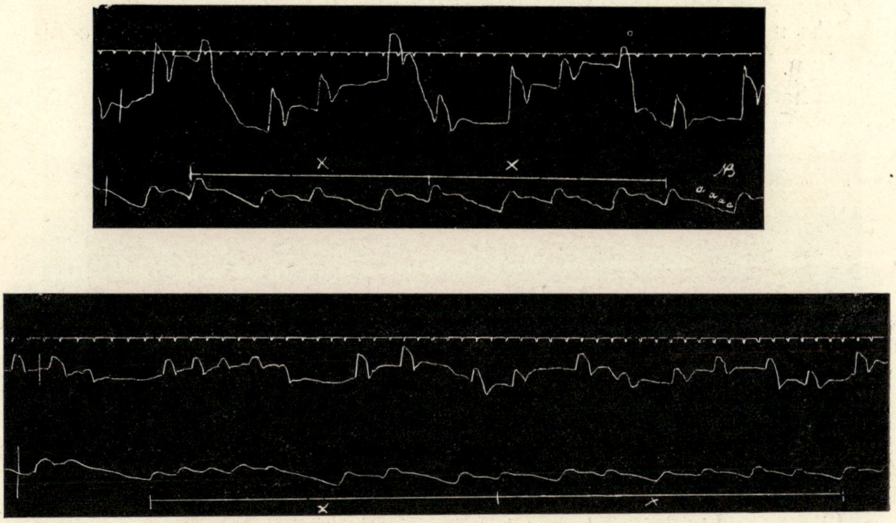

Chart 17 and 18, Case 10.—The radial curves show spacing.

Only the electrocardiograph could give a definite determination of this complex type. I think that the facts mentioned, however, indicate that the probable cause of this complex irregularity is that the original acute partial heart-block has been complicated with attacks of auricular flutter.

B. THE "LATE" TYPE

As I have mentioned already, extrasystoles were a usual finding in the convalescence after diphtheria. Five hundred and sixty-three patients with diphtheria have been examined with regard to the

[13] Mech. of Graph. Registration of Heart, 1920, p. 272.
[14] Clin. Disorders of Heartbeat, 1913.
[15] Auricular Flutter, 1914.

occurrence of extrasystoles; 113 of them had cases of grave diphtheria. Of all the 563 cases, 14% had extrasystoles during convalescence; in 61% of the 113 grave cases extrasystoles appeared. In all, 77 patients showed extrasystoles; 6 of them were adults, 71 less than 15 years old. The extrasystoles appeared at the earliest on the 18th day, at the latest on the 55th day, on an average on the 33rd day. Nine patients had extrasystoles during the 3rd week, 6 during the 4th, 32 during the 5th, 15 during the first half of the 6th, 2 during the second half of the 6th, 10 during the 7th, and 3 during the 8th week of illness. In 19 cases the extrasystoles was the first abnormal symptom from the side of the heart and in 9 of these cases it was the only one.

As mentioned, extrasystoles were diagnosed by simultaneous comparison between the pulse and the action of the heart as found by auscultation. Usually they were found for several days or weeks and

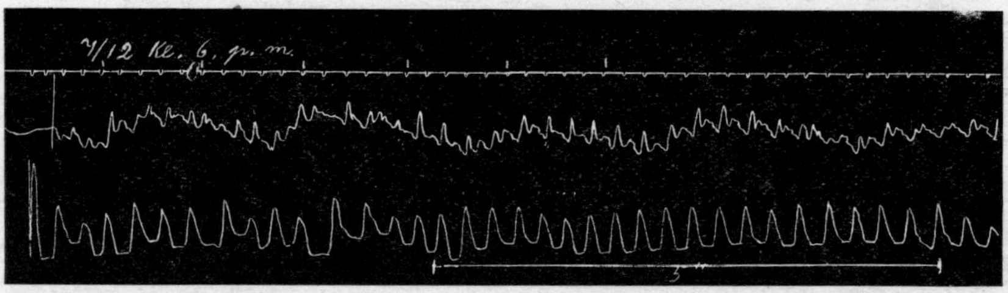

Chart 19.—The radial curve shows a regular tachycardia of about 236 per minute.

were very frequent (10 or more per 100 not uncommon); in some patients they occurred only with long intervals and during a few days; they were seldom found at only one examination. In not a few cases were found series of extrasystoles; in one case even paroxysmal tachycardia was found.

In the tracings I took in these cases I found auricular as well as ventricular extrasystoles, but as I did not take tracings in all the cases for the reasons mentioned, I cannot pass any opinion as to which is the most common type: the auricular or the ventricular, and whether they always are of the same origin in the same patient.

As an example I give a short summary of the case in which the patient had attacks of paroxysmal tachycardia:

In a girl, aged 11 years, admitted on the 5th day and discharged on the 68th day of illness, the tonsils, uvula and part of the soft palate were covered with membrane. There was some periadenitis. On the 18th day of illness the membrane had disappeared. On the 20th day a soft systolic murmur was heard at the apex. On the 30th day there were extrasystoles with long intervals. The next day she was very nervous and cried. The pulse rate was, counted by auscultation, more than 200 per minute; the action was tumultuous. While I was preparing to make the tracings she stopped crying and the tracings showed normal conditions. At 6 p. m. I obtained tracings like those shown in fig. 19. The rate, counted on the tracing, was 236 per minute. Pressure of the vagus gave no retardation. At 6:30 p. m. the character of the tracings had changed and showed a regular pulse of 144 per minute, an occasional auricular extrasystole. The day after the pulse was 140, the tracings showed extrasystoles of ventricular origin. The following day the tracings for some time were identical with those in fig. 19; then a series of extrasystoles of ventricular origin appeared (fig. 20). She had no more attacks of tachycardia, but for a fortnight she had extrasystoles. The patient was discharged without any symptom of disease of the heart.

Later I had the opportunity of examining with the electrocardiograph 31 patients who had dilatations, systolic murmurs and frequent extrasystoles during the 5th week of their illness. The electrocardio-

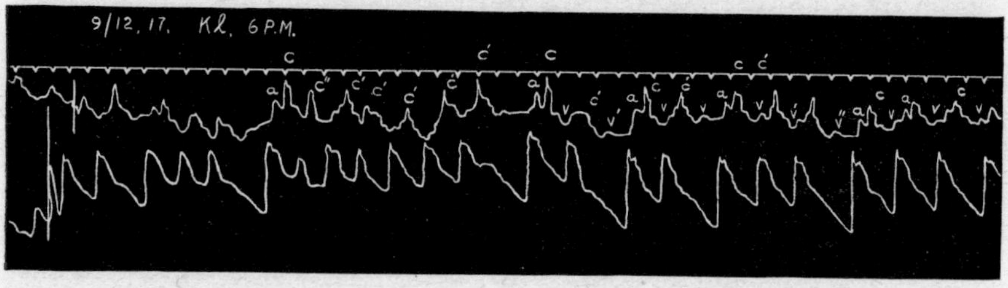

Chart 20.—There are here a series of extrasystoles of ventricular origin.

grams were taken in the ordinary way from all 3 leads. In only 3 of the patients (children) I happened to catch the extrasystoles. In 2 cases they were ordinary auricular extrasystoles while in the 3rd case there was an extrasystole arising in the junctional tissues. The electrocardiograms of the other patients were quite normal.

DETERMINATION OF THE BLOOD PRESSURE

In 4 of the fatal cases and in 69 of the grave cases I repeatedly determined the blood pressure by Riva-Rocci's apparatus with a broad cuff.

In the 4 fatal cases the systolic blood pressure fell to 60, 75, 45 and 53, respectively. In the greater part of the 69 cases I found that the systolic blood pressure decreased slowly. The minimum was reached during the 2nd or 3rd week, whereafter the pressure again rose slowly until normal heights were reached during the 4th or the 5th week. In only 3 of these cases did the pressure fall below 70. A blood pressure below 70 must therefore be considered a bad prognostic sign. These findings are in accordance with those of E. Faber.[16]

DISCUSSION

During the course of diphtheria, murmurs, dilatation and irregularity are according to my experience a usual phenomenon. These symptoms may be assumed to be the result of an acute myocarditis; the murmurs indicate not a valvulitis, but an inefficiency of the functions of the muscles around the mitral valve and of the papillary muscle (Mackenzie,[17] Krehl [18]). The great instability of the murmurs indicates that they are not caused by a valvulitis; furthermore, valvulitis is never discovered postmortem.

In 98, or 17% of my 568 cases and in 89, or 75%, of the cases of grave diphtheria, these symptoms of myocardial disease were observed.

Of these 98 cases, 60 patients had both murmurs and dilatation, 28 only murmurs but no dilatation; in 1 case the early appearing irregularity and in 9 extrasystoles were the sole heart symptoms showing disturbances of that organ.

Of the 84 patients with a grave diphtheria who survived the acute stage of illness and in whom dilatation and murmur or murmur alone were found, extrasystoles occurred later in 68, or in 81% of the cases.

The first symptom of myocarditis was found earliest on the 3rd day of illness, latest (as extrasystoles) on the 47th day, and on an average on the 15th day of illness. If we do not consider the patients in whom the extrasystoles were the first abnormal sign, the usual time for the appearance of the first symptom of myocarditis was on the 10th day of illness.

The question is whether this acute myocarditis explains all the clinical symptoms found during diphtheria or whether it will be necessary to assume vasomotor paresis or nervous influences.

It is a well-known fact that in diphtheria more than in any other acute disease there is a tendency to fatal syncope. In the cases in which death occurred in the acute stage (2nd or 3rd week) there were always found symptoms of a severe myocarditis (dilatation and murmurs). This in itself can explain the fatal course but cannot explain the frequent attacks of syncope, but when this grave acute myocarditis,

[16] Dödsaarsagene ved Difteri, 1903.
[17] Diseases of Heart, 1914, p. 304.
[18] Erkrank. d. Herzmuskels, etc., 1913, p. 373.

as I have proved, often is combined with a great disturbance of the rhythm [19] the matter is greatly simplified.

This early irregularity could, as a rule, be divided into 2 periods: in the first only varying degrees of heartblock were found, in the second was found the irregularity which I have described as the complex irregularity.

The period of heartblock makes it clear why these patients are prone to attacks of syncope and sudden death; as the result of profound slowing or prolonged standstill of the ventricle these patients have attacks of cerebral anemia.

As to the complex irregularity, Mackenzie [17] and Lewis [14] say that severe disturbance [20] of the rhythm of the heart often produces attacks of syncope as the result of cerebral anemia, especially when the muscle is damaged beforehand. Furthermore, Wenckebach [21] shows how the simultaneous contractions of the auricles and the ventricles are a hindrance in the emptying of the auricles; the blood accumulates in the central veins and in the liver; therefore there is a diminished output of the left ventricle. When the rhythm varies greatly, this abnormal mechanism may produce attacks of cerebral anemia with syncope. I have considered the consequences of the complex irregularity only as irregularity, but if these patients present cases of flutter, the attacks of syncope are only such as one usually finds in cases of flutter, in which the ventricle occasionally answers to the full call of the auricle and the heart rate leaps to its fullest. Then the blood pressure sinks rapidly, and we get syncope as a result of cerebral anemia. If these seizures are of prolonged duration, death intervenes (Lewis [20]).

Among the other important symptoms in this stage of the diphtheria the following are the most significant: enlargement of the liver, low blood pressure with coolness and pallor of the skin, vomiting, and the absence of symptoms of pulmonary stasis.

The lesser degrees of enlargement of the liver, as well as of the decrease in blood pressure, can be explained as the result of a failing heart (Sutherland [22]). In the fatal cases we often see an excessive enlargement, which appears in the course of a few hours; the liver often reaches below the umbilical-line and is very tender. This excessive enlargement can be explained by the severe irregularity of the rhythm

[19] Between Jan. 1 and Jan. 7, 1918, this abnormal rhythm was observed in 3 of the 5 patients who died in the acute stage.

[20] Lectures on the Heart, 1914.

[21] Die unregelm. Herztätigkeit, 1914.

[22] The Heart in Early Life, 1914.

of the heart (Mackenzie,[17] Wenckebach [21]), just as we often find the liver greatly enlarged in patients with paroxysmal tachycardia, especially when the heart muscle is damaged.

The low blood pressure, together with the coolness and pallor of the skin which are very serious signs in diphtheria, are a usual finding in cardial syncope and can be explained by the diminished output of the left ventricle, the blood being accumulated in the central veins and in the liver. The vomiting is a result of the cerebral anemia.

That we in these patients do not find pronounced signs of pulmonary stasis can be explained by the fact that blood is accumulated in the central veins and in the liver. For this reason the right ventricle gets very little blood, and is accordingly unable to produce a pulmonary stasis (Wenckebach [21]).

The early appearing abnormal rhythm (heartblock or "complex irregularity") which I have found in diphtheria, explains why patients die without the pathologist being able to find a sufficient cause for death; and as this abnormal rhythm is easily overlooked—if one does not specially look for it and if one examines the pulse only occasionally—it is evident that in former days there has been uncertainty as to the cause of death and that other explanations than the impairment of the heart have been sought.

For this reason the theory of vasomotor paresis or paresis of the vagal nerve has been put forward. Against this theory is the fact that instead of the increase of the pulse rate which was to be expected, we not only have bradycardia in the fatal cases with heartblock, but as mentioned before, there is in most cases a greater or smaller decrease of the rate, often a veritable bradycardia (Romberg,[23] Schmaltz,[24] Dorner [25]). This bradycardia disappears after the injection of atropine just as does the ordinary bradycardia seen during convalescence in other acute diseases. If the vasomotor paresis was the chief factor, we should furthermore find the veins of the neck empty; on the contrary, we find them distended and pulsating as the result of the simultaneous contractions of the auricle and the ventricle.

Although I am unable to prove that the vasomotor paresis, vagal paresis or the like are not present, I think that I am justified in declaring that the myocarditis, and especially the early disturbances of the rhythm explain the clinical findings during the acute stage of diphtheria.

[23] Krankh. d. Herzens, etc., 1909.
[24] Jahrb. f. Kinderh., 1897, 45, p. 89.
[25] Studien 3, Path. u. Behandl. d. Diph., 1918.

With regard to the extrasystoles, I think it is very doubtful that they are the result of an active myocarditis. The usual time for their appearance coincides with the time when the blood pressure has reached its normal height. I would rather believe that they were a symptom of convalescence and were caused by resorptive or regenerative processes (fibrous or myogenic), which might either give rise to new impulses or to an exaggerated sensibility of the tissues.

It is certain that the patients, when the extrasystoles have again disappeared, either are cured or have reached a stage in which no further progress can be expected even by prolonged staying in bed.

The extrasystoles cannot be considered as a form of diphtheric paralysis as several authors (Schmaltz,[26] Romberg,[27] Mackenzie,[17] Parkinson, Gosse and Gunson [28]) have found them during convalescence from other acute diseases (scarlet fever, typhoid fever, rheumatic fever). I have myself found them during convalescence from scarlet fever. That the extrasystole in some cases was the first, in a few even the sole, symptom of disease of the heart, can be explained by the fact that the acute lesion of the muscle was so slight that it did not give any available symptom in the acute stage, although the regenerative (resorptive) changes later gave rise to the heterogenic contractions.

REEXAMINATIONS

Mackenzie [17] says that the damage of the myocardium in acute diseases often is not stationary but progressive. The time that passes before the recognition of the cardiac impairment depends on the extent of the damage and the rapidity of its progress, and the amount of effort to which the person is subjected.

As I have showed, acute myocarditis is common in patients suffering from grave diphtheria. It is now a question of the greatest importance, whether this myocarditis disappears without leaving any available clinical symptom or whether it may be considered as the origin of chronic disease of the heart, which sooner or later may result in heart failure.

Several authors have said that the myocarditis following diphtheria gives rise to chronic diseases of the heart (Baginsky,[29] Romberg,[23] Grancher, Boulloche and Babonneix [30]). Experimentally, Mollard and Regaud have proved this.

[26] München. med. Wchnschr., 1904, 41, p. 1419.
[27] Deutsch. Arch. f. klin. Med., 1891, 48, p. 369; 1892, 49, p. 413.
[28] Quarterly Jour. Med., 1920, 13, p. 363.
[29] Diphtherie u. diph. Croup, 1913.
[30] Diphthérie, Nouv. Trait d. med.

Schmaltz[31] is the only one who has followed a greater number of patients methodically a year or more after they had diphtheria, and he found that 1 year after recovery 50% of 56 patients, 2 years after recovery 42.5% of 41 patients and 3 years after recovery 42% of 19 patients showed signs of functional inefficiency of the mitral valve. He thinks the systolic murmur is of special value for the diagnosis of the myocardial disease. Förster[32] has seen such patients develop grave heart failure 1 to 4 years after their discharge.

With the object of throwing more light on this question I have tried to examine, 2 years or more after their discharge, those of my patients who had shown signs of myocarditis. When discharged 30 (34%) of the 89 patients with myocarditis showed no abnormal heart sign; in the rest 66% either murmurs or dilatation was found.

In determining, at the reexamination, whether the patient had a normal heart I have taken into consideration the subjective symptoms of exhaustion as well as the physical signs. With regard to the former I have considered whether the patient easily tired, shortness of breath and throbbing of the heart in running or walking fast. These symptoms were often combined with pains in the precordium. As all patients who were reexamined were children—between 5 and 15 years of age—I think that these symptoms of distress must signify an impairment of the heart, especially when they occur in formerly healthy children. The parents also often told me that their children were quite changed after their attack of diphtheria; they were irritable and sulky. Often they would not play with other children as before and when allowed to choose they preferred quiet games.

As to the abnormal physical symptoms, the most interesting is the persistence of a systolic murmur or a dilatation. These murmurs cannot be accidental as they appeared in formerly normal hearts during an acute infection.

Of the 89 patients, 66 came to be reexamined; none of them had had an acute infection after discharge. In 46 were found symptoms like those in cases of mitral regurgitation. Most conspicuous was the systolic murmur, which might be soft but could be very harsh. Only in one case was a disturbed rhythm found (occasionally an extra-systole). Dilatation was often present. This mitral regurgitation must be the result not of a valvulitis, but of a progressive lesion of the myo-

[31] Festschr. 3. Feier d. 50 jähr Besteh. d. Stadtkrankheit. 3 Dresden-Friederichstadt, 1899, p. 157.

[32] Deutsch. Arch. f. klin. Med., 1906, 85, p. 11.

cardium which has given rise to a more or less pronounced impairment of the functional efficiency of the heart muscle.

In 4 of these cases there had been only a doubtful acute myocarditis during the diphtheria but on reexamination 2 years later, a pronounced impairment of the heart was found.

The question now is what the future will be for these patients. I am afraid that the more or less strenuous struggle for life with new infections, hard work and in the female, last but not least, pregnancy (delivery) will prove to be too much for the from the beginning only slightly impaired heart, so that years later heart failure will set in in many of these patients as a result of the long forgotten diphtheria in early childhood.

SUMMARY

Five hundred and sixty-eight patients with diphtheria have been examined for symptoms of cardiac impairment; 118 of them who suffered from grave diphtheria have been especially examined. Furthermore, 8 cases that were fatal in the acute stage, have been followed thoroughly.

Clinical signs of acute myocarditis were found in 17% of the 568 cases and in 75% of the cases of grave diphtheria.

Typical symptoms of myocarditis were present in all fatal cases in the acute stage.

During the course of the diphtheria two distinctly different types of disturbance of the rhythm appeared:

(*a*) An "early" type which on an average appeared on the 8th day of illness. It started as organic heartblock; in the course of a few hours to a few days the rhythm, as a rule, became very complex and varying, but still it formed a distinct, easily recognizable type (flutter?). This disturbance explains the pallor, the coolness of the skin and the frequent attacks of syncope. All these patients died of heart failure in the acute stage of the diphtheria.

(*b*) A "late" type which consisted of extrasystoles appearing on an average on the 33rd day of illness. Among the 563 cases that survived the acute stage extrasystoles were found in 14% and in 61% of the grave cases. Of the patients with symptoms of myocarditis 81% had extrasystoles during convalescence. None of these patients died of heart failure.

In 4 cases of type *a,* histologic examinations of the aterioventricular node and bundle showed that this system was attacked in the same degree as the myocardium surrounding it.

Electrocardiograms taken during the 5th week of illness were normal in 31 cases with muscular mitral insufficiency and extrasystoles. These last were found in only 3 patients; the 2 patients had extrasystoles of auricular origin while the extrasystole in the 3rd case arose from the junctional tissues.

On reexamining the patients at least 2 years after their discharge signs of impairment of the heart were found in more than two thirds of those who came to be reexamined. In some cases, in which reexamination showed pronounced impairment, there had been during the stay at the hospital only doubtful signs of myocarditis. The diphtheria must, therefore, be considered an important cause of heart failure later in life.

A STUDY OF TWO DISTINCT STRAINS OF STREPTOCOCCUS ISOLATED FROM THE SAME HEART-VALVE LESION

Katharine M. Howell

From the Nelson Morris Institute for Medical Research, Michael Reese Hospital, Chicago

Studies which have had for their aim the classification of the streptococcus group are numerous. While they have led to important additions to our knowledge of the group, they have left many questions relating to classification and to biologic reactions and variations still in doubt. The cultural studies of Andrewes and Horder,[1] Holman,[2] and Brown [3] have simplified the classification and permit ready grouping by reactions on sugar and blood mediums, but they have disregarded the immunologic relations; strains of streptococci which are culturally distinct may be immunologically identical. The application of immunologic reactions alone has yielded no more satisfactory results. In our own studies of complement-fixation reactions,[4] there was no correlation between complement fixation and the reactions on blood mediums, nor between complement fixation and grouping based on fermentative reactions; neither was there any distinct correlation between complement fixation and disease grouping. Dochez, Avery and Lancefield [5] obtained evidence of grouping by agglutination reactions. Their work, however, was limited to hemolytic strains; the results with complement fixation suggest that it is probable that some nonhemolytic strains, differing from those studied in so fundamental a property as the reaction on hemoglobin, will fall into the groups based on agglutination. The relative importance of environmental factors during the stage of parasitism, i. e., host species, tissue localization and pathologic process, and of cultural reactions during the stage of cultivation outside the body has not been sufficiently investigated.

The isolation of two morphologically and culturally distinct species of streptococci from the same lesion so deep seated as to exclude the fortuitous addition of one to the other from the surface offered an

Received for publication, Oct. 28, 1921.

[1] Lancet, 1906, 2, pp. 708, 775, 852.
[2] Jour. Med. Research, 1916, 24, p. 377.
[3] Monographs of the Rockefeller Institute for Medical Research, No. 9, 1919.
[4] Jour. Infect. Dis., 1918, 28, p. 230.
[5] Jour. Exper. Med., 1919, 30, p. 179.

opportunity to study some of these questions, and, more particularly, to determine whether the two invading organisms might have identical reactions as the result of growth in the same host, the same tissue and the same lesion. Furthermore, it appeared important to determine the fixity of the reactions by repeated investigation of the same two organisms during a prolonged period of cultivation outside the body, since several recent writers have reported the development of nonhemolytic colonies from hemolytic strains and of hemolytic variants from nonhemolytic strains.

The two strains were isolated from a vegetative growth on the aortic valve, obtained at necropsy Oct. 4, 1919. Clinically the case was a typical chronic infectious endocarditis. The lesion from which the organisms were isolated was a chronic vegetative aortic valvular endocarditis. The first cultures were obtained by grinding the vegetative growth with sterile sand, in a sterile mortar, and by streaking the fluid material thus obtained on the surface of blood agar plates. There was no growth on the blood-agar plates in 12 hours, but in 36 hours there were a number of small, round, elevated, white, moist colonies which were surrounded by a clear zone of hemolysis, 2 to 3 mm. in diameter. In 48 hours there were, in addition to the hemolytic colonies, minute, moist, elevated, green colonies, with no surrounding zone of hemolysis. The blood-agar plates were examined daily, and after 5 days, the hemolytic colonies had undergone no change, but the green colonies had turned to a brownish color.

Films made from a hemolytic colony and stained by the Gram method, showed a small, round, gram-positive coccus, in pairs and in chains of varying length (fig. 1). Films from a green colony, and similarly stained, showed a more minute gram-positive diplococcus, usually forming chains (fig. 2). The difference in the size of the two cocci is even more striking on direct visual examination than in the photomicrographs.

Which of the two streptococci was the primary cause of the heart lesion it is impossible to determine definitely. The aortic lesion was of the type usually associated with Streptococcus viridans. In the pulmonary artery, just at the bifurcation, there was a large, raised soft, warty vegetation, which on both gross and microscopic examination was more recent than the aortic lesion. From the pulmonary artery the green streptococcus alone was isolated. This would seem to indicate that the latter organism had the greater invasive powers; however, virulence tests made immediately after isolation of the two strains showed the hemolytic organism to be much more highly virulent for laboratory animals than the viridans strain. The absence of more acute ulcerative reaction in the aortic valve, such as is usually

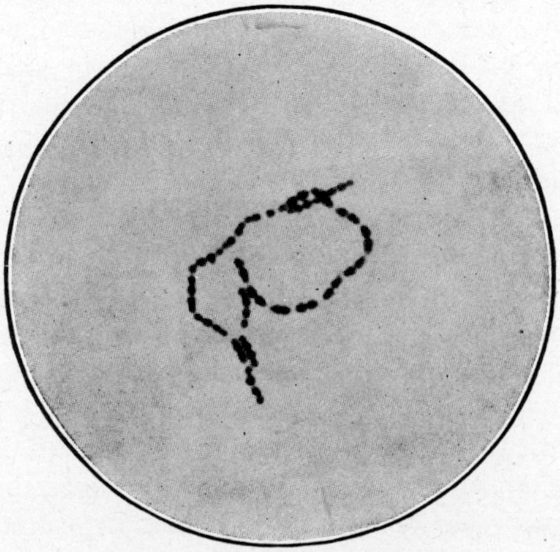

Fig. 1.—Hemolytic streptococcus; Gram stain; × 1200.

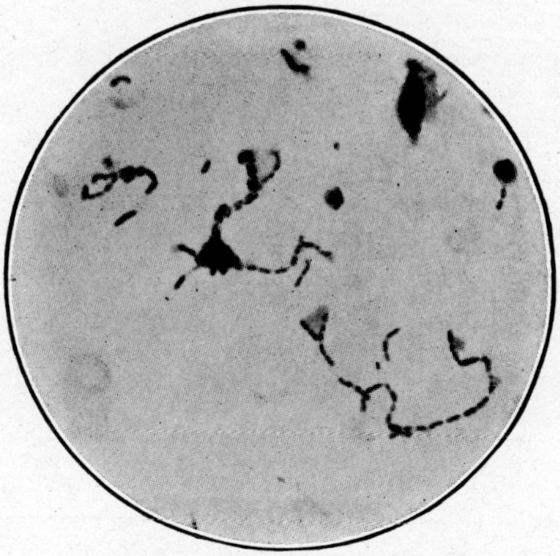

Fig. 2.—Viridans streptococcus; Gram stain; × 1200.

associated with the hemolytic streptococcus, in spite of the greater virulence of the latter, may be interpreted as evidence that this organism was a later invader of a lesion primarily due to Streptococcus viridans.

The two strains of streptococcus were subcultivated in ascites meat-infusion dextrose broth of a P_H 7.6 reaction. After 24 hours, the broth tube, inoculated with the hemolytic streptococcus, had a flocculent sediment and a cloudy supernatant; the broth tube inoculated with the nonhemolytic streptococcus had a granular sediment and a clear supernatant fluid. Neither coccus was soluble in bile nor did either ferment inulin. Classified on a basis of sugar fermentations (Andrewes and Horder,[1] or Holman[2]), the hemolytic streptococcus belonged to the Streptococcus pyogenes group, and the nonhemolytic streptococcus belonged to the streptococcus salivarius group. Neither streptococcus was a mannitol fermenter.

The virulence of the two strains was tested by intraperitoneal injection of white mice with varying doses of 18-hour growths of the bacteria in broth medium. The lethal dose of the hemolytic streptococcus was 0.06 c c of the 18-hour broth culture. The viridans streptococcus had little pathogenicity for white mice, since a whole c c of an 18-hour broth culture (having approximately the same number of organisms as did the corresponding hemolytic streptococcus) failed to kill a white mouse, although the latter was apparently quite ill for several days. Mice receiving smaller doses of this nonhemolytic streptococcus, were apparently not affected. The virulence tests were repeated after 6 weeks. The viridans streptococcus, as far as could be detected, was entirely nonpathogenic for white mice at that time. The virulent quality of the hemolytic streptococcus was almost entirely lost, since it required 1.5 c c of the 18-hour broth culture to kill a mouse. The virulence of the hemolytic streptococcus was not appreciably increased by repeated animal passage. As the hemolytic streptococcus lost its virulence, it also lost the peculiar quality, previously recorded,[6] of agglutinating instead of laking red blood cells of various species, when it was grown in broth medium.

During the two years in which the strains of streptococcus have been under observation, half-grown rabbits were immunized at different times, and agglutination, opsonic, and complement-fixation tests were made with immune serums. After a number of preliminary tests, it was decided that serum, inactivated by heating at 56 C. for 30 minutes, was more satisfactory for use in the tests than active serum, since it was less apt to be anticomplementary in the fixation tests, and at the same time it was equally good for the agglutinin and opsonin tests. Some difficulty was experienced in obtaining smooth suspensions,

[6] Jour. Infect. Dis., 1920, 27, p. 565.

since both strains were inclined to clump spontaneously in broth medium, but by transferring daily, from one ascites meat-infusion dextrose broth to another, a comparatively smooth suspension resulted. The 18-hour growths were centrifugated, the supernatant broth removed, the precipitated bacteria washed with salt solution, and resuspended in salt solution in approximately the same concentration as that of the 18-hour broth culture, shaken with sterile glass beads, centrifugated a few minutes at low speed to remove any small clumps, and the fluid removed and heated at 56 C. for 30 minutes.

Agglutination.—The macroscopic method was used. To varying dilutions of a normal rabbit serum and to varying dilutions of each immune serum was added an equal amount of killed bacterial suspension. They were mixed in tubes, and the tubes were placed in the hot water bath at 56 C. for one hour. The tests were read at once and the highest dilution of serum that agglutinated the bacteria was noted and is indicated by the figures recorded in the table. Whenever there was any clumping in the control tube that contained bacterial suspension only, or in any of the tubes containing normal serum and suspension, the tests were discarded.

Opsonic Tests.—Opsonin was estimated by the opsonic index method, and the figures are recorded in the table.

Complement Fixation.—The tests were made according to the original Wassermann test (one-tenth method). Hot water incubation was used, and the readings were made and recorded immediately after the second incubation. A normal rabbit control serum was set up with each test, and unless there was complete hemolysis with this serum, the tests were discarded. When there was complete inhibition of hemolysis with $\frac{1}{4}$ and $\frac{1}{8}$ of the anticomplementary unit of antigen, the test was considered weakly positive, and is indicated in the table by +. Fixation with $\frac{1}{16}$ and $\frac{1}{32}$ is indicated by + +, fixation with $\frac{1}{64}$ and $\frac{1}{128}$ by + + +, and fixation with $\frac{1}{256}$ or over, by + + + +

Three rabbits were immunized with the hemolytic streptococcus strain and 3 rabbits with the nonhemolytic streptococcus strain during the 2 years in which the strains were under observation. Frequent tests were made on the rabbit serums during the immunization period, but the observations recorded in the table are those in which each immune serum had the maximum reaction with the homologous suspension in the tests.

Two rabbits were immunized in 1919 with the freshly isolated strains. The hemolytic streptococcus immune serum (hemolytic streptococcus serum 1) agglutinated the hemolytic streptococcus in 1:640 serum dilution, and the nonhemolytic streptococcus in 1:80; the opsonic index to hemolytic streptococcus was 2.5, and to the nonhemolytic streptococcus 3.5; in the complement-fixation test, the immune serum gave +++ fixation with the homologous antigen, and no fixation with the heterologous antigen. The nonhemolytic immune serum (nonhemolytic streptococcus serum 1) agglutinated the nonhemolytic streptococcus suspension in 1:2560 serum dilution, but it did not agglutinate the hemolytic streptococcus suspension at all; the opsonic index to the nonhemolytic streptococcus was 3.5 and to the hemolytic streptococcus 3; in spite of the high agglutinating titer of this serum, the complement-fixation antibodies were low, + with the nonhemolytic streptococcus antigen, and negative with the hemolytic streptococcus antigen.

TABLE 1

Table of Serologic Reactions

Immune Serums	Agglutinin		Opsonic Index		Complement Fixation	
Hemolytic Streptococcus	Hemolytic Streptococcus Suspension	Nonhemolytic Streptococcus Suspension	Hemolytic Streptococcus Suspension	Nonhemolytic Streptococcus Suspension	Hemolytic Streptococcus Antigen	Nonhemolytic Streptococcus Antigen
1	640	80	2.5	3.5	+++	0
2	40	20	1.5	1.0	+	+
2A	1.280	160	4.0	1.0	++++	+
3	640	160	3.2	2.0	++	0
3A	1,280	1,280	...	...	++++*	++++*
Nonhemolytic Streptococcus						
1	0	2,560	3.0	3.5	0	++
2	10	2,560	4.0	2.0	+	++++
2A	160	2,560	4.0	2.0	+	++
3	40	640	2.0	1.0	0	+
3A	1,280	1,280	...	...	++++*	++++*

* Anticomplementary.

Two more rabbits were immunized during the spring of 1920. The hemolytic streptococcus serum was very low in antibody content; since it was impossible to raise the titer at this time, the rabbit was bled. The results of the tests with this serum (hemolytic streptococcus serum 2) were as follows: agglutination with hemolytic streptococcus suspension, 1:40, with nonhemolytic streptococcus suspension 1:20; opsonic index to hemolytic streptococcus, 1.5 and to nonhemolytic streptococcus, 1; complement-fixation was + with both antigens. It was thought that the antibody producing organs might have been overstimulated, and the rabbit was permitted to rest for about 3 months, and then it again received immunizing doses of hemolytic streptococci. A very good immune serum (hemolytic streptococcus serum 2A) resulted. Its agglutinin titer for hemolytic streptococcus was 1:1,280, for nonhemolytic streptococcus, 1:160; the opsonic index to hemolytic streptococcus was 4, and to nonhemolytic streptococcus, 1; it gave ++++ complement fixation with hemolytic streptococcus antigen, and only + with nonhemolytic streptococcus antigen. The immune serum of the second nonhemolytic streptococcus rabbit (nonhemolytic streptococcus serum 2) was as follows: Agglutination with the homologous suspension was 1:2,560, with the heterologous suspension, 1:10; the opsonic index to the nonhemolytic streptococcus was 2, and to the hemolytic streptococcus, 4; the complement-fixation with the homologous antigen was ++++, and with the heterologous antigen +. The second nonhemolytic streptococcus rabbit was also given a resting period of 3 months. There was a considerable drop in antibody content when this time had elapsed. The antibody content, after further immunization (nonhemolytic streptococcus serum 2A) was quite similar to that following the first immunization. Agglutination tests were less specific, since it now agglutinated hemolytic streptococcus bacteria in 1 : 160; the opsonic indexes were the same; the complement-fixation tests with the homologous antigen gave + + instead of + + + + fixation.

In 1921, two more rabbits were immunized with the strains (hemolytic streptococcus serum 3 and nonhemolytic streptococcus serum 3). The results were similar to those of the previous years, but the antibody content of both serums was so low that they were further immunized (hemolytic streptococcus serum 3A and nonhemolytic streptococcus serum 3A). After 3 weeks the serums became absolutely nonspecific. The agglutinin titer for all was 1 : 1,280. When the serums were used in the usual amounts all were anticomplementary in the complement-fixation tests, but when the serums were highly diluted, all gave + + + + fixation. Blood was taken several times at 2-day intervals from these rabbits, and the tests were repeated with the same results.

In the summer of 1921, the immune serums, which had been used in the tabulated tests and had been stored in the icebox, were again inactivated, and the tests were all repeated at the same time. The results were almost identical with those obtained from the former tests, an observation also made by Dochez, Avery, and Lancefield.[5]

There was no change in the morphology of the two streptococci during the two years in which they were under observation. At the end of the two years, the hemolytic streptococcus still produced hemolytic colonies on the blood-agar plates, and the nonhemolytic streptococcus still produced green colonies. This is contrary to the observations of Kuszynski and Wolf,[7] that freshly isolated nonhemolytic streptococcus cultivated on blood-agar plates yields hemolytic colonies in every generation until finally the nonhemolytic colonies are of such low vitality that they die out readily. The constancy of the hemolytic variety, noted by Dochez, Avery and Lancefield,[5] Kuszynski and Wolf,[7] Clawson [8] and others, has been widely accepted, although Rosenow [9] was able to transform a number of hemolytic strains into the viridans variety and to bring about the reverse change in strains which were nonhemolytic on isolation. This question has recently

[7] Ztschr. f. Hyg. u. Infektionskr., 1921, 92, p. 119.
[8] Jour. Infect. Dis., 1920, 26, p. 93.
[9] Ibid., 1914, 14, p. 1.

been investigated by Schnitzer and Munter,[10] who claim to have seen the development of green colonies from hemolytic strains in cultures and to have been able to cause such a change much more readily in the animal body. They interpret the loss of the hemolytic property as an evidence of decrease in virulence, those individuals of an inoculated suspension which are least resistant to the protective mechanisms of the host growing out as green, nonhemolytic colonies when subcultivated. In the hemolytic streptococcus from the heart valve, the development of green colonies was never observed, either in repeated platings or in the mouse inoculations which proved the rapid loss of virulence. The sugar fermentations of each strain remained constant throughout the two years.

Serologically, the two strains could be differentiated fairly well by the agglutination and complement-fixation tests. The opsonic tests, contrary to the results of Tunnicliff,[11] who worked with immune hemolytic streptococcus sheep serum, were less specific, since 3 of the 4 hemolytic streptococcus antiserums had higher opsonic indexes to the nonhemolytic streptococcus suspension than to the hemolytic streptococcus bacteria, and only 1 of the nonhemolytic streptococcus antiserums had a higher index to nonhemolytic streptococcus than to hemolytic streptococcus.

The cultural, agglutination and complement-fixation reactions indicate that the two organisms, supposedly distinct before their entrance into the body, maintained their original differences after a period of parasitism in the same host and did not themselves react to the host by biologic changes which might have resulted in similarity of reactions. The two strains could not be differentiated by their opsonin reactions. Whether this means that in this particular instance the phagocytic reaction is a less delicate one than the others, or that, as a result of growth in the same host, mammalian leukocytes are equally stimulated by antiserums against the two organisms, it is impossible to decide. Taking into consideration the serologic tests made with the immune serums from the two strains, the hemolytic streptococcus is a more specific and fixed strain, a conclusion agreeing with the observations of Clawson,[8] Dochez, Avery and Lancefield,[5] Howell[4] and others. If the splitting off of hemolytic variants from Streptococcus viridans occurs, as claimed by Kuszynski and Wolf,[7] one would expect it to occur in the nonhemolytic organism studied, since this strain might originally

[10] Ztschr. f. Hyg. u. Infektionskr., 1921, 93, p. 96.

[11] Jour. Am. Med. Assn., 1920, 75, p. 1339.

have been a variant of the hemolytic strain and might in later cultivation have given rise to hemolytic descendents. No hemolytic colonies ever developed from the viridans strain on frequent replatings during the course of 2 years. The reverse change, the development of nonhemolytic colonies from the hemolytic strain as reported by Schnitzer and Munter,[10] was also not observed.

The hemolytic streptococcus and the nonhemolytic streptococcus isolated from the same diseased heart valve differed in virulence when first isolated. At that time, and persistently for 2 years, they have differed in a constant manner morphologically, culturally, and to a lesser degree serologically. The virulence of each strain was rapidly lost under artificial cultivation.

SUMMARY

From the same aortic lesion in a case of chronic vegetative valvular endocarditis, two strains of streptococci were isolated.

One was a typical Streptococcus hemolyticus, the other a typical Streptococcus viridans. On the basis of sugar reactions the hemolytic organism was Streptococcus pyogenes, the nonhemolytic strain Streptococcus salivarius.

The two strains differed not only in their reactions on blood and sugar mediums, but also in their serologic reactions. A parasitic existence in the same lesion had not acted in such a manner as to tend toward similarity of biologic properties.

The characters of each organism and the differences between the two have remained fixed and constant through a period of 2 years of artificial cultivation.

When first isolated the hemolytic streptococcus was much more highly virulent than the other strain and it had the unusual property of agglutinating rather than hemolyzing red blood corpuscles when grown in fluid mediums. The latter property and the virulence were both lost under cultivation.

The viridans strain studied over a period of 2 years offers no support to the view of Kuszynski and Wolf that Streptococcus viridans gives rise to hemolytic descendents in each successive replating, or to the view of Schnitzer and Munter that viridans colonies may develop from the hemolytic variety as the virulence of the latter decreases.

THE EFFECT OF DIGITALIS IN TWO CASES OF ARRHYTHMIA IN DIPHTHERIA

V. Bie and Carl Schwensen

From Blegdams Hospital, Copenhagen

In a recent paper one of us (Schwensen[1]) has shown that a complex disturbance of the rhythm of the heart often is present in the cases that are fatal in the acute stage of diphtheria. The possibility of this abnormal rhythm being the result of attacks of auricular flutter was discussed. If this determination of the type of the irregularity is correct there should be a chance of checking this disturbance by treating the patients with full doses of digitalis. We have had the opportunity of trying this treatment in the following two cases:

Case 1.—A 6 year old girl admitted on the 4th day of illness on Oct. 11, 1920, and discharged Jan. 13, 1921, was suffering from grave diphtheria, membrane covering the tonsils, the uvula and the soft palate. In all 184,000 units of diphtheria antitoxin (8,000 units intravenously) were administered in the first 3 days in hospital.

Examination of the heart on Oct. 12 was negative with the exception of a faint systolic blowing which was heard over the whole precordial area. The liver did not extend below the costal margin in the nipple line.

The urine was examined every 3rd day and showed traces of albumin between Oct. 15 and Nov. 5.

On Oct. 19 she became pale and slightly cyanotic. Examination of the heart revealed considerable dilatation on the right side, the right border extending to the right parasternal line. The sounds were indistinct and muffled. The liver extended 3 cm. below the costal margin in the nipple line.

She was very restless. The extremities and face were cold. She talked with pronounced snuffle. The veins of the neck were much distended and pulsated much. The liver now reached the umbilical line, and was very tender on palpation. The heart beat was now felt 2 cm. to the left of the left nipple line in the 5th intercostal space. The right border extended beyond the right parasternal line. The first sound was faint and muffled at the apex, the second pulmonary sound was strongly accentuated. The rhythm was quite irregular. She was very pale and cyanotic.

On Oct. 21 the liver reached 2 cm. below the umbilical line; the veins of the neck still pulsated strongly. Examination of the heart gave the same results as on the preceding day. Tracings obtained are shown in charts 1 and 2. The blood pressure was 70. Digisolvin[2] was given three times (at 1 p. m., 6 p. m., and 11 p. m.), in doses of 1 c c.

Received for publication, August 29, 1921.

[1] Jour. Infect. Dis., 1922, 30, p. 279.

[2] Digisolvin is a physiologically standardized Danish preparation of digitalis; 1 c c corresponds to 15 centigram of fol. titrat.

On Oct. 22 she had improved slightly. The heart beat was now only 1 cm. beyond the nipple line, and the right border extended only 1 cm. beyond the right sternal margin. The liver did not quite reach the umbilical line. The rhythm of the heart was occasionally irregular; the tracings were still like those in fig. 2. At 5 p. m. the character of the tracings was still unaltered. The veins were much distended and pulsated strongly.

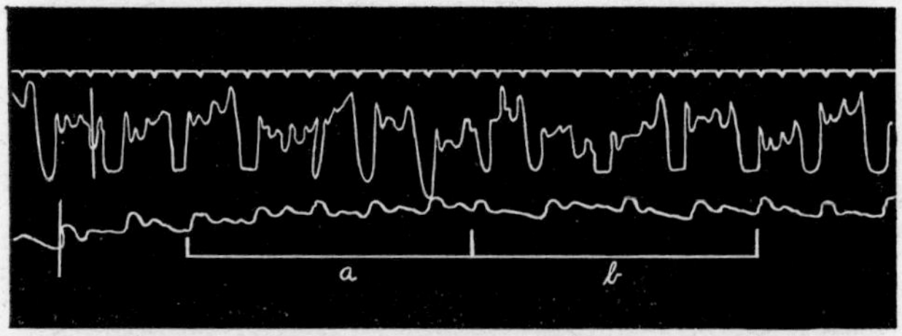

Chart 1, Case 1.—The radial pulse is irregular but with spacing. (These tracings were made with a Jacquet's polygraph. The time marking always corresponds to 1/5". The upper curve is always the jugular, the lower the radial.)

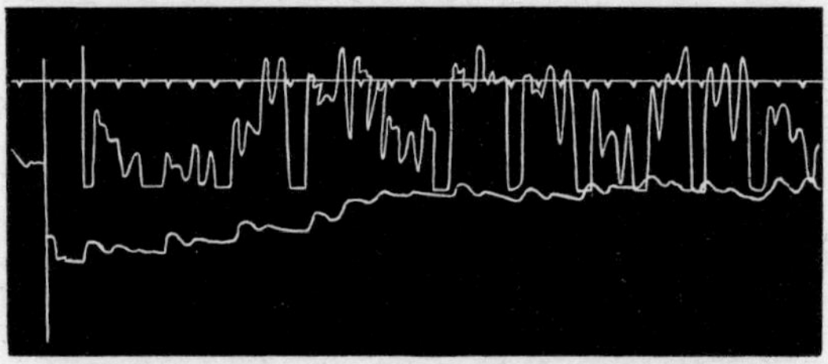

Chart 2, Case 1.—Very big waves in the jugular tracing.

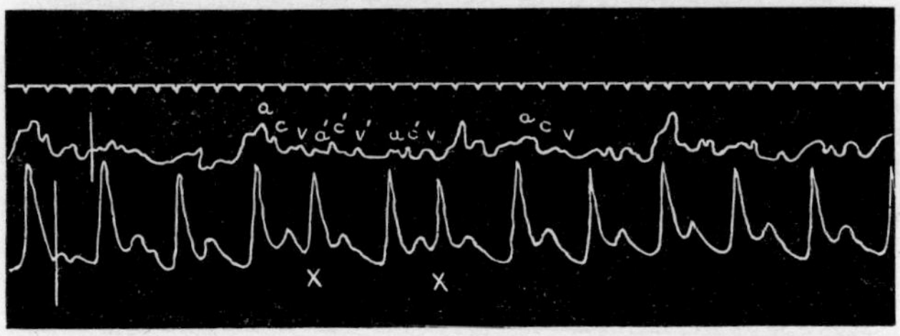

Chart 3, Case 1.—The jugular curve is now normal, the big waves have entirely disappeared. Two extrasystoles of auricular origin are seen in this chart.

On Oct. 23, the liver extended only 3 cm. beyond the costal margin. The veins of the neck were not distended and pulsated slightly. The color of her face was normal. The child was lively. Examination of the heart showed the same features as on the preceding day, only the rhythm was regular but for an occasional extrasystole (fig. 3). The blood pressure was 100.

In the following days the liver diminished and after Oct. 30 it did not reach below the costal margin. Extrasystoles were present until Nov. 17. When discharged she had a muscular mitral inefficiency (the right border did not pass beyond the border of the sternum, and the heart beat was felt inside the nipple line. Over the whole precordial area a harsh systolic murmur was heard).

CASE 2.—A 10 year old girl admitted on the 3rd day of illness, Dec. 13, 1920, died Dec. 20, 1920. She was suffering from grave diphtheria, the membrane covering the tonsils, the uvula and the soft palate, reaching the gums. In the first 3 days of the stay in hospital 340,000 units of diphtheria antitoxin were administered. The membranes diminished slowly but had not entirely disappeared on the day of death. Examinations of the heart showed that it was normal except for faint and muffled sounds until the evening of Dec. 16, when there was a great disturbance of the rhythm (fig. 4 and 5). One c c of digisolvin was then given 4 times (at 6 p. m., 10 p. m., 2 a. m., and 6 a. m.). On the following morning (Dec. 17) the tracings were normal but for an occasional ventricular extrasystole (fig. 6). The heart was normal but for muffled and faint sounds. The liver extended only 1 cm. below the costal margin. The next day (Dec. 18) the tracings showed respiratory arrhythmia. The urine contained a trace of albumin.

The following morning the liver did not extend below the costal margin. Examination of the heart showed that the heart beat was inside the nipple line. Furthermore, there was again a disturbance of the rhythm and tracings showed partial heart block. The rate was only 56. The veins of the neck were only slightly distended. At 4 p. m. the liver extended 2 cm. below the costal margin. The veins of the neck were considerably distended and pulsating. Tracings still showed partial heart block with a ventricular rate of about 50. Sometimes there were long intervals between the beats of the ventricle (the longest measured 2″). The rhythm was very irregular. The heart beat was now felt 1 cm. beyond the nipple line. The right border did not extend outside the right sternal border. As the case, according to our experience, was desperate, we administered digisolvin (1 c c) at 5 p. m. and 1 a. m. with the intention of either producing a complete heart block or of making the degree of heart block more stationary and in this way improving the circulation. At 8 p. m. she looked very ill; she was pale, cyanotic and cold. The veins of the neck were very much distended and pulsating visibly. There had not been any syncopal attacks. The liver now extended to the umbilical line. In examining the heart a pronounced dilatation was found, the right border extending to the right parasternal line; the heart beat was felt 3 cm. outside the left nipple line. The sounds were muffled, nearly inaudible. The rhythm was very irregular (fig. 7), the longest pause being more than 3″. At 11 p. m.: During the last two hours she had suffered much from pains in the right side of the abdomen. She was cold as ice and very pale with a pronounced cyanosis. The veins of the neck were unchanged. The liver extended 2 cm. below the umbilical line. The heart was in the same condition as at 8 o'clock. The rhythm was very irregular but of the same type as in fig. 7. She died at 4 in the morning.

In the 10 cases of a complex arrhythmia occurring during the first 2 weeks of the illness, which one of us [1] described, all the patients died in the course of a few hours or a few days after this irregularity had set in; the irregularity remained always of the same type until death.

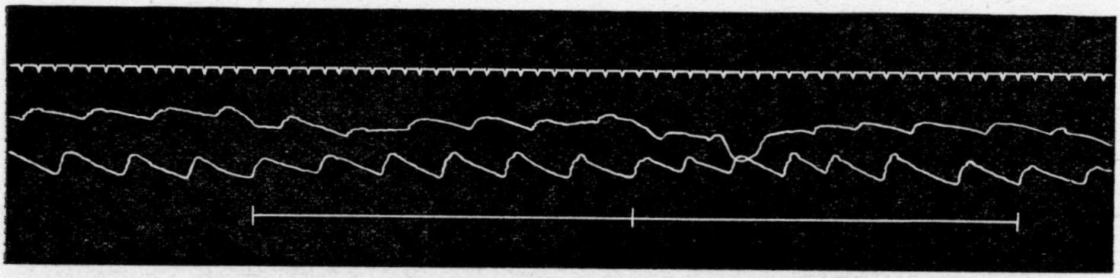

Chart 4, Case 2.—The radial curve shows irregularity with spacing.

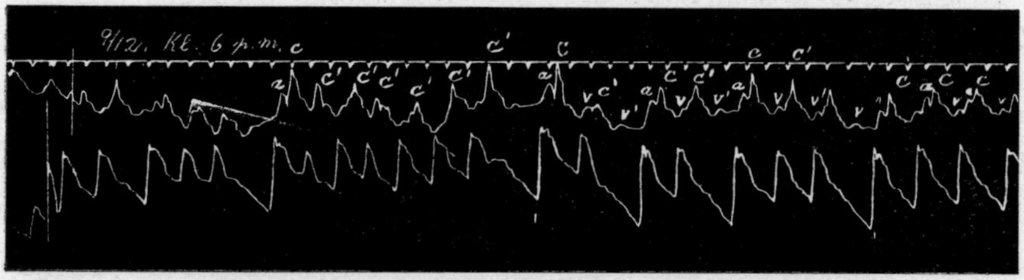

Chart 5, Case 2.—The radial curve shows attacks of regular tachycardia with a rate of about 118 per minute. This shows that the irregularity cannot be that of respiratory arrhythmia.

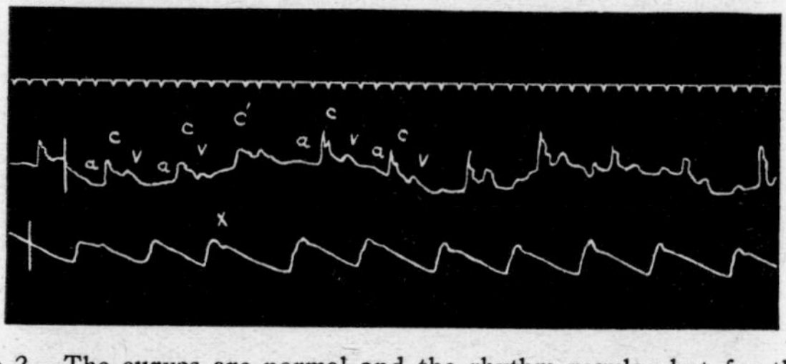

Chart 6, Case 2.—The curves are normal and the rhythm regular but for the occurrence of a **ventricular extrasystole.**

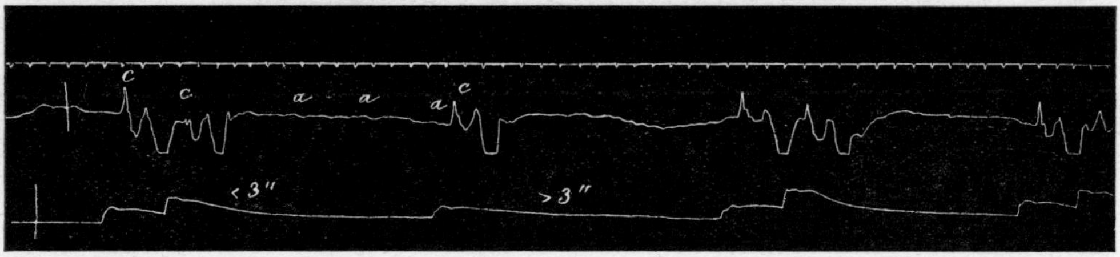

Chart 7, Case 2.—This tracing shows that the ventricle at times does not correspond to the auricle for long intervals, the longest interval being a little more than 3″.

In our two cases this irregularity set in at the usual time and was exactly of the same type as those of Schwensen.

After we had administered digitalis the arrhythmia stopped, and the tracings became normal with the exception of some extrasystoles. In the one case the child afterward recovered, in the second, death intervened a few days after as a result of the progressive acute myocarditis which attacked the atrioventricular bundle and produced partial heartblock.

The patient in our case 1 is the only one in our experience who has recovered after an attack of the complex irregularity in the acute stage of the diphtheria, and our observations are quite in accordance with those of other clinicians, who all agree that a severe irregularity in the acute stage of diphtheria in children means death in a few days.

The disappearance of this complex irregularity as a result of treatment with digitalis points to the correctness of the supposition that flutter is the cause of this irregularity.

Our two cases make it probable that in the treatment of these otherwise fatal cases with digitalis in full doses we may have a chance of curing the patient by saving the damaged myocardium from the great exertion caused by the irregularity.

Furthermore, these cases show how the greater degrees of enlargement of the liver are dependent on the disturbances of the rhythm. In case 1 the enlargement of the liver disappeared simultaneously with the disappearance of the complex arrhythmia; in case 2 the liver became very much enlarged simultaneously with the appearance of the irregular partial heartblock.

STUDIES ON COMPLEMENT FIXATION

V. THE HEMOLYTIC VERSUS FIXABILITY POWERS OF COMPLEMENT

R. L. Kahn and Ethel D. White

From the Bureau of Laboratories, Michigan Department of Health, Lansing, Mich.

INTRODUCTION

There is perhaps no element in the complement-fixation phenomenon worthy of more careful investigation than the relation between the hemolytic and fixability properties of complement. The universal employment in fixability tests of measured amounts of complement based on hemolytic potency assumes not only a qualitative relation between these two properties but a quantitative relation as well. And yet it is becoming more and more emphasized that complement of good hemolytic titer may lack the power of being "fixed" by antigen-antibody complexes. The recent studies of Wilson,[1] Ruediger,[2] Kolmer and co-workers [3] appear to lend fresh support to this view. Furthermore, according to the latter, the testing of the fixability of complement before its employment in the tests, as suggested by some workers, would appear to be of little value, as their results indicate that "a complement may be fixed by one syphilitic serum and not by another."

On the other hand, when one considers the numerous pitfalls associated with fixability tests, one is inclined to believe that the so-called nonfixability of some complement may not be due to the nature of the complement but rather to a combination of factors entering into the tests. To enumerate some of these pitfalls, we have, first, the amount of complement used. Thus a complement of good hemolytic potency used in 1:5, 1:10 or 1:20 dilutions, in nontitrated amounts, may frequently represent more than a given serum and antigen are capable of binding. And, if the amount of complement left unbound is large enough hemolysis would result and that serum would pass as negative. The titration of complement and its use, let us say, in 2 unit quantities in the tests, does not exclude the possibility of unintentionally using an excess of this ingredient, in some cases. Identical complement titrations

Received for publication Oct. 24, 1921.

[1] Jour. Immunol., 1918, 3, p. 346.
[2] Jour. Infect. Dis., 1919, 24, p. 120.
[3] Jour. Syph., 1919, 3, p. 407. This paper gives a résumé of the literature.

carried out by 2 workers sometimes vary in their results to the extent of 25% or more. When one considers the liberal amount of hemolysin commonly employed after the fixation period, we can again see why occasionally some positive serums may give the appearance of being weak or even negative.

Furthermore, the mode of fixation plays an important rôle when testing the fixability powers of a given serum and antigen. One of us has shown [4] that the rate of fixation of complement is directly proportional to the concentration of antibodies in the immune serum. A serum of high concentration will fix a considerable amount of complement immediately on mixing the ingredients, while one of low concentration will frequently fix no more than 50% of complement after an incubation period of one hour in the water bath. It is conceivable, therefore, when testing the fixability of complement with a number of syphilitic serums, that those which just approach + + + +, would be weakly positive or negative when a fixation period of one hour in the water bath is employed.

In so far as the complement fixation test in syphilis is concerned, the type of antigen employed also appears to play an important rôle when testing the fixing powers of some positive serums. When studying the potency of different Wassermann antigens, we have observed again and again that a Noguchi antigen will give a negative result with a syphilitic serum which is positive with alcoholic extract and cholesterinized antigens.

Finally, the false negative results frequently caused by the presence of natural hemolysin in human serum, and to a lesser degree in guinea-pig serum, might also incorrectly be interpreted as being due to the nonfixability of complement.

These considerations led us to investigate the relation between hemolysis and fixation of complement. More specifically, our aim was first to find some good hemolytic complement lacking fixability, and, second, to investigate the underlying cause for its nonfixability. These studies were limited to syphilitic serums and Wassermann antigens.

EXPERIMENTS

The tests were made with a sheep-cell-guinea-pig-complement system. Every effort was made in the fixability tests to overcome those factors which occasionally lead to false negative reactions. Complement was used in carefully titrated amounts and none was used which con-

[4] Kahn, R. L.: Jour. Exper. Med., 1921, 34, p. 217.

tained considerable amounts of natural hemolysin. The latter was removed from every serum tested by the method proposed by one of us.[5] Fixation was carried out for 4 hours at icebox temperature.[6] Altogether, the hemolytic and fixability powers of 478 guinea-pig complements were tested. A large number (203) of the pigs were rebled from time to time and their hemolytic titer and fixability retested. The total number of separate guinea-pig serums tested was 275.

The plan was to obtain the hemolytic unit of individual complements used in the Wassermann division of these laboratories and subsequently determine their relative fixability powers in the presence of some known syphilitic serum and antigen. Thus, if on a given day pooled complement of 4 guinea-pigs was used for the regular Wassermann tests, each of these complements was titrated for its hemolytic potency as well as for its fixability power. The syphilitic serums were those previously found to be ++++ with pooled complement from 3 to 6 guinea-pigs.

Complement was obtained by bleeding large guinea-pigs under anesthesia directly from the heart and was used after permitting the serum to remain with the clot for about 15 hours in the icebox. A hemolytic unit was taken to be the smallest quantity of complement which, in the presence of 0.1 c c (2 units) of hemolysin, laked 0.1 c c of a 5% sheep cell suspension after 15 minutes incubation in the water bath.

This unit was obtained by making a 1:10 dilution of complement with salt solution and titrating it in the following proportions:

	Tube									
	1	2	3	4	5	6	7	8	9	10
Complement (c c, 1:10).....	0.1	0.09	0.08	0.07	0.06	0.05	0.04	0.03	0.02	0.01
Hemolysin (c c, 2 units)....	0.1	0.1	0.1	0.1	0.1	0.1	0.1	0.1	0.1	0.1
Sheep cells (c c, 5%)........	0.1	0.1	0.1	0.1	0.1	0.1	0.1	0.1	0.1	0.1
Salt sol. (drops)...........	2	2	2	3	3	3	3	4	4	4

The unit was read in each case after 15 minutes' incubation in the water bath, and two units were used in the complement-fixation tests. For the sake of uniformity as well as simplicity in pipetting, the complement in each case was so diluted as to include 2 units in 0.1 c c. Thus, if the unit of complement was 0.04 c c, instead of using 0.08 c c of a 1:10 dilution in the tests, 0.1 c c of a 1:12.5 dilution was employed. The antigen was an alcoholic extract of beef hearts,

[5] Kahn, R. L.: Jour. Lab. & Clin. Med., 1921, 6, p. 218.
[6] Kahn, R. L.: Arch. Dermat. & Syph., 1921, 4, p. 358.

previously freed from ether soluble lipoids. Its mode of preparation is described in another paper.[7] The tests were read in each case after permitting the tubes to remain in the icebox over night.

TABLE 1

Relation Between Hemolytic and Fixability Powers of Complement

Guinea-Pig Complement			Syphilitic Serum, C c						
Laboratory No.	Titration Unit, C c	Dilution Representing 2 Units†	No.	Results of Fixability Tests					
				0.02	0.01	0.005	0.003	0.002	0.001
G-37	0.07	1:7		4*	4	3	1	1	—
E-24	0.04	1:12.5	1	4	4	4	1	—	—
B-19	0.08	1:6		4	4	1	—	—	—
E- 3	0.05	1:10		4	4	4	4	4	1
E-15	0.06	1:8	2	4	4	4	3	1	1
E-23	0.05	1:10		4	4	4	4	4	1
E-21	0.05	1:10		4	4	4	4	4	1
B- 4	0.04	1:12.5	3	4	4	4	4	4	1
E-16	0.05	1:10		4	4	4	4	1	—
E-20	0.04	1:12.5		4	4	4	4	4	1
E-17	0.04	1:12.5	4	4	4	4	4	3	1
E-19	0.04	1:12.5		4	4	4	4	3	1
J- 5	0.04	1:12.5		4	4	4	4	3	1
J-25	0.04	1:12.5	5	4	4	4	4	2	1
[illegible]-11	0.03	1:16.5		4	4	4	4	3	1
E-12	0.03	1:16.5		4	4	4	4	4	2
G-39	0.03	1:16.5	6	4	4	4	4	4	4
E-22	0.03	1:16.5		4	4	4	4	4	4
E- 2	0.04	1:12.5		4	4	4	4	4	4
B-13	0.04	1:12.5	7	4	4	4	4	4	1
A-50	0.03	1:16.5		4	4	4	4	4	4
A-23	0.03	1:16.5		4	4	4	4	2	—
B- 3	0.03	1:16.5	8	4	4	4	4	2	1
A-38	0.03	1:16.5		4	4	4	4	2	—
E- 8	0.04	1:12.5		4	4	4	3	1	—
E- 4	0.03	1:16.5	9	4	4	4	3	1	—
E- 7	0.05	1:10		4	4	4	3	1	—
G-39	0.04	1:12.5		4	4	4	4	2	1
G-38	0.04	1:12.5	10	4	4	4	4	3	1
G-46	0.04	1:12.5		4	4	4	4	2	1
G-22	0.07	1:7		4	4	4	4	3	1

* 4 = ++++; 3 = +++; 2 = ++; 1 = +; — = negative.

† These dilutions were determined accordingly: Titration unit : 0.05 :: (1:10) : (1:X). Thus if 0.04 is the titration unit, 0.04 : 0.05 :: 10 : X, X = 12.5.

Now, if it is true that the phenomena of hemolysis and fixation are closely related, one might expect 2 unit quantities of complement obtained from different guinea-pigs to possess the same fixability powers when used with the same serum. We found this to be largely but not entirely true. Table 1 gives an outline of the first 10 of 120 experiments. These 10 experiments represent 31 different comple-

[7] Kahn, R. L., and Olin, R. M., Jr.: Jour. Infect. Dis., 29, p. 630.

ments and illustrate the variations in fixability of 2 units of complement. It did not seem wise to present all the experiments in tabular form on account of the large space required and particularly because, in a general way, these 10 are representative of the rest of the work.

The chief reason why 2 unit quantities of different complements show varying degrees of fixability when tested with one serum, is undoubtedly that our method for titrating complement is not sufficiently precise; in other words, we believe that the comparatively small fluctuations in fixability of these quantities of complement as indicated in table 1, are due to small variations in the hemolytic potency of so-called 2 units. We hope to test the validity of this belief by developing a method for more precise titrations of complements and quantitatively test their fixability with the same serum.

The experiments in table 1 were continued until Oct. 25. The total number of complements tested to that date was 187—without finding a single one which did not possess fixability properties. Beginning with Oct. 26, these 2 changes in these experiments were made: whenever a given complement possessed a high hemolytic titer, it was used both in 2 unit quantities as well as in 1:10 quantities. Also, the methods of fixation resorted to were both, 1 hour in the water bath as well as 4 hours in the icebox. It was desired to determine whether the nonfixability of some complements reported by different investigators might not be due to brief fixation periods as well as to the employment of average amounts instead of carefully titrated amounts of complement.

Table 2 illustrates to what extent excessive amounts of complement and water-bath fixation will reduce the fixing power of syphilitic serum and antigen. Strongly positive serums did not show this tendency. These serums, as is well known, are capable of absorbing large amounts of complement and are not extensively affected by the mode of fixation. Serums which were approaching + + + +, ranged between + + and negative in practically every case, when 1:10 complement was employed with water-bath fixation.

At the time when these experiments were carried out, the routine Wassermann tests in this laboratory were carried out in duplication employing an alcoholic extract antigen with 4 hours' fixation at icebox temperature and a cholesterized antigen with a half hour fixation at water-bath temperature. Frequently, syphilitic serums were found to be + + + + with the alcoholic antigen and + + + with the cholesterinized antigen. These serums were considered as approaching ++++, and with highly potent complement used 1:10 instead of 2 units, combined with water-bath fixation, were found without exception to be weakly positive or negative.

TABLE 2

EFFECT OF EXCESSIVE AMOUNTS OF COMPLEMENT AND WATER-BATH FIXATION ON THE FIXABILITY POWERS OF FIVE DIFFERENT COMPLEMENTS WITH A FOUR PLUS SYPHILITIC SERUM

Complement No.	Titration Unit, C c	Dilutions of Complement Employed in Fixation Tests (Amount 0.1 C c)	Mode of Fixation	Results of Fixability Tests, C c					
				0.02	0.01	0.005	0.003	0.002	0.001
1	0.035	1:14.5*	4 hours in icebox.....	4†	4	4	1	1	—
		1:10	1 hour in water-bath.	2	1	—	—	—	—
2	0.03	1.16.5*	4 hours in icebox.. .	4	4	4	1	1	—
		1:10	1 hour in water-bath.	2	1	—	—	—	—
3	0.035	1:14.5*	4 hours in icebox.....	4	4	4	1	1	—
		1:10	1 hour in water-bath.	2	1	—	—	—	—
4	0.035	1:14.5*	4 hours in icebox.....	4	4	2	1	—	—
		1:10	1 hour in water-bath.	1	1	—	—	—	—
5	0.03	1:16.5*	4 hours in icebox.....	4	4	2	1	—	—
		1:10	1 hour in water-bath.	1	1	—	—	—	—

* These dilutions represent 2 units of complement.
† 4 = ++++; 3 = +++; 2 =++; 1 = +, and — = negative.

SUMMARY AND CONCLUSIONS

It has become a matter of wide acceptance among complement-fixation workers that no relation exists between the hemolytic and fixability powers of complement; that a given complement may be capable of laking corpuscles in the presence of specific hemolysin and not be capable of being "fixed" by some specific antigen-antibody complexes. This study was made with a view of finding nonfixable complements and determining the underlying cause or causes for their nonfixability. The hemolytic tests were carried out with a sheep-cell-guinea-pig-complement system and the fixability tests, with an alcoholic extract antigen of beef-heart and syphilitic serums. In these studies no complement was used which contained moderate amounts of natural amboceptor. In the fixability tests, the complement was used in carefully titrated 2 unit quantities and fixation was carried out for 4 hours at icebox temperature.

Of 478 guinea-pig complements, representing 275 separate pigs, tested for fixability, not one was found which lacked this property.

On the other hand, it was found when using an average dilution of 1:10 of highly potent complement (instead of 2 units); a 1-hour fixation period in the water-bath (instead of 4 hours in the icebox) and a positive serum which just approaches ++++, that the fixation ranged from ++ to negative in practically every case. In other words, our results indicate that so far as syphilitic serums and Wassermann antigens are concerned, the so-called nonfixability of some complements reported by some investigators may be apparent rather than real, and if all precautions are taken to overcome those factors in complement fixation which may lead to false negative results, that complements which possess hemolytic properties will also be found to be fixable.

THE PRODUCTION OF CO_2 BY THE TYPHOID BACILLUS AND THE MECHANISM OF THE RUSSELL DOUBLE SUGAR TUBE

II. FERMENTATION OR RESPIRATION. PHENOL RED AS AN INDICATOR

WITH PLATE

Henry J. Nichols and Cyrus B. Wood

From the Laboratory Division, Army Medical School, Washington, D. C.

In a previous article,[1] the production of CO_2 by the typhoid bacillus was attributed to fermentation or proteolysis, and in this sense it was stated that "this fact has apparently escaped previous observation." Our attention, however, has been called to the possibility that the CO_2 produced may be respiratory. The production of CO_2 by the typhoid bacillus as due to respiration is an old observation, dating back to Hesse,[2] in 1893. Hesse worked chiefly with glycerol agar. He estimated the O_2 used and CO_2 produced by a volumetric method after absorption with KOH and phosphorus. He tested a number of organisms, including the typhoid bacillus, and found that all use up O_2 and produce CO_2 by "breathing." The production of CO_2 in the case of the typhoid bacillus was most marked in the first three days. He advocated this method for testing the viability of a culture.

According to Gottschlich,[3] this finding was at first questioned, but has been fully confirmed by his own work and that of many others. Recently Novy[4] reached a similar conclusion that all bacteria, yeasts, molds and even protozoa produce CO_2 in their growth. Scheurlen[5] made the point long ago that the term "gas former" should be limited to gas bubble formers, as all organisms are really CO_2 producers. While in all this work it is assumed that CO_2 is respiratory, in the case of the visible gas formers it seems to have been tacitly assumed that the CO_2 is fermentative. Workers with the typhoid bacillus have apparently assumed, without sufficient reason, that the CO_2 of respira-

Received for publication Nov. 7, 1921.

1 Nichols, H. J.: Jour. Infect. Dis., 1921, 29, p. 82.
2 Ztschr. f. Hyg. u. Infectionskr., 1893, 15, p. 17.
3 Kolle u. Wassermann, 1912, 1, p. 99.
4 Personal communication.
5 Internat. Beitrage y. Inn. Med., 1902, 2, p. 205.

tion need not be taken into account in dealing with fermentation reactions.

While there is, therefore, no doubt about the production of CO_2 by the typhoid bacillus, the question of its origin is a difficult one, involving as it does the whole subject of bacterial metabolism. This subject cannot be discussed to much advantage until more is known about the endo- and exo-enzymes of the typhoid bacillus. There are certain suggestions that the CO_2 is fermentative as well as respiratory. Acid production is visible in the butt of a Russell tube a few hours after inoculation and becomes marked after 24 hours, although the evidences of growth are slight. In other words, it seems as if an exo-enzyme were present. More CO_2 is also produced in glucose than in plain mediums, although the growth is not materially different. On the other hand, the changes in a sugar-free Russell tube are the same as those in a regular tube, except in degree. The CO_2 in this case might come from proteolysis, but the fact that growth of the typhoid bacillus on any mediums produces CO_2 argues for an actual respiratory origin of some of the CO_2.

The process, whatever it is, is one in which CO_2 is produced on the slant. It escapes, leaving an accumulation of nonvolatile alkaline products. In the butt the same process occurs, but the CO_2 is retained by the medium and makes it acid. By degrees, however, the alkali from the slant diffuses downward and renders the whole tube alkaline.

As far as fermentation is concerned, formic acid may be taken as a typical example of the result of the first stages of decomposition of glucose. Under the influence of further growth, formic acid is apparently oxidized to H_2O and CO_2. Growth is, of course, favored by aerobic conditions and is more active on the slant than in the butt. Hence, the steps of fermentation are more complete on the slant than in the butt. In this sense the oxygen relations have some effect.

Phenol red has proved to be the best indicator to bring out the mechanism referred to, as it registers both on the acid and alkaline side. A pink phenol red Russell sugar tube, P_H 7.2-7.4, 24 hours after inoculation shows a yellow butt, P_H 6.8 and a red slant, P_H 7.8. In 48 hours the changes are more marked. Finally after a week, the whole tube becomes completely red from above downward. In tubes which are sealed, the butt and also the slant become and remain yellow or acid. The usual Andrade indicator shows the acid butt, but it is defective in showing an apparently unchanged slant. Litmus as an indicator shows the acid butt and also an alkaline slant, but the change is not clear cut. The reactions of phenol red are brilliant and convincing.

PREPARATION OF PHENOL RED RUSSELL DOUBLE SUGAR MEDIUM

Make extract agar (3% shred agar); clear; add 1% lactose and 0.1% glucose and 5% of a 0.02% watery solution of phenol red. Correct reaction to P_H of 7.2-7.4 hot. Tube, sterilize and slant so that there will be a deep butt and a long slant. The final reaction cold will be 7.2-7.4 as the tendency to a more alkaline reaction in cooling is overcome by a slight acidity developed in sterilization.

SUMMARY

The CO_2 produced by the typhoid bacillus in the Russell double sugar tube is probably fermentative as well as respiratory.

Phenol red is the best indicator as it shows both the acid change in the butt and the alkaline change in the slant.

The slant is not unchanged. It becomes alkaline and gradually the alkalis spread down and turn the butt alkaline.

PLATE 1

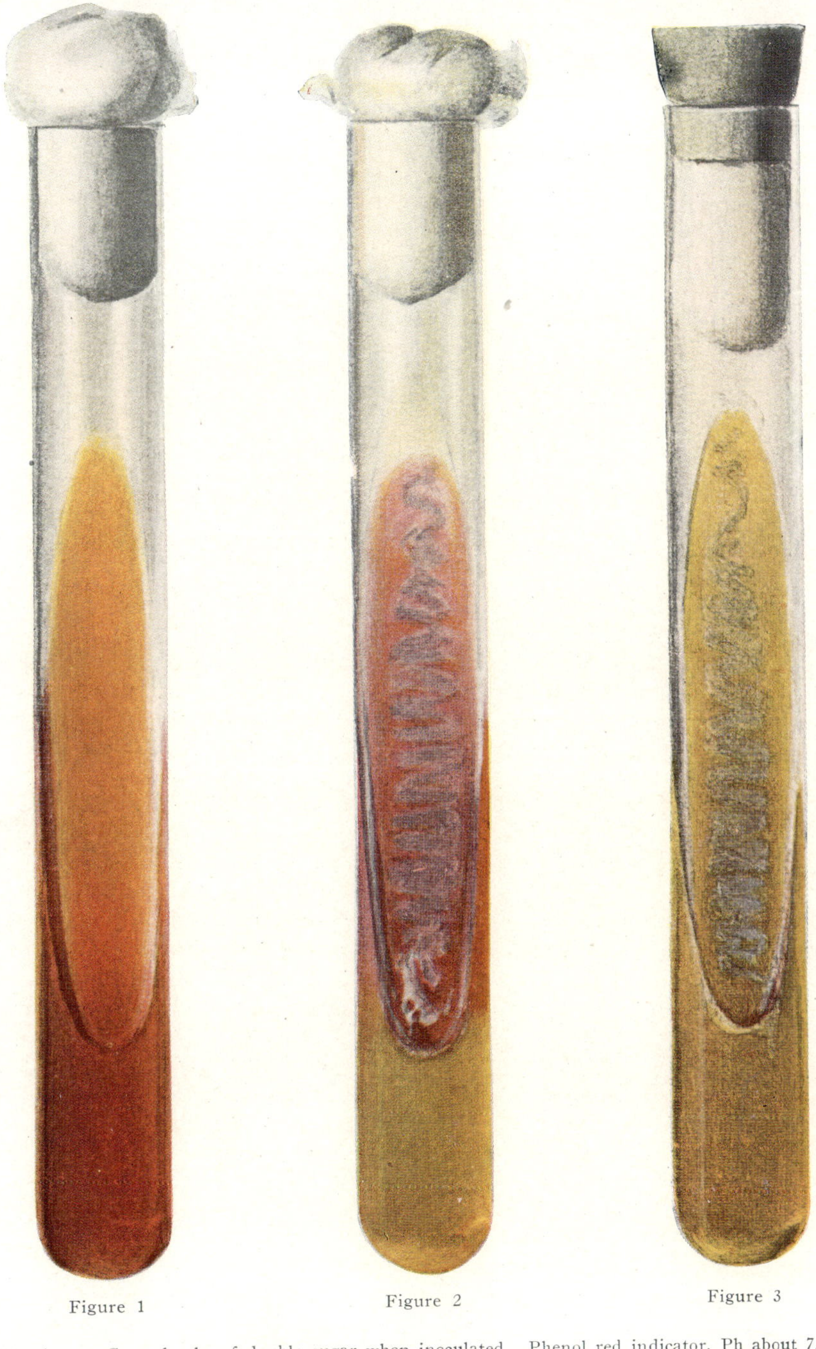

Figure 1 Figure 2 Figure 3

Fig. 1.—Control tube of double sugar when inoculated. Phenol red indicator, Ph about 7.4.

Fig. 2.—Double sugar tube inoculated with typhoid bacillus, "Rawlings" strain, after 48 hours. Ph. of butt, 6.6; Ph of slant, 7.8.

Fig. 3.—Double sugar tube inoculated with typhoid bacillus, "Rawlings" strain, 24 hours after inoculation with tube stoppered. Butt and slant have a Ph of 6.6.

EFFECTS OF PNEUMOCOCCUS TYPE I ON LEUKOCYTES AND HEMOPOIETIC ORGANS

M. S. Tongs

From the John McCormick Institute for Infectious Diseases, Chicago

THE EFFECT OF PNEUMOCOCCUS TYPE 1 ON THE BLOOD AND HEMOPOIETIC ORGANS OF RABBITS

The blood changes in croupous pneumonia have been much discussed and the occurrence of leukopenia in certain fatal cases has made it doubtful whether negative chemotaxis is the cause of leukopenia in general. Careful study of the blood and hemopoietic organs, which might give fuller information concerning the leukocytic reaction in pneumococcus and other infections, seems indicated.

Halla,[1] Kikodse,[2] and Jaksch[3] all thought that leukopenia in croupous pneumonia is a bad prognostic sign. Cabot[4] reported 6 cases of pneumonia with leukopenia and one case with leukopenia at the beginning and a progressive leukocytosis toward the end of disease, but he does not believe that there is any relation between the number of leukocytes and the severity of disease. According to Ewing,[5] a well marked leukocytosis indicates a severe infection and a leukopenia a bad prognosis. Arneth[6] states that leukopenia with a relative lymphocytosis means in general a severe infection and a doubtful, but not an absolutely bad, prognosis. Williamson[7] calls attention to the fact that a pneumococcus septicemia is usually associated with leukopenia. Rieder[8] found leukopenia with a marked relative increase in the number of polymorphonuclear neutrophils in fatal cases of lobar pneumonia. Limbeck[9] asserts that a fatal case of pneumonia is usually marked by a progressive leukocytosis. Tschistovitch[10] points out the significance of leukopenia by demonstrating experimentally that rabbits inoculated with virulent pneumococci usually die with leukopenia, but in animals inoculated with nonvirulent pneumococcus there is a leukocytosis. Billings[11] states that patients with fatal cases of pneumonia may or may not have leukocytosis, and that a continuous absence of leukocytosis indicates an unfavorable prognosis and high virulence of the pneumococcus.

Received for publication Oct. 10, 1921.

1 Ztschr. f. Heilk., 1883, 4, p. 198.
2 Path. Anat. d. Blut. b. Croup Lungenentzündung, Inaug. Diss., 1890.
3 Centralbl. f. klin. Med., 1892, 13, p. 81.
4 Bost. Med. & Surg. Jour., 1894, 130, p. 277.
5 N. Y. Med. Jour., 1893, 58, p. 715.
6 Die Neutrophilon weissen Blutkörporchen, 1904.
7 Zeigler's Beiträge, 1901, 29, p. 41.
8 Beiträge z. Kennt. d. Leukocytose, 1892.
9 Grundriss z. klin. Path. d. Blutes, Jena, 1892.
10 Ann. d. l'Inst. Pasteur, 1891, 5, p. 450.
11 Bull. Johns Hopkins Hosp., 1894, 5, p. 105.

Lambert and Samuels [12] studied the relations between the leukocytes and marrow changes in acute lobar pneumonia, and they found that in some cases there was a parallelism in the number of leukocytes and the degree of the hyperplasia of marrow, in others there was an aplastic marrow with leukocytes well above normal, and in still others there was leukopenia with a hyperplastic marrow. They explain leukocytosis with an aplastic marrow on the basis that there may be a hyperplasia in the bones that may be overlooked and a development of leukocytes in the spleen; but they could not see why there should be a leukopenia with a hyperplastic marrow. Dickson [13] found degenerative changes in the marrow of rabbits with virulent pneumococcus infection. In experimental pneumonia, Welch [14] noted that the changes in spleen and lymph nodes were somewhat dependent on the virulence of the pneumococcus, the virulent strain usually giving rise to deposits of fibrin, hemorrhage, and karyorrhexis and the nonvirulent pneumococcus to a little change or none at all.

In the experiments now reported rabbits were inoculated intravenously or intratracheally with virulent or nonvirulent pneumococcus of type I in 24 hour dextrose-broth cultures. One series of rabbits was inoculated with the filtrate of a very virulent pneumococcus culture, after being passed through a Massen filter.

The tables serve to illustrate the general results of the observations on the leukocytic reaction.

TABLE 1
EXPER. 1, RABBIT A

	Total Number of Leuko-cytes	Percentage of							
		Ampho-phils	Baso-phils	Eosino-phils	Lympho-cytes	Large Mono-nuclears	Transi-tionals	Myelo-cytes	Degen-erate Leuko-cytes
Before inoculation	8,450	52	4	0	44	0	0	0	0
Days after									
1........	9,200	50	4	0	42.6	3.4	0	0	0
2........	12,225	57	4	0	24	9.6	5.4	0	0
3........	14,475	60.2	2	0	32.2	5.6	0	0	0
4........	21,250	68.2	3	0	21.6	2.2	5	0	0
5........	22,850	72.4	3	0	20	0.6	4	0	0
6........	28,050	69	0.5	0	20.5	4	6	0	0
7........	27,800	66.2	2	0	12.4	9.4	10	0	0
8........	25,650	75.4	2	0	10	6	6.6	0	0
9........	22,725	64.2	1	0	16.8	6	12	0	0

Exper. 1.—Rabbits A and B received intratracheally 2 c c of pneumococcus strain of such virulence that about 0.2 c c of 24-hour broth culture were fatal to a mouse within 4 days. The animals died with marked leukocytosis.

[12] Jour. Infect. Dis., 1918, 23, p. 443.
[13] The Bone-Marrow, 1908.
[14] Bull. Johns Hopkins Hosp., 1892, 3, p. 125.

TABLE 2

EXPER. 1, RABBIT B

	Total Number of Leuko-cytes	Percentage of							
		Ampho-phils	Baso-phils	Eosino-phils	Lympho-cytes	Large Mono-nuclears	Transi-tionals	Myelo-cytes	Degen-erate Leuko-cytes
Before in-oculation	15,625	35.5	3.5	0.5	60	0.5	0	0	0
Days after									
1........	40,725	84.4	0	0	11	0	4.6	0	0
2........	28,025	74.2	1	0	13	4	7.8	0	0
3........	28,375	80.4	2.4	0	10	3.2	4	0	0
4........	21,275	76	3	0	14	2.4	4.6	0	0
5........	22,705	79.6	2.2	0.2	10.2	2	7.8	0	12†
6........	18,700	81.2	0	0	8	4	6.8	0	19.5†

† The granules of amphophils appeared brownish and irregular in size.

Exper. 2.—Rabbit B received intravenously 1 c c of virulent pneumococcus, about 0.01 c c being fatal to a mouse within 24 hours. The animal had a leukocytosis about 24 hours after inoculation but died with leukopenia.

TABLE 3

EXPER. 2, RABBIT B

	Total Number of Leuko-cytes	Percentage of							
		Ampho-phils	Baso-phils	Eosino-phils	Lympho-cytes	Large Mono-nuclears	Transi-tionals	Myelo-cytes	Degen-erate Leuko-cytes
Before in-oculation	13,750	45.4	5.2	0	49.4	0	0	0	0
Hrs. after									
4........	8,350	72.2	4.4	0	16	3.4	4	0	0
24........	18,750	46	5.4	0	40	5	3.6	0	19
48........	6,800	49	3.2	0	40	4.8	3	0	23
52........	4,175	35.4	5	0	45.2	4.4	7	3	22

Exper. 3.—Rabbit A received intravenously 1 c c virulent pneumococcus, about 0.001 c c being fatal to a mouse within 48 hours. The animal died within 48 hours.

TABLE 4

EXPER. 3, RABBIT A

	Total Number of Leuko-cytes	Percentage of							
		Ampho-phils	Baso-phils	Eosino-phils	Lympho-cytes	Large Mono-nuclears	Transi-tionals	Myelo-cytes	Degen-erate Leuko-cytes
Before in-oculation	9,025	31	0.5	0	67.5	1	0	0	0
Hrs. after									
24.......	4,450	48.4	3.2	0	36.4	3	9	0	12
30.......	2,250	51	4	0	34.4	3.6	7	0	All degen-erated

Exper. 4.—A series of 3 rabbits received intravenously 3 c c of the cultural filtrate of virulent pneumococcus used in exper. 3. Another rabbit used as control was also inoculated with 3 c c of sterile dextrose-broth. The number of leukocytes was counted every 2 hours within first 8 hours and thereafter every 24 hours for 3 days.

TABLE 5

RESULTS OF EXPER. 4

	Rabbit C	Control Rabbit
Before inoculation	12,450	11,250
2 hours after	8,625	11,450
4 hours after	7,945	9,500
6 hours after	4,500	9,425
8 hours after	3,250	8,225
24 hours after	5,425	10,550
48 hours after	14,500	19,250
72 hours after	12,945	15,500

Exper. 5.—By the smear method I tested the toxic action of a virulent pneumococcus on human leukocytes in vitro. The leukocytic suspension was mixed with various amounts of culture or culture filtrate of the virulent pneumococcus, and the mixtures thus made were then incubated at 37 C. and examined every 15 minutes. The smears were stained with Wright's stain. Table 6 shows the results.

TABLE 6

RESULTS OF EXPER. 5

Leukocytes, C c	Cultural Filtrate, C c	Salt Solution, C c	Results		
			15 Minutes	30 Minutes	45 Minutes
0.1	0.1	0.8	+	+	+
0.1	0.075	0.825	0	+	+
0.1	0.05	0.85	0	±	+
0.1	0.025	0.875	0	0	0
0.1	0.01	0.89	0	0	0
0.1	0.0075	0.8925	0	0	0
0.1	0	0.9	0	0	0
Leukocytes, C c	**Pneumococcus Culture, C c**	**Salt Solution, C c**	**Results**		
			15 Minutes	30 Minutes	45 Minutes
0.1	0.1	0.8	+	+	+
0.1	0.075	0.825	+	+	+
0.1	0.05	0.85	+	+	+
0.1	0.025	0.875	0	+	+
0.1	0.01	0.89	0	+	+
0.1	0.0075	0.8925	0	0	0
0.1	0	0.9	0	0	0

+ = a definite degeneration of leukocytes; ± = doubtful; 0 = negative.

In view of the foregoing results, it is evident that virulence of the pneumococcus has a direct bearing on the leukocytic reaction, a low virulence producing leukocytosis and a high virulence leukopenia. This seems to be in perfect accord with the observations of Tschistovitch and Billings, but it does not explain why there should be leukopenia in animals infected with a virulent pneumococcus. Bieganski [15] contended that the leukopenia in croupous pneumonia is brought about by the destruction of leukocytes caused by toxic substances produced by the pneumococcus. The filtrate of the very virulent pneumococcus tested in exper. 4 produced an initial leukopenia far more marked than in the control animals injected with broth. This gives rise to an assumption that the leukopenia in exper. 4 as well as in others might be in part due to the destruction of leukocytes caused by the toxic action of the pneumococcus. This is substantiated by the fact that the same filtrate produced a definite degeneration of human leukocytes in vitro. The differential count revealed that the reduction in the number of leukocytes involved a decided gain in the transitional and large mononuclear leukocytes, but the amphophils in the stage of leukopenia showed only a slight deviation from their normal percentage. In no instance were the eosinophils found increased in number.

The morphologic changes of individual cells in the peripheral circulation varied greatly, but in general the changes were practically the same as I have described in the cases of hemolytic streptococcus [16] and diphtheria toxin.[17] However, it should be borne out that the karyorrhexis observed in this study was usually followed by a pyknosis as the nuclear fragments were often seen as black globular bodies of various sizes, and that in the later stages of infection, even with less virulent pneumococci, the granules of amphophils appeared brownish and irregular in size, being in a way similar to the granules described by Alder.[18] In both rabbits in exper. 3 the blood smears made about 4 hours before death showed all the leukocytes in various stages of degeneration and also a considerable number of pneumococci free in the plasma. This seems to illustrate a close relation between the virulence of the pneumococcus and the leukocytic degeneration. The morphologic changes is leukocytes in vitro consisted of pyknosis and an increase in the acidophilia of the cytoplasm of polymorphonuclear neutrophils. The lymphocytes and other forms were less affected. The changes occurred much earlier and were more marked with the whole culture than with the filtrate.

The main changes observed in the marrow in the rabbits experimented on was hyperplasia of the leukoblastic cells which was less

[15] Deutsch. Arch. f. klin. Med., 1894, 53, p. 433.
[16] Jour. Infect. Dis., 1921, 29, p. 141.
[17] Ibid., p. 408.
[18] Schweiz. med. Wchnschr., 1921, 51, p. 437.

marked in the case of infection with virulent pneumococci. In addition to this, the virulent pneumococci also produced localized or generalized degenerative changes (Fig. 1) characterized by karyorrhexis, karyolysis, vacuolation and alteration of staining property, but cultural filtrates did not have any definite injurious effects in this respect. In one rabbit there was a leukopenia preceded by a moderate leukocytosis, the marrow showing a hyperplasia but no degenerative changes. This may be attributed to the fact that the destruction of the leukocytes in the peripheral circulation may be far beyond the power of reparation by the marrow. The sections of marrow from the rabbits in exper. 3

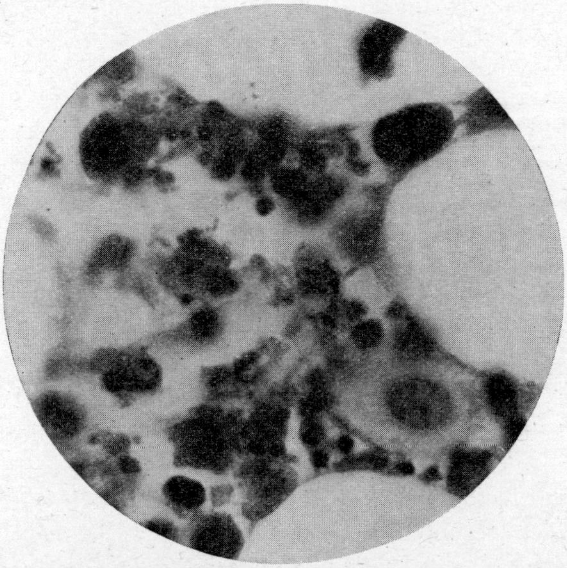

Fig. 1.—Marrow of rabbit in exper. 3; karyorrhexis of myelocytes; × 1000.

revealed, besides a very extensive degeneration, a considerable number of pneumococci. Congestion and hemorrhage were frequently encountered, but the latter was more extensive in acute cases. Megalokaryocytes often occurred in large numbers and none appeared normal.

The spleen was usually more or less degenerated and congested. The malpighian bodies were reduced in size and usually found in areas that contained fibrin, erythrocytes and nuclear fragments. In exper. 1, rabbit B, there was a marked proliferation of phagocytic cells which were crowded with degenerated erythrocytes. The lymph-nodes did not reveal many changes except congestion and sometimes distention of sinuses.

THE BEHAVIOR OF GUINEA-PIG LEUKOCYTES TOWARD PNEUMOCOCCUS TYPE 1

In spite of the great amount of work on phagocytosis, the failure of leukocytes to take up virulent bacteria remains an unsolved problem.

Virulent bacteria, as Massart[19] states, repel leukocytes, a property which is independent of toxin action. He demonstrated that leukocytes manifested a phagocytic activity toward diphtheria bacilli and hog-cholera bacilli, but were inactive in the presence of virulent anthrax bacilli. According to Bordet,[20] leukocytes have a selective action on certain bacteria, guided by chemotaxis, as shown by the fact that the same leukocytes would ingest proteus vulgaris but not virulent streptococci. He states that virulent streptococci do not paralyze

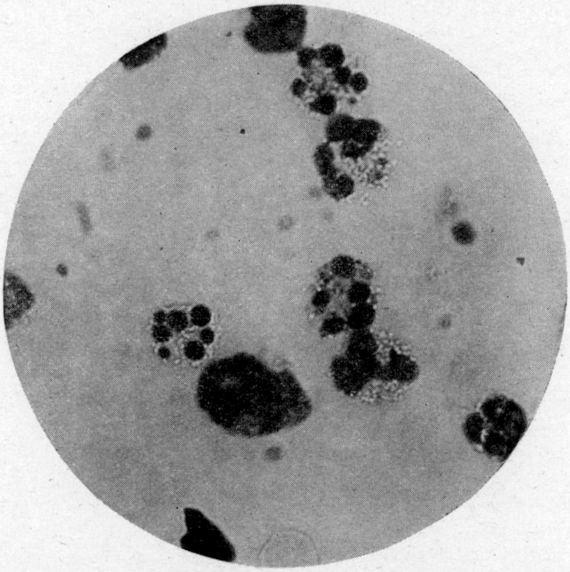

Fig. 2.—Fragmentation of nuclei of amphophils with a marked condensation of chromatin. The granules are highly refractive.

the leukocytes as the latter made ameboid movements in the presence of virulent streptococci. This is confirmed by Matalnikow[21] who found that phagocytes after coming in contact with virulent pneumococci were still able to take up carmine particles. On the contrary, Werigo[22] doubts whether virulent bacteria exert a negative chemotaxis on leukocytes as he found that even virulent anthrax bacilli were susceptible to phagocytosis.

In my experiments, guinea-pigs were inoculated intraperitoneally with virulent and nonvirulent pneumococci of type 1, and the exudate

[19] Ann. d. l'Inst. Pasteur, 1892, 6, p. 321.
[20] Ibid., 1896, 10, p. 104.
[21] Ibid., 1921, 35, p. 363.
[22] Ibid., 1894, 8, p. 1.

withdrawn at intervals. In case of a thick exudate dilution with salt solution was made in order to obtain thin smears. The smears were stained with the Wright, the Gram and the Welch capsule stains.

In the animals inoculated with less virulent pneumococci, 0.1 c c of an 18-hour broth culture being fatal to a mouse within 24 hours, there was usually a marked ingestion of pneumococci by the leukocytes. About 16 hours after inoculation the leukocytes began to undergo

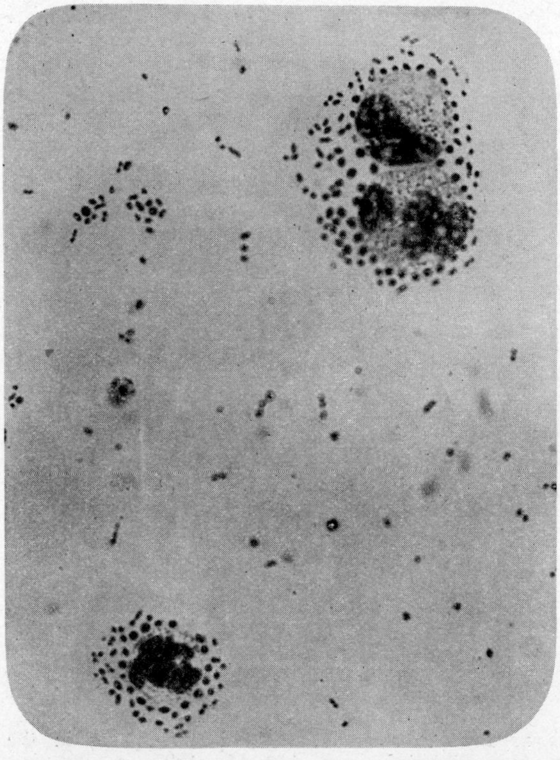

Fig. 3.—The leukocytes are surrounded by large number of pneumococci; two leukocytes are swollen and their granules have lost their refractive property and are stained dark brown with Wright stain so that they appear as cocci.

karyorrhexis and occasionally pyknosis (Fig. 2). In the presence of virulent pneumococci, 0.01 c c of an 18-hour broth culture being fatal to a mouse within 24 hours, there was little phagocytosis throughout the course of the infection, and the leukocytes soon became swollen and surrounded by pneumococci (Fig. 3.). In one case, the leukocytes obtained about 2 hours before death were surrounded by large numbers of pneumococci arranged in rows, the cocci nearest to the leukocytes undergoing involutional changes as their size had increased. Rosenow [23] found that if leukocytes were heated at 60 C. for 5 minutes, they lost their phagocytic activity but became surrounded by pneumococci, apparently by virtue of chemotaxis. In my experiments, the degenerative changes in the leukocytes seem to indicate an extreme intoxication; in the second place, the involution of the pneumococci themselves suggests the idea that the leukocytes secrete a ferment of unknown nature which is detrimental to pneumococci. One hour after inoculation with highly virulent pneumococci, 0.001 c c of an 18-hour broth culture being fatal to a mouse within 24 hours, the peritoneal exudate consisted of a few amphophils which were inactive toward the pneumococci; about 3 hours later the pneumococci and amphophils both had increased in number, but the latter presented ill-defined outlines with a swollen nucleus in most instances. Only a few leukocytes showed a little phagocytosis. There were also large numbers of so-called leukocytic shadows. If the animals remained alive longer, say 24 hours, the peritoneal exudate consisted largely of mature amphophils which were undergoing degeneration, without any indications of phagocytosis.

In an atempt to corroborate the results of Bordet and Metalnikow, I inoculated a guinea-pig with highly virulent pneumococci and 14 hours later the peritoneal exudate was withdrawn for testing the phagocytic activity of the leukocytes in vitro. To a small amount of exudate, previously diluted with citrate solution, 0.1 c c of pneumococcus was added. The mixture was then incubated at 36 C. and examined every 15 minutes for one hour. At the same time the animal was inoculated again with 1 c c of B. coli in order to observe the behavior of leukocytes toward the bacilli in the presence of virulent pneumococci. It was found that about 2 hours after inoculation with B. coli, a few leukocytes began to take up a few bacilli, but in vitro the leukocytes showed no phagocytic activity. This suggests that the leukocytes that ingested B. coli in vivo might be cells which migrated into the peritoneal cavity after inoculation with B. coli and took up B. coli before becoming intoxicated. If this supposition is true, why are the pneumococci not subjected to phagocytosis? This can be explained only by a selective action of leukocytes as Bordet advocated.

[23] Jour. Infect. Dis., 1906, 3, p. 683.

SUMMARY

The leukocytic reaction in rabbits infected with pneumococcus type 1 is somewhat dependent on the virulence of the organisms, a low virulence producing leukocytosis and high virulence leukopenia.

The leukopenia seems to be brought about by degeneration of leukocytes and of cells in the hemopoietic organs. This degeneration seems to be due to the toxic action of the pneumococcus.

After an intraperitoneal inoculation of guinea-pigs with virulent and nonvirulent pneumococci, the leukocytes as a rule show phagocystosis. In certain instances the failure of leukocytes to take up highly virulent pneumococci seems to be due to intoxication of leukocytes as evidenced by degenerative changes.

It seems that virulent pneumococci also produce a chemotactic substance, as although the leukocytes may fail to ingest virulent cocci they usually become surrounded by them.

THE SPECIFICITY OF THE DESENSITIZED STATE IN SERUM ANAPHYLAXIS *

HOWARD T. KARSNER AND ENRIQUE E. ECKER

From the Department of Pathology, School of Medicine, Western Reserve University, Cleveland, Ohio

Aside from the academic questions involved, there is an important practical problem which concerns the specificity of the desensitized state in anaphylaxis. If the occasional hypersensitiveness of man to serums which contain specific immune substances could be reduced or eliminated, the safety of employment of such serums would be much enhanced. The danger of specific desensitization lies largely in the possibility of severe or even fatal shock during desensitization. Nonspecific desensitization might eliminate this danger. Although there are certain hypersensitive states to pure or relatively pure proteins, as for example, those of the vegetable pollens, the fatalities in man have so far resulted from injections of serum. We have therefore confined this study to serum anaphylaxis in the hope that ultimately a practical method may be devised for employment in man. It does not necessarily follow that results in animals, which have been artificially sensitized, are entirely applicable to natural hypersensitiveness in man, but there are instances of the acquired state in man which seem to be identical with that of animals and it has yet to be proved that natural hypersusceptibility differs materially. If, therefore, nonspecific desensitization in the acquired serum hypersusceptibility of animals can be demonstrated satisfactorily it is worthy of further trial in human experiments.

Most studies of anaphylaxis have dealt with serum anaphylaxis and the same is true of the desensitized state. The specificity of the desensitized state has been supported by the work of Otto,[1] Rosenau and Anderson,[2] Szymanowsky,[3] Kumagai and Odaira,[4] and in particular by Besredka.[5] Nonspecific, usually transitory, reduction of shock has been produced by the injection of various substances, but the final issue as regards specificity of this phenomenon is still a matter of considerable dispute. Biedl and Kraus[6] assert

Received for publication Oct. 24, 1921.

* Aided by a grant from the Committee on Scientific Research of the American Medical Association.

[1] München. med. Wchnschr., 1907, 54, p. 1665.
[2] Hyg. Lab., Bull. 29, 1906; Bull. 45, 1908.
[3] Ztschr. f. Immunitätsf. u. Exper. Therap., 1917, 26, p. 213.
[4] Ztschr. f. Immunitätsf. u. Exper. Therap., 1912, 14, p. 391.
[5] Anaphylaxie et Antianaphylaxie, 1917.
[6] Wien. klin. Wchnschr., 1909, 22, p. 363.

that animals sensitized to serums can be desensitized with heterologous substances such as peptone, but Besredka[5] was unable to confirm their work. Kopaczevski and Vohram[7] found that sodium oleate reduces anaphylactic shock, which they assert is due to a lowering of surface tension of the blood. Even such a salt as sodium chloride has been employed with some degree of success. Richet[8] ascribes the action of this salt to a distinct influence on the nerve cells, while other investigators attribute its effect to a modification of the colloidal state of fluids and cells. Pfeiffer and Mita[9] protected sensitized animals against lethal doses of the homologous serum (horse) by previous injections of beef serum. Weil[10] desensitized guinea-pigs, passively sensitized to horse serum, with rabbit serum. More recently Calvary,[11] Bessau,[12] Benjamin and Witzinger,[13] Penna and Moreno, Penna, Cuenca and Kraus,[14] Thomson,[15] Massini[16] and also Brack[17] have examined the subject anew. According to Calvary,[11] it seems that in dogs there is an increase of lymph flow during anaphylactic shock. If, however, previous injections of beef serum are made, such an increase of lymph flow is not demonstrable. Bessau asserts that there is no difference between desensitization with homologous and heterologous serum. Bessau[18] further states that if animals are sensitized to two proteins, anaphylactic shock produced by either protein leads to reduction in the amount of precipitins for both antigens, although the homologous precipitin is the more markedly reduced. Benjamin and Witzinger,[13] who studied the problem in man, came to the conclusion that under certain conditions one antigen may modify the reaction of the other, and these authors called the phenomenon: "La competeneia de antigenos," or "antigenic antagonism." Penna and Moreno[14] were unable to desensitize in man. In animals desensitization can be more readily produced, as is known from the extensive work of Besredka, Alexandrescu and Cinca, and others. Penna, Cuenca and Kraus[14] have shown that serum disease in man is modified or prevented if beef serum is injected before the use of horse serum. Thomson[15] states that much depends on the degree of sensitiveness, that is, the relation between the period of maximal sensitization and the time of desensitization. He refers nonspecific interference in shock to a reduction in the speed of reaction between antigen and antibody whereby a greater amount of the antigen is required to induce shock. The cause of the speed reduction, however, is not explained. Massini,[16] using intestinal segments, concludes that antianaphylaxis is specific, but that there is in addition a nonspecific element. Friedberger refers this phenomenon to an aspecific resistance. Brack, using the method of Massini, found a distinct quantitative difference between specific antianaphylaxis and aspecific antianaphylaxis. The injection of heterologous serum into highly sensitized animals may lead to shock, but the reaction is a great deal less than in the case of the homologous serum. The nonspecific shock may reduce the toxic effects of the homologous serum. Of some bearing on this problem are also the

[7] Compt. rend. Acad. d. sc., 1919, 169, p. 250.
[8] Compt. rend. Acad. d. sc., 1919, 169, p. 9.
[9] Ztschr. f. Immunitätsf. u. Exper. Therap., 1910, 4, p. 410.
[10] Ztschr. f. Immunitätsf. u. Exper. Therap., 1914, 20, p. 199.
[11] München. med. Wchnschr., 1911, 58, p. 1442.
[12] Centralbl. f. Bakteriol., I, O., 1911, 60, p. 637.
[13] Ztschr. f. Kinderheilk., 1911, 3, p. 73.
[14] Rev. del Inst. Bakteriol., Dep. Nacional de Hygiene, 1919, 2, p. 1.
[15] Ztschr. f. Immunitätsf. u. Exper. Therap., 1917, 26, p. 213.
[16] Ztschr. f. Immunitätsf. u. Exper. Therap., 1918, 27, p. 194.
[17] Ztschr. f. Immunitätsf. u. Exper. Therap., 1921, 31, p. 407.
[18] Centralbl. f. Bakteriol., 2, O., 1914, 74, p. 162.

experiments of Lewis,[19] who found that if definite amounts of horse serum are slowly added to dog serum, and injected into guinea-pigs, sensitization to the horse serum is not produced. According to this author, as much as 0.1 c c horse serum in 10 c c of dog serum would not sensitize, even though 0.000,001 c c of horse serum alone will produce a high degree of sensitization. He further found that not only will dog serum inhibit sensitization to horse serum, but other serums (human, cat, beef) will do likewise, and these serums will also inhibit sensitization to dog serum if the proportions are reversed. Further experiments also showed that not only serums but also solutions of pure proteins (egg albumin) in the proper amounts will inhibit sensitization to another protein. Wells [20] claims that experiments with such hopelessly complex mixtures as are furnished by serum, organ extracts, or even egg white and milk, cannot be expected to yield much valuable information concerning specificity. He further states that "if the antigens are isolated proteins, purified as completely as possible, striking illustrations of specificity may be demonstrated both by sensitizing and by desensitizing with specific proteins." Wells' experiments are conclusive in so far as pure proteins are concerned, but the immediate problem as concerns shock in man deals principally with serum anaphylaxis.

METHOD

The experiments were undertaken to study various conditions of nonspecific reduction or elimination of anaphylactic shock. With a variety of heterologous serums we have studied the relative effectiveness of the subcutaneous, intraperitoneal and intravenous routes of injection in desensitization. We have considered the time allowed for absorption by these routes. The type of reaction in shock has been observed in relation to the various serums used for desensitization. Individual variations in animals are recognized as an important factor of error and where essentially toxic serums have been employed, the dosage has been regulated so as to reduce the factor of essential toxicity.

Guinea-pigs have been used throughout. They have been sensitized, in some series intraperitoneally, in others subcutaneously with either horse serum or human serum, or in one series with beef serum. The time allowed for sensitization has varied but in general is about three weeks. Horse, beef, goat, sheep, swine, dog, cat, rabbit and human serums have been employed in desensitization. Desensitization with homologous serums was usually in doses of about 0.05 c c, whereas the dose of heterologous serum varied between 0.5 c c and 2.0 c c. The injections varied from one to four in number and in different series were given subcutaneously, intraperitoneally or intravenously. On the day selected for producing anaphylactic shock, the minimal fatal dose of homologous serum was determined. The delicacy of the determination in our experiment permits a factor of error of 0.05 c c, not con-

[19] Jour. Am. Med. Assn., 1921, 76, p. 1342.
[20] Physiological Reviews, 1921, 1, p. 44.

sidered important in the type and number of experiments performed. Careful necropsies were made on all animals that died.

TABLE 1

THE EFFECT OF SUBCUTANEOUS DESENSITIZATION WITH HOMOLOGOUS AND HETEROLOGOUS SERUMS 24 HOURS PRIOR TO THE TOXIC DOSE *

Animals		Desensitization					Intoxication				
No.	Wt. in Gm.	Date, 1919	Serum Used	Amount Given Subcutaneously Oct. 30: A. M.	Amount Given Subcutaneously Oct. 30: P. M.	Reaction	Toxic Dose Horse Serum Intravenous	Date, 1919	Hour	Reaction	Necropsy
106	346	10/30	—	—	—	......	0.2	10/31	9:27	9:28, mod. dyspnea; 9:30, hair ruffled; 9:35, on side; 9:47, severe dyspnea; 9:47, dead	Typical
121	375	10/30	Horse	0.05	0.1	—	0.2	10/31	10:00	10:02, convulsion, severe dyspnea; 10:04, hair ruffled	
111	355	10/30	Horse	0.05	0.1	Slight	0.2	10/31	10:22	10:25, rubbed nose and body	
123	377	10/30	Beef	0.5	1.0	—	0.2	10/31	9:49	9:51, mod. dyspnea; 9:54, severe dyspnea, on side; 10:17, dead	Slight distention of lungs
108	330	10/30	Beef	0.5	1.0	—	0.2	10/31	10:16	10:20, mod. dyspnea; 10:24, severe dysp.; 10:26, on side; 10:58, dead	Slight to mod. distention of lungs; slight hemorrhages
118	365	10/30	Hog	0.5	1.0	—	0.2	10/31	9:42	9:45, slight dyspnea; 9:45, rubs nose; 10:04, convulsions; 10:05, dead	Slight distention of lungs
119	355	10/30	Hog	0.5	1.0	—	0.2	10/31	10:10	10:11, convulsions; 10:16, dead	Typical
107	295	10/30	Human	0.5	1.0	—	0.2	10/31	9:33	9:35, mod. dyspnea; 9:38, convulsions; 9:43, dead	Typical
112	275	10/30	Human	0.5	1.0	—	0.2	10/31	9:55	9:57, convulsions; 9:59, dead	Typical

* All animals were sensitized intraperitoneally with 0.05 c c horse serum, Oct. 9, 1919. Desensitizing doses of serums were given in 2 subcutaneous doses 21 days subsequently and the toxic dose intravenously the next day. Note protection by homologous serum and failure on the part of heterologous serums.

EXPERIMENTS

Series 1.—The object of this series was to determine the effect of homologous or heterologous serums given subcutaneously in 2 doses on the day preceding intoxication. With the toxic dose selected, the animal which was not desensitized in any way died in 20 minutes with typical symptoms of shock and typical necropsy findings. Those which were desensitized with homologous serum reacted severely, but survived, while all those that were desensitized with heterologous serums died. The details of this experiment are shown in table 1. The size of the doses employed in this experiment was determined by preliminary experiments. The series shows that in the doses employed the subcutaneous injection of heterologous serums does not suffice to protect the animal from anaphylactic shock.

TABLE 2

THE EFFECT OF INTRAPERITONEAL DESENSITIZATION WITH HOMOLOGOUS AND HETEROLOGOUS SERUMS 24 HOURS PRIOR TO THE TOXIC DOSE *

Animals		Desensitization				Intoxication				Necropsy
No.	Wt. in Gm.	Date, 1919	Serum Used	Dose of Serum	Reaction	Toxic Dose Horse Serum Intravenous	Date, 1919	Hour	Reaction	
117	334	—	—	—	—	0.2	10/29	9:50	9:54, mod. dyspnea; 9:58, rubbed nose, hair ruffled; 9:59, convulsions; 9:60, dead	Typical
122	330	—	—	—	—	0.2	10/29	10:20	11:22, restless, scratched nose, convulsions; 11:26, dead	Typical
100	278	10/28	Horse	0.05	Distinct	0.2	10/29	10:55	10:58, mod. dyspnea, restless; 11:00, hair ruffled; 11:06, rubbed nose	
101	255	10/28	Horse	0.5 1:1,000	None	0.2	10/29	11:08	11:09, mod. dyspnea; 11:24, on side, very sick	
102	322	10/28	Beef	0.5	None	0.2	10/29	11:00	11:03, mod. dyspnea, convulsions, on side, very sick	
103	265	10/28	Beef	1.0	None	0.2	10/29	11:12	11:15, marked dyspnea, defecation, 11:18, rubbed nose	
104	300	10/28	Swine	0.5	None	0.2	10/29	10:24	10:25, mod. dyspnea; 10:26, rubbed nose; 10:35, hair ruffled, defecation	
105	315	10/28	Swine	1.0	None	0.2	10/29	10:09	10:10, slight dyspnea, hair ruffled 10:14, marked dyspnea; 10:30, convulsions; 10:43, dead	Moderate distention of lungs

* All animals were sensitized intraperitoneally with 0.05 c c horse serum, Oct. 13, 1919. Desensitizing doses of serums were given in single intraperitoneal injections 15 days subsequently and the toxic doses intravenously the next day. Note protection by small dose of horse serum, both doses of beef serum and larger dose of swine serum.

Series 2.—This series was designed to determine the protective effect of intraperitoneal desensitization. The animals were desensitized by a single small dose of homologous horse serum and somewhat larger doses of sheep and of swine serum. The control animals which were not desensitized died typically in respectively 10 and 8 minutes following injection. Those desensitized with homologous serum showed, following the toxic injection, distinct, but not fatal, symptoms of anaphylactic shock. Of those desensitized with sheep serum both were distinctly shocked but survived. Of the two desensitized with swine serum, one died after typical symptoms but at necropsy showed only moderate distention of the lungs. It is therefore apparent that by intraperitoneal injection, and with the amount of serum used, the heterologous serums serve to protect. Even in the case of the animal that died, death was considerably postponed as contrasted with the rapid death of the control animals.

TABLE 3

THE EFFECT OF SUBCUTANEOUS AND INTRAPERITONEAL DESENSITIZATION WITH 4 INJECTIONS OF HOMOLOGOUS OR HETEROLOGOUS SERUMS IN INCREASING AMOUNTS *

Animals		Desensitization							Intoxication			
No.	Wt. in Gm.	Dates and Amounts, 1920: Nov. 9 A.M.	Nov. 9 P.M.	Nov. 10 A.M.	Nov. 10 P.M.	Serum Used	Route of Injection	Reaction	Toxic Dose Horse Serum Intravenous	Nov. 11 * Hour	Reaction	Necropsy
133	257	—	—	—	—	—	—	—	0.2	9:46	9:48, severe dyspnea; 9:50, convulsions; 9:55, dead	Moderate inflation of lungs
132	270	0.05	0.1	0.2	0.4	Horse	Subcutaneous	—	0.2	9:55	9:57, hair ruffled; 9:58, slight dysp.	
131	265	0.05	0.1	0.2	0.4	Horse	Intraperitoneal	—	0.2	9:57	9:59, restless	
127	345	0.1	0.2	0.3	0.4	Swine	Intraperitoneal	—	0.2	9:36	9:39, severe dyspnea; convulsions; 9:43, dead	Moderate nflation of lungs
115	345	0.1	0.2	0.3	0.4	Swine	Subcutaneous	—	0.2	9:43	9:44, rubbed nose; 9:45, hair ruffled; slight dysp.	
128	310	0.1	0.2	0.3	0.4	Beef	Subcutaneous	—	0.2	10:16	10:17, rubbed nose; 10:19, hair ruffled; 10:30, mod. dyspnea	
135	330	0.1	0.2	0.3	0.4	Beef	Intraperitoneal	—	0.2	10:11	10:13, dyspnea; 10:14, rubbed nose; 10:16, convulsions; 10:30, dead	Typical
113	327	0.1	0.2	0.3	0.4	Human	Subcutaneous	..	0.2	9:50	9:53, hair ruffled; 9:54, dyspnea	
129	297	0.1	0.2	0.3	0.4	Human	Intraperitoneal	..	0.2	10:23	10:25, hair ruf fled, mod. dyspnea; 10:32, rubbed nose	

* All animals were sensitized intraperitoneally with 0.05 c c horse serum, Oct. 22, 1919. Desensitization, covering 2 days, was begun 18 days subsequently and the toxic doses given the day following the second day of desensitization. Heterologous desensitization is apparent but irregular.

Series 3.—This series was undertaken in order to compare and estimate the result of desensitization intraperitoneally or subcutaneously by means of several injections of homologous or heterologous serums. The animals were all sensitized intraperitoneally and the desensitizing doses were given so that of each pair of animals one was desensitized intraperitoneally and the other subcutaneously. The toxic dose of homologous horse serum killed a pig, which had not been desensitized, in 5 minutes, with typical symptoms and typical necropsy findings. Animals desensitized with homologous serum showed relatively slight symptoms. Of the 6 animals that were desensitized with heterologous serums, 4 survived after fairly severe shock. The two that succumbed following desensitization were desensitized by the intraperitoneal route. We do not interpret this as indicating ineffectiveness of this method, but rather attribute it to individual differences in animals. Table 3 shows the protocol of this series.

Series 4.—In this series the preceding experiment was practically duplicated except that the multiple desensitizing doses were all given subcutaneously and instead of the swine, beef and horse serums we employed goat, dog and rabbit serums. The control animal, not desensitized, died in 5 minutes with typical shock. Those desensitized with homologous horse serum, although severely shocked, survived. Of those desensitized with the heterologous serums, one of each group died following typical symptoms and exhibited at necropsy typical findings. The other three were severely shocked, but survived. It is not considered necessary to submit a protocol of this series, which is essentially the same as the preceding series. It is evident, however, that by fractional desensitization it is possible to protect with homologous serum, and also it is possible to protect in a certain portion of the cases by the use of heterologous serums.

Series 5 and 6.—In these two groups of experiments the animals were desensitized subcutaneously with human serum. In both series desensitization was by the intraperitoneal route. In series 5 a single injection was given and in series 6 two injections were given 24 hours apart. In series 5, with a single desensitizing dose, the homologous human serum failed to protect in doses of 0.1 and 0.2 c c. The heterologous rabbit and horse serums were given in doses of 1 and 2 c c. Of these 5 animals, only 1 survived, namely, that which had 1 c c rabbit serum. The control animals that were not desensitized died in respectively 5 and 7 minutes with typical symptoms and typical necropsy findings. It is probable that the amount of serum used in this experiment was inadequate, but with the doses employed it appears that a single intraperitoneal injection failed to desensitize adequately, either with homologous or heterologous serums. In series VI the same experiment was performed with different serums and with 2 protecting doses. In this series 0.1 c c of the homologous human serum failed to produce fatal shock in the nondesensitized control, whereas 0.2 c c produced death in 7 minutes with typical symptoms and typical necropsy findings. Those animals protected by 2 intraperitoneal doses of homologous human serum showed only moderate symptoms following the toxic dose. Of 3 animals desensitized with ox serum, 2 succumbed, whereas of the 3 desensitized with rabbit serum all survived. It must be noted that the only survival of those desensitized with ox serum, received only one intraperitoneal injection, but in the case of this animal and in the case of that which was desensitized with only one injection of rabbit serum it is important to note that 48 hours elapsed before the toxic dose was given. Details of series 6 are found in table 4. As series 5 is simply a series of fatalities, it is not necessary to append a protocol.

Series 7.—This series was undertaken in order to determine whether there is a quantitative difference in reaction depending on the amount of serum employed for protection. In order to eliminate, in so far as possible, individual differences in absorption of the serum, the intravenous method of desensitization was employed. In desensitizing with homologous serum it was found that reaction occurred in proportion to the amount of serum employed. In spite of the fact that on the day of desensitization 0.05 c c homologous human serum killed the animal in 7 minutes, on the following day when intoxication was performed, 0.2 c c was necessary to obtain a fatal result. Even in the smallest dose for desensitization, protection was sufficient to prevent death, although with this dose the reaction was distinctly more severe than with the larger doses. Desensitization with heterologous serums was practiced with approximately 10 times the amount of homologous serum, and it is seen that the smallest doses of rabbit and horse serum failed to prevent death. The larger doses were effective in preventing death, but the reaction was practically as severe as with the homologous desensitization. Within the limits

TABLE 4

THE EFFECT OF INTRAPERITONEAL DESENSITIZATION WITH 2 INJECTIONS OF HOMOLOGOUS OR HETEROLOGOUS SERUMS *

Animals		Desensitization				Intoxication				
No.	Wt. in Gm.	Serums Used	Dates and Amounts, Intraperitoneal, 1920, Mar. 24	Dates and Amounts, Intraperitoneal, 1920, Mar. 25	Reaction	Toxic Dose Human Serum	Date	Hour, P. M.	Reaction	Necropsy
73	367	—	—	—	—	0.2	3/26	1:40	1:42, severe dyspnea, hair ruffled, scratched nose; 1:44, convulsions; 1:47, dead	Typical
90	262	—	—	—	—	0.1	3/26	1:49	1:51, scratched nose; 1:54, mod. dyspnea	
85	270	Human	0.1	0.1	—	0.2	3/26	1:57	1:59, scratched nose and body; 1:60, mod. dyspnea	
86	260	Human	0.1	0.1	—	0.2	3/26	2:05	2:08, hair ruffled	
93	315	Ox	1.0	1.0	—	0.2	3/26	2:23	2:24, scratched nose and body, mod. dysp.; 2:25, convulsions, on side; 2:27, dead	Typical
89	322	Ox	1.0	0.5	—	0.2	3/26	2:19	2:20, severe dyspnea, coughed, scratched; 2:22, hair ruffled; 2:24, convulsions; 2:27, dead	Typical
78	352	Ox	1.0	—	—	0.2	3/26	2:09	2:11, scratched nose; 2:12, coughed, hair ruffled	
77	242	Rabbit	1.0	1.0	—	0.2	3/26	2:26	2:28, hair ruffled, slight dyspnea; 2:30, scratched head; 2:33, on side	
87	287	Rabbit	1.0	0.5	—	0.2	3/26	2:30	2:33, slight dyspnea, scratched nose	
42	300	Rabbit	1.0	—	—	0.2	3/26	2:15	2:17, moderate dyspnea, hair ruffled, restless	

* All animals were sensitized subcutaneously with 0.05 c c human serum, March 10, 1920. Desensitizing doses were given 14 and 15 days subsequently and the toxic doses given the next day. Heterologous desensitization was apparent but irregular.

of the experiment, it is apparent that there is a quantitative difference in effects, depending on the amount of serum used, but this cannot be regarded as definitely proportionate to the amount of serum employed. Table 5 shows the details of this series. It will be noticed that in the amounts of serum employed, intravenous desensitization both with homologous and heterologous serums is highly effective.

Series 8.—In this series practically an identical experiment was performed except that the animals were sensitized to horse serum. The desensitization was practiced after the height of sensitization had passed, namely 50 days after sensitization. Desensitization was practiced with the homologous horse serum and heterologous sheep and human serum, the latter two in doses approximately 10 times that of the homologous serum. Desensitization was produced by the intravenous route and shock was produced 24 hours later by the same route. The same gradation of desensitizing doses was employed as in the preceding

TABLE 5

THE QUANTITATIVE EFFECT OF INTRAVENOUS DESENSITIZATION WITH HOMOLOGOUS AND HETEROLOGOUS SERUMS *

Animals		Desensitization			Intoxication				
No.	Wt. in Gm.	Serums and Amounts Intravenous, May 4, 1921		Reaction	Toxic Dose Human Serum	Date	Hour	Reaction	Necropsy
141	300	—	—	—	0.1	5/5	10:03	10:05, ruffling of hair, 10:06, mod. dyspnea; restless	
95	290	—	—	—	0.15	5/5	10:22	10:24, coughed; 10:25, hair ruffled, moderate dyspnea, scratched nose	
73	350	—	—	—	0.2	5/5	10:32	10:34, coughed; 10:35, hair ruffled, severe dyspnea, scratched; 10:47, dead	Typical
15	260	Human	0.05	Severe, dead in 7 min.	—	—	—	....	Typical
241	270	Human	0.025	Moderate to severe	0.2	5/5	10:41	10:45, restless; 10:48, hair ruffled, slight dyspnea, scratched nose	
380	275	Human	0.01	Moderate	0.2	5/5	10:48	10:50, scratched nose, moderate dyspnea; 10:57, coughed	
62	300	Human	0.005	Slight	0.2	5/5	10:37	10:40, slight dyspnea	
8	310	Human	0.001	None	0.2	5/5	10:45	10:47, slight to moderate dyspnea, hair ruffled; 10:48, coughed; 10:57, on side, very sick	
161	275	Rabbit	0.5	None	0.2	5/5	11:08	11:10, scratched nose, hair ruffled; 11:13 slight dyspnea	
54	280	Rabbit	0.25	None	0.2	5/5	11:05	11:07, ruffling of hair, scratched nose; 11:08, coughed, mod. dyspnea	
336	300	Rabbit	0.1	None	0.2	5/5	11:00	11:02, slight dyspnea, hair ruffled; 11:04, scratched nose	
42	310	Rabbit	0.05	None	0.2	5/5	—	Unsuccessful injection	
57	325	Rabbit	0.025	None	0.2	5/5	11:05	11:07, hair ruffled, scratched nose; 11:08, coughed, mod. dyspnea; 11:12, convulsions; 11:15, dead	Typical
58	280	Horse	0.5	None	0.2	5/5	11:27	11:28, scratched nose mod. dyspnea, very sick	
39	290	Horse	0.25	None	0.2	5/5	11:12	11:14, scratched nose and body	
290	295	Horse	0.1	None	0.2	5/5	11:15	11:16, scratched nose and body, hair ruffled, slight dyspnea	
106	310	Horse	0.05	None	0.2	5/5	11:30	Convulsions; 11:32, hair ruffled, mod. dyspnea, convulsions; 11:35, dead	Typical

* All animals were sensitized subcutaneously with 0.05 c c human serum, April 6, 1921. Desensitizing doses in various amounts were given intravenously 28 days subsequently and the toxic doses the next day. Although in an attempt at homologous desensitization one animal succumbed to 0.05 c c serum, the toxic dose as determined the next day was 0.2 c c. Note the failure to protect of the smallest doses of heterologous serums.

experiment. The control animal which was not desensitized succumbed to 0.2 c c horse serum in 2 minutes and another given 0.1 c c survived. Desensitization with homologous horse serum showed symptoms in proportion to the size of the dose employed, but all survived. Of the desensitized animals

TABLE 6

THE EFFECT OF INTRAVENOUS DESENSITIZATION IN PROTECTION AGAINST DOUBLE THE MINIMAL TOXIC DOSE OF HOMOLOGOUS SERUM *

Animals		Desensitization			Intoxication				
No.	Wt. in Gm.	Serums and Amounts Intravenous, July 6, 1921		Reaction	Toxic Dose Horse Serum	Date	Hour	Reaction	Necropsy
76	325	—	—	—	0.2	7/7	11:14	11:15, rubbed nose, coughed, restless, mod. dysp.; 11:16, severe dyspnea; 11:18, urinated; 11:35, convulsions, on side; 12:10, dead	Moderate inflation of lungs
63	215	Horse	0.03	Moderate	0.5	7/7	3:30	3:32, moderate dyspnea	
168	295	Horse	0.03	Slight	0.5	7/7	3:28	Slight dyspnea	
318	300	Horse	0.03	Slight	0.5	7/7	3:25	3:26, rubbed head and nose; 3:26, mod. dyspnea; 3:27, severe dyspnea; 4:05, dead	Typical
379	220	Horse	0.03	Marked	0.5	7/7	3:22	3:20, slight to moderate dyspnea, hair ruffled, rubbed nose; 3:25, severe dyspnea	
146	290	Horse	0.01	Slight	0.5	7/7	3:20	3:21, rubbed nose, slight dyspnea	
178	300	Sheep	0.5	None	0.5	7/7	3:18	Coughed; 3:10, hair ruffled, convulsions; 3:20, on side; 3:27, dead	Typical
107	275	Sheep	0.5	None	0.5	7/7	3:16	3:17, scratched nose, hair ruffled, on side; dead at 4:30	Typical
34	200	Sheep	0.5	None	0.5	7/7	3:14	Coughed, rubbed nose; 3:16, moderate to severe dyspnea	
136	275	Sheep	0.3	None	0.5	7/7	3:09	3:10, restless, severe dyspnea	
71	275	Sheep	0.3	None	0.5	7/7	3:05	Coughed; 3:08, severe dyspnea, on side; 3:10, dead	Typical
176	280	Sheep	0.3	None	0.5	7/7	3:11	Hair ruffled; 3:12, rubbed nose and head; 3:15, on side; 4:00, dead	Marked inflation of lungs
180	350	Sheep	0.1	None	0.5	7/7	2:57	2:58, restless, scratched head, mod. dyspnea, hair ruffled	
286	225	Sheep	0.1	None	0.5	7/7	3:03	3:04, coughed, scratched nose, convulsions; 3:05, on side; 3:15, dead	Typical
310	330	Sheep	0.1	None	0.5	7/7	3:00	3:01, coughed, urinated defecated, severe dyspnea	

* All animals were sensitized with 0.05 c c horse serum, June 10, 1921. Desensitizing doses were given intravenously 26 days subsequently and double the minimal toxic dose the next day. In the amounts used there is little or no quantitative desensitizing effect demonstrated against the large intoxicating dose.

all reacted severely following the shock dose, but it could not be noticed that there was much difference in reaction except that in a general way those desensitized with the larger doses of homologous horse serum were somewhat less severely shocked than those desensitized with smaller doses. Of 5 animals desensitized with human serum, all survived the subsequent shock dose. Of 5 animals desensitized with sheep serum one succumbed, namely, that which received 0.05 c c, next to the smallest dose for desensitization. The details of this experiment are essentially the same as those of the preceding experiment, and it is not considered necessary to append a protocol. All animals which received the smallest desensitizing doses reacted with distinctly greater severity than those receiving larger desensitizing doses except in the case of the fatality noted. The fact that the smallest doses in this series sufficed to protect, may be because the height of sensitization had passed, whereas in the preceding experiment it was maximal.

Series 9.—This series was undertaken in order to determine whether the protection afforded against a single minimal toxic dose would suffice to protect against a considerably increased toxic dose. In the control animal, not desensitized, death occurred 55 minutes after injection of 0.2 c c of homologous horse serum, but the animal reacted severely and promptly and death was delayed apparently only by marked individual resistance. Of those desensi-

TABLE 7

THE EFFECT OF LAPSE OF VARIOUS TIME INTERVALS BETWEEN DESENSITIZATION AND INTOXICATION *

Number of Hours of Shock After Desensitization	Desensitization					
	Homologous Horse Serum		Heterologous			
			Human Serum		Sheep Serum	
	No. of Animals	Deaths	No. of Animals	Deaths	No. of Animals	Deaths
24	2	0	2	0	4	1
72	2	0	2	0	4	3
120	3	0	3	2	3	2

* All animals were sensitized subcutaneously with 0.05 c c horse serum, April 15, 1921. All were desensitized May 6, and shocked in groups May 7, 9 and 11.

tized with homologous serum, one died following the large toxic dose of 0.05 c.c. Nine animals were desensitized with various doses of heterologous sheep serum. Five of these animals, a relatively high percentage, died with typical symptoms and with typical necropsy findings. Death occurred without any noticeable reference to the size of the desensitizing doses. It is probable that the differences in shock doses are not sufficiently marked to make any difference in response, or that all the doses employed are really maximal. Those animals which did not die had severe reaction regardless of whether the desensitization was with homologous or heterologous serums. As will be seen from table 6, the desensitizing doses of heterologous serums were approximately 10 times those of the homologous serum. As compared with other experiments, the doses in both the groups of animals were sufficiently large to insure adequate protection against a single toxic dose of the homologous serum, but it is apparent that with a larger toxic dose the protective effect of these doses is insufficient.

Series 10.—This group of experiments was undertaken to determine the duration of desensitization by heterologous and homologous serums. The series comprises 32 animals and is too long for a detailed protocol. Table 7, however, gives a summary of the results. The animals were all desensitized on the same date with 0.05 c c homologous horse serum and 1 c c of the heterologous sheep and human serums. The animals were divided into groups and the members of each group were given the toxic dose of horse serum 24, 72 and 120 hours subsequently. The control animal, not desensitized, died following a dose of 0.12 c c homologous serum. According to the summary, all the animals that were desensitized with homologous serum survived. A large intravenous dose of sheep serum gave fairly adequate protection over the course of 24 hours, but after 72 and 120 hours the effect was greatly reduced. In the case of desensitization with human serum the effect was noticed for 72 hours after desensitization, but had almost disappeared at the end of 120 hours. An examination of the clinical symptoms manifested by the animals shows no important difference either as regards the length of time elapsed following desensitization or as regards the different serums used. The conclusion which may satisfactorily be drawn from this experiment is that heterologous desensitization is distinctly shorter in duration than is homologous desensitization.

DISCUSSION

A detailed statistical study of the experiments is subject to many factors of error, such as individual resistance or susceptibility of animals, the toxicity for guinea-pigs of some of the serums employed, and the relatively small number of animals in each series and in the entire group. The discussion of the experiments is therefore undertaken with a realization of its limitations. Although no exactly comparable experiments were made with intraperitoneal and subcutaneous methods of sensitization, no difference in effect is observed, and in view of preceding work on the subject it is safe to assume that the method of sensitization does not affect the attempts at desensitization.

A summary of the attempts at desensitization shows that of 5 animals desensitized by subcutaneous injection of homologous serums, none died as the result of the toxic dose. Of 19 animals desensitized subcutaneously by heterologous serums, 10 died. Following intraperitoneal desensitization with homologous serums, 1 of 6 animals died of the subsequently induced shock; with heterologous serums, 9 of 18 animals died. These figures do not indicate any practical advantage in the intraperitoneal as compared with the subcutaneous route. This result might well be altered in a larger series. Following intravenous desensitization with homologous serum, only 1 of 20 animals died of the subsequently induced shock, whereas with heterologous serums 20 of 56 animals died of subsequent shock. Including the total number of animals employed, it appears that intravenous desensitization with homologous serum is slightly superior to the subcutaneous or intraperitoneal routes. With the use of heterologous serum, the intravenous route is decidedly superior. Our examination of the question of multiple doses by the intraperitoneal or subcutaneous routes as contrasted with single doses is too small to be of service, but the work of Besredka and others leaves no doubt that multiple subcutaneous injections are superior to single subcutaneous injections. Our small series of 35 animals shows no superiority of multiple intraperitoneal injections over single injections by the same route. The number is too small, however, for accuracy or reliance.

Including all the series, it is found that of 31 animals desensitized with homologous serum only 2 died subsequently of anaphylactic shock. Of 93 animals desensitized with heterologous serums, 39 died of the subsequently produced shock. By the methods employed homologous desensitization is not necessarily prophylactic but gives, as will be seen from the preceding paragraph, apparently better results by the intravenous than by the subcutaneous or intraperitoneal routes. Heterologous desensitization saved more than half the animals in which it was employed. Here the intravenous method is decidedly superior; it shows 36% fatalities as compared with 51% fatalities by the intraperitoneal and subcutaneous routes.

It is apparent that a considerably larger quantity of heterologous serum than of homologous serum is required to protect. Preliminary experiments not reported in the protocols indicated that the ratio is approximately 10: 1, and it is for this reason that this ratio was employed in many of the experiments. In both homologous and heterologous desensitization, larger doses are more effective than very small doses, although this does not follow, as far as we can demonstrate, in any definite proportion. Protection is not so well assured against large intoxicating doses as against the minimal fatal dose. This lesser degree of protection is more evident in the case of heterologous, than of homologous, desensitization.

It is well known that the desensitized state in anaphylaxis is of comparatively short duration. The experiments in our last series indicate that the duration of protection is quite definitely shorter following heterologous than following homologous desensitization. It is true that symptoms of shock often appear as the result of homologous desensitization, whereas they are unusual following heterologous desensitization. If minor shock or shocks be the essential element of desensitization, then the reason for greater protection by homologous serums is apparent, but the fundamental nature of anaphylaxis is as yet unexplained and theories of desensitization must depend on a satisfactory explanation of the fundamental phenomena of sensitization and shock.

Antigenic antagonisms have been referred to in our review of the literature. Brack has shown that in highly sensitized animals actual shock may be produced by otherwise nontoxic heterologous serums, but is less marked than with the homologous serum. Lewis suggests that this phenomenon is due to a protein common to all the serums employed. It must be apparent, however, that the specificity of serum sensitization is not absolute, the specificity of serum anaphylactic shock is only relative, and the desensitized state may be produced by a wide variety of heterologous serums. Further studies are in progress with reference to the influence of colloidal disturbances on desensitization, but our present studies offer no explanation for the phenomena observed.

CONCLUSIONS

Animals sensitized to serum may be desensitized by the use of heterologous serums. The most effective desensitization is by the use of homologous serums.

Heterologous desensitization is most effective by the intravenous route. It develops with apparently the same rapidity as homologous desensitization but is of distinctly shorter duration.

Reactions appear in intoxicated animals following either form of desensitization, but are apparently somewhat less severe following homologous desensitization. The latter rule has many exceptions.

Heterologous desensitization becomes less effective as larger intoxicating doses of serum are used to produce shock. Homologous desensitization is more effective than heterologous in protection against large shock doses.

ANTIBODY PRODUCTION AFTER INTRATRACHEAL INJECTION OF ANTIGEN

RIGNEY D'AUNOY

From the Department of Pathology, Tulane University, and The Rathbone Memorial Laboratories of the Charity Hospital, New Orleans, Louisiana

The importance of the intratracheal route of inoculation as a possible practical measure for the production of antibodies was first suggested by Besredka.[1] During his studies on anaphylaxis he observed that rabbits and guinea-pigs withstood large intratracheal injections of serum, and that the intratracheal inoculations of B. tuberculosis occasioned the production of specific antibodies for this organism. Recently Pfenninger [2] has recorded the production of agglutinins for B. paratyphosus, of lysins for sheep erythrocytes, and of lysins for Vibrio cholerae after intratracheal injections.

It is not surprising that the intratracheal route for introducing an antigen should be followed by ready antibody response when we consider the high vascularity of the mucous membrane of the whole of the respiratory tract, and especially that of the trachea. Due to the numerous infoldings of various parts of this mucosa, considerable surface for absorption exists. Goodwin, Segalos and Mayer [3] have observed practically instantaneous absorption of water injected intratracheally in dogs and rabbits. Colin [4] introduced eighteen liters of water within three hours in the trachea of horses without ill results. He also showed that salts of strychnine can be demonstrated in the jugular vein four minutes after their intratracheal injection. Guieysse-Pellissier [5] has shown that olive oil is readily absorbed by the respiratory mucosa.

During the course of this investigation an attempt was made to record the comparative antibody production achieved in guinea-pigs and rabbits by the injection of various antigens by diverse routes. Thus, agglutinin production after intraperitoneal, intravenous, and intratracheal injections of B. typhosus and B. dysenteriae (Flexner) was studied; production of precipitins for horse and human serums, of lysins for sheep and human red blood cells, and of bacteriolysins and bactericidins for Vibrion cholerae were similarly investigated.

Received for publication Oct. 24, 1921.

[1] Ann. de l'Inst. Pasteur, 1919, 33, p. 882; 1920, 34, p. 361.
[2] Ibid., 1921, 35, p. 237.
[3] Halliburton, Handbook of Phys., 1905.
[4] Traite de Phys. Comp., 1888.
[5] Congress de Phys., 1920.

METHODS

The animals used throughout the experiments were full grown healthy rabbits and guinea-pigs that had been isolated in thoroughly cleansed pens for three weeks before being used.

All bacterial antigens were prepared by suspending 48-hour agar growths of the various organisms in normal salt solution. No attempts at standardization of these suspensions were made, inoculations being accomplished with such unkilled suspensions and with organisms killed by 60 C. as indicated in the protocols.

Horse and human serums were obtained by venipuncture and diluted with equal parts of normal salt solution before inoculation; no preservatives were added, the various portions of such serum being aseptically handled and stored at 40 C.

Sheep cells and human cells were secured in the usual manner and washed 6 times with normal salt solution, 10% suspensions being used for inoculation.

Agglutination tests were made macroscopically with living organisms, the usual precautions as to control for each dilution in the presence of homologous serum being always observed. Final readings were made after 2 hours at 45 C. and overnight in the icebox. Precipitins were demonstrated by overlaying 0.2 c c portions of various dilutions of the serum to be tested with the antigen in question. Readings were made after 45 minutes at room temperature (25-35 C.). The hemolytic titer of serums was determined by allowing decreasing dilutions of serum to be tested to act on 0.5 c c portions of alexin (guinea-pig serum 1: 10) and 5% washed homologous erythrocytes. Final readings were made after 2 hours at 45 C. and after over night in the icebox. Bacteriolysins were studied by causing various dilutions of serum to be in contact with salt suspensions of viable organisms in the peritoneal cavity of normal guinea-pigs. Stained and unstained preparations of material secured by peritoneal puncture of such animals at varying intervals were observed, the technic being essentially that of Pfeiffer. Agar poured plates were also prepared with immune serum; in this manner relative determination of bactericidal power of serums was possible.

Intravenous and intraperitoneal inoculations were made in the usual manner. Intratracheal inoculations were made under ether anesthesia; the skin of the neck was incised in the midline and the trachea exposed. After steadying the trachea, the inoculating needle (usually a 24 gage)

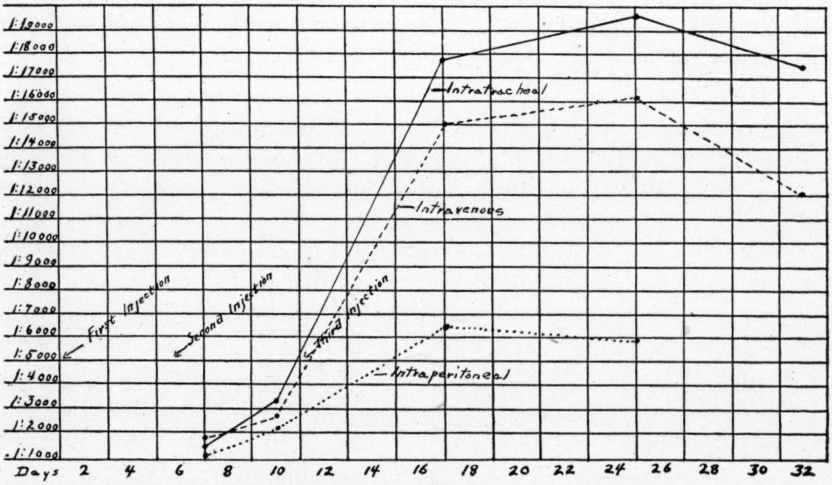

Chart 1.—Production of agglutinin for B. typhosus.

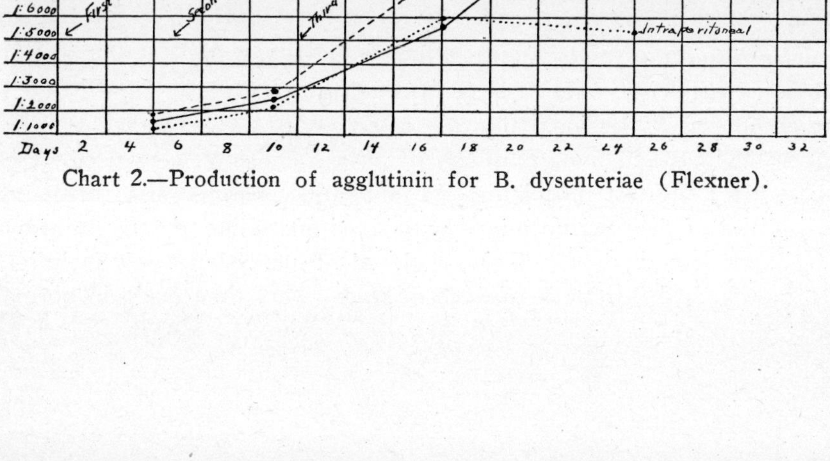

Chart 2.—Production of agglutinin for B. dysenteriae (Flexner).

was thrust into the organ between the cartilaginous rings, and the inoculating material introduced slowly. By this method 15 c c of fluid were readily injected into the trachea of full grown rabbits, with no inconvenience to the animal. The wounds were iodinized and the lips held together by a single catgut suture.

EXPERIMENTAL

Agglutinins.—For the production of these antibodies two bacterial species were employed, namely, B. typhosus and B. dysenteriae (Flexner). With each antigen 9 rabbits were injected, 3 intraperitoneally, 3 intratracheally and 3 intravenously, with intervals of 5 days between the inoculations. The first inoculation consisted of one half agar slant killed organisms, the second and third inoculations of one agar slant live organisms. Four days after the first, 4 days after the second, 6, 14 and 21 days after the last, inoculations the agglutinating power of the various serums was determined. Charts 1 and 2 illustrate the results obtained.

Precipitins.—Human and horse serums were employed as antigens, 9 rabbits being used for each type of serum. Three intraperitoneal, intravenous and intratracheal inoculations of 4 c c of serum diluted with equal parts of normal salt solution were made at intervals of 6 days. Precipitin content of the immune serum was determined 5 days after the first and second injections and 5, 10, and 20 days after the last injection (charts 3 and 4).

Hemolysins.—Here again 3 series of 3 rabbits each were used for intraperitoneal, intravenous and intratracheal injections of sheep and human erythrocytes. Four c c of 10% suspensions were inoculated at 6 day intervals on 3 different occasions. The hemolytic power of the serum was determined 5 days after the first inoculation, 5 days after the second inoculation and 5, 10, 20 and 40 days after the last inoculation (charts 5 and 6).

Bacteriolysins and Bactericidins.—Six guinea-pigs were used in these experiments. Three were injected intraperitoneally and 3 intratracheally on 3 occasions, allowing 6 days to elapse between the injections. Killed and living cultures of Vibrio cholerae were used. Six days after the last inoculation the animals were bled and increasing quantities of their serum mixed with fixed quantities of actively growing agar cultures of Vibrio cholerae suspended in salt solution. Intraperitoneal injections of such mixtures were then made in normal guinea-pigs, and at suitable intervals portions of the peritoneal exudates were secured for study along the lines indicated by Pfeiffer. In addition, plating of mixtures of actively growing cultures and immune serums were made (table 1).

TABLE 1

BACTERIOLYTIC AND BACTERICIDAL POWERS OF PRODUCED SERUMS

Guinea-Pigs	Method of Inoculation	Hanging Drop Preparation of Peritoneal Fluid After Intraperitoneal Inoculation of 2 C c Actively Growing Bouillon Culture V. Cholera		Stained Preparation of Peritoneal Fluid After Intraperitoneal Inoculation of 2 C c Actively Growing Bouillon Culture V. Cholera		Colonies per C c 24-Hour Agar Plates (1 C c Serum + 1 C c 24 Hr. Bouillon Culture Plated After 4 Hours Incubation)
		Fluid Removed 30 Minutes After Inoculation	Fluid Removed 60 Minutes After Inoculation	Fluid Removed 30 Minutes After Inoculation	Fluid Removed 60 Minutes After Inoculation	
1	Intraperitoneal	Few motile forms; few granular organisms.	No motile forms; granular, disintegrating organisms only	Many bizarre shaped granular organisms; few comma shaped forms	Many granular organisms	110,000
2	Intraperitoneal	Few motile forms; few granular organisms	Markedly granular forms only	Many bizarre shaped granular organisms-few comma shaped forms	Few granular rod shaped organisms	225,000
3	Intraperitoneal	No motile forms; granular organisms only	No organisms recognizable	Many granular forms; occasional normal appearing organisms	No organisms recognizable	360,000
4	Intraperitoneal	Many motile organisms; few granular forms	Occasional motile organisms; most forms granular	Many normal appearing organisms; few granular forms	Few comma shaped forms; many attenuated granular organisms	98,000
5	Intratracheal	Many granular forms only	No organisms recognizable	Granular rod shaped organisms only	No organisms recognizable	100,000
6	Intratracheal	Many granular forms only	No organisms recognizable	Granular rod shaped organisms only	No organisms recognizable	1,000
7	Intratracheal	Organisms completely disintegrated	No organisms recognizable	Few granular attenuated rod shaped organisms	No organisms recognizable	55,000
8	Intratracheal	Organisms completely disintegrated	No organisms recognizable	Few granular attenuated rod shaped organisms	No organisms recognizable	162,000
9	Control	Actively motile, comma shaped organisms	Actively motile, comma shaped organisms	Organisms present; no morphologic changes	Organisms present; no morphologic changes	Innumerable

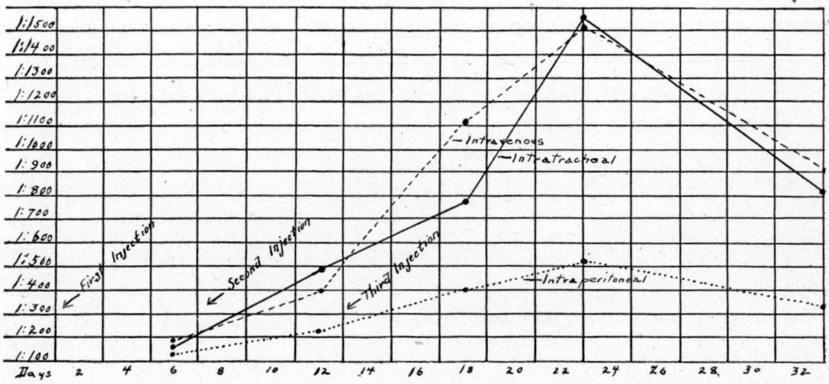

Chart 3.—Production of precipitin for human serum.

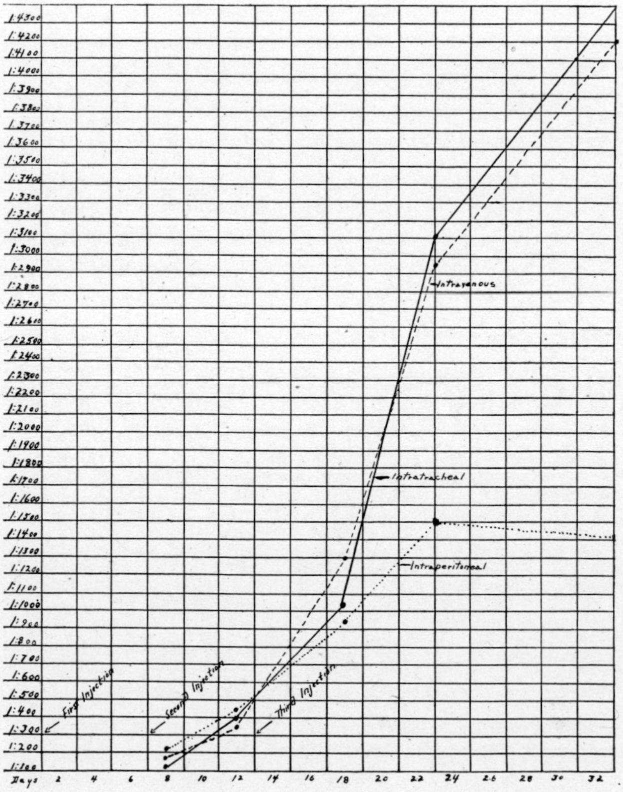

Chart 4.—Production of precipitin for horse serum.

DISCUSSION

The data secured shows that the agglutinins produced by the intratracheal innoculation of B. typhosus appear in as large quantities and as early as when the intravenous route for injection is chosen. Considerably more of these immune bodies can be demonstrated after intratracheal inoculations than after intraperitoneal injections of similar amounts of antigen. Of the 3 animals inoculated intraperitoneally, the average agglutinin titer, 14 and 21 days after the last injection of antigen, was 1 : 5,200 and 1 : 3,500 with averages of 1 : 15,000 and 1 : 11,000 for the one surviving animal after intravenous injection and averages of 18,600 and 16,600 for the 3 animals injected intratracheally. Although 2 animals injected intravenously succumbed with no discernible lesions at necropsy, as happens so frequently with rabbits used for production of antiserum, no deaths occurred in the series inoculated intratracheally. With B. dysenteriae (Flexner) as antigen the results obtained were practically similar to those for B. typhosus. Here the average agglutinating titer, 14 and 21 days after intraperitoneal injections was 4,500 and 4,800 for 3 animals in comparison with 14,500 and 13,000 for 2 animals after intravenous injections and 11,000 and 11,000 for 3 animals following intratracheal inoculations. It would then appear to be fairly well established that for certain organisms, agglutinins can be produced by intratracheal inoculations with results, judged by titer of serums and time of appearance of immune bodies, as good and probably with more safety than by intravenous injections.

With precipitin production the results secured after intratracheal injection were generally as good as those following intravenous inoculations. Here the titer of intravenously produced antihuman serums averaged 1,500 and 800, 10 and 20 days after final injections as compared to averages of 1 : 1,500 and 1 : 700 for intratracheally produced serums. After injections of horse serum the comparative titers were 1 : 2,800 and 1 : 4,100 for intravenous serums and 1 : 3,000 and 1 : 4,300 for intratracheal serums, 10 and 20 days, respectively, after injections of similar doses of antigen. With both of these antigens intraperitoneal injections consistently resulted in serum of very low precipitin titer.

For hemolysins produced by human and sheep erythrocytes; the results were slightly different. Consistently these antibodies would appear in lesser amounts and later in the animals injected intratracheally than in those injected intravenously. The ultimate titers, however, of the serums were practically identical. Thus the average titer for 3 animals injected intratracheally with human cells 5, 10, 20

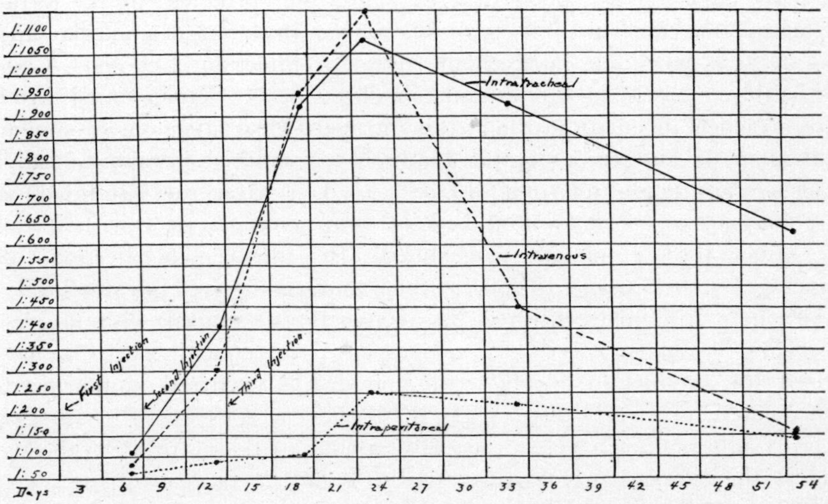

Chart 5.—Production of hemolysin for human erythrocytes.

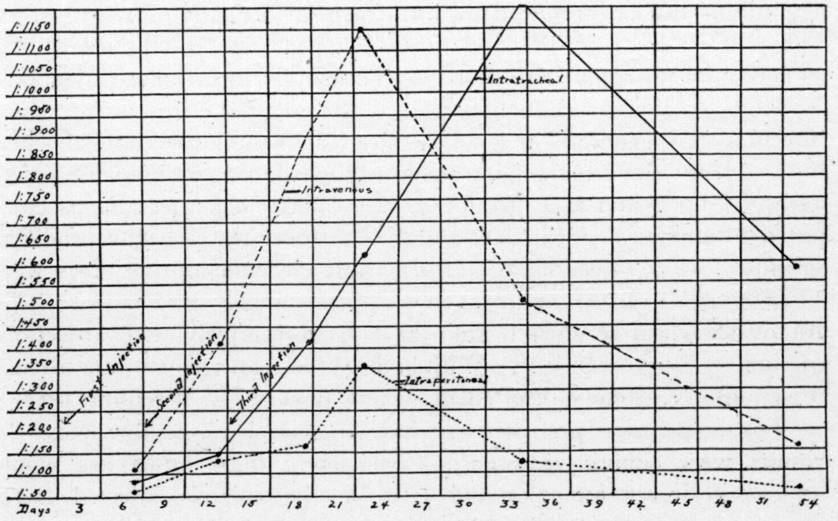

Chart 6.—Production of hemolysin for sheep erythrocytes.

and 40 days after the last inoculation were 1:860, 1:1,030, 1:860 and 1:560 as compared to averages of 1:900, 1:1,100, 1:400, 1:100 obtained for one animal successfully injected intravenously. With sheep cells, the averages for 3 animals injected in the vein were 1:830, 1:1,100, 1:460 and 1:100 as compared with averages of 1:360, 1:560, 1:1,160 and 1:530 for the intratracheally injected animals, 5, 10, 20 and 40 days after final injections. Again it is to be noted that no accidents occurred in the series of animals injected intratracheally with human erythrocytes in contradistinction to the 2 fatalities reported after intravenous injection and the well-known accidents so often attendant on the intracirculatory injection of heterogenous hemic material.

The production of bacteriolysins and bactericidins after intratracheal injections of Bibrio cholerae compares most favorably with the production noted after intravenous injections of these organisms. Most of the animals in the intratracheally inoculated series produced lytic serum far more powerful and possessing bactericidal powers far more marked than did the animals injected intravenously.

The practicability of antibody production by intratracheal injections of some antigens seems established. That such a method may offer decided advantages in the production of antiserum for organisms to which ordinary laboratory animals are highly susceptible seems plausible. Again, in the production of lytic serums, especially for human erythrocytes, the method appears to be especially promising.

CONCLUSIONS

Antibodies are produced in animals by the intratracheal inoculation of various antigens.

Agglutinins for B. typhosus and B. dysenteriae are as readily produced by this method as by the intravenous method.

Precipitins can be demonstrated in as high titer in animals injected intratracheally with human and horse serums as when such injections are made intravenously.

Lysins for human and sheep erythrocytes are produced by intratracheal injections, but such production requires a greater length of time before being evidenced than following the intravenous injections of similar quantities of antigens.

Bacteriolysins for Vibrio cholera are elaborated earlier and in larger quantities following intratracheal injections than following intraperitoneal injections.

No fatal results followed attempts at producing various antibodies by intratracheal methods.

The further study of this apparently safe and efficient method of antibody production is suggested especially with virulent organisms for which the ordinary laboratory animals are highly susceptible as antigens.

A STUDY OF AMMONIA PRODUCTION BY A CERTAIN STRAIN OF AVIRULENT HUMAN TUBERCLE BACILLUS

Alfred W. Bosworth; Marion G. Elkins,

and

Marguerite E. Blanchard

The Boston Floating Hospital, Boston

Kendall, Day and Walker[1] say: "A study of the nitrogenous metabolism of certain rapidly growing acid-fast bacteria, so-called saprophytic human tubercle bacilli, in plain glucose, mannitol and glycerol broths, revealed the fact that the organisms produced moderate amounts of ammonia. . . . The maximum production of ammonia was reached about the third week in plain glucose and mannitol cultures, the reaction becoming progressively alkaline during this period. In glycerol medium, on the other hand, the increase in ammonia was progressive to the fourth week, although the rate of production was slower and the reaction became acid, contrasting sharply in this respect with the alkalinity of the other cultures. The ammonia curve gradually diminished from the maximum, particularly in plain, glucose and mannitol mediums, until scarcely half the amount remained in solution at the end of the sixth week. . . . A definite explanation for this phenomenon of waxing and waning of ammonia production is not apparent, but available evidence points to a coincidence between luxuriance of growth and ammonia increase followed by autolysis of the organisms and a decrease in ammonia." They go on to state that "total nitrogen determinations of the bacteria-free cultures show a small but unmistakable decrease at the height of bacterial development, indicating the incorporation of this element in the bacterial bodies, followed later by an increase in nitrogen, suggesting a gradual autolysis of the organisms with the liberation of some of the nitrogen in soluble form."

In this connection Kendall, Day and Walker apparently have not determined the total nitrogen of the bacterial bodies themselves (merely of the clear underlying broth) to see whether there actually was an increase in the nitrogen content of the bacteria which would be necessary to prove their statement.

In our first experiment the organism was inoculated into a sufficient number of Erlenmeyer flasks, each containing 100 c c of 1% dextrose broth, so that duplicate flasks could be studied at weekly intervals for a period of 6 weeks. In this and the following experiments an avirulent culture of the tubercle bacillus obtained from the American Museum of Natural History, New York, designated as "597" was

Received for publication Oct. 28, 1921.

[1] Jour. Infect. Dis., 1920, 26, p. 45.

used. The analysis comprised the determination of a titratable reaction using phenolphthalein as an indicator, the measure of ammonia by Folin's method, the determination of the total nitrogen content of the medium plus the bacterial growth in contrast to Kendall's method of determining only the total nitrogen in the bacterial free broth.[2]

The data obtained are given in table 1, and bring out the following points: The medium, which is acid toward phenolphthalein at the beginning of the experiment, gradually undergoes a change in reaction until it becomes quite strongly alkaline toward phenolphthalein. After the medium becomes alkaline the ammonia and the total nitrogen contents both decrease. The steady gradual decrease in the amount of nitrogen in the total contents of the flasks shows that the loss of nitrogen noted by Kendall, Day and Walker, cannot be wholly attributed to the incorporation of nitrogen within the bacilli.

TABLE 1

Metabolism of Tubercle Bacillus

	Dextrose Broth			Glycerol Broth		
Age in Days	Reaction Toward Phenol-phthalein	Total Nitrogen	Nitrogen Present as Ammonia	Reaction Toward Phenol-phthalein	Total Nitrogen	Nitrogen Present as Ammonia
Control	+1.8*	0.3346	......	+1.00	0.3892	
7	+0.8	0.3206	0.0300	+0.9	0.3547	0.0243
14	−2.0	0.2905	0.0435	+1.7	0.3554	0.0238
21	−3.0	0.2748	0.0120	+0.5	0.3561	0.0305
28	−2.3	0.2619	0.0020	+0.6	0.3511	0.0282
35	.....	0.2459	0.0025	No reading made	0.3512	0.0252
42	.....	0.2213	......	No reading made	0.3270	0.0242

* Figures represent the acidity (+) or alkalinity (−) of 100 c c of medium expressed as cubic centimeters of normal acid or alkali.

A similar experiment was made with glycerol broth as a medium and these data also are given in table 1. In this case the acid reaction of the medium persisted longer than in the case of the dextrose broth. The total nitrogen content remains constant during this period of acid reaction while the ammonia content increased during the same period. When the amount of total nitrogen began to decrease the ammonia also began to decrease. Unfortunately the inadvertent absence of the reaction data does not permit us to determine in this instance whether the decrease of total nitrogen and loss of ammonia are coincident with

[2] Ibid., 1914, 15, p. 423.

the advent of an alkaline reaction of the medium. Experiments reported in another table in this paper, however, show this to be the case.

From the results obtained with dextrose broth we were led to suspect that the decrease in the nitrogen and ammonia contents was due simply to volatilization of ammonia caused by the alkaline reaction of the medium and the heat of the incubator. If nitrogen were lost in this fashion, the trapping and measuring of the escaping ammonia would prove or disprove this assumption. In order to do this the following experiments were performed:

Four culture mediums were used, plain broth, 1% mannitol broth, 1% dextrose broth and 3% glycerol broth. The plain broth (sugar-free broth made from meat juice) was used as a basis for the other 3. The apparatus for growing the organism and collecting the volatilized ammonia was set up

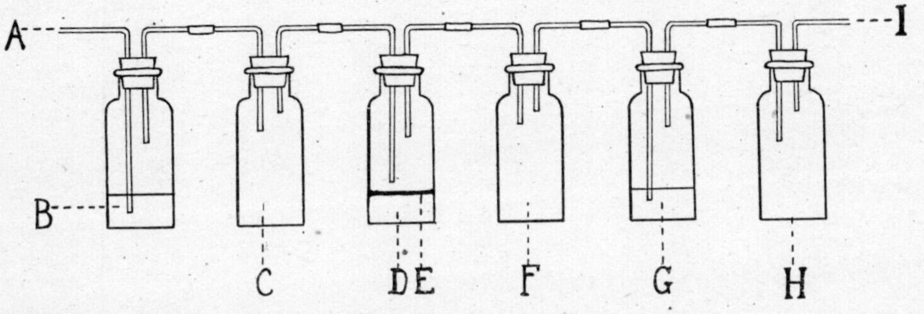

Fig. 1.—A, open to air; B, diluted sulphuric acid (5%); C, empty bottle; D, culture medium; E, pellicle; F, empty bottle to save culture from possible back flow of acid; G, trap bottle containing standardized acid; H, empty trap bottle connected with suction pump at I. (Any number of sets, D, F. G, may be inserted in the series.)

in the following manner: 18 clean and sterile 8 ounce, wide mouthed bottles, each containing 50 c c of culture medium were inoculated with the bacillus; 18 similar bottles, each containing 15 c c of normal hydrochloric acid, 40 c c of distilled water (or sufficient water to cover the end of the glass tube), and 3 drops of alizarin, were paired with the culture bottles and connected by means of glass tubes and rubber stoppers. The 36 bottles, culture and acid bottles alternating, were then connected with each other in an incubator kept at a temperature of 37, one terminal joined to a wash bottle containing diluted sulphuric acid and the other terminal to a suction pump. In this manner a constant stream of ammonia free air passed over the cultures, at the same time drawing any volatilized ammonia from each culture bottle into the succeeding acid trap bottle.

The experiment was set up to cover a period of 6 weeks, 3 pairs of bottles being removed each week. The acid in each trap bottle was titrated with standard sodium hydroxide to determine the amount of volatilized ammonia which had been trapped. The contents of 2 culture bottles were used for total nitrogen determinations in duplicate according to the Kjeldahl method. It may be noted here that the entire contents of the bottles, broth and pellicle, were used. From the third culture bottle were taken two 10 c c portions of the medium for duplicate ammonia determinations according to the Folin air method, and portions for the determination of the reaction of the medium toward phenolphthalein and alizarin. The data collected are summarized in table 2.

TABLE 2

Ammonia Production by Tubercle Bacillus in Plain, Dextrose, Mannitol and Glycerol Broths

Age in Days	Broths	Reaction Toward Alizarin	Reaction Toward Phenolphthalein	1 Grams Nitrogen in Culture Bottle	2 Grams Nitrogen Caught in Trap as Ammonia	3 Total Nitrogen 1 + 2	4 Grams Nitrogen in Medium as Ammonia	5 Total Ammonia Produced by Organism in Terms of Nitrogen 2 + 4
Control	Plain.......	—3.0*	+1.7*	0.1937	0	0.1937		
	Dextrose...	—3.05	+1.2	0.1563		0.1563		
	Mannitol...	—3.0	+1.6	0.2098		0.2098		
	Glycerol....	—4.0	+0.5	0.1836		0.1836		
7	Plain.......	—6.4	—0.75	0.1901	0.0031	0.1932	0.0266	0.0297
	Dextrose...	—5.1	—1.2	0.1602?	0.0065	0.1667?	0.0202	0.0267
	Mannitol...	—4.8	—0.2	0.2062	0.0031	0.2093	0.0185	0.0216
	Glycerol....	—3.9	0.00	0.1752	0.0074	0.1826	0.0021	0.0095
14	Plain.......	—5.5	—1.7	0.1611	0.0338	0.1949	0.0168	0.0506
	Dextrose....	—6.1	—1.1	0.1359	0.0204	0.1563	0.0239	0.0443
	Mannitol...	—6.8	—1.2	0.2091?	0.0023	0.2114?	0.0261	0.0284
	Glycarol....	—5.1	—0.8	0.1830	0.0041	0.1875	0.0056	0.0097
21	Plain.......	—7.8	—1.2	0.1539	0.0402	0.1941	0.0360	0.0762
	Dextrose....	—6.2	—1.35	0.1325	0.0234	0.1559	0.0221	0.0455
	Mannitol...	—8.8	—1.0	0.2005	0.0094	0.2099	0.0396	0.0490
	Glycerol....	—4.4	—0.75	0.1834	0.0031	0.1865	0.0084	0.0115
28	Plain.......	—6.2	—1.1	0.1367	0.0567	0.1934	0.0208	0.0775
	Dextrose....	—4.6	—1.2	0.1121	0.0439	0.1560	0.0029	0.0468
	Mannitol...	—6.35	—0.95	0.1644	0.0463	0.2107	0.0136	0.0599
	Glycerol...	.....	.....	......	......	......	......	......
35	Plain.......	—7.7	—0.2	0.1329	0.0607	0.1936	0.0229	0.0836
	Dextrose....	—3.9	—0.9	0.1111	0.0460	0.1570	0.0035	0.0495
	Mannitol...	—4.45	—1.05	0.1386	0.0743	0.2129	0.0010	0.0753
	Glycerol....	—4.9	—1.2	0.1737	0.0135	0.1872	0.0155	0.0290
42	Plain.......	—5.0	—1.0	......	0.0744	......	0.0044	0.0826
	Dextrose....	—4.3	—0.8	0.1118	0.0440	0.1558	0.0028	0.0468
	Mannitol..	.....	.....	......	......	......	......	......
	Glycerol....	—4.6	—0.4	......	0.0409	......	0.0242	0.0651

* Figures represent the acidity (+) or alkalinity (—) of 100 c c of medium expressed as cubic centimeters of normal acid or alkali.

Reaction.—The reaction of the medium to phenolphthalein is variably alkaline in every case, though the mediums were at first acid. The alkalinity of the glycerol broth during the activity of the bacilli is at variance with the results obtained by Kendall [2] for saprophytic human tubercle bacilli and the Theobald Smith [3] reaction, according to

[3] Am. Jour. Med. Sc., 1904, 128, p. 216.

which human tubercle bacilli cultures become pronouncedly acid in glycerol broth. It also differs from the results obtained in our first experiment (table 1).

Total Nitrogen.—Our suspicion in regard to the evaporation of ammonia seems to have been justified. A study of the accompanying table shows that in every case, with the exception of the glycerol broth, there is a decrease, from week to week, in total nitrogen content of the bottles (clear broth and pellicle). Accompanying the loss of nitrogen from the bottles there is a compensating increase of nitrogen (in the form of ammonia) in the acid of the trap bottles. This simple statement scarcely needs any elaboration. It is most clearly shown in the experiment with plain broth as a medium, but it is just as evident in the other cases.

Ammonia Production.—If we consider the production of ammonia in the culture medium alone, we find, except in the case of glycerol broth, the "waxing and waning" phenomenon noted by Kendall. However, the total ammonia actually produced by the organism must be sought for both in the culture medium and in the acid of the trap bottle. The sum of these two ammonias will reveal the true ammonia production of the tubercle bacillus. We have expressed it in terms of grams of nitrogen. In no case do we find a fall in the ammonia curve. The maximum amount is produced in plain broth, with mannitol broth a close second; the least is found in dextrose broth. While there is a steady increase in total ammonia in plain broth, mannitol broth and glycerol broth, in dextrose broth there seems to be little increase after the fifteenth day. In glycerol broth the early production of ammonia is very slight.

SUMMARY

A study of the nitrogenous metabolism, during six weeks, of a certain avirulent culture of human tubercle bacilli revealed the fact that there is a continuous production of ammonia in plain, dextrose, mannitol and glycerol broths.

Over 30% of the nitrogen originally present in the medium may be converted to ammonia.

The ammonia produced is partly retained in the medium but the greater part is lost through volatilization.

The loss of ammonia is coincident with an alkaline reaction of the medium.

There was no recession in the production of ammonia by the organisms during the period covered by our experiments (6 weeks).

The "waxing and waning" of ammonia as noticed by Kendall is due to two factors: a continuous production of ammonia by the organism, and a loss of ammonia from the medium into the air by volatilization.

So long as the medium remains acid (see especially the glycerol broth) both the total nitrogen and the ammonia contents of the broth show no decrease.

When the broth becomes alkaline both the total nitrogen and ammonia contents show a decrease.

If ammonia is utilized by the tubercle bacilli the amount is extremely small in comparison with the amount lost by volatilization.

THE INHIBITORY ACTION OF CERTAIN ORGANIC MERCURY COMPOUNDS ON THE GROWTH OF HUMAN TUBERCLE BACILLI

STUDIES ON THE BIOCHEMISTRY AND CHEMOTHERAPY OF TUBERCULOSIS. XXII

LYDIA M. DEWITT

From the Otho S. A. Sprague Memorial Institute and the Pathological Laboratory of the University of Chicago

Of all the chemicals so far tested by me during my study of the chemotherapy of tuberculosis, certain organic compounds of mercury have been found the most promising. About a year ago, a report [1] was made of the results so far obtained with about 20 mercury compounds used in experimental tuberculosis and the present report is based on work with 10 organic mercury compounds of phenol, nitro and nitroso phenols and saligenin or phenol carbinol; also on work with about 14 organic mercury compounds of aniline, the nitranilins, and methyl and ethyl anilins and nitranilins. A few other mercury compounds of the benzene nucleus have been used and the results are included in this report. Most of these preparations have been made for me in the Chemical Laboratory of the University of Chicago by Maurice Kharasch, Isadore Jacobsohn and Lyman Chalkley, to all of whom I am indebted for faithfulness and interest.

While my experiments with the organic mercurials were proceeding, Schamberg, Kolmer and Raiziss [2] published a report of a mercurial preparation made by them and called mercurophen or oxy-mercury-ortho-nitro phenolate. This is an interesting compound since it is freely soluble, contains about 53% of mercury, yet is several times as germicidal as mercuric chloride which contains 74% of mercury. Its phenol coefficient for different organisms is from 700 to 3,600 and even 10,000 in some reports. It is nonirritant to the skin, does not tarnish metallic instruments and is much less toxic than mercuric chloride. It was represented as especially valuable for the sterilization of the hands, skin, instruments, tubes, etc.[3] Since some of this compound was sent to me through the kindness of Dr. Schamberg, and since it is of the same type as some of my mercury nitro-phenol compounds, it was tested in the same way and is included in table 1 of this report.

In 1919, Young, White and Schwartz [4] developed an organic mercury compound of the dye fluorescein and called it mercurochrome-220. It contains

Received for publication Oct. 29, 1921.

[1] Jour. Infect. Dis., 1921, 28, p. 150.

[2] Ibid., 1919, 24, p. 547.

[3] Jour. Am. Med. Assn., 1917, 68, p. 1458.

[4] Ibid., 1919, 73, p. 1483. Lancaster, Burnett and Gaus: Ibid., 1920, 75, p. 721. Jour. Urol., 1921, 5, p. 353.

about 26% of mercury, is readily soluble and quite nonirritant and nontoxic. It kills B. coli in 15 minutes in a dilution of 1:5,000 and staphylococcus in a dilution of 1:10,000. It has been used with good effect in washing[4] out infected bladders, in open wounds, sinuses, and in treatment of infections of the throat, nose, ear and eye. Although unlike the other preparations here reported, it is, with mercurochrome 205 and 253, samples of which were also sent me by the kindness of Dr. White, included in table 3 of this report. A preliminary report on mercurophen and mercurochrome 220 in their action on tubercle bacilli and on experimental tuberculosis was made by me about a year ago.[5]

Hirschfelder[6] has made several organic mercury compounds of saligenin or phenol carbinol and has kindly furnished me with quantities sufficient for testing in my work. The results of my tests with these compounds also will be found in table 1.

In all my chemotherapeutic work it has been my custom to test first the power of the chemical being studied to inhibit the growth of the human tubercle bacillus in the test tube, not because we believe that therapeutic value is necessarily closely associated with inhibitory efficiency, but because it is the simplest method of getting a "lead" on the possible value of the compound and the advisability of testing it further. The chemicals which show a high inhibitory power are afterward tested on animals for their bactericidal and therapeutic efficiency. This paper reports only the inhibitory experiments. In every case, human tubercle bacilli of different degrees of virulence have been used, so that many of the tests have been repeated ten or twelve times. The tables give the extremes of variation when the different tests gave different results.

My method has been to add to tubes containing 10 c c of a sterile glycerol agar enough of the compound or of a stock solution of the compound to make dilutions from 1:100 up to 1:1,000,000. The tubes were then well shaken, slanted, cooled, and inoculated; they were examined after 15 days in the incubator, again after 30 days, and sometimes again after 45 days. The highest dilutions on which there was no growth at the end of the longest period allowed is recorded as the limit of "complete inhibition."

The mercury compounds of phenol in this table are all soluble in an alkaline solution so dilute that it does not itself prevent the growth of tubercle bacilli. Phenol itself has been found to inhibit growth of the human tubercle bacillus in a dilution of 1:1,000 but not at 1:5,000. Phenol with HgCl in the ortho position is 100 times as efficient in the

[5] Jour. Am. Med. Assn., 1920, 75, p. 1422.
[6] Jour. Am. Chem. Soc., 1920, 42, p. 2678.

TABLE 1

PHENOLS

Name	Formula	Percentage of Mercury	Complete Inhibition
Phenol	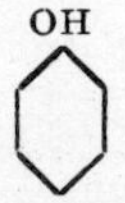	0	1: 1,000
Phenol o–mercuric chloride	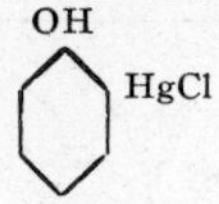	64.07	1: 100,000
Ortho–nitro phenol	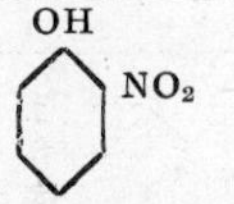		1: 40,000 to 1: 50,000
Meta–nitro phenol	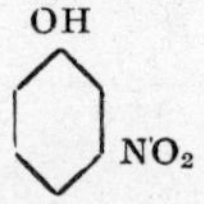		1: 5,000
Para–nitro phenol	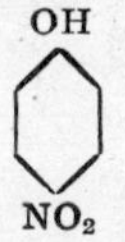		1: 10,000 to 1: 20,000
Mercurophen Sodium o–nitro Phenol p–mercuric hydroxide	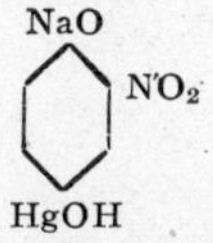	52.8	1: 50,000 to 1: 80,000
No. 9 Sodium p–nitro phenol o–mercuric chloride	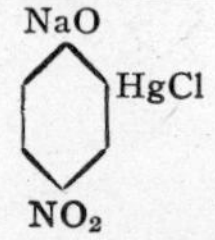	52.8	1: 50,000 to 1: 100,000
No. 15 2,2′ mercuric bis p–nitro phenol	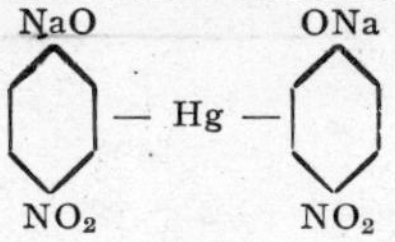	42	1: 100,000
P–nitroso phenol	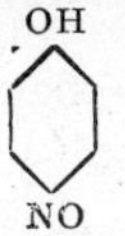		1: 1,000 to 1: 5,000

TABLE 1—*Continued*

Phenols

Name	Formula	Percentage of Mercury	Complete Inhibition
P–nitroso phenol O–mercuric chloride	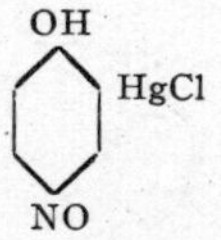	55.9	1: 80,000 to 1: 100,000
No. 20 2,2′ hydroxy 4–nitroso–mercury diphenyl	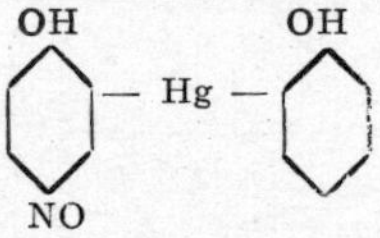	48.2	1: 100,000 to 1: 300,000
Saligenin phenol o–carbinol	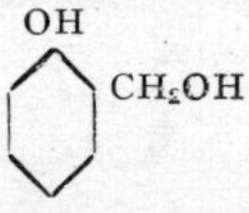		1: 1,000
Phenol o–carbinol 2, 4 mercuric acetate	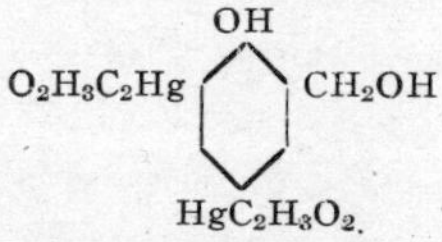	45.5	1: 20,000
Phenol o–carbinol 2, 4 mercuric hydroxide	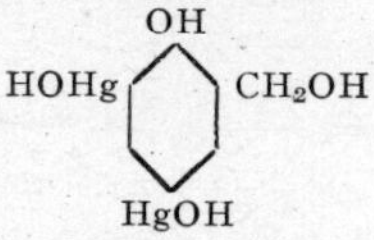	74.4	1: 50,000 to 1: 60,000
O–nitro phenol P–carbinol O–mercuric acetate	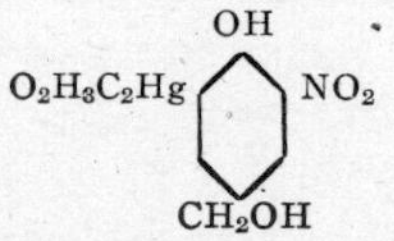	46.9	1: 100,000

prevention of growth of the human tubercle bacillus as phenol and two and one half times as efficient as mercuric chloride, which inhibits in a dilution of 1:40,000. We find that the nitro-phenols are more efficient than phenol, the ortho-nitro-phenol being from 40 to 50 times as strong, the para-nitro-phenol from 10 to 20 times as strong and meta-nitro-phenol only 5 times as strong in its inhibitory action on the tubercle bacillus. The quinoidal change which is supposed to take place in the phenol molecule on the substitution of NO_2 for hydrogen probably accounts for this, since that change occurs most readily with NO_2 in the ortho position and least readily with it in the para position

Mercurophen and Na9 are isomers and the ortho position of the mercury in the latter seems more favorable than the para position. Na15 in which mercury forms a bridge between two sodium nitro phenols is stronger in its action than either of the other compounds, although its content of mercury is considerably less. In this, also, the bridge occupies the ortho position. Although p-nitroso phenol has lower inhibitory power than p-nitro-phenol, p-nitroso-phenol o-mercuric chloride has about the same power as Na9 which has the same chemical formula except that it has NO_2 in place of NO. Number 20, in which a phenol ring is substituted for the Cl and is connected to the p-nitroso-phenol by a mercury bridge in the ortho position, has greater inhibitory power than any of the other phenol compounds so far studied. The mercury saligenin compounds inhibited at from 1 : 20,000 to 1 : 60,000, although containing 45 to 74% of mercury, while the saligenin mercury compound which had one nitro group in the ortho position completely inhibits at 1 : 100,000.

Table 2 contains the results of my inhibitory tests with a number of organic mercury compounds of aniline, nitro-anilines and methyl or ethyl anilines and nitranilines. Most of these compounds are insoluble except in dilute alcohol, which itself has considerable inhibitory power. Several of the mercury aniline and mercury methyl and ethyl anilines were combined with tartaric acid or acetic acid to form salts which are readily soluble in an alkaline solution so dilute that it does not itself check the growth of the organisms. The nitranilines, however, would not form soluble salts with any acids tested. The results as shown in table 2, seem to indicate that the addition of one or two methyl or of one or two ethyl groups does not materially affect the efficiency of these compounds as antiseptics and that the mercury is mostly, if not wholly, responsible for the fact that the mercury compounds of aniline are from 20 to 80 times as strong in their inhibitory action on the tubercle bacillus as aniline itself. On account of their insolubility, it has been necessary to use the nitro-compounds of aniline and mercury in alcoholic solutions, and even in alcohol they have not always been completely soluble down to dilutions of 1 : 1,000. At 1 : 10,000, however, they were soluble and in this dilution, the alcohol was sufficiently dilute to have very little if any antiseptic action, and growth has been completely prevented at 1 : 100,000. The nitro group in the aniline molecule has not increased the inhibitory action of this substance as much as it did that of the phenol molecule, but the increase amounts to 5 to 10 times that of aniline. In the nitranilines, the meta

TABLE 2

Anilines

Name	Formula	Percentage of Mercury	Complete Inhibition
Aniline	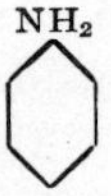	0	1: 1,000
Aniline p–mercuric tartrate	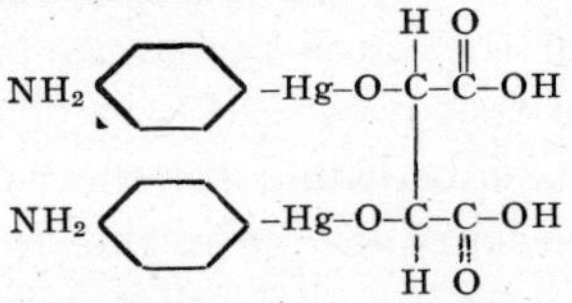	53.9	1: 20,000 to 1: 40,000
Mono methyl aniline p—mercuric tartrate	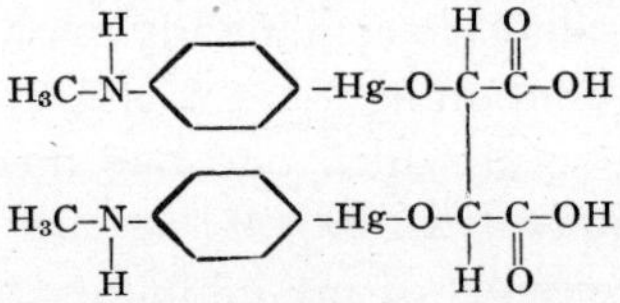	50.7	1: 40,000 to 1: 80,000
Mono ethyl aniline p–mercuric acetate	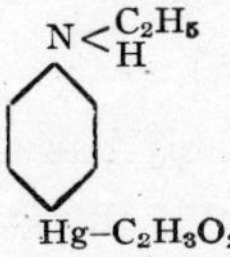	52.8	1: 40.000 to 1: 60,000
40 A di methyl aniline p–mercuric tartrate	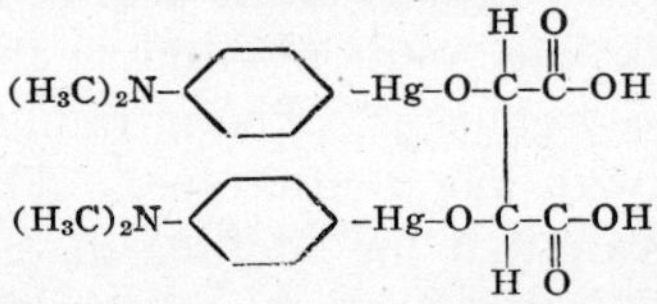	49.1	1: 20,000 to 1: 40,000
No. 37 Di methyl aniline p–mercuric acetamide	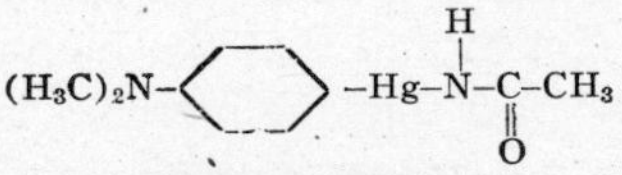	53.0	1: 40,000 to 1: 60,000
4, 4′ mercury bis di methyl aniline	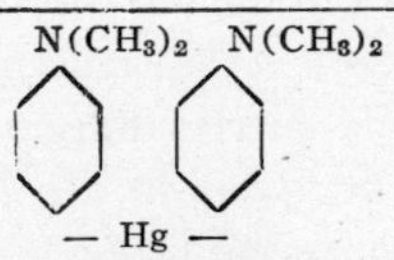	45.5	1: 20,000
Di methyl aniline p–mercuric acetate	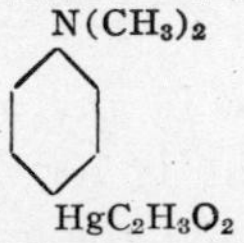	52.8	1: 20,000 to 1: 40,000
O–nitraniline	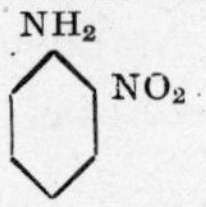	0	1: 5,000

TABLE 2—*Continued*

ANILINES

Name	Formula	Percentage of Mercury	Complete Inhibition
M–nitraniline	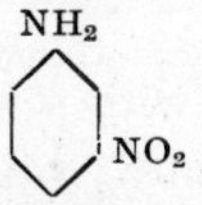	0	1: 10,000
P–nitraniline	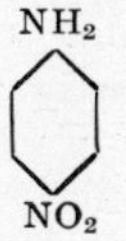	0	1: 1,000 to 1: 5,000
O–nitraniline P–mercuric chloride	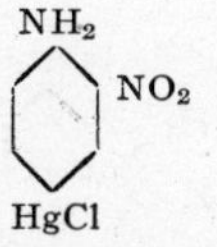	57.8	1: 100,000
M–nitraniline P–mercuric chloride	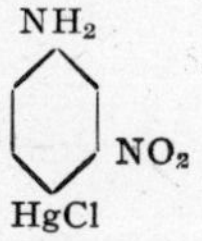	57.8	1: 100,000
P–nitraniline o–mercuric acetate	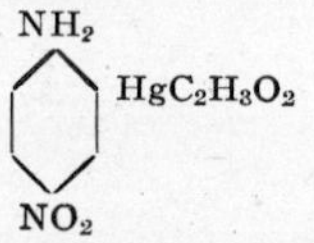	50.6	1: 50,000 to 1: 60,000
(14 M) Mono ethyl p–nitro aniline o–mercuric acetate	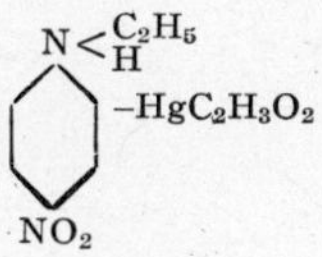	47.2	1: 100,000
No. 26 Di methyl m–nitro aniline p–mercuric acetate	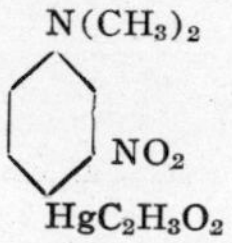	47.2	1: 100,000
No. 27 Di methyl o–nitro aniline p–mercuric acetate	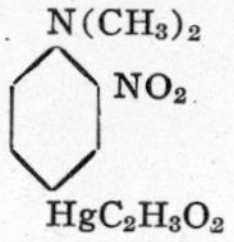	47.2	1: 100,000
No. 29 Mono methyl p–nitraniline o–mercuric acetate	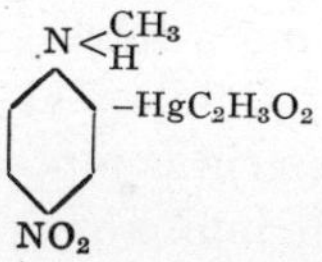	48.8	1: 80,000 to 1: 100,000

position of the nitro group is most favorable instead of the ortho position as in the nitro-phenols. This is probably due to the fact that the quinoidal change in the ring does not easily take place in the aniline molecule.

Table 3 presents my results with several unrelated organic mercury compounds of the benzene nucleus. L. C. 27 is a very soluble mercury

TABLE 3

Other Mercury Compounds of the Benzene Nucleus

Name	Formula	Percentage of Mercury	Complete Inhibition
L. C. 27 Mercuric-bis 3-hydroxy phenyl trimethyl ammonium acetate	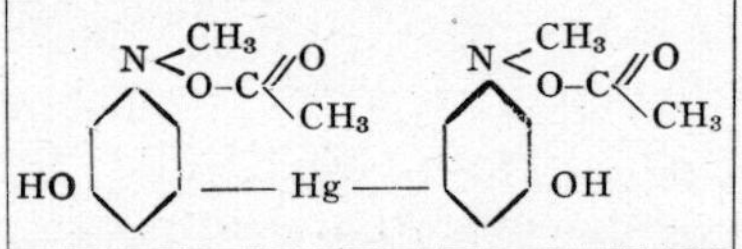	32	1: 1,000 to 1: 5,000
No. 55 Phenoxyl acetic acid o-mercury hydroxide	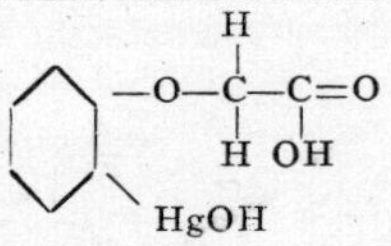	55.2	1: 10,000
No. 62 3 nitro – 4 hydroxyl 5-mercury-hydroxide benzoic acid	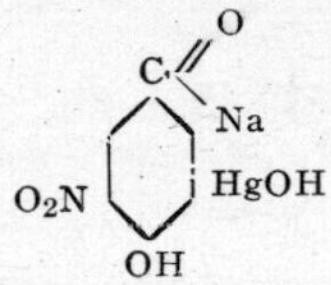	48.2	1: 20,000 to 1: 80,000
Mercurochrome-220	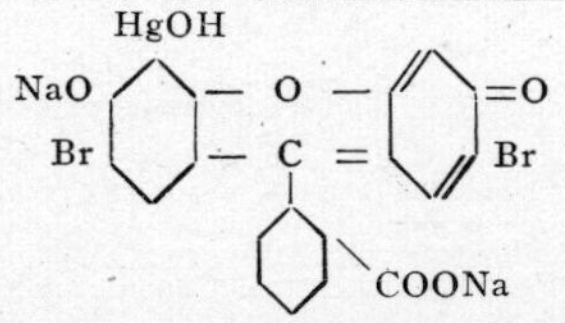	26.7	1: 10,000
Mercurochrome-205			1: 10,000
Mercurochrome-253			1: 10,000

bridge compound containing only 32% of mercury. It shows, however, very little more inhibitory action than phenol. Number 55 is soluble, contains 55% of mercury and inhibits at 10,000, while No. 62, a similar compound but having a nitro group ortho to the hydroxyl and with only 48% of mercury, inhibits at 1:80,000. Three modifications of the mercurialized fluorescein compound made by Young, White and Schwartz all have the same inhibitory power, 1:10,000.

SUMMARY

The power of phenol to inhibit the growth of the human tubercle bacillus is greatly increased by the substitution of a mercury salt in place of one of the hydrogens,—hence a mercury united by one bond to carbon.

It is also increased by the substitution of one NO_2 group for one hydrogen in the ring.

The position of the NO_2 group has much to do with the degree of increase of the inhibitory power, the ortho position being most favorable and the para position next. This is probably due to a quinoidal change in the phenol nucleus.

The position of the mercury group also has much influence on the degree of increase of inhibitory power, the ortho position seeming most favorable.

The mercury bridge compounds seem also to have a high inhibitory power, at least in the two compounds tested, in both of which the bridge occupies the ortho position.

Although saligenin or phenol carbinol has the same inhibitory power as phenol, the mercury derivatives of this have a greatly increased efficiency, varying somewhat with the percentage of mercury; one compound, however which has less mercury but in which both a nitro and a mercury group occupy the ortho position with respect to the hydroxy group, has a higher inhibitory power.

In the aniline compounds also the substitution of a mercury group greatly increases the efficiency.

The nitro group also increases the inhibitory efficiency but not in the same order of position as in the nitro-phenols, since the quinoid change does not readily take place in the aniline nucleus. However, the aniline compounds having the nitro group in the ortho position and the mercury salt in the para position seem more efficient than if the order is reversed.

Methyl and ethyl groups do not materially affect the antiseptic power of the aniline compounds, although these compounds having methyl or ethyl groups plus nitro groups plus mercury groups have a very high antiseptic power, not apparently varying much either with the percentage of mercury or with the relative position of the different groups.

A SORE THROAT EPIDEMIC OF UNUSUAL TYPE

INFLUENZA STUDIES. VIII.

William B. Sharp; John F. Norton,
and
John E. Gordon

From the Department of Hygiene and Bacteriology of the University of Chicago

An unusual disorder involving the upper respiratory tract was observed among the students of the High and Elementary Schools of the University of Chicago during March, 1920, and continued more or less in evidence for the following three months. The condition was noted by the school physician, Dr. Monilaw, to whom we are indebted for valuable assistance in connection with routine throat examinations, first in grades 3 A and 3 B (children 9 to 10 years old), subsequently in grade 2 B (6 to 7 years), in grade 7 B (12 to 13 years) and in many high school students. Subjective symptoms were slight although some of the children at times reported slightly sore or irritated throats with a general loss of ambition. The teachers noticed that during March the younger children were below par physically and less bright than usual. The school quarter was nearing its end, however, and such observations are not infrequent at that time.

Objectively, the children had sometimes a general lassitude, often a degree or two of fever, usually a mild but distinct reddening, more persistent and pronounced than in the average throat, of tonsillar pillars, soft palate, uvula or pharynx and occasionally enlargement of the cervical lymph nodes. In no instance were the tonsils intensely inflamed. The most striking clinical feature and the one which led to our study of what appeared to be an epidemic was the extension of redness along the tonsillar pillars toward the uvula. This redness about the tonsillar region, together with the fact noted in our early laboratory tests that the bacterial growth in material from the tonsils was more abundant than in that from the pharynx, suggested that we were dealing with an unusual chronic tonsillitis, although many of the children gave a history of tonsillectomy.

The Respiratory Disease Commission was asked to investigate grade 2 B from which 9 children were selected for intensive study. This

Received for publication Nov. 2, 1921.

study was extended and to a certain degree controlled by examination of 7 children from grade 3 B in which conditions had been observed similar to those found in grade 2 B, of 7 children from grades 5 and 6 in which conditions were thought to be normal and of 8 high school students who were convalescent from sore throats of a different clinical character than that just described.

Our work with grade 2 B was started on March 17 (1920) and observations were made for 3 consecutive days before the spring vacation (March 20 to April 2) intervened. After the return of the children to school weekly or biweekly examinations were conducted until the close of the spring quarter about the middle of June. A final observation was made after the children resumed their school work in the autumn.

The number of examinations made, together with the laboratory designation of each subject and the location in school was as follows: In Grade 2 B (intensively studied): E 1, 2; E 2, 9; E 3, 10; E 4, 11; E 5, 10; E 6, 7; E 7, 9; E 8, 10; E 9, 9; in Grade 3 B (probably involved in the epidemic): E 25, 1; E 26, 1; E 27, 1; E 28, 1; E 29, 1; E 30, 1; E 31, 1; in Grade 5 A-B (probably normal): E 21, 1; E 22, 1; E 23, 1; E 24, 1; in Grade 6 A-B (probably normal): E 18, 1; E 19, 1; E 20, 1; in high school (sore throat convalescents): E 10, 1; E 11, 1; E 12, 1; E 13, 1; E 14, 1; E 15, 1; E 16, 1; E 17, 1.

The clinical symptoms tended to persist as first observed among the children of grade 2 B. Elevated temperature was found in all cases at least once, in subject E 4 nine times in 11 observations, in E 5 nine in 10 observations, in E 6 six in 7 and in E 8 eight in 10. Redness of the pharynx and tonsillar pillars was continuously observed in this group for one month and in four subjects for 12 weeks. Redness of the uvula was found only in the early examinations. The children in grade 3 B, with the exception of subject E 31 to be described later, were free from any marked symptoms except slight temperature elevations. Those in grades 5 A-B and 6 A-B were normal in all respects. On the other hand, the high school students (sore throat convalescents) showed in all instances a distinct redness of the pharynx accompanied in 4 subjects by tonsillar redness and a slight temperature elevation.

Epidemiology.—In any elementary school there is opportunity for more or less intermingling of children from all classes both inside the school and at play. Conditions, therefore, exist for the spread of respiratory infections. The laboratory data obtained in this study furnished further evidence, although not conclusive, of such intermingling. The records of both the high and elementary schools showed that there were more absences than usual during the month of April (1920) on account of "sore throats," "pharyngitis" and "tonsillitis" and that throat infections were unusually prevalent during the entire spring quarter (April 2 to June 10).

There were also indications of a connection between high school students and those in the elementary grades. For example, W.P., a high school student, was the brother of J.P., a child in grade 2 B. About April 10 W.P. developed a sore throat much more severe than that prevalent among the younger children, though also atypical in character. On returning to school (April 21) hemolytic streptococci and type 4 pneumococci belonging to the same biologic groups as those present in the throats of the children in grade 2 B were isolated from his throat. The mother of W.P. and J.P. and a sister and brother home from another college for the holidays also had an infection giving, as did that of W.P., the following clinical picture: a sore throat which their family physician found unusual and unlike follicular tonsillitis, difficulty in swallowing, a temperature of 102 F. and in two cases accompanied by a rash.[1] Hemolytic streptococci were found in the throats of 5 others in the high school group and type 4 pneumococci in 3, but the biologic grouping of these organisms was not determined in all cases.

Laboratory Studies.—The clinical observations were accompanied each time by laboratory studies on the bacterial flora of the tonsillar region. Swabs were made from the tonsils and streaked on blood-agar plates in the usual manner. The swabs were then placed in 5% sheep blood dextrose broth and incubated 6-8 hours. One c c of the blood broth culture was then injected into a white mouse. If the animal died within 24 hours the peritoneal cavity was washed and the presence or absence of fixed type pneumococci determined by agglutination and precipitin tests. Cultures were made on blood-agar plates from the peritoneal fluid and heart blood and the usual confirmatory tests made for pneumococci. The blood-agar plates made from the original tonsillar swabs were incubated for 24 hours and then studied in the usual manner.

The first examination of cases E 1 to E 9, made on March 17, 1920, showed the presence of a hemolytic streptococcus on all plates and of a type 4 pneumococcus in all instances. These two organisms were the

[1] Scarlet fever was considered as a possibility but the symptoms did not warrant such a diagnosis.

principal ones sought for in subsequent examinations of all subjects, those serving as controls as well as those having pathologic throats. Table 1 gives the number of times these organisms were found in comparison to the attempts made in the selected group from grade 2 B.

TABLE 1

HEMOLYTIC STREPTOCOCCI AND PNEUMOCOCCI IN GROUP 2 B

Case	Number of Examinations for Streptococci	Number of Times Hemolytic Streptococci Found	Percentage Positive	Number of Examinations for Pneumococci	Number of Times Type 4 Pneumococci Found	Percentage Positive
E1	2	2	100	2	2	100
E2	9	5	56	6	5	83
E3	11	8	73	5	4	80
E4	12	11	92	7	4	57
E5	12	9	75	5	4	80
E6	7	4	57	4	4	100
E7	9	7	78	6	6	100
E8	9	7	78	6	5	83
E9	9	6	67	7	5	71
Totals........	80	59	...	48	39	
Average......	..	..	74	..	..	81

The laboratory examinations show that hemolytic streptococci were isolated in 74% of attempts made and type 4 pneumococci in 81%.

The control group, including 8 convalescents from sore throat, gave hemolytic streptococci in 9 instances (41%) and type 4 pneumococci in 10 instances (45%). Eight of the 9 strains of hemolytic streptococci and 4 of the 10 strains of pneumococci were isolated from the group of convalescents.

TABLE 2

AGGLUTINATION OF HEMOLYTIC STREPTOCOCCI

Strain	Serum 4 (5) TH1 Dilutions					Serum 7 (8) TH1 Dilutions				
	1:160	1:320	1:640	1:1,280	1:2,560	1:80	1:160	1:320	1:640	1:1,280
1 TH 1	+	+	+	+	+	+	+	—	—	—
4 (5) TH 1	+	+	+	+	+	+	+	—	—	—
4 (5) TH 2	+	+	+	+	+	+	+	+	—	—
4 (5) TH 5	+	+	+	+	—	+	+	—	—	—
4 (6) TH 5	+	+	+	+	+	+	+	—	—	—
7 (5) TH 1	+	+	+	+	+	+	+	+	—	—
7 (6) TH 1	+	+	+	+	+	+	+	+	+	—
12 TH 2	+	+	+	+	+	+	+	+	—	—
17 TH 2	+	+	+	+	+	+	—	—	—	—

The hemolytic streptococci found on the blood plates were difficult to grow on transfers made to blood-agar slants. We were able to obtain them only from subjects E 1, E 4, E 7, E 12, E14, and E 17. All strains from E 1, E 4, E 7, E 12 and E 14 fermented lactose, mannite and salicin, thus falling in Holman's group S. infrequens. Strains from E 17 did not ferment mannite. Immune serums for 2 strains [4(5)TH 1 and 7(6)TH 1] were prepared by injection of rabbits and agglutination tests made against a number of strains with the results recorded in table 2.

Three strains from influenza cases gave no agglutination in any dilution with either serum. The strains from case E 1 was isolated at the first examination. Three strains from case E 4 were obtained 3 weeks after the first observation and one strain after 4 weeks. The two strains from case E 7 were isolated after 3 and 4 weeks, respectively. The strains isolated were thus biologically identical, including the strain from subject E 17 which was culturally different.

The type 4 pneumococci were likewise tested with an immune serum prepared with one of the strains (E 4-6). Table 3 gives the results of agglutination.

TABLE 3

AGGLUTINATION OF TYPE 4 PNEUMOCOCCI

Strain	Dilutions (Serum E 4-6)								
	1:10	1:20	1:40	1:80	1:160	1:320	1:640	1:1,280	1:2,560
E 2-5	+	+	+	+	+	+	+	+	+
E 2-7	+	+	+	+	+	+	—	—	—
E 3-5	+	+	+	+	+	—	—	—	—
E 3-6	+	+	+	+	+	—	—	—	—
E 4-6	+	+	+	+	+	+	+	+	+
E 5-5	+	+	+	+	—	—	—	—	—
E 5-6	+	+	+	—	—	—	—	—	—
E 6-3	+	+	+	+	+	—	—	—	—
E 8-5	+	+	+	+	—	—	—	—	—
E 9-4	+	+	+	+	+	—	—	—	—
E 10	+	+	+	+	+	—	—	—	—
E 12	+	+	+	+	—	—	—	—	—
E 15	+	+	+	—	—	—	—	—	—
E 16	—	—	—	—	—	—	—	—	—
E 24	—	—	—	—	—	—	—	—	—
E 27	+	+	+	—	—	—	—	—	—
E 31	+	+	+	+	+	+	+	—	—

Strains from cases of common colds gave no agglutination with this serum. As with the hemolytic streptococci the strains were obtained at various times—from 2 days to 4 weeks after our work was started. A biologically identical type 4 pneumococcus was thus isolated from all the cases of grade 2 B except 2 from which the strains failed to survive, from 3 high school students and from 2 children of grade 3 B.

The persistence of clinical symptoms in some cases led to a study of the length of time that hemolytic streptococci and type 4 pneumococci remained in the throats of the children of grade 2 B. Unfortunately it was not possible to complete this part of the investigation because of the withdrawal from school of some of the children and the closing of school for the summer. Table 4 gives the available data correlated with the appearance of tonsils and pharynx.

These results show a close correlation between clinical observations and the presence of hemolytic streptococci, pneumococci or both.

An examination made October 25, after the autumn opening of the school, revealed the persistence of clinical symptoms in group 2 B. These, however, were less severe in character than those noted 7 months previously. Hemolytic streptococci were absent from all throats while type 4 pneumococci were isolated in 2 instances. It is not known that these 2 strains were identical with those previously studied.

TABLE 4

PERSISTENCE OF HEMOLYTIC STREPTOCOCCI AND PNEUMOCOCCI (PRESENCE AFTER 8 WEEKS)

Subject	Redness of Pharynx	Redness of Tonsils	Hemolytic Streptococci	Type 4 Pneumococci
E 2	+	Slight	+*	+
E 3	0	Doubtful	+*	+
E 4	+	+	+	+
E 5	+	+	+*	—
E 6	0	0	—	+
E 7	+	+	+	+
E 8	0	0	—	—
E 9	0	0	+*	—

* Numbers very few.

Subject E 31, a member of grade 3 B, proved to be of some interest. This child had an attack about June 9 and presented a clinical picture of a more severe character than observed in the other children. The pharynx became so acutely inflamed, edematous and painful that the head was retracted. The temperature rose several degrees. We isolated from the tonsils a type 4 pneumococcus serologically identical with the others studied but failed to find a hemolytic streptococcus. Whether or not the pneumococcus was the etiologic factor is unknown, but the finding of a specific serum strain of this organism in connection with a distinct pathologic condition is worth noting.

SUMMARY

The data here presented show the occurrence of a sore throat epidemic of an unusual clinical type. A hemolytic streptococcus and a type 4 pneumococcus were found simultaneously in the tonsillar regions of a group of children with the symptoms described. The streptococcus was of an unusual cultural type, belonging to Holman's group S. infrequens. The hemolytic streptococcus is known to be at times the etiologic factor in sore throats. That the type 4 pneumococcus present in our group might be pathogenic is suggested by its presence unaccompanied by hemolytic streptococci in one case of acute inflammation.

One of the most striking features was the carrier condition. It is impossible to say how long this was maintained, but in 5 of 8 instances it persisted for not less than 8 weeks as shown by finding immunilogically identical organisms continually on the tonsils during this period. Hemolytic streptococci were found after 12 weeks. The proportion of hemolytic streptococci in the tonsillar flora as indicated on blood-agar plates varied considerably, some examinations being negative. It is well recognized that the technic usually employed may yield discrepancies. The reappearance of these organisms on blood-agar plates does not necessarily mean that a new invasion has occurred. We had no way of determining the relative numbers of the pneumococcus.

The finding of specific strains of hemolytic streptococci and of type 4 pneumococci, biologically identical with those from the group of children intensively studied, in convalescents among high school students and in children in other grades of the elementary school indicated the prevalence of these organisms throughout the whole school. The possibility of contact among the children existed and was substantiated by certain well established instances.

The persistence of clinical symptoms closely paralleled the occurrence of the two specific strains of the organisms (see table 4). These symptoms were so mild after the earliest examinations as almost to escape attention.

This epidemic may have been caused by one of the organisms isolated or by their simultaneous action.

PHENOL AND CRESOL AS PRESERVATIVES IN BIOLOGIC PRODUCTS

Peter Masucci

From H. K. Mulford Co. Biological Laboratories, Glenolden, Pa.

In the manufacture of serums, vaccines and other biologic products, it is customary to add phenol or cresol as a preservative. When added to serums, a precipitate forms, due to the interaction of the phenol or cresol with the serum proteins. Krumwiede and Banzhaf [1] developed a method of adding cresol to antitoxins which eliminated the precipitation of the serum proteins. They used equal parts of cresol and ether. The addition of this mixture to serums in a concentration of 0.4%-0.5% cresol caused little or no precipitation. The authors state that subsequent precipitation is not necessarily limited by the ether but is never greater than in cresol alone. They also claim that the mixture of ether and cresol is more strongly antiseptic than cresol alone.

Experiments were made to determine (1) the effect of cresol and ether-cresol with time on serums in relation to the amount of precipitate formed, (2) the influence of ether in the ether-cresol mixture as to (a) germicidal value, (b) hemolytic power of cresol, and (3) the mechanism of the ether-cresol action on serums. A somewhat similar study was made on the action of phenol and ether-phenol on serums.

THE ACTION OF CRESOL AND ETHER-CRESOL ON SERUMS

In order to study the comparative action of cresol and ether-cresol on serums the following experiment was performed:

(a) One hundred c c amounts of fresh horse-serum previously candle filtered were placed in nonsoluble flint bottles. To some was added cresol ranging from 0% as control to 0.6% and to others was added ether-cresol solution 1:1 in amounts from 0.2% to 1%. All the ether-cresol solution used in this experiment consisted of equal parts of ether and cresol. A series of bottles containing citrated plasma was treated in exactly the same manner as the normal serum.

It was noted that the serum and plasma receiving the straight cresol were "burned" at the point of contact between the cresol and the serum in question. This was more pronounced when the cresol was

Received for publication Nov. 7, 1921.

[1] Jour. Infect. Dis., 1921, 28, p. 367.

added at once in a continuous stream. If, however, the cresol was added drop by drop the behavior was somewhat different. The first drop spread on the surface of the serum while additional drops gradually sank to the bottom in separate "oily" globules having on the outside a coating of albuminous material. When these were shaken, solution took place but not with much "burning" action. This behavior of cresol suggested at once that surface tension and surface phenomena played a part.

The bottles treated with ether-cresol solution did not show the destructive burning action of the straight cresol; those serums receiving 0.2% to 0.6% ether-cresol solution remained clear, while the 0.8% and 1.0% bottles showed a turbidity and opalescence resembling colloidal solutions.

The normal serum and citrated plasma were kept at room temperature and observed at various intervals for precipitated protein, change of color and formation of fibrin. In order to determine the amount of precipitate somewhat quantitatively, the normal serum was centrifuged at constant high speed for 30 minutes, the supernatant siphoned off carefully, and the sediment tested for total nitrogen by the Kjeldahl method. This procedure does not give strictly quantitative results, but would show any great variations in the amount of precipitate formed.

The same method was not used for the citrated plasma because the fibrin formed in some of the bottles shortly after adding the preservative.

Tables 1 and 2 give a summary of the serums described after eight months' standing at room temperature.

Discussion of Results.—The data in tables 1 and 2 bring out these facts: 1. Cresol changes the color of serum or plasma from yellow with a reddish tinge to yellow with a definite greenish or greenish yellow tinge. 2. Although the method used for determining the amount of precipitate formed on standing is only approximately quantitative, there is no marked difference between the amount of precipitate in the serums treated with straight cresol and those treated with ether-cresol. 3. The action of cresol or ether-cresol on citrated plasma is to accelerate the formation of fibrin. Those bottles containing 0.2% or more cresol showed complete fibrin formation in a month, whereas the controls, without preservative, did not coagulate completely until after 7 months. 4. The precipitate in normal serum formed on standing was insoluble in water, cold solutions of acids and alkalis, or in salt solution. Apparently it was mostly finely divided fibrin. On shaking the precipitate went into suspension giving the serums a milky opalescence.

TABLE 1

NORMAL SERUM

Percentage of Preservative	Color	Appearance	Precipitate as Mg. Nitrogen
0 cresol	Reddish-yellow	Clear	8.5
0.1 cresol	Reddish-yellow	Clear	7.6
0.2 cresol	Greenish-yellow	Slight opalescence	9.2
0.3 cresol	Greenish-yellow	Marked opalescence	8.7
0.4 cresol	Greenish-yellow	Colloidal; muddy	9.0
0:5 cresol	Greenish-yellow	Colloidal; muddy; opaque	11.6
0.2 ether-cresol	Reddish tinge	Clear	8.2
0.3 ether-cresol	Reddish tinge	Clear	6.7
0.4 ether cresol	Greenish tinge	Clear	7.8
0.5 ether-cresol	Greenish tinge	Slight opalescence	8.5
0.6 ether-cresol	Greenish tinge	Slight opalescence	8.9
0.7 ether-cresol	Greenish tinge	Marked opalescence	9.5
0.8 ether-cresol	Greenish tinge	Colloidal; muddy	9.0
0.9 ether-cresol	Greenish tinge	Colloidal; muddy	9.8
1.0 ether-cresol	Greenish tinge	Colloidal; muddy; opaque	10.8

TABLE 2

CITRATED PLASMA

Percentage of Preservative	Color	Appearance	Fibrin
0 cresol (control)	Yellow	Coagulated	Completely formed
0.1 cresol	Yellow	Coagulated	Completely formed
0.2 cresol	Greenish-yellow	Coagulated	Completely formed
0.3 cresol	Greenish-yellow	Coagulated	Completely formed
0.4 cresol	Greenish-yellow	Turbid and coagulated	Completely formed
0.5 cresol	Greenish-yellow	Turbid and coagulated	Completely formed
0.2 ether-cresol	Greenish-yellow	Clear and coagulated	Completely formed
0.3 ether-cresol	Greenish-yellow	Clear and coagulated	Completely formed
0.4 ether-cresol	Greenish-yellow	Clear and coagulated	Completely formed
0.5 ether-cresol	Greenish-yellow	Clear and coagulated	Completely formed
0.6 ether-cresol	Greenish-yellow	Clear and coagulated	Completely formed
0.7 ether-cresol	Greenish-yellow	Turbid and coagulated	Completely formed
0.8 ether-cresol	Greenish-yellow	Turbid and coagulated	Completely formed
0.9 ether-cresol	Greenish-yellow	Turbid and coagulated	Completely formed
1.0 ether-cresol	Greenish-yellow	Turbid and coagulated	Completely formed

Another experiment was made in which a lot of normal serum was divided into 3 parts: One portion had no preservative added, a second portion had 0.3% cresol, and a third portion had 0.6% ether-cresol. The three portions were candle-filtered and placed in the refrigerator for aging. At the end of 10 months, the 3 portions were tested quantitatively for precipitate. Instead of using the previous method of determining the amount of precipitate by centrifuging and running a Kjeldahl on the sediment, the following procedure was adopted, which we think is more accurate:

One hundred c c samples of the 3 serums were centrifuged for the same length of time and same speed. The supernatant clear serum was carefully poured off, and the sediment suspended in 200 c c of distilled water. The resulting turbidity was then measured by a Jackson turbidimeter, such as is used for determining sulphates in water. The results representing the average of 3 readings and expressed as SO_3 pts. per million were as follows: (a) normal serum — no preservative, 52.0; (b) normal serum + 0.3% cresol, 63.0, and (c) normal serum + 0.6% ether-cresol, 64.0. These results are striking and show conclusively that the amount of precipitate in the ether and ether-cresol samples is the same.

THE MECHANISM OF ETHER-CRESOL SOLUTION ON PREVENTING THE BURNING OF SERUMS

As the ether-cresol solution did not "burn" the serum to the same degree as the straight cresol, it was thought important to study the reason for this behavior. Various cresol solvents were used in the proportion of 1:1. Glycerol, benzene, carbon bisulphide, chloroform, ethyl alcohol and amyl-alcohol were tried. Of these, only the amyl-alcohol behaved similarly to the ether-cresol solution, that is, it failed to "burn" the serum. A consideration of surface tension phenomenon suggested itself. Accordingly, the surface tension of normal serum without preservative was found and compared with that of normal serum containing straight cresol or ether-cresol.

In all surface tension determinations a Traube stalagmometer was used, that is, the average weight of a drop of the fluid from a standardized pipette was found. Taking the surface tension of water as unity, the surface of a solution is given by the formula:

$$\frac{\text{Specific gravity of solution} \times \text{number of drops of water}}{\text{Number of drops of solution}}$$

The result obtained is relative and not absolute; to express the tension in dynes per cm. it is necessary to multiply the ratio in the formula by 73.3, the surface tension of pure water at 18° C.

The surface tension of 6 normal serums without preservatives and with 0.3% cresol or 0.3% phenol was determined, and it was found that the cresol lowered the surface tension considerably more than the phenol. The results are given in table 3. (Surface tension of water equals 1.)

TABLE 3
THE EFFECT OF CRESOL ON THE SURFACE TENSION OF SERUM

Serum No.	Without Preservative	With 0.3% Cresol (Redistilled)	With 0.3% Phenol (Redistilled)
91,563	0.94	0.70	0.82
92,183	0.86	0.64	0.76
91,693	0.83	0.63	0.74
92,399	0.90	0.66	0.78
3,932	0.83	0.64	0.73
4,953	0.92	0.67	0.79

Table 3 shows that cresol lowers the surface tension markedly, an average of about 25%, whereas, phenol lowers it only about one-half that amount.

Lowering of surface tension and concentration was then studied. It was found that small amounts of cresol lowered the tension a certain amount while each additional quantity lowered it less and less.

TABLE 4
THE EFFECT OF CRESOL ON THE SURFACE TENSION OF SERUM

Percentage of Cresol	Tension
0 (no preservative)	0.86
0.1	0 80
0.2	0.70
0.3	0.67
0.4	0.65
0.5	0.64
0.6	0.62

The surface tension of serum containing 0.6% ether-cresol was found to be more or less the additive effect of cresol and ether, thus

TABLE 5
THE EFFECT OF ETHER-CRESOL ON THE SURFACE TENSION OF SERUM

Serum	Tension
No preservative	0.85
0.3% cresol	0.64
0.3% ether	0.74
0.6% ether-cresol	0.58

Before discussing the significance of the lowering of surface tension by cresol and phenol it is well to attempt to explain the reason why straight cresol "burns" the serum while the ether-cresol does not. According to Gibb's theorem, a substance which lowers the surface tension of a solvent becomes more concentrated in the surface film than in the interior. We are dealing with a system of two phases, serum and ether. For simplicity's sake we may assume that ether is immiscible in serum, then the cresol which lowers the surface tension of the serum concentrates in the surface layer next to the ether. As cresol is much more soluble in ether than in serum and as it does not lower the surface tension of ether, it will diffuse into the layer of ether until an equilibrium is established in the surface layer of the serum. Expressed in general terms a fluid 3 spreads over the common boundaries of two fluids, 1 and 2, whenever

$$\sigma \tfrac{1}{2} > \sigma \tfrac{2}{3} - \sigma \tfrac{3}{1}$$

where $\sigma 1/2$ = surface tension of serum against ether
$\sigma 2/3$ = surface tension of ether against cresol
$\sigma 3/1$ = surface tension of cresol against serum

Therefore, when the ether-cresol is added to the serum the cresol concentrates in the layer of ether. However, by constant shaking and on standing an equilibrium is established between the cresol in the ether and that in the serum. Ether itself is soluble to some extent in the serum, so that the final effect of the ether on the cresol is to distribute the latter more intimately in the serum. Hence, we have the action of the cresol on the serum evenly distributed with a resulting colloidal opalescence, instead of the selective "burning" of the straight cresol which acts in a concentrated form on that part of the serum with which it comes in contact.

PHENOL COEFFICIENT OF CRESOL AND ETHER-CRESOL SOLUTION

Banzhaf and Krumwiede [1] state that ether-cresol is more strongly antiseptic than cresol alone. We have not been able to confirm their results. The phenol coefficient of an ether cresol solution 1:1 and straight cresol was determined according to the U. S. Hygienic Laboratory method, using distilled water for diluting. The results are shown in table 6. The experimental data shows that ether-cresol is not more strongly germicidal but slightly less germicidal than cresol alone. It is true that ether has antiseptic properties but that depends on the concentration used. If the concentration is high, the ether exerts its germicidal action on bacteria by its power to penetrate their cell membrane. A concentration of 0.3%, the amount used in serums, is not strong enough to exert any germicidal action.

If we take a suspension of bacteria and regard it as a dispersed phase, the suspension must obey certain physical laws. A suspension of organisms has large surface development, and therefore it will adsorb with great affinity those substances which lower the surface tension of water. The amount adsorbed is greater, the more the dissolved substance lowers the surface tension. Therefore, cresol should be adsorbed much more than phenol. When ether cresol is added to a bacterial suspension, the adsorption equilibrium is disturbed. The cresol is less adsorbed by the bacteria due to the fact that the ether increases the surface tension between the bacterial suspension and cresol. As a result the cresol is less adsorbed and its antiseptic power diminished. Paul and Krönig[2] found this to be true with

TABLE 6

HYGIENIC LABORATORY TEST WITH B. TYPHOSUS

Substance	Dilution	Time in Minutes						Date
		2½	5	7½	10	12½	15	
Cresol	250	—	—	—	—	—	—	1/12/21
	300	—	—	—	—	—	—	
	350	—	—	—	—	—	—	
	400	—	—	—	—	—	—	
	450	+	—	—	—	—	—	
Cresol-ether	250	—	—	—	—	—	—	1/12/21
	300	—	—	—	—	—	—	
	350	—	—	—	—	—	—	
	400	+	+	—	—	—	—	
	450	+	+	+	—	—	—	
Cresol	300	—	—	—	—	—	—	6/7/21
	350	—	—	—	—	—	—	
	400	+	+	—	—	—	—	
	450	+	+	—	—	—	—	
	500	+	+	+	+	+	+	
Cresol-ether	300	—	—	—	—	—	—	6/7/21
	350	—	—	—	—	—	—	
	400	+	+	+	—	—	—	
	450	+	+	+	+	—	—	
	500	+	+	+	+	+	—	

anthrax. Their results showed that phenol was far more germicidal on the spores when used as an aqueous solution than as an alcoholic solution.

SURFACE TENSION AND HEMOLYSIS

Woodward and Alsberg[3] showed that the lowering of surface tension by saponins and their hemolytic power did not run parallel. As phenol and cresol are known to hemolyze blood corpuscles, it was decided to study the comparative hemolytic power of phenol and cresol and the relation to the lowering of surface tension.

[2] Colloids in Biology and Medicine, p. 395.

[3] Jr. Pharm. and Expt. Therap., 1920, 16, p. 237.

The cytolytic power of disinfectants varies with their penetrating power, and should vary also with their power to lower surface tension. Therefore, cresol should be more effective than phenol.

Experiments showed this to be true. The technic employed for determining hemolysis was that of Woodward and Alsberg.[3] Different percentages of phenol or cresol in Locke solution were made. Ten c c of the solution at 37 C. were placed in test tubes, and then 2 drops of washed sheep erythrocytes were added to each. The tubes were mixed by inverting and then placed in the incubator at 37 C. The relative hemolytic activity was noted every 10 minutes, for one hour. With higher concentration of cresol hemolysis took place within less than 5 minutes.

The surface tension of each solution was determined at 18 C. although the hemolysis took place at 37 C. This introduces an error but as we are interested in comparative results, the error plays no part in the final conclusion. The results obtained are given in table 8 for cresol, ether-cresol, phenol and ether-phenol. The tubes containing the ether were stoppered to prevent evaporation.

TABLE 7

RESULTS OF EXPERIMENTS

Substance	Tension	10 Min.	20 Min.	30 Min.	40 Min.	50 Min.	60 Min.
Water	1.00						
Locke solution	1.00	0	0	0	0	0	0
Locke solution + 0.1% cresol	0.91	0	0	0	0	0	0
Locke solution + 0.2% cresol	0.80	0	0	+	+++	+++	+++
Locke solution + 0.3% cresol	0.74	++	+++	+++	C	C	C
Locke solution + 0.4% cresol	0.70	+++	+++	C	C	C	C
Locke solution + 0.5% cresol	0.65	+++	+++	C	C	C	C
Locke solution + 0.3% ether	0.90	0	0	0	0	0	0
Locke solution + 0.2% ether-cresol	0.80	0	0	0	0	0	0
Locke solution + 0.4% ether-cresol	0.75	0	0	0	0	++	+++
Locke solution + 0.6% ether-cresol	0.70	+	++	+++	+++	C	C
Locke solution + 0.8% ether-cresol	0.65	+++	+++	C	C	C	C
Locke solution + 1.0% ether-cresol	0.60	+++	C	C	C	C	C

0 = no lysis; + = slight lysis; ++ = considerable lysis; +++ = complete lysis; C = complete lysis with coagulation of protein.

* The composition of the Locke solution was as follows: NaCl, 9.0 gm. per liter; KCl, 0.42 gm. per liter; $CaCl_2$, 0.24 gm. per liter; $NaHCO_3$, 0.10 gm. per liter.

A study of table 7 brings out that (1) cresol produces hemolysis of the erythrocytes much more rapidly than phenol; (2) the rate of lysis is directly proportional to the concentration of the cresol or phenol and to the lowering of the surface tension; (3) ether-cresol produces hemolysis just as readily as cresol; (4) the same relation is true for phenol and ether-phenol; (5) although ether lowers the surface tension, it in itself does not produce hemolysis.

Discussion of Results.—The fact that ether itself lowers the surface tension without producing hemolysis is significant. Merely lowering the surface tension does not necessarily mean hemolysis, but on the other hand substances which lower the surface tension are easily adsorbed by the erythrocytes. Cresol, therefore, produces hemolysis more rapidly than phenol because it is adsorbed more than phenol and is thus more effective in bringing about cytolysis.

Another important difference in the behavior of the two substances is that cresol acts on the erythrocytes in two distinct ways: (1) it causes cytolysis with production of hemolysis, and (2) it acts on the liberated hemoglobin and coagulates the protein faction or globin. Phenol in a concentration of 0.5% produces hemolysis in one hour but does not destroy the globin. This means that cresol is far more active on proteins than phenol.

Summary.—A study of preservatives including cresol, ether-cresol, phenol and ether-phenol on serum and plasma brings out that: (1) cresol or ether-cresol changes the color of serum or plasma from a light yellow to a greenish yellow; (2) there is no marked difference in the amount of precipitate formed on standing between serums treated with straight cresol or ether-cresol; (3) the precipitate formed in normal serum is mostly finely divided fibrin; (4) cresol hastens the formation of fibrin in plasma; (5) cresol lowers the surface tension of serum much more markedly than phenol; (6) ether-cresol does not "burn" serum on account of a surface tension phenomenon; (7) cresol produces hemolysis rapidly with destruction of the hemoglobin while phenol produces only slight hemolysis with no effect on the hemoglobin under the conditions of the experiment; (8) ether does not alter the course of hemolysis in itself or as ether-cresol or ether-phenol; (9) the lowering of surface tension in itself does not produce hemolysis, but substances which lower the surface tension are adsorbed by the erythrocytes to a greater degree.

CONCLUSION

Experimental data do not show that ether-cresol has any advantages as preservative of serum over straight ether in the total precipitate formed on standing or in germicidal value.

DIFFERENTIATION OF HEMOLYTIC STREPTOCOCCI FROM HUMAN AND BOVINE SOURCES BY THE HYDROLYSIS OF SODIUM HIPPURATE

S. Henry Ayers and Philip Rupp

From the Research Laboratories of the Dairy Division, United States Department of Agriculture

The close resemblance between hemolytic streptococci of human and bovine origin has led to extensive studies of these organisms. Hemolytic streptococci are commonly found in the udders of cows and are therefore present in the milk from such animals. Since these streptococci are so similar to the human hemolytic types in cultural characteristics, varying practically only in the vigor of their growth, milk containing them has been looked on as a potential source of infection for human beings.

The appearance of hemolytic colonies gives occasion for alarm to those familiar with the use of blood plates in connection with the examination of material from pathologic sources but unaccustomed to the plating of fresh milk on blood agar. However, those who have observed large numbers of samples of fresh milk plated on blood agar have been impressed with the fact that the hemolytic streptococci commonly found must be different from the human types. If such were not the case streptococcal infection from milk might be very widespread.

Hemolytic streptococci from the udder of the cow are mentioned specially because there are types found in pasteurized milk which are somewhat hemolytic, but which because of their characteristics should not be confused with the hemolytic types of human origin. Such organisms have been studied by Salter.[1]

In recent years tests have been devised which have helped materially to separate the human and bovine hemolytic streptococci. On blood plates, both produce hemolytic zones about the colonies, but usually the zone of hemolysis is larger about the colonies of the human type. Careful measurement of their hemolytic activity in our laboratories has shown that the human type is approximately 100 times as active as the bovine streptococcus. This extreme difference is easily overlooked on plates, but the difference has been recognized by Brown,[2]

Received for publication Nov. 25, 1921.

[1] Am. Jour. Hyg., 1921, 1, p. 154.
[2] Jour. Exper. Med., 1920, 31, p. 35.

who has made use of it in a method of testing for hemolysis in order to separate the two types.

Another test which has served to distinguish between hemolytic streptococci of human and bovine origin is the difference in their final hydrogen-ion concentration. The difference in final P_H among streptococci as pointed out by one of us (Ayers)[3] was applied by Avery and Cullen[4] to differentiate between the hemolytic human and bovine types. The bovine type gives a higher acidity in dextrose broth than the human type and the difference in P_H, while small, is quite definite and characteristic in the proper medium.

There are two tests, therefore, the hemolysis test of Brown and the final hydrogen-ion concentration, which can now be used to distinguish between the human and bovine types of hemolytic streptococcus. These tests are valuable, but of course the difference in hemolytic activity and acid-producing power may be considered only a matter of difference in degree and not a fundamental difference. While we do not believe that such a view should be taken, it seemed desirable to find other differences, if possible.

HYDROLYSIS OF SODIUM HIPPURATE

In another paper[5] we mentioned the fact that certain streptococci gave indication of fermenting organic acids, and further work has given definite proof. While engaged in this study it was found by one of us (Rupp) that one of our cultures of hemolytic streptococci of human origin did not hydrolyze sodium hippurate, while a culture of bovine origin split it into benzoic acid and glycocoll. The significance of this was at once obvious, and more cultures were studied and the same results obtained.

There is nothing new in the hydrolysis of sodium hippurate by bacteria, for it was observed as early as 1864 by Van Tieghem[6] and since that time numerous investigators have observed this action by various bacilli and cocci. After the completion of our work a paper by Stapp[7] was found in which he refers to some work by Crisafulli in 1895 which showed that Streptococcus erysipelatis could split sodium hippurate. The original paper by Crisafulli has not been seen by us.

[3] Jour. Bacteriol., 1916, 1, p. 84; Jour. Infect. Dis., 1918, 23, p. 290.
[4] Jour. Exper. Med., 1919, 29, p. 215.
[5] Jour. Infect. Dis., 1921, 29, p. 235.
[6] Compt. Rend. Acad. Sc., 1864, 58, p. 210.
[7] Centralbl. f. Bakteriol., II, 1920, 51, p. 11.

In order to show the hydrolysis of sodium hippurate two cultures were selected, A-34 of human origin and 90H-1 from the udder of a cow. These cultures were grown in the following medium for 7 days at 37 C. with and without sodium hippurate:

10 gm. peptone (Parke-Davis)
5 gm. pepsin
0.03 gm. calcium chloride
1 drop of 1 per cent. solution of ferric chloride
1000 c c of distilled water
NaOH to give PH 7.1

After incubation the cultures were made acid, then distilled, and the volatile acid titrated. The amino-nitrogen was determined by formol titration.

From table 1 it will be seen that the streptococcus of human origin A-34 gave practically the same results with and without the sodium hippurate. But culture 90H-1 from the udder of a cow showed a large increase in volatile acid and in amino-nitrogen in the medium with sodium hippurate. Tests showed that about 96% of the volatile acidity from this medium was benzoic acid. Since hippuric acid is easily decomposed by chemical agents, by an enzyme of the kidney (histoenzym), and by bacteria, into benzoic acid and glycocoll, an increase in amino-nitrogen should be expected. Such was the case, as may be seen from the table.

TABLE 1

ACTION OF REPRESENTATIVE CULTURES OF HEMOLYTIC STREPTOCOCCI OF HUMAN AND BOVINE ORIGIN ON SODIUM HIPPURATE

Culture of Hemolytic Streptococcus	No Hippurate		1% Hippurate	
	C c N/10 Volatile Acid*	Amino-N Mg. per 100 C c Excess over Control	C c N/10 Volatile Acid*	Amino-N Mg. per 100 C c Excess over Control
A-34 (of human origin)..........	7.72	15.12	8.21	15.40
90H-1 (of bovine origin)..........	6.03	8.68	53.35	69.73

* Volatile acid in 1,000 c c of distillate from 100 c c of medium.

This hydrolysis may be expressed as follows:

$$\begin{matrix} \text{Hippuric Acid.} & & \text{Benzoic Acid.} & & \text{Glycocoll.} \\ \left.\begin{matrix} C_6H_5CO. \mid NH.CH_2COOH \\ + \quad OH \mid H \end{matrix}\right\} & = & C_6H_5COOH & + & NH_2CH_2COOH \end{matrix}$$

The amount of sodium hippurate used was 1%, and to show the approximate amount hydrolyzed the following calculation has been made from the results obtained with culture 90H-1: The excess of amino-nitrogen (69.73 mg.) corresponds to 373.9 mg. of glycocoll, while the excess of volatile acid in 1,500 c c of distillate (50.29 c c $\frac{N}{10}$) corresponds to 613.8 mg. benzoic acid. In order to form hippuric acid 373.9 mg. glycocoll would require 608.1 mg. benzoic acid. This shows that the hydrolyzed products are present in the proportion to form hippuric acid and furthermore that, in this case, the hippuric acid was completely hydrolyzed.

RATE OF HYDROLYSIS OF SODIUM HIPPURATE

The rate of the hydrolysis and its relation to simple and complex mediums was of interest because of the effect on the development of a satisfactory test. It was determined therefore in a simple peptone medium and also in a more complicated broth medium containing dextrose.

Peptone Medium

10.0 gm. peptone (Parke-Davis)
1.5 gm. potassium diabasic phosphate
10.0 gm. sodium hippurate
1000 c c distilled water
PH 7.2

Dextrose Broth Medium

1000 c c infusion broth
10.0 gm. peptone (Parke-Davis)
1.5 gm. potassium diabasic phosphate
10.0 gm. sodium hippurate
2.0 gm. dextrose
PH 7.2

Flasks containing 100c c of medium were prepared and inoculated with culture 90H-1, a bovine udder type of hemolytic streptococcus.

TABLE 2

RATE OF HYDROLYSIS IN SIMPLE AND COMPLEX MEDIUMS

Days	Volatile Acid from Hippurate	
	Peptone and Sodium Hippurate C c	Infusion Dextrose Broth and Sodium Hippurate C c
1	25.72*	41.21
2	42.93	41.29
3	42.74	41.40
4	42.47	42.20
5	42.65	41.43

* C c N/10 volatile acid in 1,000 c c distillate from 100 c c medium.

The volatile acid produced in medium without sodium hippurate was determined and subtracted, so table 2 shows the amount of volatile acid (benzoic acid) from the hippurate during 5 days of incubation at 37° C. It will be observed that the hydrolysis proceeded at a greater rate in the dextrose broth medium during the first 24 hours of incubation, but after that the results were practically identical. This was undoubtedly due to the more rapid growth in the more complex medium during the first 24 hours.

From these results it is evident that the presence of dextrose or beef broth does not interfere with the hydrolysis, and that 48-hours' incubation is sufficient, at least for the culture studied.

INFLUENCE OF HYDROGEN-ION CONCENTRATION ON THE HYDROLYSIS

The well-known influence of hydrogen-ion concentration in accelerating or retarding enzyme action suggested the possibility of similar effects on the splitting of sodium hippurate.

In order to determine the effect of acidity on the hydrolysis two mediums were prepared, one being heavily and the other lightly buffered. The sugar content was also adjusted so that in the lightly buffered medium the acidity would rapidly increase.

The composition of the mediums was as follows:

Medium A

1,000 c c infusion broth
10 gm. peptone (Parke-Davis)
10 gm. sodium hippurate
2 gm. dextrose
10 gm. potassium diabasic phosphate
P_H 7.2

Medium B

1,000 c c infusion broth
10 gm. peptone (Parke-Davis)
10 gm. sodium hippurate
5 gm. dextrose
P_H 7.2

Flasks containing 100 c c of these mediums were inoculated with culture A-34, a hemolytic streptococcus of human origin, and culture 90H-1 of bovine origin.

TABLE 3

EFFECT OF THE DEVELOPMENT OF ACIDITY IN THE MEDIUM ON THE HYDROLYSIS

Medium	Culture	No Hippurate		Hippurate		Volatile Acid from Hippurate C c*
		N/10 Volatile Acid, C c*	P_H	N/10 Volatile Acid, C c*	P_H	
A	A-34	22.76	6.4	22.60	6.4	0.0
	90H-1	19.44	6.4	64.15	6.4	44.71
B	A-34	12.35	4.9	12.30	5.1	0.0
	90H-1	11.65	4.6	56.53	5.1	44.88

* In 1,000 c c distillate from 100 c c culture medium.

The results given in table 3 again show that A-34 did not split sodium hippurate and that the increase of acidity in the medium had no effect on the hydrolysis by culture 90H-1. In medium A, 44.71 c c $\frac{N}{10}$ volatile acid (benzoic acid) was formed from the hippurate, while the acidity had increased from P_H 7.2 to P_H 6.4. In medium B, the acidity increased from P_H 7.2 to P_H 5.1, and 44.88 c c $\frac{N}{10}$ volatile acid was found.

This experiment, of course, does not show directly the effect of acidity on the hydrolyzing enzyme, because the original P_H was on the alkaline side and the hydrolyzing action may have taken place during the bacterial development and while hydrogen-ion concentration was increasing.

The experiments show, however, that the development of acidity in the medium did not interfere with the hydrolysis of the hippurate and consequently need not be given consideration in connection with tests for this reaction.

The effect of an alkaline reaction was determined in a little different manner in the following medium:

10 gm. peptone (Parke-Davis)	0.03 gm. calcium chloride
5 gm. pepsin	1,000 c c distilled water
1 gm. sodium chloride	NaOH to give the required P_H

Two series of 2 flasks each were prepared, each flask containing 100 c c of this medium, one series without sodium hippurate and the other with 1% of this substance. In each series one of the flasks was adjusted to P_H 8.0 and the other P_H 9.0, and all were inoculated with culture 90H-1. Table 4 shows no growth occurred at P_H 9.0 while the alkaline reaction of P_H 8.0 showed no influence on the hydrolysis. The amount of $\frac{N}{10}$ volatile acid found was 39.0 c c, as compared with the usual amounts which ranged generally from 40 to 44 c c. While the amount in this reaction was slightly lower, it will be seen that only 500 c c of distillate was obtained, against the usual volume of 1,000 c c.

TABLE 4

EFFECT OF INITIAL ALKALINE REACTION ON HYDROLYSIS

Culture	No Hippurate		1% Hippurate	
	P_H 8.0	P_H 9.0	P_H 8.0	P_H 9.0
90H-1............................	C c* 3.76	C c* No growth	C c* 39.00 P_H after growth 8.0	C c* No growth

* N/10 volatile acid in 500 c c distillate from 100 c c of medium.

These experiments indicate clearly that if a medium is suitable for a good growth of a streptococcus capable of splitting sodium hippurate, its composition or reaction has no effect on the hydrolysis.

APPLICATION OF THE HYDROLYSIS OF SODIUM HIPPURATE TO THE DIFFERENTIATION OF HEMOLYTIC STREPTOCOCCI OF HUMAN AND BOVINE ORIGIN

The value of any tests which will help to differentiate between hemolytic streptococci of human and bovine origin will be readily appreciated by a careful comparison of the cultural characteristics shown in tables 5 and 6. The greatest difference was the more active hemolysis of the human types on blood-agar plates. Both human and bovine cultures showed the beta type of hemolysis. Practically the only other difference was in the fermentation of salicin and mannite. These differences in fermentation were not at all constant and are apparently of no real value.

TABLE 5

Cultural Characteristics of Hemolytic Streptococci (beta type) from the Udder of Cows

Culture No.	Fermentations							NH_3 from Peptone	CO_2 from Peptone	CO_2 from Dextrose
	Dextrose	Lactose	Saccharose	Salicin	Mannite	Raffinose	Inulin			
8H	+	+	+	+	—	—	—	+	+	—
8H-1	+	+	+	+	—	—	—	+	+	—
8H-2	+	+	+	+	—	—	—	+	+	—
11H	+	+	+	—	—	—	—	+	+	—
16H-2	+	+	+	—	—	—	—	+	+	—
16H-3	+	+	+	—	—	—	—	+	+	—
20H	+	+	+	+	—	—	—	+	+	—
20H-1	+	+	+	+	—	—	—	+	+	—
20H-3	+	+	+	+	—	—	—	+	+	—
25H-1	+	+	+	—	—	—	—	+	+	—
28H-1	+	+	+	+	—	—	—	+	+	—
28H-2	+	+	+	+	—	—	—	+	+	—
28H-3	+	+	+	+	—	—	—	+	+	—
28H-4	+	+	+	+	—	—	—	+	+	—
32H-3	+	+	+	+	—	—	—	+	+	—
32H-4	+	+	+	+	—	—	—	+	+	—
32H-x	+	+	+	+	—	—	—	+	+	—
37H-4	+	+	+	+	—	—	—	+	+	—
37H-S	+	+	+	+	—	—	—	+	+	—
38H	+	+	+	—	—	—	—	+	+	—
39H-3	+	+	+	—	—	—	—	+	+	—
41H-1	+	+	+	+	—	—	—	+	+	—
41H-2	+	+	+	+	—	—	—	+	+	—
41H-3	+	+	+	+	—	—	—	+	+	—
41H-x	+	+	+	+	—	—	—	+	+	—
42H-3	+	+	+	—	—	—	—	+	+	—
54H	+	+	+	—	—	—	—	+	+	—
54H-1	+	+	+	—	—	—	—	+	+	—
59H	+	+	+	—	—	—	—	+	+	—
59H-1	+	+	+	—	—	—	—	+	+	—
67H-1	+	+	+	+	—	—	—	+	+	—
80H	+	+	+	—	—	—	—	+	+	—
80H-2	+	+	+	—	—	—	—	+	+	—
83H	+	+	+	—	—	—	—	+	+	—
90H	+	+	+	+	—	—	—	+	+	—
90H-1	+	+	+	+	—	—	—	+	+	—
96H	+	+	+	—	—	—	—	+	+	—
97H	+	+	+	—	—	—	—	+	+	—
103H-2	+	+	+	+	—	—	—	+	+	—
106H-4	+	+	+	—	—	—	—	+	+	—
108H-2	+	+	+	—	—	—	—	+	+	—
113H-1	+	+	+	—	—	—	—	+	+	—
115H-2	+	+	+	—	—	—	—	+	+	—
126H-1	+	+	+	—	—	—	—	+	+	—

TABLE 6

CULTURAL CHARACTERISTIC OF HEMOLYTIC STREPTOCOCCI (BETA TYPE) OF HUMAN ORIGIN

Culture No.	Source	Fermentations							NH_3 from Peptone	CO_2 from Peptone	CO_2 from Dextrose
		Dextrose	Lactose	Saccharose	Salicin	Mannite	Raffinose	Inulin			
A 32	Sputum, postinfluenzal pneumonia	+	+	+	+	+	—	—	+	+	—
A 34	Abscess in myocardium	+	+	+	+	—	—	—	+	+	—
A 38	Throat, tonsillitis	+	+	+	+	+	—	—	+	+	—
A 42	Throat, measles	+	+	+	+	+	—	—	+	+	—
A 43	Throat, measles	+	+	+	+	—	—	—	+	+	—
A 45	Throat, measles	+	+	+	+	+	—	—	+	+	—
A 46	Throat, measles	+	+	+	+	+	—	—	+	+	—
A 47	Throat, measles	+	+	+	+	+	—	—	+	+	—
A 49	Throat, measles	+	+	+	+	+	—	—	+	+	—
A 51	Throat, measles	+	+	+	+	+	—	—	+	+	—
A 52	Throat, measles	+	+	+	+	—	—	—	+	+	—
A 56	Normal throat	+	—	+	+	—	—	—	+	+	—
A 59	Normal throat	+	—	+	+	—	—	—	+	+	—
A 60	Normal throat	+	+	+	+	—	—	—	+	+	—
A 63	Normal throat	+	+	+	+	—	—	—	+	+	—
A 64	Normal throat	+	+	+	+	—	—	—	+	+	—
A 65	Throat, pharyngitis	+	+	+	+	—	—	—	+	+	—
A 66	Normal throat	+	+	+	+	—	—	—	+	+	—
A 67	Throat, tonsillitis	+	+	+	+	—	—	—	+	+	—
A 69	Throat, bronchitis	+	+	+	+	—	—	—	+	+	—
A 73	Throat, tonsillitis	+	+	+	+	—	—	—	+	+	—
A 74	Throat, normal	+	+	+	+	—	—	—	+	+	—
A 78	Throat, normal	+	+	+	+	—	—	—	+	+	—
A 79	Throat, normal	+	+	+	+	—	—	—	+	+	—
A 80	Throat, normal	+	+	+	+	—	—	—	+	+	—
A 81	Throat, normal	+	+	+	+	—	—	—	+	+	—
A 82	Throat, normal	+	+	+	+	—	—	—	+	+	—
A 94	Throat, normal	+	+	+	+	—	+	—	+	+	—
A 95	Hemolytic streptococcus, army strain	+	+	+	+	—	—	—	+	+	—
R 2	Lung necropsy	+	+	+	+	—	—	—	+	+	—
R 24	Bronchopneumonia	+	+	+	+	—	—	—	+	+	—
R 66	Throat, measles	+	+	+	+	+	—	—	+	+	—
R 271	Blood, septicemia	+	+	+	+	—	—	—	+	+	—

The ability of these hemolytic cultures from human and bovine sources to hydrolyze sodium hippurate was determined in the most simple medium which would support growth, in order to minimize the formation of volatile acid from anything but the hippurate. For this purpose the following peptone medium was quite satisfactory:

10 gm. peptone (Parke-Davis)
10 gm. sodium hippurate
1.5 gm. potassium diabasic phosphate
1,000 c c distilled water
Reaction adjusted to PH 7.2

The medium was put up in 100 c c amounts in flasks, and after inoculation was incubated 7 days at 37 C. Growth was slow in starting with some cultures and moderate in amount in all cases. Therefore it was considered advisable to allow 7 days for incubation. After incubation the cultures were made acid, and the volatile acidity was determined in 500 c c of distillate from 100 c c of culture.

All our 33 hemolytic cultures of human origin and 44 hemolytic cultures of the beta type of bovine origin were examined for their ability to split sodium hippurate. From the results in table 7 it is evident that the hydrolysis of the hippurate by the hemolytic streptococci of bovine origin separated them perfectly from those of human origin. All of the bovine types split the hippurate, while none of the

TABLE 7

DIFFERENTIATION OF HEMOLYTIC STREPTOCOCCI OF HUMAN AND BOVINE ORIGIN BY MEANS OF THE HYDROLYSIS OF SODIUM HIPPURATE SHOWING HOW A POSITIVE REACTION CORRELATES WITH A LOW PH

Hemolytic Streptococci, Udders of Cows				Hemolytic Streptococci, Human Sources			
Culture No.	C c N/10 Volatile Acid	Hydrolysis	PH Dextrose Yeast Broth	Culture No.	C c N/10 Volatile Acid	Hydrolysis	PH Dextrose Yeast Broth
8H	40.52*	+	4.5	A 32	3.65*	—	5.5
8H-1	41.51	+	4.5	A 34	3.37	—	5.4
8H-2	44.73	+	4.5	A 38	3.50	—	5.3
11H	41.17	+	4.5	A 42	3.31	—	5.4
16H-2	38.00	+	4.5	A 43	3.64	—	5.4
16H-3	39.08	+	4.5	A 45	3.19	—	5.5
20H	39.51	+	4.5	A 46	3.50	—	5.5
20H-1	42.36	+	4.6	A 47	3.52	—	5.5
20H-3	40.71	+	4.5	A 49	3.31	—	5.5
25H-1	41.42	+	4.5	A 51	3.49	—	5.5
28H-1	40.14	+	4.5	A 52	2.84	—	5.5
28H-2	44.14	+	4.6	A 56	3.53	—	5.3
28H-3	39.61	+	4.5	A 59	3.22	—	5.4
28H-4	39.96	+	4.5	A 60	2.90	—	5.5
32H-3	43.89	+	4.5	A 63	3.24	—	5.5
32H-4	35.64	+	4.5	A 64	3.11	—	5.6
32H-x	42.27	+	4.6	A 65	3.40	—	5.6
37H-4	42.12	+	4.5	A 66	2.47	—	5.6
37H-5	36.22	+	4.5	A 67	3.05	—	5.5
38H	41.01	+	4.6	A 69	3.10	—	5.6
39H-3	39.45	+	4.5	A 73	3.13	—	5.5
41H-1	42.52	+	4.5	A 74	3.37	—	5.5
41H-2	44.27	+	4.5	A 78	3.08	—	5.4
41H-3	39.73	+	4.5	A 79	3.31	—	5.3
41H-x	41.83	+	4.5	A 80	3.27	—	5.6
42H-3	40.24	+	4.6	A 81	3.54	—	5.6
54H	42.72	+	4.5	A 82	3.56	—	5.6
54H-1	43.10	+	4.5	A 94	1.44	—	4.6
59H	40.32	+	4.5	A 95	2.60	—	5.5
59H-1	41.23	+	4.5	R 2	3.39	—	5.4
67H-1	38.36	+	4.5	R 24	1.36	—	5.5
80H	41.02	+	4.5	R 66	3.46	—	5.6
80H-2	41.79	+	4.5	R 271	2.32	—	5.4
83H	39.03	+	4.5				
90H	43.07	+	4.5	A 34	No hippurate 4.86		
90H-1	36.69	+	4.5				
96H	44.70	+	4.5				
97H	38.63	+	4.5				
103H-2	40.08	+	4.6				
106H-4	39.07	+	4.5				
108H-2	40.07	+	4.5				
113H-1	20.07	+	4.5				
115H-2	37.28	+	4.5				
126H-1	41.04	+	4.6				
90H-1	No hippurate 3.28						

* C c N/10 volatile acid in 500 c c distillate from 100 c c of medium.

human type possessed this ability. The hemolytic streptococci from both human and bovine sources produced from 3 to 4 c c $\frac{N}{10}$ volatile acid in the medium without sodium hippurate. When there was a hydrolysis the volatile acidity was increased to about 40 c c; both qualitative and quantitative tests showed the excess to be benzoic acid.

A further study of the results shows that all of the bovine types reached a final hydrogen-ion concentration is dextrose yeast broth of P_H 4.5-4.6, while all the human types reached only P_H 5.3-5.6, with one exception. This exception is interesting, since by P_H it might be considered a bovine type, or by the lack of power to hydrolyze hippurate it could be considered a human type. This culture (A-94) was isolated from a normal throat and varied from the other human types in its ability to ferment raffinose. It does not appear to be of the ordinary human type either in its fermentations or in final P_H, yet it is clearly not a bovine udder organism because of its inability to hydrolyze sodium hippurate.

The use of sodium hippurate should materially assist in the proper placing of cultures of this type which are found in normal throats.

Our results indicate that the hemolytic B types of streptococci of human origin can be separated from similar types of bovine origin by the inability of the human type to hydrolyze sodium hippurate. We realize, however, that a larger number of cultures must be examined before definite statements regarding this can be made.

TESTS FOR THE HYDROLYSIS OF SODIUM HIPPURATE

In our work we used a simple peptone medium and distilled each culture for volatile acidity in order to determine the hydrolysis. This process has the advantage of giving clear-cut results, but it is too long for routine work.

Several rapid tests have therefore been worked out and are suggested for the routine examination of cultures. It is important that a simple medium be used, which will show good growth, and for this purpose the following medium is recommended.

Peptone Pepsin Medium

10 gm. peptone (Parke-Davis)	1 drop of 1 per cent. ferric chloride solution
5 gm. pepsin	1,000 c c distilled water
.03 gm. calcium chloride	NaOH to give P_H 7.1
10 gm. sodium hippurate	

If cultures are found which will not grow in this medium, the usual beef-infusion peptone broth with or without dextrose may be used, but the tests are not quite so satisfactory with this complex medium.

The presence of benzoic acid in the medium can be demonstrated by the addition of either a ferric-chloride solution or an inorganic acid, the ferric-chloride test being the more delicate of the two. The protein, the hippurate, and the benzoate are precipitated by ferric chloride, the difference between them being that the protein and the hippurate precipitates are more readily soluble in an excess of ferric chloride than the benzoate. If, therefore, we add a definite amount of ferric chloride solution to a fixed quantity of the medium, the reaction can be so balanced that the protein and hippurate precipitate redissolve in the excess of the reagent while the benzoate remains as an insoluble precipitate.

Ferric-Chloride Test.—The amount of ferric chloride required depends on the medium used. In the case of the peptone pepsin medium, 0.5 c c of a 7% solution of ferric chloride is added to 2 c c of the medium. When it is thoroughly shaken, an insoluble precipitate remains in the mixture if the hippurate has been split into benzoate and glycocoll, whereas the mixture becomes clear on standing 5 or 10 minutes if the hippurate has not been hydrolyzed. The precipitate of ferric benzoate is well marked when one-fifth or more of the hippurate has been split, while only a turbidity is produced when less has been hydrolyzed.

Udder hemolytic streptococci hydrolyze the hippurate completely or nearly so, and the test is sharp and distinct. A slight opalescence is generally present in the medium containing only hippurate which is not acted on by the hemolytic streptococci of human origin, and this becomes somewhat more marked when some of the growth is transferred to the test tube, but neither turbidity nor precipitate is produced.

If the medium contains phosphates, it is necessary to add a small amount of hydrochloric acid to the ferric-chlorid solution, so as to redissolve the phosphate of iron formed.

In the case of a beef-infusion peptone medium, it is necessary to use a 12% ferric chloride solution containing from 2.0 to 2.5 c c concentrated hydrochloric acid per liter, and it requires a longer time for the medium to become clear when the hippurate has not been hydrolyzed.

ACID TEST

On adding an excess of an inorganic acid to the medium, the benzoic acid separates as a white crystalline precipitate. About one-half of the hippurate must be split in order to give a well-marked precipitate, the protein in the solution preventing the separation of the acid if present in only small amounts.

Test: Five-tenths c c of 50% sulphuric acid is added to 2 c c of the medium; the mixture is well shaken and allowed to stand. In cultures of hemolytic streptococci of bovine origin a large amount of benzoic acid is always present.

Hydrolysis Indicated by Increase in Amino-Nitrogen.—As hippuric acid is split into benzoic acid and glycocoll, there should be an increase in the amino-nitrogen content of the medium unless the glycocoll is utilized by the bacteria.

Our results idicate that there is such an increase with the streptococci during hydrolysis. A formol titration therefore shows a considerable increase in amino-nitrogen in cultures which hydrolyze hippuric acid, and this increase may be as high as eight times the amount found in control cultures without the hippurate, as is shown in table 1.

This large increase in amino-nitrogen therefore constitutes another test for the hydrolysis.

SUMMARY

It has been shown that hippuric acid is hydrolyzed by the 44 hemolytic streptococci from the udders of cows, but not by the 33 hemolytic streptococci of human origin which are in our collection of cultures.

As much as 1% of hippurate may be split into benzoic acid and glycocoll.

The hydrolysis is not affected by the hydrogen-ion concentration of the medium, at least under the experimental conditions of our work.

The composition of the medium does not appear to affect the hydrolysis, provided it is suitable for the growth of the streptococci.

Simple tests have been devised for the detection of the hydrolysis routine work.

The hydrolysis of sodium hippurate seems to separate the hemolytic beta streptococci of the bovine udder from those of human origin, but should be used at present only with beta hemolytic types. It is hoped this reaction will be equally valuable after large numbers of cultures have been examined.

Particular attention is called to the fact that the usefulness of the hydrolysis of sodium hippurate is discussed only in its relation to the beta hemolytic streptococci of human and bovine origin. Our studies have shown that the ability of streptococci to split sodium hippurate is not limited to the hemolytic types. Some of the alpha types from the udder of the cow do not produce the hydrolysis, while, on the other hand, the hydrolyzing property is common among the lactic type of streptococci. The test must not be applied indiscriminately, therefore, to all groups of streptococci.

STREPTOCOCCI IN CHRONIC RESPIRATORY INFECTIONS

W. Ray Hodge and Cecile Cohen

From the Connaught Antitoxin Laboratories, Research Division, University of Toronto, Toronto, and the Laboratory Division of the Chest Clinic of the Department of Soldiers' Civil Reestablishment

The clinical material for the present study was made available through the Chest Clinic of the Department of Soldiers' Civil Reestablishment at Toronto. Ideal conditions for repeated examinations of sputum were obtained as many of the cases were pensioners returning for periodic examination and many were attending for vaccine treatment, while others still were held in observation wards for varying periods of time.

The chief aim of the study was to determine the constancy or inconstancy of types of streptococci occurring in chronic nontuberculous respiratory infections. In the determination of this first objective, many points of interest occurred and many questions of doubt arose, necessitating extensive collateral investigations; the apparently simple problem proved complex and an attempt was made to solve questions of doubt by frequent specially conducted experiments which are incorporated in this paper. It was hoped that strains constantly present on closely repeated examinations of sputum might be isolated; that vaccines might be prepared from strains so isolated, and that in this way vaccine treatment might be rendered less haphazard and the results more uniformly encouraging. Roughly, our idea was to examine three samples of sputum collected at two day intervals from selected cases. The cases of bronchial asthma in this series include only those which failed to show any evidence of sensitization with extensive percutaneous protein tests. Streptococci in these samples were to be identified by Brown's method of classification. The choice of this classification was made chiefly because of convenience and uniformity of terminology; and though at first sight somewhat confusing and complicated was justified by the ease with which the flora in various samples of sputum from the same source could be compared. The effect of vaccine therapy on the patient and on the streptococcal flora was to be observed. The numerous sidepaths of investigation have, however, prevented the fulfilment of this aim; it soon became apparent

Received for publication Nov. 25, 1921.

that the streptococcal flora in these cases was not simple, and that the preparation of vaccines by the suggested method would be too laborious. Accordingly, attention was finally focused on the flora alone and an attempt made to discover precisely how complex this aspect of the problem was.

METHODS

The streptococcal reactions in blood agar were determined by the use of Brown's [1] standard deep plates substituting citrated human blood for defibrinated horse blood. Repeats made with citrated human and defibrinated horse blood were found to give parallel results. In blood agar the organisms were thus identified as falling into one of 4 types: beta (complete hemolysis), alpha prime (partial hemolysis), alpha (green production), and gamma (no change). For further identification the fermentative reactions were determined in the 6 carbohydrates: mannite, lactose, salicin, raffinose, inulin, and saccharose. The information obtained in this way was used to place the organisms in Brown's classification. In this classification streptococci are placed according to types in blood agar: groups, with respect to fermentation of mannite, lactose and salicin; and subgroups, with respect to fermentation of saccharose, inulin and raffinose. The types are alpha, alpha prime, beta and gamma; the groups are numbered 1 to 8, and the subgroups 0.1 to 0.8, inclusive. By this means the hemolytic and fermentative properties of a streptococcus can be referred to by a letter, a number, and a decimal. Hence α 1.2 indicates a green-producing streptococcus which ferments lactose, salicin, saccharose and raffinose, but does not ferment mannite or inulin. This classification was found to be very convenient for the work in hand for the reasons mentioned. It is, however, unfortunately handicapped because of the confusion attending such a complete revolution in terminology. It should be emphasized that this classification in many instances simply introduces new terms for streptococcus groups already known under more familiar name. For instance, a beta type streptococcus simply means a strongly hemolytic streptococcus; an alpha type streptococcus is what is characterized as Streptococcus viridans in ordinary terminology.

Thus	β 1.1 is S. pyogenes	(Rosenbach)
	β 2.1 is S. anginosus	(Andrews and Horder)
	β 3.1 is S. equi	(Schultz)
	β 4.1 is S. subacidus	(Holman)

[1] Use of Blood Agar for Study of Streptococci, Rockefeller Monograph 9.

β 5.1 is	S. infrequens	(Holman)
β 7.1 is	S. alactosus	(Smith and Brown)
α 1.1 is	S. mitis	(Andrews and Horder)
α 2.1 is	S. salivarius	(Andrews and Horder)
α 3.1 is	S. equinus	(Andrews and Horder)
α 4.1 is	S. ignavus	(Holman)
α 5.1 is	S. fecalis	(Andrews and Horder)

TECHNIC

Particles of sputum were washed twice in sterile saline, planted in serum broth, and after 6 hours' incubation, a loopful of this broth culture was plated on blood agar. After 24 hours' incubation single colonies were picked and streaked on the surface of blood agar and after further incubation, the culture so obtained was planted in a tube of serum broth; after 18 hours' incubation a loopful of properly diluted broth culture was sown in deep blood agar plates. Care was taken to have the agar cooled to 45 C. before the blood was added, thus preventing hemolysis due to heat. From the deep plate single colonies were picked under the microscope, carved out with a wire loop and emulsified in a tube of broth (beef infusion broth P_H 7.6 with 3 or 4 drops of sterile, citrated human blood added to each tube). After 18 hours, films were made and the appearance noted. The blood broth culture, in which growth was invariably heavy, was used for seeding the sugar tubes. Medium for fermentations was beef infusion broth, P_H 7.6 previously fermented with B. coli and so rendered sugar-free. The reaction was adjusted colorimetrically and checked by electrolytic methods. Electrolytic determinations were done by Mr. Moloney of the Connaught Laboratories. The sugars were dry sterilized, suspended in thin glass bulbs [2] over a small amount of water in a flask; the water contained sufficient Andrade's indicator for final concentration of 1%. These flasks were sterilized in the autoclave for half an hour at 15 pounds. After sterilization the glass bulbs were broken against the bottom of the flasks and the sugars dissolved. The sugar and indicator was added to the sugar-free broth, to which 10% sterile horse serum had been added. The completed fermentation medium was poured into a sterile funnel covered with sterile gauze and tubed through a hooded pipet. In this way a second sterilization of the sugar was avoided. The tubes were paraffined and incubated

[2] A method devised by Dr. D. T. Fraser of these laboratories to prevent hydrolysis of the sugars.

for 48 hours and those not contaminated stored in the ice-chest until required. Contamination of any of the tubes was infrequent. Mediums so prepared with a final P_H of 7.6 and stored in the ice-chest for eight months showed a P_H of 7.42. The seeded fermentation tubes were incubated for 6 days at 37 C. and the results read. Films invariably revealed good growth.

In the preliminary work, using these methods, it was found that sputum collected at 2 or 3 day intervals from the same source showed marked variations in the strains isolated. It was not possible to pick out any particular strain which occurred in succeeding samples and which might be considered pathogenic on account of the constancy of its appearance. It seemed possible that this might be due to three causes: (1) inaccuracy of the methods employed or inconstancy of appearance of organisms on blood agar or inconstancy of fermentations; (2) an insufficient number of organisms were being picked from the preliminary plates so that the determination of flora present was haphazard; (3) an actual variation in flora from day to day. These three possible causes were investigated in detail and the results obtained form the bulk of the material of this paper.

Owing to lack of space it is not possible to give in detail the work dealing with the accuracy of these methods. Briefly, we found that under constant conditions the appearance produced in blood agar was constant. An interesting variation was encountered in certain alpha prime strains (α' 2.1); it was found that in lightly seeded plates the alpha prime appearance was constantly produced. In heavily seeded plates, however (over 200 colonies), these organisms produced green zones and on repeated refrigeration and incubation alternate green and hemolytic rings. The fermentations were found to be rather less accurate. Lyall [3] found that on repetition less than 5% of his strains showed variations. Holman [4] has pointed out that supposed variations in fermentative reactions may be due to the use of inferior mediums. Streptococci grew well in our sugar-free broth before the addition of carbohydrate. One hundred strains after storage were replated for purity, and the fermentative reactions determined with variations in 10 strains. There were 2 apparent types of variation; (a) certain alpha and alpha prime strains, although showing quite good growth, failed to ferment a sugar which they had fermented previously. In these instances by increasing the amount of seed

[3] Jour. Med. Research, 1914, 30, p. 487.
[4] Ibid., 1916, 35, p. 151.

culture and producing abnormally heavy growth fermentation resulted. This was evidently a marginal type of fermentation. (b) Certain beta strains seemed to lose completely their power to ferment certain sugars —this latter finding is in agreement with Clawson [5] who found considerable variation on repeated titrations of certain strains of hemolytic streptococci after storage. We found that repeated subculture in the sugar showing variation leads to greater ease of fermentation of this sugar.

Having determined that the methods employed were sufficiently accurate, the remaining two possibilities were investigated, namely, the possibility of an extensive flora and the possibility of a daily variation in the strains present. Walker and Adkinson [6] investigated the sputum of patients with bronchial asthma and concluded that the thick sputum of these cases, provided it was washed, contained few types of streptococci. The classification adopted by these authors was that suggested by Holman. It should be remembered that in the present work Brown's classification was used throughout and that the possible number of variations in this classification is much greater than in that of Holman.

INVESTIGATION OF VARIATIONS IN FLORA

The early experiments of this part of the investigation cannot be given in detail. It was necessary first of all to reassure ourselves that the colonies were picked clean from the surface plates and that the cultures in the deep plates were pure. This was carefully checked, and the results showed that the strains were pure in every instance. We were now in a position to proceed with the problem in hand; the early work at this stage soon showed an occasional marked variation in flora in succeeding samples of sputum collected at short intervals from the same source. Such a variation is shown in table 1. In these samples the sputum was surface plated in 4 ways. Direct particle, wash saline, 6-hour broth and 24-hour broth.

Here the variation of flora in the first and second specimens is marked. One cannot pick out any strain which occurs in considerable numbers in both specimens. There are no beta organisms in the first specimen, but a beta organism appears several times in the second specimen. Has the flora actually changed so considerably in three days or have the variations in flora not been exhausted in each sample?

[5] Jour. Infect. Dis., 1920, 26, p. 93.
[6] Jour. Med. Research, 1919, 40, p. 229.

The next experiment is an attempt to answer this question. Here the number of organisms picked from the surface plates was greatly increased, in this way an attempt was made to exhaust completely the variations in flora in the various samples examined.

TABLE 1

CHRONIC BRONCHITIS. STREPTOCOCCI FROM SAMPLES OF SPUTUM COLLECTED AT TWO DAY INTERVALS

Material Plated	Specimen 1	Specimen 2
Washed Direct Particle	Alpha 2.4 Alpha 1.2 Alpha 6.1 Alpha′ 2.3 Alpha′ 2.1	Beta 1.1 × 2 Alpha 1.5 Alpha 1.2 Alpha′ 3.1 Gamma 3.1
Wash Saline	Alpha 6.1 × 2 Alpha′ 2.1	Beta 1.1 × 2 Alpha 1.1 Alpha 1.2 Gamma 1.2
Broth, 6 hours incubation	Alpha 1.2 Alpha′ 2.1 × 2 Alpha′ 3.1 × 4	Alpha 1.2 Alpha′ 3.1 Gamma 1.2
Broth, 24 hours incubation	Alpha′ 3.1 × 3	Beta 1.1 Alpha′ 3.1 Alpha 3.1 Alpha 1.2 × 2

TABLE 2

BRONCHIAL ASTHMA. ONE HUNDRED AND TWELVE DIFFERENT STREPTOCOCCI ISOLATED FROM FOUR SAMPLES OF SPUTUM SHOWING TYPES ISOLATED FROM VARIOUS SAMPLES

Sputum Sample			
1. 7/12/20	2. 18/12/20	3. 27/1/21	4. 31/1/21
Total number of strains......... 18	Total number of strains......... 22	Total number of strains......... 39	Total number of strains......... 33
Number of different types....... 11	Number of different types....... 8	Number of different types....... 8	Number of different types....... 10
Beta 1.1 × 2 Beta 2.2 × 1 Alpha′ 2.1 × 5 Alpha′ 2.2 × 1 Alpha 1.1 × 2 Alpha 1.2 × 1 Alpha 1.3 × 1 Alpha 2.1 × 1 Alpha 2.2 × 2 Alpha 3.3 × 1 Gamma 5.4 × 1	Beta 2.1 × 2 Alpha′ 2.1 × 4 Alpha 1.1 × 2 Alpha 1.2 × 3 Alpha 2.1 × 6 Alpha 2.2 × 3 Alpha 3.1 × 1 Gamma 1.1 × 1	Beta 2.1 × 4 Beta 3.1 × 1 Alpha′ 1.1 × 2 Alpha′ 2.1 × 5 Alpha 1.1 × 6 Alpha 1.2 × 8 Alpha 2.1 × 7 Alpha 2.2 × 6	Beta 2.1 × 1 Beta 3.1 × 1 Alpha′ 1.1 × 3 Alpha′ 2.1 × 2 Alpha′ 5.1 × 2 Alpha 1.1 × 10 Alpha 1.2 × 8 Alpha 1.3 × 2 Alpha 2.1 × 3 Alpha 2.2 × 1

In table 2 are shown the results obtained by picking large numbers of colonies from the preliminary plates; four different samples of sputum from the same patient (a bronchial asthmatic) were examined.

In this experiment 112 strains were isolated from 4 samples of sputum with 19 different types. Thirty-one strains were rechecked for appearance in blood agar and fermentation reactions with constant results. It will be seen that the flora appears fairly constant—the number of different types in various samples varies from 8 to 11. The organism appearing most frequently is α 1.2. There are various beta and alpha prime types in each sample, and as far as these groups of the flora are concerned, the parallelism between samples 3 and 4 is almost complete, not quite so complete between samples 2 and 3, or 2 and 4, and still less complete between samples 1 and 2, 1 and 3, and

TABLE 3

BRONCHIAL ASTHMA. ONE HUNDRED AND THIRTY-ONE DIFFERENT STREPTOCOCCI ISOLATED FROM TWO SAMPLES OF SPUTUM, SHOWING TYPES ISOLATED FROM TWO SAMPLES

Sputum Sample			
1. 2/3/21		2. 3/5/21	
Total number of strains	58	Total number of strains	73
Number of different types	12	Number of different types	16
Beta 2.1 × 2		Beta 1.1 × 6	
Alpha′ 1.1 × 5		Alpha′ 1.1 × 10	
Alpha′ 2.1 × 2		Alpha′ 2.1 × 4	
Alpha 1.1 × 10		Alpha′ 4.5 × 1	
Alpha 1.2 × 4		Alpha 1.1 × 8	
Alpha 1.4 × 1		Alpha 1.2 × 2	
Alpha 2.1 × 16		Alpha 1.3 × 2	
Alpha 2.2 × 6		Alpha 1.4 × 2	
Alpha 2.4 × 6		Alpha 2.1 × 13	
Alpha 3.1 × 3		Alpha 2.2 × 6	
Alpha 4.1 × 2		Alpha 2.4 × 5	
Alpha 5.1 × 1		Alpha 5.1 × 1	
		Alpha 5.2 × 1	
		Alpha 6.4 × 1	
		Alpha 4.5 × 2	
		Gamma 5.1 × 9	

1 and 4. This probably indicates a gradual change in flora as samples 1 and 4 with the largest time interval (almost 2 months) show the most marked divergence of types, while samples 3 and 4 with only 4 days interval show almost complete parallelism. α′ 2.1, although not occurring as frequently as α 1.2, occurs most persistently, from 4 to 5 times in each sample.

This experiment was repeated on the sputum of another patient with bronchial asthma. The results are shown in table 3.

In this experiment 131 strains were isolated from 2 samples of sputum (with 2 days intervening) with 19 different types. The number of types in each sample varied from 12 to 16. Here again there is an essential parallelism of types in the 2 samples, broken most conspicuously by the beta types, β 2.1 being recovered twice in sample

1, and β 1.1 being recovered 6 times in sample 2. The variation in these beta types is of considerable interest; it is difficult to reconcile the variations in these types with the relatively high pathogenicity which they possess. As the agglutination results do not place these types in a single immunologic group we can only conclude that these variations are real and that the beta group is at least not a supreme etiologic factor in these cases. The organism occurring most frequently in these samples is α 2.1, and next in frequency α 1.1.

The influence of the type of particle on the flora developed is shown in table 4.

It is immediately apparent that the flora does not vary appreciably in particles of different appearance in the same sample of sputum—the

TABLE 4

BRONCHIAL ASTHMA. FLORA IN THREE DIFFERENT PARTICLES FROM THE SAME SAMPLE OF SPUTUM

Gray Feathery Particle That Floated	Heavy Greenish Particle	Light Mucoid Particle
Beta 1.1 × 1	Beta 1.1 × 3	Beta 1.1 × 2
Beta 2.1 × 1	Beta 2.1 × 1	Alpha′ 1.1 × 4
Alpha′ 1.1 × 8	Alpha′ 1.1 × 4	Alpha′ 2.1 × 1
Alpha′ 2.1 × 1	Alpha′ 2.1 × 3	Alpha′ 4.5 × 1
Alpha 1.1 × 5	Alpha 1.1 × 7	Alpha 1.1 × 6
Alpha 1.2 × 3	Alpha 1.2 × 3	Alpha 1.3 × 1
Alpha 1.3 × 1	Alpha 2.1 × 7	Alpha 1.4 × 1
Alpha 1.4 × 1	Alpha 2.2 × 4	Alpha 2.1 × 10
Alpha 2.1 × 12	Alpha 2.4 × 5	Alpha 2.2 × 2
Alpha 2.2 × 5	Alpha 3.1 × 1	Alpha 2.4 × 3
Alpha 2.4 × 3	Alpha 4.1 × 1	Alpha 5.1 × 2
Alpha 3.1 × 4	Alpha 5.1 × 1	Alpha 4.1 × 1
Alpha 4.1 × 1	Gamma 5.1 × 1	Gamma 5.1 × 5
Gamma 5.1 × 1		

growth is apparently homogeneous throughout the sputum; hence the choice of particle has little effect on the flora ultimately developed in the culture.

The method of making the preliminary plate was similarly investigated. The results are shown in table 5.

In table 5 it is seen that the 3 methods employed give essentially parallel results. The beta organisms are not apparently overgrown by the alphas in a 24-hour broth culture. These observations have an important bearing on the method of preparation of vaccines.

It is obvious, from the results obtained by an exhaustive exploration of the flora in these cases, that the classification adopted distinguished many different groups of streptococci in single specimens of sputum. The immunologic relationship of these various groups was a question of interest which we felt demanded investigation. The agglutination reaction was chosen as being the reaction most likely to bring out sharply the differences sought. Kligler [7] found that there was a distinct parallelism between groups of streptococci distinguished by fermentations and by agglutinations. He concluded that fermentation reactions tended to divide streptococci into broad, distinct species. Floyd and Wolbach [8] found that agglutination reactions supported the value of fermentation tests. Dochez, Avery and Lancefield, in an investigation of hemolytic streptococci isolated during the course of an epidemic of bronchopneumonia, distinguished by the agglutination reaction 4 distinct types. They found that all members of their type S_{60} fermented mannite. The agglutinations in the present work were undertaken

TABLE 5

BRONCHIAL ASTHMA. INFLUENCE OF METHOD OF PLATING ON FLORA DEVELOPED

Plating Washed Particle Direct	Six-Hour Broth Culture Plated	Twenty-Four-Hour Broth Culture Plated
Total number of strains.... 50	Total number of strains.... 40	Total number of strains.... 42
Number of different types.. 15	Number of different types.. 13	Number of different types.. 12
Beta 1.1 × 1	Beta 1.1 × 1	Beta 1.1 × 4
Beta 2.1 × 1	Alpha′ 1.1 × 5	Beta 2.1 × 1
Alpha′ 1.1 × 8	Alpha′ 2.1 × 1	Alpha′ 1.1 × 2
Alpha′ 2.1 × 2	Alpha 1.1 × 8	Alpha′ 2.1 × 3
Alpha 1.1 × 3	Alpha 1.3 × 1	Alpha′ 4.5 × 1
Alpha 1.2 × 3	Alpha 1.4 × 1	Alpha 1.1 × 7
Alpha 1.3 × 1	Alpha 2.1 × 8	Alpha 1.2 × 4
Alpha 1.4 × 1	Alpha 2.2 × 6	Alpha 1.4 × 1
Alpha 2.1 × 13	Alpha 2.4 × 2	Alpha 2.1 × 8
Alpha 2.2 × 6	Alpha 3.1 × 4	Alpha 2.4 × 6
Alpha 2.4 × 3	Alpha 4.1 × 1	Alpha 4.1 × 1
Alpha 3.1 × 2	Alpha 6.4 × 1	Gamma 5.1 × 4
Alpha 5.1 × 2	Gamma 5.1 × 1	
Alpha 5.2 × 1		
Gamma 5.1 × 3		

simply for the further elucidation of the problems we were trying to solve and not to attempt an immunologic classification of streptococci, hence relatively few animals were immunized.

AGGLUTINATIONS

Rabbits were immunized with 7 different strains of streptococci, all of which had been isolated from the sputum of the 2 patients with bronchial asthma, intensively investigated by the other methods. The immune serums obtained in this way were used for agglutinations with 62 strains from various specimens of sputum and one strain from a case of erysipelas.

[7] Jour. Infect. Dis., 1915, 16, p. 327.
[8] Jour. Med. Research, 1913, 29, p. 493.

TABLE 6

RESULTS OF AGGLUTINATION TESTS

		Serums								
Strain number		Boy 1	Boy 2	Day 1	Boy 3	Boy 4	Boy 5	Boy 6	Normal Human and Rabbit Serum	Control
Classification		Beta 2.1	Beta 1.1	Alpha′ 3.1	Alpha′ 2.1	Alpha′ 2.1	Alpha 1.1	Alpha 2.2		
Dilutions		1:20 1:40 1:80	1:20 1:40 1:80	1:50 1:100 1:200	1:50 1:100 1:200	1:50 1:100 1:200	1:50 1:100 1:200	1:50	1:20 1:40 1:80	
Strain Number	Classification									
Boy 1	Beta 2.1	CA 1:80 ACA 1:160 SA 1:320	—	—	—	—	—	—	—	—
Boy 2	Beta 1.1	—	CA 1:320 ACA 1:640	—	—	—	—	—	—	—
Day 1	Alpha′ 3.1	—	—	CA 1:8000 SA 1:64,000	—	—	—	—	—	—
Boy 3	Alpha′ 2.1	1:400	CA 1:200 ACA 1:400	1:1600	CA 1:12,000	CA 1:12,800	CA 1:5120	1:80	—	—
Boy 4	Alpha′ 2.1	1:400	CA 1:200 ACA 1:400	1:1600	CA 1:12,000	CA 1:12,800	CA 1:5120	1:80	—	—
Boy 5	Alpha 1.1	—	—	—	—	—	CA 1:3200 ACA 1:5120	—	—	—
Boy 6	Alpha 2.2	—	—	—	—	—	—	CA 1:400 SA 1:800	—	—
Boy 7	Alpha′ 5.1	—	—	—	—	—	—	—	—	—
Boy 8	Alpha′ 1.1	—	—	—	—	—	—	—	—	—
Boy 9	Alpha 1.1	—	—	—	—	—	—	—	—	—
Boy 10	Alpha 1.2	—	—	—	—	—	—	—	—	—
Boy 11	Alpha′ 1.1	—	—	—	—	—	—	—	—	—
Boy 12	Beta 3.1	—	—	—	—	—	—	—	—	—
Boy 13	Beta 2.1	+	+	+	+	+	+		+	+
Boy 14	Alpha′ 2.1	+	+	+	+	+	+	+	—	—
Boy 15	Alpha′ 2.1	+	+	+	+	+	+	+	—	—
Boy 16	Alpha′ 2.1	+H	+H	+	+	+	+	+	—	—
Boy 22	Alpha′ 2.1	+H	+H	+H	+H	+	+	+	—	—
Boy 25	Alpha′ 2.1	+H	+H	+H	+H	+H	+H		—	—
Boy 26	Alpha 1.1	—	—	—	—	—	+	—	—	—
Boy 19	Alpha 1.1	—	—	—	—	—	+		—	—
Boy 17	Alpha′ 1.1	—	—	—	—	—	—			—
Boy 18	Alpha 1.2	—	—	—	—	—	—			—
Boy 20	Alpha 1.3	—	—	—	—	—	—			—
Boy 21	Alpha 2.2	—	—	—	—	—	—	1:80,		—
Boy 23	Alpha 2.1	—	—	—	—	—	—		—	—
Boy 24	Beta 2.1	±	—	—	—	—	—		—	—
Day 2	Alpha′ 3.1	—	—	+	—	—	—			—
Day 3	Alpha′ 3.1	—	—	+	—	—	—			—
Day 4	Alpha′ 3.1	—	—	+H	—	—	—			—
Day 5	Alpha′ 3.1	—	—	+	—	—	—			—
Day 6	Alpha′ 3.1	—	—	+H	—	—	—			—
Day 7	Alpha′ 3.1	—	—	+	—	—	—			—
Day 8	Alpha′ 3.1	—	—	+	—	—	—			—
Day 9	Alpha 2.1	—	—	—	—	—	—			—
Day 10	Beta 1.1	—	—	±	—	—	—			—
Day 11	Beta 1.1	—	—	±	—	—	—			—
Day 12	Alpha′ 2.1	+	+	+	+	+	+	—	+	+

TABLE 6—Continued

RESULTS OF AGGLUTINATION TESTS

		Serums								
Strain number.......		Boy 1	Boy 2	Day 1	Boy 3	Boy 4	Boy 5	Boy 6	Normal Human	Con-
Classification........		Beta 2.1	Beta 1.1	Alpha′ 3.1	Alpha′ 2.1	Alpha′ 2.1	Alpha 1.1	Alpha 2.2	and Rabbit Serum	trol
Dilutions............		1:20 1:40 1:80	1:20 1:40 1:80	1:50 1:100 1:200	1:50 1:100 1:200	1:50 1:100 1:200	1:50 1:100 1:200	1:50	1:20 1:40 1:80	
Strain Number	Classification									
SMP 1	Alpha 2.2	—	—	—	—	—	—	—	—	—
SMJ 2	Alpha′ 2.1	+H	+H	+H	+H	+	+H			—
SHJ 3	Alpha 1.1	—	—	—	—	—	+	—		—
SMJ 4	Alpha 2.1	—	—	—	—	—	—	—		—
SMJ 5	Alpha 2.1	—	—	—	—	—	—			—
SMJ 6	Alpha′ 1.1	—	—	—	—	—	—			—
SMJ 7	Alpha 2.1	—	—	—	—	—	—			—
Kel 1	Alpha′ 5.1	—	—	—	—	—	—			—
Kel 2	Alpha′ 1.1	—	—	—	—	—	—			—
McAl 1	Beta 3.1	—	—	—	—	—	—			—
McAl 2	Alpha 1.2	—	—	—	—	—	—			—
SC 2	Beta 3.1	—	—	—	—	—	—			—
S.Erysip.	Beta 1.1	—	—	—	—	—	—			—
Car 2	Alpha′ 2.1	+	+H	+H	+	+	+			—
Faw 1	Alpha′ 2.1	+H	+H	+H	+H	+H	+H			—
Faw 2	Alpha′ 2.1	+H	+H	+H	+H	+H	+H			—
Faw 3	Alpha′ 2.1	+H	+H	+H	+H	+H	+H			—
Faw 4	Alpha 1.1	—	—	—	—	—	+			—
Faw 5	Alpha 1.1	—	—	—	—	—	+			—
Faw 6	Alpha 1.1	—	—	—	—	—	+			—
Faw 7	Alpha 1.2	—	—	—	—	—	—			—
Faw 8	Alpha 2.2	—	—	—	—	—	—	+		—
Faw 9	Alpha 3.1	—	—	—	—	—	—			—
Faw 10	Alpha 1.2	+H	+H	+H	+H	+H	+H			—
Faw 11	Alpha′ 1.1	+H	+H	+H	+H	+H	+H			—

— = no agglutination; + = complete agglutination in three tubes; H = held over night; CA = complete agglutination; SA = slight agglutination; ACA = almost complete agglutination.

The organisms were grown in calcium carbonate broth and rabbits injected intravenously on 3 successive days at 5-day intervals. At first cultures heated to 55 C. for one hour were used for immunization. Later living cultures were employed. Immunization was carried on over a period of from 2 to 3 months. The loss of 1 or 2 animals through anaphylactic shock led to a preliminary intravenous desensitizing dose being given as routine.

The organisms were grown for 24 hours in calcium carbonate broth, centrifugalized at high speed for half an hour, the supernatant fluid poured off and the sediment resuspended in calcium carbonate broth to make an emulsion of the required density. Clumps were broken up by drawing the sediment in and out through a fine hypodermic needle till an even emulsion was obtained.

In each tube was placed 0.2 c c of suspension and 0.2 c c of the diluted serum, giving an ultimate dilution of twice that of the serum added. Final dilutions are the ones tabulated. Results were read after incubation in a water bath for one hour at 45 C., and again in certain instances after standing over night. The results are shown in table 6.

Beta Strains.—Rabbits immunized against β 2.1 and β 1.1 showed a relatively low titer (β 2.1 complete 1:160 and β 1.1 complete 1:320) so that the grouping here cannot be considered perfectly satisfactory. There is however, satisfactory evidence to show that there is no close inter-relationship between any of the beta strains tested with these serums. In each case the homologous strain is agglutinated and heterologous strains are not completely agglutinated even in 1:20 dilution. In one case β 2.1 strain from the same source as that used for immunizing the β 2.1 rabbit was completely agglutinated only in a 1:10 dilution of the serum. This seems to indicate the presence of immunologic subgroups in the broader groups outlined by the fermentation.

Alpha Prime Strains.—Rabbits were immunized against 3 alpha prime strains, α′ 3.1 and two α′ 2.1 strains with the production of a high titer serum in each case (α′ 3.1 complete 1:8,000, α′ 2.1 complete 1:12,000, α′ 2.1 complete 1:12,800). The α′ 3.1 serum agglutinates all of the heterologous α′ 3.1 strains but fails to agglutinate such strains as α′ 5.1 and α′ 1.1. The α′ 2.1 serums agglutinate all the α′ 2.1 strains and no other organisms in the series with the exception of a single α 1.2 and α′ 1.1 strain. These 3 serums in no case agglutinate any of the beta or alpha strains; one might expect to find an α′ 2.1 immune serum of high titer agglutinating a β 2.1 or α 2.1 strain in the lower dilutions; this, however, does not occur, so that one finds no evidence of an immunologic relationship between separate members of each of Brown's 3 types which have identical fermentation reactions. These alpha prime immune serums therefore demonstrate a high degree of specificity in agglutinative power, and there is a striking parallelism between the fermentative grouping of this type and the immunologic grouping. There is, however, a curious apparent loss of specificity when α′ 2.1 emulsions are combined with the various immune serums. Two of these α′ 2.1 strains behaved capriciously at times, emulsions more than one or two days old becoming inagglutinable. The α′ 2.1 immune serum also after storage for 4 months showed a great diminution in agglutinative power. In every case (12 strains) this class of organism was universally agglutinated by the immune serum, but not by normal human, normal rabbit serum, nor by antityphoid immune rabbit serum, or high titer type 1 antipneumococcus serum; it was, however, occasionally agglutinated by a 1:20 dilution of normal horse serum but not in higher dilutions. In every case the agglutination of these α' 2.1 emulsions by the heterologous immune serums occurred in high dilutions of the immune serum. The identification of these α' 2.1 strains in better known classifications is difficult because the alpha prime group was not formerly recognized as an entity. These organisms, owing to their occasional green production, might have been classed as S. salivarius (Andrewes and Horder) or on account of their hemolytic properties as S. anginosus (Andrewes and Horder). In the case of the α 1.1 immune serum the homologous organism was completely agglutinated in a 1:3,200 dilution and the α' 2.1 strain in a 1:5,120 dilution. The immunologic relationship of these strains was of considerable interest so that absorption tests were carried out, the results of which are shown in table 7.

Alpha Strains.—Rabbits were immunized with two alpha strains—alpha 1.1 and alpha 2.2. The titer of the α 1.1 immune serum was 1:3,200 complete and of the α 2.2 serum 1:400 complete (this rabbit was lost through anaphylactic shock before immunization was complete). With these immune serums the same striking parallelism is maintained between the fermentative grouping and the agglutinations. The α 1.1 immune serum agglutinated six α 1.1 strains from various sources and no other strains with the exception of all the α' 2.1 strains, and a single α 1.2 and α' 1.1 strain. With the lower titer α 2.2 serum, three α 2.2 strains from various sources were agglutinated and no other strains, with the usual exception of the α' 2.1 strains.

ABSORPTION EXPERIMENTS

The immune serum chosen for absorption was that produced against the α 1.1 strain. This serum was of a suitable titer, and agglutinated the α' 2.1 strains in high dilutions.

The α 1.1 immune serum was absorbed with the homologous strain, with another α 1.1 strain, with an α' 2.1 strain and with the α 1.2 and α' 1.1 strains which showed cross agglutination. The various batches of absorbed serums were tried out with selected emulsions.

The technic adopted for absorption was a modification of that described by Gordon.[9] A measured amount of broth diluted serum (1/32 of its full titer) was mixed with an equal quantity of heavy emulsion (1 c c=50,000 million) and placed in a water bath at 45 C. for 2 hours with frequent shaking and then left in an incubator over

[9] Brit. Med. Jour., 1921, I, p. 632.

night. After this period of contact, the mixture was centrifugalized and the supernatant fluid used for the agglutinations. The method followed for agglutinations was that previously described. The lowest dilution of absorbed serum was therefore 1/64 of the full titer and the final dilution, after addition of the emulsion, 1/128 of the full titer. The results are shown in table 7.

The chief interest of this experiment lies in the relationship revealed between the α 1.1 strain and the α' 2.1 strains. It has already been shown that the various α' 2.1 strains encountered have been agglutinated

TABLE 7

ABSORPTION EXPERIMENTS

Serum	Absorbing Emulsion	Emulsion	1:400	1:800	1:1,600	1:3,200	1:6,400	1:12 800
Boy 5 (Alpha 1.1)	Not absorbed	Boy 5 (Alpha 1.1)	+	+	+	+	±	—
	Not absorbed	Boy 4 (Alpha′ 2.1)	+	+	+	+	±	±
	Not absorbed	Boy 22 (Alpha′ 2.1)	+	+	+	+		
	Not absorbed	Faw 1 (Alpha′ 2.1)	+	+	+	+		
	Not absorbed	Boy 26 (Alpha 1.1)	+	+	+	±		
	Not absorbed	Faw 10 (Alpha 1.2)	+	+	+	+		
	Not absorbed	Faw 11 (Alpha′ 1.1)	+	+	+	+		
	Boy 5 (Alpha 1.1)	Boy 5 (Alpha 1.1)	±	—	—	—	—	
	Boy 5 (Alpha 1.1)	Boy 4 (Alpha′ 2.1)	+	+	±	—	—	
	Boy 5 (Alpha 1.1)	Boy 22 (Alpha′ 2.1)	—	—	—	—	—	
	Boy 5 (Alpha 1.1)	Faw 1 (Alpha′ 2.1)	—	—	—	—	—	
	Boy 5 (Alpha 1.1)	Boy 26 (Alpha 1.1)	±	—	—	—	—	
	Boy 5 (Alpha 1.1)	Raw 10 (Alpha 1.2)	+	+	+	+		
	Boy 5 (Alpha 1.1)	Faw 11 (Alpha′ 1.1)	+	+	+	+		
	Boy 4 (Alpha′ 2.1)	Boy 5 (Alpha 1.1)	Some +	Traces ±	—	—	—	
	Boy 4 (Alpha′ 2.1)	Boy 4 (Alpha′ 2.1)	+	±	±	—	—	
	Boy 4 (Alpha′ 2.1)	Boy 22 (Alpha′ 2.1)	±	—	—	—	—	
	Boy 4 (Alpha′ 2.1)	Faw 1 (Alpha′ 2.1)	+	±	—	—	—	
	Faw 10 (Alpha 1.2)	Faw 10 (Alpha 1.2)	±	—	—	—	—	
	Faw 11 (Alpha′ 1.1)	Faw 11 (Alpha′ 1.1)	±	—	—	—	—	
	Faw 11 (Alpha′ 1.1)	Faw 10 (Alpha 1.2)	+	+	+	+		
	Boy 26 (Alpha 1.1)	Boy 26 (Alpha 1.1)	±	—	—	—		
	Boy 26 (Alpha 1.1)	Boy 5 (Alpha 1.1)	±	—	—	—		

+ = complete agglutination; ± = partial agglutination; — = no agglutination.

by all the immune serums in our series, but that they are not agglutinated by normal human, normal rabbit or antityphoid immune rabbit serum, and that the serum produced by these strains is quite specific, agglutinating only α' 2.1 strains. Table 7 shows that the α 1.1 serum, absorbed by the homologous α 1.1 strains has lost agglutinating power for both the α 1.1 and α' 2.1 strains to an almost equal degree; and that the α 1.1 serum absorbed by an α' 2.1 strain shows not only greatly diminished power of agglutinating the α' 2.1 strains, but also a comparable loss of power for agglutinating the homologous α 1.1 strain. On this basis of absorption therefore these strains are immunologically identical

—yet there is a great difference, for although the α 1.1 strain will produce an immune serum capable of agglutinating the α' 2.1 strains in as high dilutions as its homologous strain, the α' 2.1 strains produce an antiserum quite specific and incapable of agglutinating the α 1.1 strains. The position of these α' 2.1 strains is further considered in the discussion which follows. The position of the single α 1.2 and α' 1.1 strains included in the table is quite different. It is seen (table 6) that these organisms are universally agglutinated like the α' 2.1 strains; in table 7 it is seen that these strains are capable of absorbing the substances responsible for their agglutination, but that this agglutination is unaffected by the absorption of the α 1.1 immune serum with its homologous strain. The agglutination of these strains must therefore be considered to be due to the production of group agglutinins.

DISCUSSION

The results of the experiments detailed justify the conclusion that the streptococcal flora in the sputum of patients with bronchial asthma is fairly constant. There is a gradual but slight change of flora (chiefly noticed in the beta types) over long periods (2 months; see table 2). It is true that the evidence in table 1 does not support this conclusion, but this experiment was not conducted on a sufficiently extensive scale. The evidence in table 2 and 3 shows a quite conclusive parallelism in the various samples, with certain exceptions in the beta types, when sufficient colonies are picked from the preliminary plates. The flora in these cases is not simple as there were from 8 to 14 different types of streptococcus in each sample of sputum examined. It was thought that the variations in flora encountered in the earlier work might have been due to the choice of particle from the sample of sputum under examination. The results in table 4 show that the flora is remarkably constant in dissimilar particles of sputum in the same sample. The conclusion therefore seems inevitable that apparent variations in flora are due to picking an insufficient number of colonies on the preliminary plates.

Ample confirmation of the complexity of the flora in these cases is contained in the agglutination results in table 6. It is seen that there is a quite striking parallelism between the grouping by fermentations and by immunologic methods. This is best seen in the results obtained with immune serums α' 3.1, α' 2.1, α 1.1 and α 2.2, which agglutinate only organisms of a like type and grouping, with a few exceptions noted earlier. The grouping of the beta types is less clearly discernable as the titer of the two immune serums was low; there is an indication, however, that in this type the broad groups based on the fermentation reactions show further immunologic subdivisions. For instance, a heterologous β 2.1 strain is only slightly agglutinated by the β 2.1 immune serum, and 2 heterologous β 1.1 strains are only doubtfully agglutinated by the β 1.1 immune serum.

The position of Brown's suggested alpha prime type is interesting; the evidence for considering this a distinct type seems ample as the members of this group (with the exception of the α' 2.1 strains) show no immunologic relationship with either the beta or alpha types of similar fermentation reactions. The α' 2.1 strains are the most interesting members of the alpha prime group that we have encountered. We have seen that these strains under varying conditions produce radically different appearances in human blood agar, at one time producing green zones (heavy seeding) and at another time producing definite partial hemolytic zones without a shade of green (light seeding). The immunologic relationship of these strains is of still greater interest; all the α' 2.1 strains encountered were agglutinated by all our immune antistreptococcal serums but not by immune antityphoid serum; the α' 2.1 immune serums, however, agglutinate only α' 2.1 strains. These findings are somewhat comparable to those of Kinsella and Swift.[10] These authors, using the complement fixation reaction as a basis for grouping nonhemolytic streptococci, found that strains of streptococci producing antiserums of wide reacting capacity (extensive cross fixation) will not themselves react with a serum of narrow reacting capacity (fixing only its homologous strain), and a strain which produces an antiserum of narrow reacting capacity will usually react with many serums of a wider reacting capacity than its own. Kinsella and Swift base their explanation of this phenomenon on a consideration of the complexity of the chemical nucleus in various strains. A rabbit injected with a streptococcus of complex chemical nucleus will produce an antiserum capable of fixing this streptococcus and such other strains as contain the same or some of the same structural units. A rabbit injected with an organism containing only one of these units will present an antibody incapable of union with the more complex structures and will fix only streptococci of corresponding simplicity. The α' 2.1 strains in our series, on this explanation, would represent streptococci of relatively simple nuclei but this simple structural unit is apparently one occurring in the more

[10] Jour. Exper. Med., 1917, 25, p. 877.

complex nuclei of the other strains used for immunization of our rabbits. Hence, these types are universally agglutinated but produce an antiserum which agglutinates only this single type. This conception is supported by the absorption experiments conducted with the α 1.1 immune serum and the α' 2.1 strains. It is found that absorption of this serum with its homologous strain removes not only the agglutinins for that strain, but also, and to the same extent, for the α' 2.1 strains. It is further found that absorption of the α 1.1 immune serum with an α' 2.1 strain not only removed the agglutinins for this strain but also, and to the same extent, for the α 1.1 strains. Absorption of the α 1.1 immune serum with the α' 2.1 emulsion must therefore remove some fraction of the agglutinins without which agglutination of the α 1.1 strains cannot occur.

The position of the other alpha prime organisms is more definite. For instance the α' 3.1 immune serum does not agglutinate the β 3.1 organisms nor does it agglutinate the single α 3.1 strain present in the series, also the α' 1.1 strains are not agglutinated by the β 1.1 antiserum nor by the α 1.1 antiserum. It may be assumed then that the members of this alpha prime group possess distinctive cultural and immunologic characteristics.

The immediate practical importance of these observations is related to the method of preparation of vaccines from sputum. With 8 to 14 different types of streptococci in single specimens of sputum, the difficulty of identifying the offending organism is great. It seems to be established that the beta type includes the most actively pathogenic streptococci, yet these organisms are in the minority in the types of sputum which we have studied and the flora of this type is not completely constant in successive samples of sputum from the same source; hence a vaccine including only this type and leaving out the many strains of the other types would seem to be incomplete. The best plan, as far as the streptococcal flora is concerned, appears to be to include all the types which are present, and as far as possible, in the same proportions as they appear in the sputum itself. This can be most simply done by using a 24-hour broth culture of a washed particle of sputum as the basis for the vaccine. Our observations have shown that practically all the organisms are present here and in the same proportion as they are in the particle of sputum itself (table 5). In the preparation of these vaccines, organisms other than streptococci must not be neglected; it has been our experience that these are best isolated on surface plates made from 6-hour broth cultures. These seem to develop optimum conditions for the isolation of hemoglobinophilic bacilli which if present may be incorporated in the vaccine.

CONCLUSIONS

The streptococcal flora in various samples of sputum from the same source, is, in patients with bronchial asthma, fairly constant and quite complex, from 8 to 14 types of streptococci occurring in single specimens.

The streptococcal flora in various particles from the same sample of sputum does not vary.

The simple method of using a 24-hour serum broth culture of a washed particle of sputum as a basis for vaccine preparation seems as efficient as any, the streptococcal flora in such a culture being approximately parallel to that in the sputum itself.

There is, in general, a close parallelism between the grouping of streptococci arrived at through biochemical (fermentation) and serologic (agglutination) reactions.

Certain members (α' 2.1) of Brown's suggested alpha prime group of streptococci are of particular interest; these α' 2.1 strains are universally agglutinated by all of our 7 antistreptococcal serums, but produce agglutinins active against their own type of strain only. Absorption experiments indicate that this organism contains a fundamental unit which occurs in each one of the more complicated streptococci used for immunization in our series.

ANAPHYLAXIS PRODUCED BY EYE TISSUES

PRIMARY TOXICITY OF EYE TISSUES—ORGAN SPECIFICITY AND GROUP REACTIONS OF EYE TISSUES—ANAPHYLACTIC THEORY OF SYMPATHETIC OPHTHALMIA

Ryuzo Kodama

From the John McCormick Institute for Infectious Diseases, Chicago

The biologic differentiation of animal, vegetable and bacterial species is established, but many questions in regard to organ specificity and group reactions of the proteins of animal tissues are still unsolved.

Uhlenhuth first showed the existence of organ specificity, differentiating the lens of beef[1] from the vitreous and other proteins of the same animal by the method of precipitation. This remarkable fact was confirmed by anaphylactic reactions by Kraus, Doerr and Sohma.[2] The lack of species specificity, here revealed, was studied further by Andrejew and Uhlenhuth[3] by anaphylaxis and confirmed by Peiffer and Mita.[4] Uhlenhuth and Haendel,[5] Mita,[6] and Krusius[7] discovered also a new fact, namely, that guinea-pigs may be sensitized and intoxicated by their own lens, but Roemer and Gebb[8] did not confirm this. Though the serologic peculiarity and equality of lens protein through vertebrate animals is well recognized, the coexistence of some species specificity is indicated in the results of anaphylactic experiments, especially of Andrejew[4] and Kapsenberg,[9] while the precipitin reactions do not seem to reveal any species specificity in lens protein, as emphasized recently by Hektoen.[10]

When other tissues are considered, it is to be noted that Ranzi,[11] who worked with the liver, kidney and testicle of beef, horse and man as well as with malignant tumors, concluded that the anaphylactic state produced by organ extracts is not organ specific; the animals treated with one organ reacted with the same organ and other organs, also with the serum of the same species, giving no stronger reaction with the homologous organ than with other organs or the serum. Extracts of malignant tumors also sensitized to tumor and normal tissues and serum. However, Pfeiffer's[12] investigation on anaphylaxis with spermatozoa, kidney and blood led to the conclusion that injections with the pure proteins of those materials produced different anaphylactic states, which are to be regarded as organ specific, that is, there is a closer relation between

Received for publication, December 1, 1921.

1 Koch Festschrift, 1903, p. 49.
2 Wien. Klin. Wchnschr., 1908, 21, p. 1084.
3 Arb. a. d. k. Gsndhtsamte., 1909, 30, p. 450.
4 Ztschr. f. Immunitätsf., 1911, 8, p. 358.
5 Ibid., 1910, 4, p. 61.
6 Ibid., 1910, 5, p. 297.
7 Arch. f. Augenh., 1910, 67, p. 6.
8 Arch. f. Ophth., 1912, 31, p. 367.
9 Ztschr. f. Immunitätsf., 1912, 15, p. 518.
10 Jour. Am. Med. Assn., 1921, 77, p. 32.
11 Ztschr. f. Immunitätsf., 1909, 2, p. 12.
12 Ibid., 1911, 8, p. 358.

spermatozoa and kidney than between spermatozoa and blood. Guerrini[13] worked with the nucleoprotein of liver, spleen and serum of dog and horse and found that the anaphylactic reaction was organ specific, as only weak reactions could be obtained occasionally with the different organs of the same animal, but not between the same organs of different animals.

The eye tissues, especially uvea pigment, have interested ophthalmologists especially since Elschnig's[14] pioneer work in which he applied the anaphylactic theory to sympathetic ophthalmia. His complement-binding experiments led to the conclusion that uvea antibody is not sharply organ specific and not species specific and that uvea pigment in its antigenic action is species specific. Weichardt and Kümmel[15] obtained a strong but not absolute organ specificity with the serum of rabbits injected with beef uvea in experiments with the epiphanin reaction. Arisawa[16] reports that immune serum for sheep and calf uvea reacted with homologous organs distinctly, but not at all or slightly with heterologous tissues, in short, a distinct species specificity and a weak organ specificity were observed in complement fixation tests, while in the precipitin tests the organ specificity appeared stronger and the species specificity weaker. Rados[17] immunized rabbits with homologous uvea and cornea and demonstrated iso-antibodies which were neither organ nor species specific by the method of complement fixation. Szily,[18] in his anaphylaxis experiments, found that his chemically pure uvea pigment did not give any reliable general anaphylaxis and gave no trace of local anaphylaxis by reinjection. Woods[19] made perfusion experiments to study the local reaction and concluded that organ specificness was shown by uvea and its pigment in beef and dogs. Nakamura,[20] by complement fixation found that the uvea was organ specific and not absolutely species specific.

Uhlenhuth[1] observed that in precipitin tests the vitreous reacts with serum, contrary to the lens. Possek[21] could find no organ or species specific properties in the vitreous. Trubin[22] made intra-ocular anaphylactic reactions with beef and sheep vitreous as antigen and obtained certain degenerative changes of the retina, pigment epithelium and choroid, which differed from the typical form of sympathetic ophthalmia with plastic uveitis. Nakamura[20] found that in complement fixation vitreous reacts with homologous vitreous and uvea and slightly with homologous lens, but not with homologous serum and heterologous vitreous.

Concerning the other eye tissues, Hess and Roemer[23] found that the retinal rods have particular antigenic properties and produce antibodies that are lytic and agglutinating for rods, and recently Hektoen[9] observed that beef cornea reacts with beef serum, vitreous and aqueous, but not with lens in precipitin reactions. Roemer and Gebb[24] made anaphylactic reactions with several eye tissues, but they withheld any conclusion for other tissues than lens, saying that the results were too inconstant and that more extended experiments were needed to determine the antigenic properties of the rest of those tissues.

13 Ibid., 1912, 14, p. 70.
14 Ibid., 1916, 20, p. 305.
15 München. med. Wchnschr., 1911, 58, p. 1714.
16 XXXVIII Vers. J. ophth. Gesells., Heidelberg, 1912, p. 253.
17 Ztschr. f. Immuntätsf., 1913, 19, p. 579.
18 Seventeenth Intern. Med. Congress, 1913, 9, p. 289.
19 Jour. Am. Med. Assn., 1921, 77, p. 1317.
20 J. Komoto, Festschrift, 1919, p. 211.
21 Klin. Monatsbl. f. Augenheilk., 1907, 45, p. 329.
22 Graefe's Arch. f. Ophthalmol., 1915, 89, p. 227.
23 Arch. f. Augenheilk., 1906, 54, p. 13.
24 Graefe's Arch. f. Ophthal., 1912, 81, p. 367.

My earlier experience with the precipitin reactions of beef lens, cornea, vitreous, retina, uvea, optic nerve and serum as well as of horse and rabbit lens, which led me to the present work with anaphylaxis, indicated that strong antibeef-lens rabbit serum reacted distinctly with homologous and heterologous lens, and not at all with serum and that there were some quantitative differences between the reactions of lenses of different species. Such immune serums gave also weakly positive reactions with homologous cornea, vitreous and retina, especially at the acme of immunization; on the other hand, antibeef-cornea rabbit serum at the acme showed distinct reaction with cornea and weakly positive reactions with homologous vitreous, retina, optic nerve and serum.

From the review of the literature we see that the problems of the organ and species specificity of the tissues are far from solved and that the group reactions of tissues, particularly the relations between important eye tissues, have not been studied extensively. Moreover, the question of anaphylactic origin of sympathetic ophthalmia is still problematic. As stated before, V. Szily [18] failed to substantiate Elschnig's conclusions, concluding from anaphylactic tests that the pigment is without antigenic properties; Woods,[19] on the contrary, came to the conclusion that the uvea pigment has antigenic property, substantiating Elschnig's [14] view that the pigment is responsible for the antigenic properties of uvea tissue. It seemed, therefore, of interest at this time to reinvestigate the antigenic properties of certain eye tissues.

GENERAL TECHNIC

The difference in the results obtained by various workers on organ specificity seems to be due partly to the admixture of blood constituents to the tissue proteins, partly to different methods of preparation of materials, determination of biologic reactions and estimation of the results obtained. The materials in this work were obtained from the fresh normal eyes of cattle killed by bleeding. The tissues were prepared aseptically, each tissue was isolated cautiously from the others and washed carefully with sterilized normal salt solution, and ground with quartz sand in mortar, after being cut in small pieces, then mixed with normal salt solution, and kept at 37 C. for 2 hours and shaken by machine for from 3 to 5 hours. All suspensions were filtered to secure fine emulsions. To obtain the uvea pigment pure, it was washed three times with salt solution and centrifugated carefully. For conservation a few drops of thymol solution were added. All materials were kept in the icebox. The lens and vitreous of other animals (horse, rabbit, guinea-pig and mouse) were prepared by the same method; blood serum was obtained in the usual way. Fine emulsions were made of cornea, retina, uvea and optic nerve (intra-orbital part) in dilutions of 1 to 20; of lens in dilution of 1 to 100, and of uvea pigment in dilution of 1 to 1,000. The vitreous was used in full strength. The cornea, lens and vitreous body were absolutely free from blood and for the retina, uvea and optic nerve, it may be said that they were almost or nearly free from blood.

According to our knowledge, anaphylaxis is a most delicate and complicated biologic reaction which is open to sources of confusion and errors, if carried out without great caution. The action of surgical shock and the primary toxicity of the materials injected have not been considered carefully enough always. In the present work all possible care has been used to obtain reliable results, and I have estimated the results quantitatively on the basis of the fall of temperature by applying the Pfeiffer and Mita formulas: Shock units $= \frac{\text{temperature} \times \text{time}}{2}$. Thus, if in a given case the temperature falls 1.5 C. and returns to normal in 140 minutes, the calculation would be $\frac{15 \times 140}{2} = 1050$ shock units.

In fatal cases the formula used by Pfeiffer and Mita is as follows: Shock units $= 30{,}000 + (20{,}000 - \frac{\text{temperature} \times \text{time}}{2})$. Thus, if we assume that the temperature falls 4.5 C. and 60 minutes elapse before death, the calculation would be $30{,}000 + (20{,}000 - \frac{45 \times 60}{2}) = 48{,}650$ shock units. At the same time the general symptoms were studied carefully.

Guinea-pigs were sensitized by intraperitoneal injection, the intoxicating dose being given intravenously: After the animal was fixed on a board, the hair was cut, the skin sterilized and cut, the jugular vein then separated carefully and two threads placed under it; after the injection, these were tied firmly and the wound closed.

In our tables, the doses are given by weight in grams for the cornea, lens, retina, uvea and optic nerve, and in cubic centimeters for the vitreous body and serum.

PRELIMINARY EXPERIMENTS ON SURGICAL SHOCK

In many of the reports on anaphylactic experiments no attention seems to have been given to the influence of the operative procedure on results of the experiments. Some investigators have endeavored to account for this factor or have used some harmless route for the intoxicating dose. While the subcutaneous or intraperitoneal injection seems to be practically harmless, the intravenous (jugular vein), intracardial or intracerebral injection may cause more or less shock by itself in a sensitive animal like the guinea-pig. This is especially important when one wishes to make a quantitative estimation of anaphylactic reactions. As stated, I chose the intraperitoneal injection for the sensitizing dose and the intrajugular route for the intoxicating injection, but first an effort was made to determine exactly the effect of such injections by themselves.

TABLE 1

EFFECTS OF INTRAJUGULAR AND INTRAPERITONEAL INJECTIONS OF SALT SOLUTION IN GUINEA-PIGS

Temperature	Intrajugular Injections					Intraperitoneal Injections		
	Weight 430 gm. Amount Injected 2 c c	Weight 460 gm. Amount Injected 1 c c	Weight 265 gm. Amount Injected 0.5 c c	Weight 330 gm. Amount Injected 0.1 c c	Weight 225 gm. Amount Injected 0	Weight 435 gm. Amount Injected 10 c c	Weight 400 gm. Amount Injected 5 c c	Weight 2 5 gm. Amount Injected 1 c c
Before injection.....	40.0	39.8	39.1	38.5	38.8	39.0	39.0	39.3
Min. after injection								
10................	39.0	39.0	37.6	36.7	38.1	38.7	38.8	39.3
20................	39.0	39.5	37.8	36.9	38.4	38.7	38.7	39.3
30................	39.1	39.6	38.0	37.1	38.8	38.6	38.7	39 3
60................	39.5	39.6	39.1	38.3	39.1	38.8	39.0	39.6
90................	40.0	39.5	39.7	38.9	39.2	39 0	39 8	39.9
120................	40.5	39.7	39.6	39.3	39.5	39.0	40.2	40.1
150................	40.7	39.9	40.1	39.4	39.7	39.5	40.1	39.7
180................	41.1	40.0	40.1	38.9	39.8	40.3	40.1	39.6
210................	41.0	40.1	40.4	39.1	39.6	40.2	40 0	39.6
240................	40.9	39.8	40.3	30.2	39.7	40.1	39.6	39 6
270................	40.8	39.9	40.5	39.0	40 0	40 0	39.6	39.5
300................	40.9	39.8	40.3	39.0	39.9	39.6	39.7	39.6
330................	40.8	39.9	40.6	39.2	39.8	39.4	39.6	39.5
360................	40.9	39.8	40.6	39.1	39.9	39.2	39.6	39.4
390................	40.8	39.9	40.5	39.8	39 8	39.2	39.4	39.4
420................	40.8	39.8	40.4	40.4	39.9	39.1	39.3	39.3
Shock units..........	450	540	450	675	158	180	90	0
	Average 455					Average 90		

Normal guinea-pigs, weighing from 225 to 460 gm., were used. Five pigs were injected, respectively, into the jugular vein as described with 2.0, 1.0, 0.5, 0.1 and 0 c c of sterilized normal salt solution, and 3 pigs were injected with 10.0, 5.0, and 1.0 c c, respectively, of normal salt solution into the intraperitoneal cavity.

As the direct results of the intrajugular injection itself, the animals remained quiet for a while, the hair being ruffled, and sometimes trembling and increased tear secretion appeared. A short period of quiet, sometimes slight epiphora and a short apnea were noted after the intraperitoneal injection of a relatively large dose. The rectal temperature was tested in the same way as the anaphylactic temperature measurements are made, and I have estimated the shock value by the Pfeiffer and Mita formula. The results are given in table 1, which shows that the intravenous injection itself caused the temperature to fall from 0.8 to 1.8 C., and that 60 to 150 minutes were needed to recover; thus the calculated shock values fluctuated from 150 to 675 units, the average value being 455 units. In the intraperitoneal injections, in which neither dissection nor bleeding occurs, the amount of fluid injected (1.0 to 10.0 c c) was apparently the only influence to account for the change of the temperature. The injection of 5.0 c c and 10 c c of normal salt solution caused the temperature to decrease 0.3 C. and 0.4 C., respectively, and the time for recovery was from 60 to 90 minutes, giving the shock values of 90 and 180 units; the injection of 1.0 c c of salt solution caused no fall in temperature.

PRELIMINARY EXPERIMENTS ON THE PRIMARY TOXICITY OF EYE TISSUE EMULSIONS AND OF SERUM

In the literature on anaphylaxis the relation between the general primary toxicity and the anaphylactic reaction is a subject of much discussion. There are many articles concerning the primary toxicity of normal and pathologic tissues and of normal and immune serums, but comparatively few observations of this kind have been made on eye tissues, and on this account a preliminary study was made of their primary toxicity.

For this purpose normal healthy pigs weighing from 260 to 450 gm. were used, 4 for the cornea, 13 for the lens, 4 for the vitreous body, 3 for the retina, 3 for the uvea, 3 for uvea pigment, 3 for the optic nerve and 2 for serum. The cornea, retina, uvea and optic nerve were injected in 5% emulsions, the lens in 1%, and uvea pigment in 0.1% emulsions, the vitreous body and serum in full strength. The injections were made mostly into the jugular vein and partly intraperitoneally. The reactions were carefully studied by observation of the general symptoms and the temperature changes as well as by postmortem examination.

The general manifestations caused by the primary toxic action of the cornea, lens, vitreous body, retina, uvea and optic nerve were similar. Though some differences were noted, they seemed to be due to differences in quantity, in solubility and the individuality of the animals rather than to the inherent difference in the materials injected.

Generally speaking, guinea-pigs injected with one of the eye tissues mentioned showed the following phenomena: they became quiet, the hair rough, the body trembled, tears flowed, and there was more or less scratching, lapping and chewing; first slow, depressed, then quickened and sometimes labored breathing was constant; relaxation of the muscles, paresis of the hind legs and drowsiness with narrowed lids often followed; the temperature first fell and later increased, but in the case of grave intoxication the latter did not occur; the lids and pupils were dilated and the eyeballs protruded when grave respiratory distress and convulsions came on; congestion of the ear lobes and of the conjunctivae and epiphora were common, but white discharge from the eyes was rare; convulsions were also rare; conjunctival hemorrhage was noted once. These are all principally similar to general protein toxicity and delayed anaphylaxis.

The anatomic lesions caused by the primary toxic action of eye tissues were similar, although some variations were noted, probably owing to the difference of concentration of the material injected and the individuality of the animal. Generally speaking, the lungs were often distended, with congestion usually and sometimes with petechiae, but pale lungs were found also, though rarely; the heart was often dilated, but not always; the myocardium was usually congested, the right side of the heart and vena cava usually holding soft coagula, while the left ventricle was empty; the abdominal organs usually showed congestion, but its grade varied; the intestines, especially the duodenum, the stomach, suprarenal, pancreas, liver, testicles and uterus usually showed marked congestion about in the order named; the skull, the pia, the subcutaneous tissue and muscles were also often found congested. These lesions were more or less similar to those of delayed anaphylactic death.

The temperature fall, fever reaction, absolute shock values (after deducting the surgical shock) and the outcome in each instance are shown in table 2, which shows that the cornea, lens, vitreous body, retina, uvea, uvea pigment and optic nerve of the beef and the lens of guinea-pigs may cause fatal intoxication in guinea-pigs due to primary toxicity, death occurring within from 5 to 73 hours. The minimal fatal dose per 100 gram body-weight for each eye tissue tested is as follows:

Beef cornea	0.322	Beef uvea	0.0357
Beef lens	0.000666	Beef uvea pigment	0.00329
Beef vitreous	0.938	Beef optic nerve	0.0313
Beef retina	0.0294		

Hence, the order of beef eye tissues according to primary toxicity is lens, uvea pigment, retina, optic nerve, uvea, cornea, and vitreous body. Taking the vitreous body as the base, the scale of the primary toxicity of the tissues of the beef is as follows:

Crystalline lens	1408	Uvea	26
Uvea pigment	285	Cornea	3
Retina	32	Vitreous body	1
Optic nerve	30		

Heating at 56 C. for 1 hour 2 times reduced greatly the primary toxicity (uvea, optic nerve), and the fresh materials (rabbit lens and vitreous) gave higher fever reaction.

TABLE 2

PRIMARY TOXICITY OF EYE TISSUES AND SERUM OF BEEF AND OTHER ANIMALS

Guinea-Pigs, Number and Weight	Materials Injected		Place of Injection	Fall in Temperature in 0.1 C.	Minutes Before Return of Temp. to Normal or Death Caused by Shock	Absolute or Net Shock	Results and Fever in Centigrade Degrees
	Kind	Amount					
1-285	Beef cornea	0.25	Jugular	21	150	1,120	Survived, 1.2
2-310	Beef cornea	0.1	Jugular	15	210	1,120	Survived, 1.9
3-285	Beef cornea	1.0	Peritoneum	12	180	900	Died in 5 hours
4-310	Beef cornea	1.0	Peritoneum	1	30	0	Died in 7 hours
5-385	Beef lens	0.1	Jugular	32	660	38,985	Died in 11 hours
6-260	Beef lens	0.05	Jugular	28	1,440	29,385	Died in 24 hours
7-350	Guinea-pig lens	0.02	Jugular	41	540	38,475	Died in 9 hours
8-500	Rabbit lens (fresh)	0.02	Jugular	21	600	5,845	Survived, 2.4
9-370	Beef lens	0.02	Jugular	33	300	4,495	Survived, 0 9
10-355	Mouse lens	0.02	Jugular	20	210	1,645	Survived, 0 6
11-345	Beef lens	0.01	Jugular	19	330	2,680	Died in 21 hours
12-390	Beef lens	0.01	Jugular	6	120	0	Died on third day
13-390	Beef lens	0.005	Jugular	17	150	825	Died in 21 hours
14-375	Beef lens	0.0025	Jugular	7	240	385	Died in 6 hours
15-310	Beef lens	0.0025	Jugular	9	150	220	Survived, 1.5
16-250	Beef lens	0.001	Jugular	24	60	265	Survived, 0.4
17-410	Beef lens	0.001	Jugular	10	60	0	Survived, 0.6
18-320	Beef vitreous	3.0	Jugular	14	240	1,230	Died in 24 hours
19-380	Rabbit vitreous (fresh)	3.0	Jugular	13	70	0	Survived, 1.4
20-410	Beef vitreous	2.0	Jugular	12	180	625	Survived, 0 6
21-405	Beef vitreous	2.0	Jugular	14	150	595	Survived, 0.5
22-285	Beef retina	0.2	Jugular	13	600	7,345	Survived, 0.5
23-340	Beef retina	0.1	Jugular	14	1,260	40,625	Died in 21 hours
24-450	Beef retina	0.1	Jugular	16	390	2,665	Survived, 0 2
25-280	Beef uvea	0.1	Jugular	32	390	43,305	Died in 6½ hours
26-400	Beef uvea (heated)	0.1	Jugular	29	180	4,765	Survived, 0.4
27-300	Beef uvea (heated)	0.05	Jugular	2	60	0	Survived, 0.0
28-390	Beef uvea pigment	0.05	Jugular	8	1,290	44,385	Died in 21½ hours
29-380	Beef uvea pigment	0.0125	Jugular	11	120	205	Died on third day
30-300	Beef uvea pigment	0.01	Jugular	5	90	0	Survived, 0.8
31-280	Beef opticus	0.1	Jugular	44	360	41,625	Died in 6 hours
32-320	Beef opticus (heated)	0.1	Jugular	26	180	1,885	Died on third day
33-300	Beef opticus (heated)	0.05	Jugular	3	60	0	Survived, 0.1
34-285	Beef serum	2.0	Jugular	22	180	1,525	Survived, 0 3
35-350	Horse serum (11 months old)	2.0	Jugular	12	67	0	Survived, 0.4

In mice and rabbits the intraperitoneal injection of suspensions of eye tissues may also cause severe symptoms of intoxication.

According to Wissmann,[25] human and beef eyes as a whole are toxic for guinea-pigs, but the lens, vitreous body, uveal tract and retina, injected separately, are harmless. The carrier of the toxic action of the eye seems to be the uvea and the retina which become active by the action of the lens and vitreous, which by themselves are not toxic; his results differ from mine and apparently they are not in accord with generally accepted principles. Dold and Ogata [26] studied the toxic action of watery extracts of rabbit tissues for rabbits, and they assert that the uvea plus the retina contain the most toxic substance, next the sclera and cornea, the lens and vitreous body not being toxic enough to cause death. Their results also differ from mine, but as their materials, methods of preparation and animals are also different, the results are not comparable.

ANAPHYLACTIC REACTION WITH EMULSIONS OF EYE TISSUES AND WITH SERUM

For this purpose normal healthy guinea-pigs weighing from 250 to 450 gm. were used in 7 different groups. The animals of each group were sensitized with one of the 7 materials prepared: the cornea, lens, vitreous body, retina, uvea, optic nerve, or beef serum. The sensitizing dose—0.05 gm. of cornea, retina, uvea, or optic nerve, 0.005 of lens, 1.0 c c of vitreous—was injected 3 times at short intervals into the peritoneal cavity; 1.0 c c of serum was injected once intraperitoneally. Between 18 and 25 days after the last injection, the intoxicating injection was made into the jugular vein; usually 0.01 or 0.02 gm. of lens, 0.1 gm. of cornea, retina, uvea and optic nerve, 2.0 or 3.0 c c of vitreous and of serum. The general symptoms, the change in temperature, and anatomic changes were carefully observed. The animals which escaped acute death were tested by subsequent injections as to refractoriness. The anaphylactic shock value was estimated by the fall in temperature, and the shock values due to surgical shock and primary toxicity were deducted for each case.

GENERAL CLINICAL PHENOMENA AND ANATOMIC CHANGES OF ANAPHYLAXIS CAUSED BY EYE TISSUES AND BEEF SERUM

The reactions of the animals which received reinjections of eye tissue, heterologous and homologous, and of serum after the sensitiza-

[25] Graefe's Arch. f. Ophth., 1912, 80, p. 437.
[26] Ztschr. f. Immunitätsf., 1912, 13, p. 667.

tion with one of our seven antigens may be classified as acute anaphylactic death, severe and moderate anaphylactic reactions and mild symptoms.

Acute Anaphylactic Death.—A few animals died instantaneously owing to respiratory stoppage in about 30 seconds, sometimes with a few agonal respirations. In these cases the lungs were usually distended typically, but sometimes there was no distention, which suggests a particularly severe intoxication of central origin; the heart usually beat strongly with dilatation and injection of the myocardium and contained fluid blood; the pia, cutis and abdominal organs sometimes showed some congestion. Many animals suffered typical acute anaphylactic death with great respiratory distress, violent convulsions and unconsciousness, which developed soon after injection, with defacation and micturition, death usually occurring in from 2 to 5 minutes. In these cases the lungs were greatly distended, emphysematous and mostly pale with more or less petechiae; the heart was dilated always, the walls congested and the blood fluid; the pia and abdominal organs usually showed more or less congestion, more marked when death was delayed; among the abdominal organs, the intestine, especially the duodenum, showed most intensive congestion, then the stomach, suprarenal, pancreas and sexual organs.

Severe Anaphylactic Reaction.—Many reinjected animals reacted with acute or delayed development of respiratory distress followed by convulsions, relaxation, paralysis, drowsiness, marked fall of temperature, congestion of the ear lobes and conjunctivae and an abundant white discharge from the eyes. Some died after several hours, up to 24 hours, and others survived. The postmortem examination gave less typical lung and heart findings, usually there was marked congestion of the pia, cutis, muscles and abdominal organs, generally resembling the changes caused by the primary toxicity of eye tissues.

Moderate Anaphylactic Reaction.—The animals became nervous, scratching and chewing, trembling, sometimes shaking the head, weeping and coughing, with roughening of the hair; the respiration first quickened, then slowed; partial relaxation and paresis, moderate fall in temperature and epiphora developed. These cases were not fatal directly.

Mild Symptoms.—The animals became a little nervous; slight respiratory changes and fever were observed; there were no fatal results.

TABLE 3

ANAPHYLACTIC REACTIONS OF GUINEA-PIGS TO TISSUES OF BEEF EYE AND OF BEEF SERUM

Sensitizing Injections (Intraperitoneal)	Weight	Reactions to Intoxicating Injections (Intrajugular)						Tests of Refractory State of Survivors					
		Days Since First Injection	Material Injected Intrajugularly	Fall in Temperature in 0.1 C.	Minutes Before Return of Temperature to Normal or Death from Shock	Aboslute or Net Shock	General Reaction	Hours Since Intoxicating Injection	Material of Third Injection (Intrajugular)	Fall in Temperature in 0.1 C.	Minutes Before Return to Normal Temperature or Death Caused by Shock	Absolute or Net Shock	General Reaction
Beef cornea..... 0.15	360	21	Beef cornea.. 0.1	7	2	48,418	Fulminant, death						
	390	21	Beef lens..... 0.01	10	30	0	Slight............	½	Beef cornea.... 0.1	11	2	48,414	Acute, death
	375	22	Beef vitreous 2.0	28	450	5,250	Moderate.........	24	....	28	540	5,985	Moderate
	355	22	Beef retina... 0.1	44	540	35,000	Severe, death						
	370	22	Beef uvea.... 0.1	21	200	0	Moderate.........	4	....	12	1,440	7,065	Moderate
	290	23	Beef opticus. 0.1	23	390	2,145	Moderate.........	24½	....	28	330	3,045	Moderate
	270	23	Beef serum... 2.0	27	2	47,993	Fulminant, death						
Beef lens....... 0.015	335	21	Beef lens..... 0.005	21	2	48,704	Acute, death						
	350	21	Beef lens..... 0.0025	11	45	0	Moderate.........	26	Beef lens....... 0.02	11	2	45,039	Acute, death
	335	23	Beef cornea.. 0.1	20	840	6,825	Moderate.........	26½	Beef lens....... 0.01	17	90	0	0
	400	23	Beef vitreous 3.0	18	2,700	24,650	Severe, death						
	360	25	Beef vitreous 2.0	20	270	1,650	Moderate.........	6	Rabbit lens.... 0.02	20	200	41.700	Severe, death
	310	23	Beef retina... 0.1	10	2	46,870	Acute, death						
	[illegible]	25	Beet uvea.... 0.1	10	120	0	Moderate.........	3½	Guinea-pig lens 0.02	10	3	11,055	Acute, death
	380	25	Beef opticus. 0.1	7	20	0	Slight............	2½	Mouse lens..... 0.02	30	1,740	21,800	Moderate
	410	21	Beef serum... 2.0	12	120	0	Slight............	24	Beef lens....... 0.0025	14	60	0	Slight
Beef vitreous... 3.0	450	21	Beef vitreous 3.0	23	4	48,274	Acute, death						
	390	23	Beef vitreous 2.0	42	440	38,710	Severe, death						
	450	22	Beef cornea.. 0.1	27	4	48,371	Acute, death						
	370	22	Beef lens..... 0.02	6	3	45,041	Acute, death						
	385	23	Beef retina... 0.1	9	2	46,871	Fulminant, death						
	410	22	Beef uvea.... 0.1	44	540	32,900	Severe, death						
	370	21	Beef opticus. 0.1	3	540	0	Moderate.........	28	Beef vitreous.. 2.0	13	1,020	5,550	Moderate, death
	380	23	Beef serum... 2.0	27	210	855	Moderate.........	3½	Rab't vitreous 3.0	19	1,440	13,225	Slight
Beef retina...... 0.15	390	21	Beef retina... 0.1	24	470	2,520	Severe............	8	Beef retina.... 0.125	17	2	46,863	Acute, death
	430	24	Beef retina... 0.1	6	1½	46,875	Fulminant, death						
	320	24	Beef retina... 0.1	38	1,260	22,440	Severe, death						
	340	21	Beef cornea.. 0.1	41	540	26,285	Severe, death						
	340	21	Beef lens..... 0.01	23	470	3,657	Severe............	8	Beef retina.... 0.125	16	2	46,844	Acute, death
	250	23	Beef vitreous 2.0	38	1,350	24,700	Moderate.........						
	385	23	Beef uvea.... 0.1	16	150	0	Slight............	5	Beef retina.... 0.1	16	2	46,844	Acute, death
	370	23	Beef opticus. 0.1	36	1,620	26,820	Severe............	29	Beef retina.... 0.1	17	2,430	17,535	Severe, death
	350	24	Beef serum... 2.0	33	150	495	Moderate.........	5	Beef retina.... 0.1	19	2	46,860	Acute, death
Beef uvea....... 0.15	240	21	Beef uvea.... 0.1	46	1,440	27,900	Severe............	26	Beef uvea...... 0.1	49	1,260	13,910	Slight
	290	21	Beef cornea.. 0.1	37	420	6,195	Severe............	23	Beef uvea...... 0.1	41	1,800	31,680	Severe, death
	220	21	Beef lens..... 0.02	36	360	1,530	Moderate.........						
	235	19	Beef vitreous 2.0	17	5	48,907	Acute, death						
	480	19	Beef retina... 0.1	13	300	0	Slight............	24½	Beef uvea...... 0.1	47	360	3,240	Severe, death
	450	19	Beef opticus. 0.1	40	15	47,360	Acute, death						
	300	20	Beef serum... 2.0	25	5	47,957	Acute, death						
Beef optic nerve 0.15	270	21	Beef opticus. 0.1	22	3	47,627	Acute, death						
	450	20	Beef cornea.. 0.1	26	420	3,885	Moderate.........	24	Beef optic N... 0.1	47	35	46,837	Severe, death
	300	20	Beef lens..... 0.02	15	180	0	Slight............	24	Beef optic N... 0.1	52	1,260	14,500	Severe, death
	450	21	Beef vitreous 2.0	18	5	48,875	Acute, death						
	350	21	Beef retina... 0.1	44	1,320	17,840	Severe, death						
	270	22	Beef uvea.... 0.1	43	570	32,525	Severe, death						
	280	22	Beef serum... 2.0	21	5	47,967	Acute, death						
Beef serum...... 1.0	435	21	Beef serum... 2.0	20	2	48,000	Acute, death						
	350	24	Beef cornea.. 0.1	18	240	585	Slight............	4½	Beef serum.... 2.0	14	5	47,985	Acute, death
	440	22	Beef lens..... 0.02	10	25	0	Slight............	2½	Beef serum.... 0.5	15	3	48,702	Acute, death
	435	24	Beef vitreous 2.0	13	5	48,917	Acute, death						
	435	28	Beef vitreous 2.0	40	900	30,950	Severe, death						
	[illegible]	25	Beef retina... 0.1	14	540	660	Moderate.........	23¼	Beef serum.... 2.0	11	4	47,998	Acute, death

Generally speaking, there is no principal difference between the anaphylactic reactions of different eye tissues and of serum, except that with materials from eye tissues there may be some irregularity of development of reactions as compared with serum anaphylaxis.

QUANTITATIVE ESTIMATION OF ANAPHYLACTIC REACTIONS BY THE TEMPERATURE FALL AND THE CLINICAL CLASSIFICATION

The rectal temperature of all animals which were used in anaphylactic experiments was measured exactly according to same method. The temperature was taken 3 times successively to begin with, then measurements were made three times at 10 minute intervals, then at 30 minute intervals. Thus the maximum temperature-fall in tenths of centigrade degrees and the time to recover or before death caused by shock in minutes were found, and the extent of shock was estimated by the formulae of Pfeiffer and Mita as explained already. Then the shock caused by the primary action of the eye tissue materials and the shock caused by the injection itself was deduced. The results are shown in table 3.

The tests of refractoriness or antianaphylaxis show that the animals reacted moderately or not at all on the third injection of the homologous antigen after the reinjection of homologous tissue or serum or tissue which is regarded as probably containing homologous anaphylactogen; on the contrary, the animals which received as second injection eye tissue, which is supposed to have little or no homologous antigen, died from typical anaphylactic shock on the third injection of homologous tissue or serum.

In the results we find rarely that the intoxicating injection of serum or of a different, but closely related, tissue gave a little more intensive reaction than the homologous tissue. This irregularity of reaction may be considered as due to differences of solubility and to the individuality of the animals.

THE ORGAN-SPECIFIC AND GROUP-REACTIONS OF EYE TISSUES AND SERUM

The results in the animals tested with emulsions of eye tissues and with serum have been recorded in the same terms and the results are summarized in table 4.

We see that there is no absolute organ-specificity in the narrow sense as commonly defined in any of eye tissues tested, although some of them may be organ-specific as concerns tissues outside the eye. Within the eye itself there are complicated interreactions or group reactions of the embryologically, functionally and metabolically closely related tissues to a much greater degree than indicated in the previous investigations of these problems. In this respect my results may appear somewhat strange, but we know now that specificness does not depend on histologic structure but on chemical constitution.[28] According to my results, the general anaphylactogenic activities of the tissues of the beef eye and of beef serum as represented in table 5 indicate that the cornea and the vitreous body contain in greater or less degree all

TABLE 4

SUMMARY OF NET SHOCK VALUES OF ANAPHYLACTIC REACTIONS PRODUCED IN GUINEA-PIGS BY EYE TISSUES AND SERUM OF BEEF

Sensitizing Antigens	Shock Values from Intoxicating Injections of						
	Cornea	Lens	Vitreous Body	Retina	Uvea	Optic Nerve	Serum
Cornea	48,418	0	5,250	35,000	0	2,145	47,993
Lens	6,825	48,704	13,120	46,870	0	0	0
Vitreous body	48,371	45,041	39,710	46,871	32,900	0	855
Retina	26,285	3,657	24,700	24,112	0	26,820	495
Uvea	6,195	1,530	48,907	0	27,900	47,360	47,957
Optic nerve	3,885	0	48,875	17,840	32,525	47,627	47,967
Serum	585	0	39,934	660	0	44,660	48,000

TABLE 5

THE GENERAL ANAPHYLACTIC EFFECTS OF TISSUES OF BEEF EYE AND OF BEEF SERUM

Sensitizing Injection	Intoxicating Injections						
	Cornea	Lens	Vitreous Body	Retina	Uvea	Opticus	Serum
Cornea emulsion	+++	0	++	+++	0	++	+++
Lens emulsion	++	+++	+++	+++	0	0	0
Vitreous	+++	+++	+++	+++	+++	0	+
Retina emulsion	+++	++	+++	+++	0	+++	+
Uvea emulsion	++	++	+++	0	+++	+++	+++
Opticus emulsion	++	0	+++	+++	+++	+++	+++
Serum	+	0	+++	+	0	+++	+++

+++ = strong reaction; ++ = moderate reaction; + = mild reaction; 0 = no reaction.

anaphylactogens of the eye tissues, while the lens and uvea contain the least number of associate anaphylactogens, the retina and optic nerve standing between.

Considering the anaphylactic theory of sympathetic ophthalmia on this basis, it is clear that uvea pigment is not the only possible source of the hypothetic active agent; the other elements of the uvea as well as constituents of other eye tissues may play a certain rôle, especially

[28] Abderhalden, E.: Ztschr. f. Physiol. Chem., 1912, 81, p. 322. Wells and Osborne, Jour. Infect. Dis., 1913, 12, p. 341.

in that form of sympathetic ophthalmia in which papilloretinitis is the prominent feature; here at least anaphylactogens of retinal and optic nerve origin might be the primary factors.

SUMMARY AND CONCLUSIONS

This work was undertaken to study the organ specificity and the group reactions of the eye tissues. As pure materials as possible were prepared. The cornea, lens, and vitreous body were used free from blood; the retina, uvea, uvea pigment and optic nerve were carefully washed as free from blood as possible.

The part played by surgical shock in the anaphylactic reaction was determined, and it was found that intrajugular injection itself causes a shock of from 150 to 675 units, according to the grade of injury to sensory nerves, the amount of bleeding and the individuality of the animals. The intraperitoneal injection causes a smaller degree of shock, varying from 0 to 180 units according to the amount of fluid injected.

The primary toxic effects of the tissues of the eye were determined for each tissue and they were found to be similar to the effects of protein toxicity in general and to delayed anaphylactic reactions.

Contrary to Wissmann, the lens, cornea, vitreous body, retina, uvea, uvea pigment and optic nerve of the beef and guinea-pig lens were found to be fatally toxic to guinea-pigs, mice and rabbits, death resulting in from 5 to 72 hours in guinea-pigs after intravenous or intraperitoneal injections. According to the minimal fatal dose the eye tissues stand in the following order according to primary toxicity: lens, uvea pigment, retina, optic nerve, uvea, cornea and vitreous body. Heating at 56 C. for one hour twice reduced the primary toxicity considerably, the fresh tissue materials producing a higher febrile reaction.

The specific anaphylactic reactions caused by the tissues of the beef eye were determined by studying the general symptoms, the anatomic changes, and the resulting refractory states; the shock values were estimated on the basis of fall in the temperature. Generally speaking, there is no essential difference between the anaphylactic reactions of the different eye tissues and of serum, but there may be some irregularity in the development of the reactions caused by ocular tissues, probably connected with questions of solubility and individuality.

The specific anaphylactic shock in each case was determined by deducing the effects of the primary toxicity of the material and quantity used and the shock produced by the injection itself. In this way the organ-specific and group reactions of the eye tissues and serum were studied carefully. No absolute organ-specificity in the narrow sense as commonly defined since Uhlenhuth's discovery of the organ-specificity in precipitin reactions, was found in any of the eye tissues studied, not even the lens, though some may be specific for the eye. The results indicate that there are complicated group reactions within the eye tissues as might be expected of tissues that are related embryologically, functionally and metabolically. The facts at hand lead to the conclusion that the specific reacting units of anaphylactogens are not cells but chemical constituents of the tissues.

It appears that each eye tissue studied contains several antigens (anaphylactogens) in varying amounts, in addition to a specific or chief antigen peculiar to itself. The cornea and vitreous body contain in greater or less degree anaphylactogens that are common to all the different tissues of the eye. On the other hand, the lens and uvea contain the smallest number of associate anaphylactogens, the retina and optic nerve standing between.

If we apply these results to the anaphylactic theory of sympathetic ophthalmia, we must conclude that the active agent of that disease needs not to be uvea pigment alone as believed at present, as other elements in the uvea and in other eye tissues may play the same rôles as the uvea pigment is assumed to play. This enlargement of the anaphylactic theory of sympathetic ophthalmia readily takes in the form in which papilloretinitis develops, a process that the present pigment theory does not explain.

INOCULATION OF WHITE MICE WITH PFEIFFER'S BACILLUS

INFLUENZA STUDIES. IX *

N. Paul Hudson

From the Department of Hygiene and Bacteriology, University of Chicago

Some investigators have reported that Pfeiffer's bacillus is nonpathogenic for white mice, others that the organism can be recovered from the heart blood of a mouse only when injected with other bacteria, while yet others assert that even in pure culture it is distinctly pathogenic for these animals.

Spooner, Scott, and Heath,[1] using cultures isolated at Camp Devens early in the influenza outbreak of 1918, stated that Pfeiffer's bacillus is nonpathogenic for white mice, basing their conclusions on more than 100 intraperitoneal injections. A description of the technic and a statement of the amounts injected were not given.

Jacobson[2] was not able to kill white mice by intraperitoneal injections in amounts of one slant of Pfeiffer's bacillus in pure culture, and he concluded that the organism was nonpathogenic for white mice. But when he grew it "symbiotically," or mixed it with streptococci, the virulence was sufficiently raised for smaller doses to cause the death of this animal. Wolf[3] likewise declared that this organism did not invade the blood stream of the mouse even when large amounts of pure culture were injected intraperitoneally, and since he was never able to demonstrate the bacillus in the heart blood, he was of the opinion that in these cases death was due to intoxication. But when he injected a broth culture of streptococcus intraperitoneally or subcutaneously together with one slant of Pfeiffer's bacillus, a fatal septicemia followed, and both organisms were recovered from the heart blood. Roos[4] obtained similar results in experiments on simultaneous intraperitoneal injections into white mice of Pfeiffer's bacillus with streptococcus or with sputum. The exact dosage used is not recorded. After such injections, Pfeiffer's bacillus was often demonstrable in the heart blood, and Roos thought that "the symbiosis of these organisms increased the virulence of B. influenzae about ten-fold."

Albert and Kelman[5] agree with Roos on the question of increase of virulence of Pfeiffer's bacillus in mixed culture with streptococcus or pneumo-

Received for publication Nov. 15, 1921.

* This is one of a series of studies carried out in connection with the Influenza Commission established and financially aided by the Metropolitan Life Insurance Company of New York. Part of the expense of these studies has been met by a grant from the University of Chicago.

[1] Jour. A. M. A., 1919, 72, p. 155.

[2] Arch. de Med. Exper., 1901, 13, p. 425.

[3] Centralbl. f. Bakteriol., I, O., 1920, 84, p. 241.

[4] Jour. Immunol., 1919, 4, p. 189.

[5] Jour. Infect. Dis., 1919, 25, p. 433.

coccus, but consider the organism even in pure culture to be distinctly pathogenic for white mice. They base their conclusion on a series of 24 mice, among which there was a mortality of 83% following intraperitoneal injections, the amount injected not being stated. Similar results were reported by Ferry and Houghton,[6] who found that the strains used in their investigation of the toxin of Pfeiffer's bacillus all proved pathogenic for white mice, and that these animals were "invariably susceptible." Wollstein,[7] found that mice were highly susceptible to small injections of either spinal fluid of influenzal meningitis or pure cultures therefrom. The 8 cases reported by her at that time were all fatal, and hence the virulence of the strains may be considered high.

These differences in the findings as to pathogenicity by various workers may be due to differences in the dosages used, as Albert and Kelman[5] conclude, but they might also conceivably be due to differences in the source of the cultures and, perhaps as a result, the virulence of the strains.

The experiments reported here were undertaken to throw some light not only on the pathogenicity of Pfeiffer's bacillus for white mice, but also to relate the pathogenicity to the source of the strain. Other questions investigated were the invasiveness of the bacillus in pure and mixed culture, the possibility of increase in virulence by passage through white mice, and the presence of immunity in those mice that have recovered from a sublethal dose.

The strains used in these experiments were obtained from various sources. They were repeatedly examined and identified in this laboratory as Pfeiffer's bacillus. They had been cultivated on chocolate agar for varying lengths of time, although they had been isolated within a period of five months. In a short preliminary investigation it was found that the length of cultivation on artificial mediums within the limits of several weeks had no marked effect on the comparative pathogenicity of the bacillus for white mice, comparing strains from the same source. This allowed for reliable grouping of results from strains of one source and also for comparison of results from strains of different sources. All injections were made intraperitoneally. In the experiments on pathogenicity a 22-24 hour culture on chocolate agar slant suspended in 1 c c saline solution was injected into each mouse. A standard slant was adopted and adhered to closely. It was a slant about 8 cm. long in an ordinary 5/8 by 6 inch test-tube. An even growth was obtained by gently smearing the entire surface of the slant when inoculating.

[6] Jour. Immunol., 1919, 4, p. 233.
[7] Am. Jour. Dis. Child., 1911, 1, p. 42.

Early in the investigation on pathogenicity it was found that white mice had considerable individual susceptibility or resistance to this organism, and hence the plan was adopted of injecting the same strain into a series of 5 mice. This could not be done in every case because of the loss in the laboratory stock of some of the cultures before the adoption of this scheme and before the series of 5 mice for each strain was complete. This had little effect, however, on the final results as table 1 shows. One slant each of the 44 strains used was injected intraperitoneally into 146 mice, of which 120 died with the resulting mortality of 82%, which is in near agreement with the mortality of 83% which Albert and Kelman [5] found in a series of 24 mice similarly injected. The average period of survival among the 120 mice that died was about 19 hours. Considering only those strains that were injected in a series of 5 mice (4 mice in one case), we find nearly the same results, namely a mortality of 80% among 119 mice injected with 24 strains, and an average period of survival of about 18 hours after injection. It is worthy of note that one strain of Pfeiffer's bacillus isolated from a case of influenzal meningitis killed 3 out of 5 mice injected in the routine manner. The average period of survival was about 25 hours. This strain had been cultivated on artificial mediums for the same length of time as the other strains, and, although the results are comparable, they are not included in the figures presented since this was the only strain from influenzal meningitis.

Heart blood cultures of the mice that died usually showed the presence of Pfeiffer's bacillus either in pure culture or mixed with a postmortem invading organism, which was commonly a bacillus of the colon group. Pfeiffer's bacillus was recovered in pure culture from the heart blood in 68%, and either in pure culture or with another organism in 86%, of the fatal cases. The presence of Pfeiffer's bacillus was determined by cultivating the heart blood on chocolate agar and identifying the bacillus by its colony, morphology, and staining reaction. The peritoneal fluid was cultivated regularly also and Pfeiffer's bacillus was often found in the peritoneal fluid in pure culture, but another organism usually belonging to the colon group occurred with it about twice as often as in the heart blood. Gram-positive cocci were rarely found in the cultivation of either the heart blood or peritoneal fluid, being found 4 times in the cultures from 146 mice. Hence these cocci could not be considered an important factor in causing the death of the mice. These cultural findings are contrary to those of Wolf [3] who reported a repeatedly sterile heart blood even in fatal cases following injections of pure cultures. The high mortality following intraperitoneal injections of pure cultures of Pfeiffer's bacillus and the recovery of the same organism from the heart blood favor the view that the Pfeiffer's bacillus invades the blood stream and is pathogenic for white mice, irrespective of the source.

The original cultures came from several sources: throats of normal persons, throats of persons with common colds, and throats of military

TABLE 1

RESULTS OF INJECTIONS OF STRAINS OF PFEIFFER'S BACILLUS FROM VARIOUS SOURCES

I. Strains Tested in 1 or More Mice

Source of Original Cultures	Number of Cases from Which Strains Came	Number of Strains Tested in 1 or More Mice	Total Number of Mice Injected with All Strains	Number of Mice That Died	Number That Recovered	Percentage That Died	Average Hours of Survival After Injection
1. Normal respiratory tract........	8	10	31	25	6	80	19.8
2. Persons with common colds........	6	7	35	31	4	88	19.2
3. Influenza cases—civilian..........	7	8	36	22	14	61	22.4
4. Influenza cases—military..........	8	19	44	42	2	95	16.0
Totals.........	29	44	146	120	26	82	19.3

II. Strains Tested in Series of 5 Mice Each

Source of Original Cultures	Number of Cases from Which Strains Came	Number of Strains Tested in Series of 5 Mice	Total Number of Mice Injected in Series	Number of Mice That Died	Number That Recovered	Percentage That Died	Average Hours of Survival After Injection
1. Normal respiratory tract........	4	4	20	16	4	80	18.1
2. Persons with common colds........	6	7	35	31	4	88.6	19.2
3. Influenza cases—civilian...........	7	7	35	21	14	58	23.0
4. Influenza cases—military..........	5	6	29	28	1	96.5	13.8
Totals.........	22	24	119	96	23	80.6	18.5

and civilian patients with influenza. The observations gave an opportunity to determine the relation of the source of the strain to its pathogenicity for white mice. Correlation of the results of these experiments, as indicated in table 1, shows that the strains from the influenza epidemics at the Great Lakes Training Station and at Camp Grant early in 1920 were the most highly pathogenic with a mortality of 96.5% and an average period of survival of only 13 hours among 29 mice injected. The strains from persons with common colds, from normal throats, and from throats of influenza patients among civilians followed in that order in decreasing mortality rate and a corresponding lengthening of the period of survival after injection. While the evidence here is interesting, and indicative of the high virulence of strains of Pfeiffer's bacillus coming from epidemics in military camps, it cannot be taken as meaning that there is a definite etiologic relation of this organism to such an epidemic; nor can it be taken as conclusive that the virulence of Pfeiffer's bacillus is increased in epidemics of influenza, since the strains from typical civilian cases of influenza furnished the lowest mortality rate among white mice with the longest average period of survival. On the other hand, the conditions in the military camps, especially during a respiratory epidemic, were conducive to rapid transfer of respiratory organisms, which might tend to increase their virulence irrespective of the existence of an influenza epidemic. Likewise this might explain the lower virulence of the strains from civilian cases of influenza. The less crowded conditions in the civilian populace would give less opportunity for rapid transfer of respiratory organisms. The small difference between the mortality of mice injected with strains from normal throats and from throats of persons with common colds is not enough to give any significance to the presence of more virulent strains of Pfeiffer's bacillus in connection with common colds. The experimental evidence on these points is summarized in table 1.

Experiments were made to show the result of simultaneous injections of Pfeiffer's bacillus together with Streptococcus viridans and the pneumococcus. Strains of these cocci were taken at random from the laboratory stock cultures and had been grown on artificial mediums for some time (at least several months). Amounts of these gram-positive cocci were standardized for injection by growing them on whole blood-agar slants of the same size as for Pfeiffer's bacillus.

Streptococcus viridans was injected in amounts of 1 slant and one-half slant with the same doses of Pfeiffer's bacillus. The pneumococcus was injected in one-half and one-eighth slant amounts with equal doses of Pfeiffer's bacillus. The control and mixed culture tests of the pneumococcus and the bacillus were made in series of at least 5 mice of each amount, and the results presented are averages of such tests (table 2).

In no instance did the mouse survive when injected with both Pfeiffer's bacillus and a gram-positive coccus. Both organisms were invariably isolated from the heart blood in approximately equal numbers, although one-eighth slant of the same strain of Pfeiffer's bacillus used in pure culture was previously found always sublethal. The control mice injected with both amounts of Streptococcus viridans alone recovered. Pure cultures of pneumococcus were repeatedly fatal, but the simultaneous inoculations with Pfeiffer's bacillus were more rapidly fatal.

Streptococcus viridans was recovered from the heart blood of mice inoculated with mixed cultures of the coccus and Pfeiffer's bacillus, although the same dosages of the coccus in pure culture were innocuous. Likewise, sublethal doses of Pfeiffer's bacillus (one-eighth slant) with

TABLE 2

SIMULTANEOUS INJECTIONS OF PFEIFFER'S BACILLUS WITH STREPTOCOCCUS VIRIDANS AND PNEUMOCOCCUS TYPE 3.

	Amount Injected, in Slants	Period of Survival After Injections of Pure Cultures	Period of Survival After Injections of Pfeiffer's Bacillus with Gram-positive Coccus in Equal Amounts	Findings in Culture of Heart Blood Following Injections of Mixed Cultures
Pfeiffer's bacillus........	1	16 hours		
	½	22 hours		
	⅛	All recovered		
Streptococcus viridans..	1	Recovered	14 hours	Pfeiffer's bacillus and Streptococcus viridans
	½	Recovered	30 hours	Pfeiffer's bacillus and Streptococcus viridans
Pneumococcus Type III.	½	13 hours	11 hours	Pfeiffer's bacillus and pneumococcus
	⅛	18 hours	11 hours	Pfeiffer's bacillus and pneumococcus

the same amount of pneumococcus resulted in the death of all the mice so injected and in the recovery of both organisms from cultures of heart blood. It seems from these experiments that the invasiveness of both Pfeiffer's bacillus and Streptococcus viridans was increased by simultaneous mixed inoculations. A definite conclusion cannot be drawn, however, as to whether the coccus or the bacillus had the more active part in causing the death of the mouse since they were found on culture in approximately equal numbers.

The question whether an increase in virulence of Pfeiffer's bacillus was produced by passage through white mice was studied by a series of injections in decreasing doses of the heart blood culture of a fatal case. In the first group of experiments, 11 mice were fatally injected each with 1 slant of stock cultures. One-half slant of pure cultures from the heart blood of these 11 mice was injected into 11 other mice. As a result, only 4 mice succumbed with an average period of survival of 14 hours, while the 11 original mice injected with full slants had averaged about 13 hours of survival. The virulence was not sufficiently raised in one passage for half the original dose to be regularly fatal. In another group of experiments, repeated injections were made of pure cultures from the heart blood of the mouse dying with the minimal lethal dose and at the same time furnishing a pure culture of the bacillus in the heart blood. Decreasing doses of the pure subculture were given to several mice, fractions of a slant being injected as parts of a salt suspension of that slant. Variations in results presented themselves which were probably due to differences in resistance and susceptibility of the mice. The lethal amount of bacterial suspension was not reduced to any marked extent by such repeated transfers. Each series of tests was blocked after 3 or 4 transfers, however, either by inability to recover Pfeiffer's bacillus from the heart blood, or failure to recover it in pure culture.

These results are comparable to those of Roos [4] who found that the virulence of this organism is not increased by passage through rabbits. They also agree with the findings of Wollstein [7] who reported that "it was not found possible to increase the virulence appreciably by passing the organisms through series of mice, although the average dose was found to be reduced in the ninth passage to about one half the original fatal dose." Ferry and Houghton,[6] on the other hand, found the virulence "increased four-fold, and over" by repeated injections. The kind of animal used, however, is not specifically named. Jacobson [2] found that by repeatedly injecting mixed cultures of Pfeiffer's bacillus and streptococcus, he recovered from the heart blood, after 5 or 6 transfers, the Pfeiffer's bacillus which had increased in virulence sufficiently to kill a mouse even in pure culture, whereas originally the same strain was nonlethal. The brief experiments summarized in table 3 suggest that there was no marked increase in the virulence of Pfeiffer's bacillus by passage through white mice as many as 3 or 4 times. The arrow in the table indicates the mouse from whose heart blood was cultivated the bacillus for injection into the next group in the stated amounts. The hours refer to the period of survival after injection.

Observations were made on the degree of immunity possessed by those mice that had recovered from sublethal doses of Pfeiffer's bacillus. Eleven mice recovered from injections of sublethal doses of strains picked at random from the stock cultures on hand. The doses varied from 1/16 to 1/4 slant in amount. To these mice was added a control mouse that recovered from a dose lethal to 5 other mice. These 12 mice were then inoculated with doses found to be lethal to control mice. One-sixteenth to 1/4 slant of the strains used were sublethal and immunizing in effect, and 1/2 slant generally lethal to the nonimmunized mice. Seven of the 12 mice were injected with lethal and then twice

TABLE 3

EXPERIMENTS ON THE INCREASE IN VIRULENCE OF PFEIFFER'S BACILLUS BY PASSAGE THROUGH WHITE MICE

Strain	Amount Injected				
	1 Slant	½ Slant	¼ Slant	⅛ Slant	1/16 Slant
GL 6 NPBc	9 hours ↓				
	10 hours	10 hours	5 hours ↓		
		24 hours ↓	Recovered	Recovered	Recovered
	17 hours	17 hours	29 hours ↓	Recovered	Recovered
	17 hours	26 hours	Recovered	1 hour*	Recovered
GL 1 TBc	4 hours ↓				
	25 hours ↓	12 hours	Recovered	Recovered	Recovered
	26 hours	11 hours	Recovered	Recovered	Recovered
GL 10 TBc	26 hours	19 hours ↓			
	8 hours ↓	Recovered	Recovered	Recovered	Recovered
	21 hours ↓	Recovered	Recovered	Recovered	Recovered
	42 hours	26 hours	Recovered	Recovered	Recovered

* Died in convulsions at end of 1 hour.

lethal doses of the same strain. Six of the 7 mice recovered from the lethal dose, and 5 of the remaining 6 recovered from the twice lethal dose. These 5 mice and the other 5 of the original 12 immunized mice were then injected successively with 2 other strains of Pfeiffer's bacillus taken at random from the stock cultures. The dose of the first strain was lethal and of the second strain twice lethal. All the mice but 1 recovered from these two injections. Several control injections of these 2 strains were fatal in every case. The injections throughout the experiments on immunity were made at intervals of a few days and extended over a period of 40 days. The immunized mice showed no signs of sickness when injected with lethal doses and were plainly protected by previous sublethal doses. The mice were protected not only against the strain used in immunization, but they possessed immunity also against lethal doses of other strains. During the following 8 weeks, 2 of the immunized mice died of unknown cause. At the end of that time the 6 remaining mice were injected with a twice lethal dose of one of the immunizing strains. Only 1 mouse succumbed. This indicated that the specific and cross immunity lasted at least for the period of 8 weeks. The results of these experiments are given in table 4.

TABLE 4

EXPERIMENTS ON IMMUNITY ACQUIRED BY WHITE MICE AGAINST PFEIFFER'S BACILLUS

Strain..........	GL 10 TBc						GL 6 TOa	N 18 NPOb		N 9 NPOb	C 225 NPB	GL 10 TBc
Nature of dose.	Immunizing			Lethal		Twice Lethal	Lethal	Immunizing	Lethal	Lethal	Twice Lethal	Twice Lethal
Amount of dose in slants......	¼	⅛	1/16	½	½	1	½	⅛	½	½	1	1
Mouse 284......	L	..	..	L	L	L	L	..	..	L*		
Mouse 285......	L	..	..	L	L	L	L	..	..	L	L	D
Mouse 272......	L	..	..	L	L	L	L	..	..	D		
Mouse 277......	L	..	..	D								
Mouse 273......	..	L	..	L	L	D						
Mouse 278......	..	L	..	L	..	L	L	..	..	L	L	L
Mouse 274......	..	..	L	L	L	L	L	..	..	L	L†	
Mouse 296......	..	..	..	..	..	..	..	L	..	L	L	L
Mouse 297......	..	..	..	..	..	..	..	L	..	L	L	L
Mouse 298......	..	..	..	..	..	..	..	L	..	L	L	L
Mouse 299......	..	..	..	..	..	..	..	L	..	L	L†	
Mouse 291...... (a control that lived)	..	..	..	..	..	..	..	L	L	L	L	L
Control mice— Died..........	..	..	..	10	..	5	4	..	..	5	5	10
Recovered....	..	..	..	1	..	0	1	..	..	0	0	1

L = lived; D = died.
* 284 died of unknown cause 4 days after complete recovery from previous injection.
† 274 and 299 died several weeks after complete recovery from previous injection.
Note: Eight weeks elapsed between the injections of C 225 NPB and GL 10 TBc.

SUMMARY

Pfeiffer's bacillus when injected intraperitoneally in pure culture was found to be pathogenic for white mice irrespective of the source, and was readily recovered from the heart blood by cultivation on chocolate-agar medium. Strains isolated during influenza epidemics at military camps were more pathogenic for white mice than strains from other sources.

The invasiveness of both Pfeiffer's bacillus and Streptococcus viridans seemed to have been increased by injections in mixed cultures: the bacillus by injection with pneumococcus, and the coccus by injection with Pfeiffer's bacillus.

Pfeiffer's bacillus was not found to be appreciably increased in virulence by passage three or four times through white mice.

Sublethal doses (one-fourth to one-sixteenth slant of the strains used) of Pfeiffer's bacillus conferred immunity to white mice against lethal (one-half slant) and twice lethal (one slant) doses of heterologous as well as homologous strains. This immunity lasted at least eight weeks.

STUDIES ON THE FORMOL AND WASSERMANN REACTIONS

Manuel Armangué and Pedro Gonzales

From the Municipal Laboratory of Barcelona, Spain

Recently Gaté and Papacostas [1] reported a new reaction of syphilitic serum. According to these authors, positive serums gel under the influence of formol while negative serums remain fluid. It was of interest to study this reaction on account of the simplicity of technic and its excellent results. We have followed the exact method applied by the authors with this difference, that the readings were taken after the lapse of 40 to 48 hours instead of 24 to 30 hours, because negative reactions have been observed to become positive at the end of 40 hours. In one instance (a positive case) complete coagulation of the serum was observed in 10 minutes following the addition of the reagent. This is exceptional because ordinarily the reaction is slow. We have also noted, in certain serums, following addition of formol, an increased viscosity with flocculation but without the formation of a gel; the mixture remains semifluid so that it runs along the side of the inclined tube. These false or doubtful positives will be referred to subsequently. Tubes and pipets used in this reaction should be dry and tubes containing the serum and formol should be well stoppered. The reason for this will be found in some experiments to be discussed.

The following table gives the results of the Wassermann and formol reactions in 174 serums of suspicious cases.

We obtained positive formol reactions in 67% of cases of malignant tumors which gave negative Wassermann reactions. We have, therefore, a higher percentage of positive reactions among patients with malignant tumors than among syphilitic patients. The serum of a woman, taken 8 days after the extirpation of a sarcoma of the neck, reacted only moderately. We were unable to obtain serum of this case subsequently. The serums of pregnant women (7 to 9 months) always gave a negative formol reaction.

Serums of normal dogs, rabbits, guinea-pigs, hogs, etc., were always negative, but often positive in pathologic conditions. In cases of dogs, 28% positive reactions were obtained, and this was practically constant

Received for publication, Dec. 1, 1921.

[1] Compt. rend. Soc. de biol., 1920, 83, p. 1432.

in tenia infestations. In rabbits affected with coccidiosis of the peritoneal cavity, 34% gave a positive reaction, while 100% positive reactions were obtained if the spleen harbored coccidia or other parasites. A rabbit with hydatid cysts also gave a positive reaction.

Formol positive serums are rendered negative by dilution with water to more than 1 : 5 or 1 : 6. Dilution of the serum leads to the development of false positives in which there is increased viscosity with flocculation. Concentration of serums to ¾ or ⅘ their original volume (depending on the species of animal) changes negative serums so that they give positive reactions.

TABLE 1

RESULTS OF WASSERMANN AND FORMOL TESTS

Wassermann Reaction	Formol Reaction
41 strongly positive	11 positive 4 doubtful 26 negative
6 weakly positive	1 positive 1 doubtful 4 negative
127 frankly negative	5 positive 1 doubtful 121 negative

It seems to us fair to conclude that the formol reaction is not due to some specific substance but to a relative increase of the usual constituents of normal serum, possibly globulins. As is well known, various authors have shown that an increase of globulins in syphilis and malignancy exists.

While our work was under way, Pauzat[2] reported results entirely different from those of Gaté and Papacostas, and more recently Ecker[3] also obtained results identical with those of Pauzat and ourselves.

[2] Ibid., 1921, 84, p. 503.
[3] Jour. Infect. Dis., 1921, 29, p. 359.

DIFFERENTIATION AND IDENTIFICATION OF THE SPORULATING ANAEROBES *

Ivan C. Hall

From the Department of Hygiene and Bacteriology, University of Chicago, Chicago, Ill., and the Department of Bacteriology and Experimental Pathology, University of California, Berkeley, Calif.

This paper undertakes a taxonomic organization of the anaerobic bacteria. It is based on a study of 73 pure strains, all but 4 of which belong to 15 species. A new species, B. centrosporogenes, is described from 4 cultures. Much use has been made of the excellent contributions of the Medical Research Committee [1] and of Weinberg and Seguin [2] and other recent investigators who have appreciated the necessity of purity of culture as a fundamental premise in the description of bacterial species. Three species that have not been recognized in my work are included in the differential key (chart 1) solely on a basis of the published descriptions. The 4 unidentified cultures in the collection have not been included, pending a more thorough study.

THE PURITY PROBLEM

The building of the collection had not proceeded far when it was realized that many of the cultures were impure and more were improperly named, owing perhaps to the survival of a contaminant. The solution of the taxonomic problem was conceived to involve absolute purity of the cultures; impurity appears now to have been the most serious former obstacle to progress in the taxonomy of the anaerobes.

After several years of study, two methods of purification were selected as being of greatest utility, namely, deep agar dilution (depth colonies) and the blood agar slant (surface colonies) method.[3] Further experience teaches that while the latter has its limitations, so also has the former; there are advantages in the consecutive use of both. All new cultures should be regarded as possibly contaminated or mis-

Received for publication Dec. 1, 1921.

* This work was sustained in part by a grant under the Logan Fellowship at the University of Chicago in 1919-20, and by grants from the National Canners' Association, and from the Board of Research at the University of California in 1920-21.

1 Reports of the Committee upon Anaerobic Bacteria and Infection, Special Report Series 39, 1919.

2 La Gangrene gazeuse, 1918.

3 Jour. Infect. Dis., 1920, 27, p. 576.

named. Cultures received bearing labels are first tested for the salient characters of the organisms indicated, then repeatedly passed through the routine of purification, using first the deep agar, then the blood agar surface, culture method. Sometimes several attempts have to be made before securing well separated colonies. Always a careful scrutiny is made for differences in colony type that might indicate the presence of more than one species. Colonies of different appearance are picked separately with a view to differentiation. In several instances more than one species came from a single culture. On the contrary, in some instances differently appearing colonies later proved identical. In the latter the colony differences were rarely constant and may have been due to differences in age of the individual colonies in a single tube. Thus, while colony differences may indicate contamination in some cases, in others they do not. It has been my practice generally to subject each culture to one or the other or both purification processes repeatedly, until it has shown no dissimilar colonies in a single tube on at least three successive occasions. In the detailed discussion the total time occupied in purification is stated as an index of the labor involved, daily examination being made in order to push the procedure as rapidly as possible.

The necessity of extreme care regarding the purity and identity of named stock cultures received from other laboratories was shown recently.[4] Cultures of anaerobes require exceptional care to avoid contamination and loss of identity; no culture can be accepted on its face value.

Once a culture is purified it must be watched constantly for recurrent contamination. Imperfect sterilization is the chief cause of anaerobic contamination, but one still has to guard against aerobic contamination. I test every transplant by subculture on aerobic agar in slants or Petri dishes which must remain barren on incubation.

The stock cultures in the collection are kept in duplicate in deep brain medium without any seal other than that provided by the depth of the medium itself. The cultures are inoculated by loop, incubated at 37 C. for 24-48 hours, tested for aerobic contamination and placed in a clean, dark cupboard at room temperature. Especial care is exercised to have good cotton stoppers wrapped in gauze. Transplants are made at intervals of 1-2 months or oftener if needed. None of the cultures has been handled since purification by any other person than

[4] Proc. Soc. Exper. Biol. & Med., 1921, 18, p. 314.

the writer during the past six years. Some unfortunate experiences in depending on assistants previous to that time taught the necessity of assuming the whole burden of responsibility.

IDENTIFICATION

Little attention was paid to identification until approximately 50 strains had been purified. Certain strains had never shown any evidence of contamination and were possessed of such outstanding characteristics that there could be no question of their identity. Thus our conceptions of the non-motility and stormy milk fermentation of B. welchii, and of specific toxin formation of B. tetani and B. botulinus were sufficient to identify. More difficult were the "blackleg bacillus," Vibrion septique, and "bacillus of malignant edema," whose tangled history and nomenclature were so ably unraveled by Weinberg and Seguin,[2] and the terminally spored organisms. I was fortunate in having at hand cultures of B. chauvœii, Vibrion septique, and "bacillus of malignant edema" in which no evidence of impurity had been found and which had been made the subjects of careful record by Meyer.[5] Some of the more recently described species were obtained from Messrs. Weinberg and Seguin in Paris and from the Lister Institute, London.

The first step was to separate the proteolytic from the nonproteolytic cultures as judged by the action on brain medium. The next involved the production of agglutinating serums for the known strains with which it was thought that certain of the unknown strains could be identified. But while agglutinating serums were made for every species except B. egens, B. aerofetidus, B. novyi, B. multifermentans-tenalbus, and B. fallax, only that for B. bifermentans failed either to subdivide the species or to react simply with the culture used in immunization. Notwithstanding the successful segregation of 3 strains of B. bifermentans, of 19 out of 24 strains of B. sporogenes, of 3 type "B" strains of B. botulinus, of certain strains of B. tetani and of Vibrion septique by specific agglutination, this means of identification is subject to such limitations as to be of little practical value.

Adequate identification may be based on certain criteria which should be applied, as far as possible, in order, as follows: Morphology, vegetative forms, spores, flagella (motility); cultural reactions; action on proteins, coagulated albumin (brain or meat mediums), gelatin; action on carbohydrates; pathogenicity.

[5] Jour. Infect. Dis., 1915, 17, p. 458.

These points were utilized in setting up the appended differential key (chart 1).

CHART 1.

A DIFFERENTIAL KEY FOR THE SPORULATING ANAEROBES

1. Spores central (rarely subterminal); not swelling the rod; often difficult to demonstrate in the nonputrefactive forms (No record for B. egens).
   Nonmotile rods.
      Coagulated albumin liquefied; brain blackened; gelatin liquefied; lactose not fermented........................B. bifermentans
      Coagulated albumin not liquefied; brain not blackened (except in presence of iron by B. welchii); gelatin liquefied (no record for B. egens).
         Lactose fermented ....B. welchii
            Glycerol and inulin fermented...................type 1
            Glycerol fermented; inulin not fermented.....type 2
            Glycerol not fermented; inulin fermented.......type 3
            Neither glycerol nor inulin fermented.........type 4
         Lactose not fermented...........................B. egens
   Motile rods.
      Coagulated albumin liquefied; brain blackened; gelatin liquefied ....B. centrosporogenes, N. Sp.
      Coagulated albumin not liquefied; neither plain nor iron brain blackened; gelatin not liquefied (or only tardily)..B. butyricus

2. Spores subterminal (rarely central); always when mature swelling the rod into clostridiums.
   Motile rods.
      Coagulated albumin liquefied; brain blackened; gelatin liquefied.
         Lactose fermented ....B. aerofetidus
         Lactose not fermented:
            Filtrates toxic for guinea-pigs on feeding....B. botulinus
               Toxic for chickens............................type A
               Slightly or nontoxic for chickens..............type B
            Filtrates nontoxic on feeding:
               Cultures pathogenic on injection in doses of 1 cc or less; lytic action peculiar to this species ....B. histolyticus
               Cultures nonpathogenic except in large doses........ ....B. sporogenes
      Coagulated albumin not liquefied; brain not blackened.
         Gelatin liquefied; usually pathogenic for guinea-pigs (see B. novyi).
            Lactose fermented:
               Saccharose fermented; salicin not fermented ....B. chauvœi
               Saccharose not fermented; salicin fermented ....Vibrion septique
            Lactose not fermented..........................B. novyi
         Gelatin not liquefied:
            Lactose and glycerol fermented.B. multifermentans-tenalbus
            Lactose and glycerol not fermented.............B. fallax

3. Spores terminal.
   Spores round or nearly round; rods motile.
      Coagulated albumin slowly liquefied; plain brain slightly, iron brain markedly blackened; gelatin liquefied; glucose not fermented.
         Toxic on injection, causing tetanus....................B. tetani
         Nonpathogenic ....B. putrificus
      Coagulated albumin not liquefied; neither plain nor iron brain blackened.
         Gelatin liquefied slowly; lactose and salicin not fermented....... .... B. tetanomorphus
         Gelatin not liquefied; lactose and salicin fermented..B. sphenoides
   Spores elongate:
      Motile rods; coagulated albumin not liquefied; neither plain nor iron brain blackened; gelatin not liquefied....................B. tertius

This key is to some extent still in a formative stage; perhaps additions will be necessary to include properly described organisms that may have been omitted, and new organisms that may be described hereafter. It follows admittedly the beginning made by the Medical Research Committee but undertakes a greater detail.

MORPHOLOGY AS A CRITERION IN IDENTIFICATION

Morphology should be utilized just as far as possible as the primary means of differentiating living organisms. In the study of a given culture, an early emphasis on morphology serves to some extent as a check against otherwise undetectable contamination.

VEGETATIVE FORMS

While each species of anaerobe presents certain tendencies in the morphology of its vegetative forms, differences in the vegetative morphology are not of great differential value owing to pleomorphic tendencies. Most of the known forms are gram-positive rods. The gram stain has therefore only a limited usefulness for differentiation. The breadth of the vegetative rods in a given species is to some degree subject to less variation than their length and is therefore fairly characteristic.

FORM OF THE SPORES

The form of the spores appears to be constant and characteristic for the species. Three distinct groups may be differentiated—one with central spores which do not swell the rods, a second with subterminal or clostridial spores, and a third with terminal or plectridial spores. The last may be again subdivided as the spore is round or elongate.

Spores are formed most abundantly in mediums not containing fermentable carbohydrates in excess. Deep brain medium, Robertson's alkaline egg broth,[6] deep meat infusion agar and blood-agar slants provide excellent conditions for sporulation.

The use of spores as the criterion for the primary subdivision of the anaerobes is distinctly limited in that certain species, such as B. welchii, and B. aerofetidus, produce spores only sparsely under cultural conditions. Certain strains even of species known to produce abundant spores, may produce few or none. Thus two strains of B. botulinus have as yet failed to reveal spores with certainty, after the most diligent and prolonged search. It so happens that this species may be recognized beyond a doubt by the specific action of its filtrable toxin. So in some cases it is necessary to pass on to other features in the identification, but the search for spores concentrates the attention early in the study of a given culture on one of its most important idiosyncrasies.

FLAGELLA AND MOTILITY

Flagella may be postulated on the demonstration of motility. Ultimately a staining method may prove superior, but an intensive study of flagella staining has not yet developed any technic that justifies the assumption that flagella are absent when they cannot be stained.

While the inhibition of motility of some strains by exposure to air or the loss of motility after a few hours of incubation present difficulties in technic and fallacies of interpretation, motility constitutes a satisfactory criterion if too much confidence is not placed in negative results.

Suitable material for motility tests may be secured with a minimum of exposure from the closed arm of the writer's new fermentation tube with marble seal, by means of a pipet. Only young cultures should be examined for motility, as old cultures are frequently nonmotile. Motility in most strains may be determined at 24 hours but nonmotility should be recorded finally, if ever, for cultures examined as early as growth becomes evident (see B. centrosporogenes N.Sp.). Age of culture is unquestionably one of the most important elements in the determination of this function.

Hollow ground slides are not recommended; plain slides provide more nearly a single plane of distribution of the organisms and give better protection from the air. The complicated device of Dunham[7] is not practical.

[6] Jour. Path. & Bacteriol., 1916, 20, p. 327.
[7] Bull. Johns Hopkins Hosp., 1897, 8, p. 74.

A preliminary test may be made by placing the liquid culture on a plain glass slide under a coverslip with the high power lens. If definitely motile, no further examination is necessary; if apparently nonmotile, further tests should be made in which the culture is better protected from the air by means of a ring of petrolatum. Final decision as to nonmotility should be made only after testing very young cultures in various liquid mediums, with and without glucose and with a warm (37 C.) stage or with the microscope in a warm box.

PROTEOLYSIS AND PUTREFACTION AS CRITERIA IN IDENTIFICATION

Fischer[8] defined putrefaction as "the biochemical decomposition of nitrogenous organic compounds by the action of microorganisms," and this definition was accepted by Kendall,[9] who considers that most aerobic as well as anaerobic bacteria, produce putrefaction in this sense in mediums free from fermentable carbohydrates, as shown by their increased ammonia production. Rettger,[10] holds that putrefaction is a function peculiar to certain obligate anaerobes, the criterion of putrefaction being a foul odor. Rettger failed to find indol and skatol in sufficient quantity to serve as a criterion for putrefaction, an observation confirmed by my strains of B. sporogenes and B. botulinus, using the delicate Ehrlich test. B. bifermentans, however, produces indol. Rettger would not admit liquefaction of albumins as a criterion of putrefaction and distinguished the decomposition of albumins due to certain aerobes as nonputrefactive and pointed out that "decomposition of albumin by the aerobes is never accompanied by the foul odors which are so characteristic of putrefaction."

Acceptance of the latter statement depends to some extent on one's conception of a "foul odor." We have to distinguish between various grades of proteolysis. Few investigators regard streptococci as proteolytic, yet they liberate distinctly more ammonia in sugar free mediums than in mediums containing glucose,[9] but they never produce foul odors. Bact. coli liberates much more ammonia and, in the writer's opinion, produces a distinctly foul odor in nonsugar mediums. But neither organism liquefies gelatin or coagulated albumins. Proteus vulgaris and Pseudomonas pyocaneus, on the contrary, produce abundant ammonia, liquefy both gelatin and coagulated albumins, and produce foul odors in mediums not containing fermentable carbohydrates in excess.

What is acceptable evidence of proteolysis? One aspect of the question concerns those phenomena that attend the destruction of protein without regard to the special products formed, the other the

[8] Vorlesungen über Bakterien, 1903, 2, p. 206.

[9] Jour. Med. Res., 1911, 20, p. 140; also Bacteriology, General, Pathological, Intestinal, 1916.

[10] Jour. of Biol. Chemistry, 1908, 4, p 45.

production of various end products, proteoses, albumoses, amino acids, mercaptan, sulphuretted hydrogen, indol, skatol, etc. The products undoubtedly vary according to the organism, and, furthermore, require special chemical tests for their demonstration; it is preferable, therefore, in the beginning, to utilize criteria of proteolysis that are generally applicable without highly specialized procedures. Odor alone, however, is unsuitable owing to the difficulty of its objective interpretation. Liquefaction, on the contrary, offers a criterion of proteolysis that is easily interpreted and described; it presents only this difficulty, that some organisms liquefy coagulated proteins so slowly and so slightly that some qualification is necessary to distinguish them from nonproteolytic organisms. Proteolysis in this sense is a narrower term than in Fischer's definition of putrefaction since a number of organisms deaminize proteins in order to get at the carbon for their energy requirements, without carrying the destruction of the protein to the point of liquefaction. In this narrower sense such organisms are regarded as nonproteolytic, while proteolytic micro-organisms are those that liquefy coagulated albumins, egg white, blood serum, meat, brain tissue, etc.

Certain conditions must be provided in testing for proteolysis. Some micro-organisms require a fermentable carbohydrate in order to grow; on the contrary, an excess of fermentable carbohydrate tends to inhibit proteolysis. I observe proteolysis in a brain medium [3] containing 0.1% added glucose. The modicum of fermentable sugar stimulates the growth but is soon exhausted so that it does not interfere with protein splitting.

DISCOLORATION OF BRAIN AND MEAT MEDIUMS

All of the actively proteolytic anaerobes blacken brain and chopped meat mediums under proper conditions, owing apparently to the precipitation of a sulphur compound by sulphuretted hydrogen, as can be proved by the lead acetate test. The addition of a few drops of ferric chloride or lead acetate solution to brain cultures that show liquefaction throws down an intense, heavy, granular, or flaky metallic black deposit, but no such result can be secured with cultures of B. butyricus, B. chauvœi, B. novyi, B. tetanomorphus, B. sphenoides or B. tertius, which have little or no digestive action on proteins and do not blacken brain mediums.

An excess of fermentable carbohydrate, say 5% glucose, inhibits the blackening by putrefactive anaerobes, and smaller quantities distinctly delay it through a very evident protection of the protein. But a modicum of glucose, i. e., less than an excess, is of value in the initiation of a heavier development of bacteria, and the black deposit is distinctly more marked with peptone present.

The discoloration is greatest near the top of the medium, which von Hibler [11] explained as due to the greater concentration of gas there. He believed that iron sulphid was formed and that the iron was derived from traces of hemoglobin in the tissues. But this seems improbable since the addition of blood failed to increase the blackening of brain medium by B. sporogenes, B. botulinus, or B. tetani, or to cause its production by B. welchii. It seems likely that the iron responsible for the blackening of brain and meat mediums by putrefactive anaerobes is derived from those compounds in the tissues in which iron is less firmly bound than in hemoglobin.[12]

The addition of metallic iron and of some iron salts to these mediums greatly increases the blackening; a most striking result is obtained by the inclusion of a clean iron nail. The strongly proteolytic and putrefactive anaerobes, such as B. bifermentans, B. sporogenes, B. centrosporogenes, and B. botulinus, produce a much earlier and heavier deposit, but no difference is to be seen in cultures of the nonputrefactive B. butyricus, B. chauvœi, Vibrion septique, B. novyi, B. tetanomorphus, B. sphenoides and B. tertius.

Intermediate between these are B. welchii, B. tetani, and B putrificus, for while these weakly proteolytic organisms do not ordinarily blacken brain mediums, they produce sulphuretted hydrogen according to the lead acetate test. But metallic iron and certain iron salts cause distinct blackening in all three. According to von Hibler, a distinctly alkaline reaction is necessary, and B. welchii, being only weakly proteolytic, fails ordinarily to produce a sufficient OH- ion concentration to blacken. My experiments suggest that the failure of B welchii, B. tetani, and B. putrificus, to blacken ordinary brain and meat mediums hinges in part on their inability to liberate the iron from the tissues in sufficient quantity to precipitate the sulphid.

The presence of metallic iron does not lead to any marked discoloration of the medium without bacterial growth. Copper does, however, and must be avoided in the utensils employed in the preparation of the medium.

[11] Untersuchungen über pathogene Anaëroben, 1908.
[12] Chemical Pathology, 1918.

The fact that quite a number of proteolytic anaerobes, including B. bifermentans, B. centrosporogenes and B. histolyticus, produce crystals of tyrosine suggested, in view of the supposed oxidation of tyrosine to melanin by tyrosinase,[12] that the black coloring matter in meat and brain cultures of proteolytic anaerobes might be identical with melanin. This was disproved by the observations that various proteolytic anaerobes produce tyrosine abundantly in salmon flesh without blackening, although they blacken meat and brain mediums. The digestive action of these organisms in salmon was evident, and the H_2S test was strongly positive with lead acetate. The reaction of the salmon cultures became alkaline as in meat. Furthermore, sulphuretted hydrogen passed through uninoculated salmon medium failed to discolor it while it darkened the beef. The darkening of beef and brain mediums seems to be due to the precipitation by sulphur of some cation, probably iron, that is absent from salmon flesh, for the inclusion of an iron nail insures an abundant black discoloration in salmon medium. The blackening of brain and meat mediums is therefore independent of the formation of tyrosin and is perfectly correlated with the production of H_2S in the presence of iron.

In a strict sense, an increase in alkalinity (OH- ion concentration) should be regarded as the criterion of proteolysis, but many bacteria that have only the mildest action on proteins would then have to be classed as proteolytic.

Liquefaction and the blackening of brain medium either with or without added iron are therefore the most convenient macroscopic criterions of proteolysis.

GELATINOLYSIS

All the organisms that liquefied coagulated proteins also liquefied gelatin. But gelatin liquefaction is not peculiar to the liquefiers of coagulated proteins. It extends to all organisms that produce H_2S as well as to some that do not. Gelatin liquefaction has therefore no differential value among proteolytic anaerobes, but its usefulness is limited to differentiation of nonproteolytic organisms. However, the prominence given gelatin in Chester's "Manual of Determinative Bacteriology" in the differentiation of anaerobes is wholly unjustified and misleading.

The usual principles regarding the presence of fermentable sugars apply; a modicum is necessary to insure growth but an excess in some cases inhibits or retards liquefaction. I add 0.2% glucose to 12%

gelatin, 2% peptone meat infusion ($P_H = 7.0$). Perfect clarity is not necessary.

The first report of the Medical Research Committee on Classification and Study of the Anaerobic Bacteria of War Wounds in 1917 considered gelatin liquefaction "highly unsatisfactory" as a criterion of differentiation; the second report in 1919 made use of gelatin as a means of subdividing those anaerobes that do not liquefy coagulated serum. The method of securing anaerobiosis was not mentioned, but the tubes were incubated at 37 C. for 48 hours and then tested by immersion in cold water.

Weinberg and Seguin [2] tested gelatin liquefaction in deep tubes, presumably at room temperature since the form of the colonies was described.

In my experience, gelatin at 37 C., like broth, unless provided with a definite seal, must be quite deep to secure satisfactory growth on account of convection currents which aid oxygen absorption; at room temperature accurate results may be secured in deep culture if one waits several days or weeks. The records are based on tests in constricted tubes with marble seals, with incubation at 37 C. and daily cooling in the ice chest to determine liquefaction.

It is necessary to control gelatin liquefaction tests carefully for satisfactory growth, for aerobic contamination and for failure of liquefaction in uninoculated tubes. Some difficulty in securing satisfactory growth in gelatin might be attributed to the instability of the reaction which tends to become too acid during sterilization. Vigorous growth usually leads to gas formation, and a darkening of the sediment in the base of the tube, which appears as an all but constant accompaniment of anaerobic growth in gelatin.

With vigorous growth, liquefaction occurred, if at all, as a rule during the first 48 hours, although certain cultures required several weeks. Further work on the conditions that govern liquefaction by anaerobes is desirable.

FERMENTATION TESTS AS CRITERIA IN IDENTIFICATION

The use of differential fermentation tests in anaerobic bacteriology has been retarded by lack of agreement as to criteria and by inadequate methods of technic. My efforts to solve some of the problems of the fermentation tests have already resulted in the extension of the mechanical seal principle to the fermentation tube,[13] the advocacy of B. welchii in the preparation of sugar-free culture mediums,[14] and the

[13] Jour. Infect. Dis., 1921, 29, p. 317.
[14] Ibid., p. 344.

conclusion that an increase in H + ion concentration constitutes the best single criterion of fermentation.[15] The designation of an increase in dissociated hydrogen as the criterion of fermentation caused me finally to disregard gas production in the fermentation tests. There is, however, evidence to show that in some cases large gas production may compensate for a slight increase in H + ion concentration and vice versa, so that perhaps both should be taken into account. The tests reported were made with meat infusion 2% peptone broth fermented out with B. welchii, readjusted to $P_H = 7.0$ when necessary, and sterilized in constricted tubes with marble seals. The carbohydrates were chemically pure; they were sterilized by autoclave in 10% solution in neutral distilled water, and added aseptically to make 1% final concentration. Uninoculated controls of each sugar and inoculated sugar-free broth controls were included in every test. The earlier tests utilized azolitmin as indicator; it decolorizes below the seal, but shows acidity changes readily above. Recently, owing to difficulty in securing good azolitmin, I have pipetted out from below the seal about 1 c c of culture into a white porcelain test plate and added 2 drops of brom-thymol blue. Acidity is shown by a yellow color.

CULTURES

The various strains are discussed in the order of appearance of the species to which they were assigned in the diagnostic chart. The date of original receipt is given in each case to show the length of time they have been under study.

Anaerobes with Centrally Located Spores

This group comprises B. bifermentans, B. welchii, B. egens, B. centrosporogenes N.Sp., and B. butyricus.

BACILLUS BIFERMENTANS

This species was first recognized by Tissier and Martelly[16] in 1902 when they recovered it from tainted meat and designated it B. bifermentans sporogenes. Tissier[17] again encountered it in 1916 in war wounds. Weinberg and Seguin[2] recovered B. bifermentans twice from among 91 cases of gaseous gangrene, but did not consider it an impor-

[15] Ibid., p. 321.
[16] Ann. de l'Inst. Past., 1902, 16, p. 865.
[17] Ibid., 1916, 30, p. 681.

tant factor in this infection; it probably plays a rôle similar to that of B. sporogenes in mixed wound infections.

I have isolated 3 strains as follows: 1 from the heart blood of a rabbit at necropsy, 1 from a carious tooth, and 1 from the liver of a rabbit at necropsy. These cultures were first grouped with other proteolytic anaerobes in the collection, notably B. sporogenes and B. botulinus, which they resemble culturally. They were separated from the latter on the basis of their nonpathogenicity, from the former through their failure to be agglutinated by a specific serum prepared against B. sporogenes 10, and from both by the central position of their spores and nonmotility, and were finally grouped by means of a specific serum prepared against culture 50.

B. bifermentans 50 was recovered in May, 1916, from the heart blood of an adult female rabbit that died suddenly from an undetermined cause. Intravenous injection of a rabbit with 1 c c of an 8-day brain culture plus 5 c c glucose broth culture failed to establish a suspected etiologic relation; it was regarded therefore as a postmortem invader.

This culture has never shown any evidence of anaerobic impurity; hay bacillus contaminations were twice eliminated by selective bacteriostasis.[18] It was reisolated twice from single colonies by the surface culture method in 1917. There was some difficulty in securing well separated surface colonies with this culture owing to a tendency to form a lace-like confluent growth on the surface of blood agar, but well separated depth colonies were secured in 1% meat infusion agar without difficulty.

B. bifermentans 70.—This was recovered Dec. 6, 1917, from the packing of a carious tooth. The initial culture was apparently pure and free from aerobes, although examination of other packings from the same tooth showed streptococci in addition.

The culture was easily repurified 3 times from well separated surface colonies on plain agar slants under alkaline pyrogallol, and 3 times from blood agar slants within the time of about one month. There was no essential difference in the form of the colonies on plain agar and blood-agar slants. The isolated culture possessed the properties of the initial culture.

B. bifermentans 102.—March 3, 1920, a normal rabbit was killed by a blow on the head and then placed in the incubator at 37 C. as a control in a test of the ability of various anaerobes to simulate the well-known effect of B. welchii. At 24 hours the abdomen was only slightly inflated; incubation was continued to 48 hours. The belly was then greatly inflated, and the hair slipped easily. There was no subcutaneous emphysema as with the inoculated animals. The distention of the belly was due to gas in the intestinal tract, not in the tissues or body cavities, but the heart chambers contained some gas. No heart blood could be secured. The gas burned with a blue flame. The liver was not foamy though considerably softened; impression smears from its cut surface showed large gram-positive single rods.

The initial culture secured from the liver in deep brain medium was apparently pure; well separated deep colonies in meat infusion agar were all alike. The culture was repurified on three successive occasions from such deep colonies, and the purified culture was shown to be identical with the original.

In addition a culture labeled "B. bifermentans No. 506, Strain F," from the Lister Institute, London, like 3 other strains of central spored proteolytic anaerobes, while nonmotile in cultures of 24 hours' or more incubation, is actively motile at 8 hours, and must therefore be excluded as constituting another species. There was no evidence of impurity in the English culture (see B. centrosporogenes N.Sp., No. 145).

Morphology. — B. bifermentans cultures consist of large gram-positive nonmotile rods forming oval spores that do not swell the vegetative form. Free spores are slightly barrel-shaped, their location

[18] Hall, Jour. Am. Med. Assn., 1919, 72, p. 274.

in the vegetative cell being best determined in young cultures. Vegetative forms are usually single or in chains of 2-3 cells and are always nonmotile.

Colony Form.—The form of blood-agar surface colonies is not sufficiently constant to have diagnostic value. Those of culture 50 were always irregular, ameboid, or even lace like, spreading over the surface of the medium. Those of cultures 70 and 102 were always round like dew drops. All were hemolytic.

In deep 1% meat infusion agar the colonies were granular, diffusely opaque globules, tending to break up as they became older.

Physiology.—All 3 cultures are highly proteolytic, liquefying the coagulated albumin in deep brain and meat mediums and coagulated egg white, with marked blackening. Gelatin is actively liquefied. Indol is formed in suitable sugar-free mediums.

The action on milk is characteristic of putrefactive anaerobes, slow coagulation with little or no gas formation at first followed by liquefaction with slight gas production.

Glucose and glycerol were fermented by all 3 cultures; lactose saccharose, salicin, inulin and sugar-free broths were not fermented.

Pathogenicity.—There is no evidence of pathogenicity in pure cultures of B. bifermentans, either in the literature or in our own records. At various times guinea-pigs were injected subcutaneously with 1-2 c c and rabbits intravenously with 2-5 c c without any demonstrable effect.

BACILLUS WELCHII

This species is perhaps one of the best understood anaerobes, especially since the able reviews of Simonds,[19] Jablons [20] and Esty.[21] B. welchii is readily defined as the only nonmotile anaerobic bacillus producing a stormy fermentation in milk, although the latter is somewhat irregular and varies, as Simonds [22] showed, according to the perfection of anaerobiosis provided. The following 6 strains came: One from human feces, 1 from a stock laboratory culture labeled B. tetani, 1 from a guinea-pig inoculated with soil, 1 from a spoiled can of Swiss chard, 1 from the stomach of a woman dead of botulism, and 1 from the tissues of a cow dead of a disease of unknown etiology.

[19] Monograph 5, Rockefeller Inst. for Med. Res., 1915.
[20] Jour. Lab. & Clin. Med., 1920, 5, p. 374.
[21] Jour. Bacteriol., 1920, 5, p. 375.
[22] Compt. rend. Soc. de biol., 1916, 79, p. 904; Trans. Chicago Path. Society, 1917, 10, p. 167.

B. welchii 2, type 2.—May 2, 1916, "B. welchii B. 521" was received from the American Museum of Natural History. Dr. Simonds had recovered it from stools in 1912 and designated it No. 16 in his series.

When received it was free from areobes and gave a typical stormy fermentation in milk, but the blackening of brain medium and the finding of motile rods and clostridial spores pointed to contamination with a putrefactive anaerobe. When isolation was first undertaken in March, 1918, there were clearly on a plain agar slant under alkaline pyrogallol 2 types of small round colonies, one more transparent in appearance than the other. The transparent colony was isolated and later proved to be B. sporogenes (see No. 72). The more opaque type was 4 times repeatedly picked from well isolated colonies on the surface of blood-agar slants during a period of 10 days.

Subsequent to identification, an erroneous suspicion of contamination owing to certain variations of morphology in a glucose-broth culture led to 4 more successive resiolations from deep agar colonies and a repetition of the identification tests. This culture ferments glycerol with acid production but not inuline, and is therefore assigned to Simonds' type 2. Only a trace of gas appears in either medium. It is moderately pathogenic for guinea-pigs, pigeons and rabbits.

B. welchii 20, type 4.—This type was received from the Cutter Laboratories, Berkeley, Calif., about 1915, labeled B. tetani. Kept in a collection of stock cultures, it did not come into the writer's hands until Dec. 15, 1916. It was then free from aerobes, but a deep brain culture blackened notably, indicating the presence of a proteolytic anaerobe. Morphologically, there were 2 forms present, large nonmotile gram-positive vegetative rods (B. welchii undoubtedly) and slender, motile gram-positive rods with terminal oval spores attached. There were also numerous free oval spores. One c c of a 13-day brain culture suspension was injected subcutaneously into a rabbit without result. There was thus neither morphologic nor toxicologic evidence of B. tetani in the culture.

Purification consisted in thrice repeated picking of well separated colonies from the surface of blood-agar slants under alkaline pyrogallol during the interval from March 24 to April 2, 1918. These were always hemolytic round smooth-edged dew-drop-like colonies. None of the picked cultures blackened brain medium, and the putrefactive contaminant was never isolated.

Testing the purified culture for B. tetani in week old and 11-day old glucose broth cultures, there was no action of 1 c c injected subcutaneously into guinea-pigs of 450 gm. weight.

This culture was identified as B. welchii in March, 1920, on morphologic and cultural grounds. Without any record of spores in this strain, the vegetative morphology is characteristic; it is always nonmotile, and it gives a typical "stormy" fermentation in milk. It ferments neither glycerol nor inulin and therefore belongs to Simonds' type 4. The strain is also moderately pathogenic for guinea-pigs, as discussed later. Undoubtedly the initial tests for pathogenicity with this culture when we were searching for B. tetani in it, were conducted with cultures too old to show any virulence for B. welchii.

B. welchii 26, type 1.—May 15, 1917, Professor J. Traum of Div. of Vet. Sc., Univ. of Calif., sent me a guinea-pig recently dead following symptoms of tetanus after the inoculation of earth treated with sodium hydroxide in a study of tubercle bacilli in soil. The muscle tissues at the site of inoculation had undergone considerable necrosis and digestion. The bloody exudate contained many gram-positive rods but no visible spores.

Primary culture in a glucose-broth constricted tube produced much gas; it was free from aerobes. A brain medium culture blackened showing the presence of putrefactive anaerobes.

Purification did not start until March 9, 1918, when a variety of colonies on a blood-agar slant indicated the presence of several forms. A pure culture was probably secured in the second picking for none of the brain medium transplants thereafter showed the black pigmentation. There were 4 repeated pickings of well separated colonies during a period of 14 days.

The culture was identified as B. welchii, on the basis of morphology, nonmotility, and stormy fermentation of milk.

This culture is atypical in respect to its failure to blacken iron brain, to liberate H_2S, and in its fermentation of salicin. It forms acid, but only a trace of gas from glycerol and considerable gas but little or no acid from inulin;; it is assigned to Simonds' Group 1.

B. welchii 36, type 4.—Oct. 15, 1918, two tins of commercially canned spinach were received from Dr. Albert Schneider. Both were greatly swelled; one had been opened (see B. centrosporogenes 82); the other was allowed to remain in the room and burst 2 days later from the pressure.

The contents of the latter were softened and full of gas but not foul in odor.

Microscopically there were gram-negative rods and filaments but no spores. Glucose broth culture showed gas and turbidity and gram-positive rods without spores. No aerobes were present. Brain medium produced abundant gas but failed to blacken.

Purification started at once and occupied about 10 days during which time 4 repeated successive isolations from well separated blood-agar surface colonies were carried out. From the first the colonies were all alike, round, moist, dew-drop-like, and hemolytic. The initial culture is considered to have been pure.

Identification was made on the basis of morphology, nonmotility, and stormy fermentation of milk. It ferments neither inulin nor glycerol and therefore belongs to Simonds' type 4. This culture is highly pathogenic and produces certain peculiar lesions in guinea-pigs on subcutaneous inoculation.

B. welchii 129, type 4.—Oct. 22, 1920, the writer received a small portion of the stomach contents of Dr. E. S., dead 3 days previously with symptoms of botulism at St. Anthony's Hospital in Oakland from eating canned spinach. The body had been embalmed and the stomach contents had stood in glass for 48 hours.

The material was liquid and strongly acid. Microscopically the only distinguishable organisms were large gram-positive rods. A 370 gm. guinea-pig was inoculated subcutaneously with 1 c c without harm.

Deep brain cultures produced abundant gas, did not blacken, and showed gram-positive rods and cocci; milk gave a stormy fermentation. Aerobic cocci were eliminated by selective heating at 75 C. for 20 minutes.

Purification occupied 8 days and consisted in 3 repeated successive transfers of the well isolated compact disk-like depth colonies in deep meat infusion agar.

The purified culture was readily identified as B. welchii by its morphology, nonmotility, and action in milk. It was nonpathogenic in a dose of 1 c c of a 24-hour glucose broth culture inoculated subcutaneously into a 500 gm. guinea pig.

B. welchii 135, type 4.—This strain was received from Dr. F. W. Wood of the Cutter Laboratories of Berkeley, Calif., Dec. 10, 1920, having been recovered from the tissues of a cow dead of a disease of unknown etiology that is prevalent in the Sierra Nevada mountains. This disease is known locally as "red water cattle disease" because of the blood tinged urine.

The culture was apparently pure but had not been identified. It presented at once all the typical features of B. welchii, in morphology, nonmotility, and action on milk and brain cultures. One c c of a 24-hour glucose-broth culture inoculated subcutaneously into a 320 gm. guinea-pig produced in about 7 hours a typical severe gaseous edema associated with marked intoxication followed shortly by death. At necropsy the usual slightly sanguinous subcutaneous emphysematous edema was found showing the gram-positive short thick rods characteristic of B. welchii.

The original culture was repurified twice by the blood-agar surface colony method, purification occupying about 10 days.

Identity was fully established by the usual morphologic and cultural criteria.

Virulence for guinea-pigs has not been tested since purification. One c c of a 24-hour glucose-broth culture injected intravenously into a rabbit was without effect. This animal was subsequently immunized and made to produce a specific agglutinating serum, which, however, was not effective against any other strain of B. welchii.

In addition to culture 2, which was contaminated with B. sporogenes when received, I have studied 2 other contaminated cultures undoubtedly containing B. welchii, from which only B. sporogenes was isolated (see Nos. 42 and 66) also 2 cultures labeled B. welchii that apparently consisted only of B. sporogenes (see Nos. 113 and 114).

Morphology.—Vegetative rods are usually short, thick, and stubby and strongly gram-positive. Chains of 2-3 rods, rarely more, may form, especially in the tissue of injected animals. Such organisms are frequently capsulated. There may be considerable variation in the morphology of a single strain according to the medium on which growth is obtained. They are never motile. Spores are not easily demonstrated visually with most strains. As Simonds [19] showed, sporulation is inhibited in mediums with an excess of fermentable sugar; Noguchi [23] pointed out that acids, preformed or due to fermentation, prevent sporulation. According to Esty [21] and my own experience, spores are never formed in living animal tissues but cultural tests indicate that they are formed readily in the intestine. Spores were observed in Robertson's [6] alkaline egg medium after about 3 weeks' incubation, sparsely with strain 2, more abundantly with 36. Blood-agar surface culture under alkaline pyrogallol appears to be one of the best means for demonstrating spores, but one may establish the identity of B. welchii without seeing the spores.

Colony Form.—Blood-agar surface colonies of B. welchii are strikingly hemolytic, dewdrop in form, transparent at first but becoming

[23] Trans. N. Y. Path. Soc., 1907, 7, p. 196.

opaque in 2-3 days. On soft mediums lobulate colonies may occur or they may be typhiform, i. e., flat.

In deep meat infusion 1% agar compact opaque disks are formed.

Physiology.—Welch cultures are only mildly proteolytic. Brain medium is neither blackened nor liquefied but is slightly softened. In the presence of an iron nail, however, brain medium was distinctly blackened by all cultures except 26.

The blackening of brain medium is correlated perfectly with a separate test for the production of H_2S in lead acetate peptone agar; culture 26 alone failed to produce dark colonies in this medium.

Gelatin was blackened and actively liquefied by all cultures. Indol was not produced by cultures 2, 20, 26 or 36 (the only Welch cultures tested) in a meat-infusion broth containing 1% Armour's peptone according to the Ehrlich test made after 4 days' incubation. That the conditions were right for the test with certain organisms was shown in positive results obtained with B. tetani 1 and 3 strains of B. bifermentans.

All strains fermented glucose, lactose, and saccharose, with acid and gas production; culture 26 alone fermented salicin.

In the presence of fermentable sugars, at least a trace of which seems to be necessary for the growth of this species,[14] B. welchii typically forms acid and gas. In some cases only a little acid, in others only a little gas is formed. The acid results in the coagulation of casein in milk which is then torn to shreds by the gas, providing conditions of anaerobiosis are suitable, giving the well-known "stormy fermentation." Such coagulated casein is only slightly, if at all, digested by pure cultures. The characteristic stormy fermentation of B. welchii is greatly aided by the addition of a small amount of sterile blood.

In Robertson's alkaline egg medium the action of B. welchii is somewhat distinctive. While with Vibrion septique, B. botulinus, and B. tetani, the medium only becomes slightly opaque, with B. welchii it becomes almost milky, owing perhaps to the greater acid production.

Glucose broth cultures of B. welchii 2 and 20 were always mucoid; cultures of the other strains, never.

Pathogenicity.—The statement is sometimes made that the bloating effect in the tissues of a rabbit inoculated intravenously with B. welchii and then killed and incubated, represents the characteristic pathology of gaseous gangrene. It would seem rather to represent more nearly the result of postmortem changes in an animal that had either a septicemic or agonal invasion by this organism. This curious phenomenon is by no means peculiar to B. welchii, although undoubtedly it is most strikingly displayed by this species according to my experiments, A similar result may be produced with Vibrion septique (see also B. bifermentans 102) so that this reaction should not be accorded diagnostic significance.

The pathogenicity of our different strains of B. welchii varied considerably just as other investigators have found; while with virulent cultures the pathology is to some degree characteristic, as both English and French writers have pointed out, it is scarcely differential. Thus No. 36 never produces the characteristic slightly blood tinged emphysematous edema but always separates the skin from the muscles by what seems to be a digestion of the subcutaneous connective tissue leaving the skin and muscles of a pale color.

A single comparative test of cultures 2 and 36 on pigeons showed the former to be more virulent than the latter but culture 36 has repeatedly proved to be unusually virulent for guinea-pigs. Arranged in order of virulence for guinea-pigs, these cultures may be aligned as follows: 26, type 1, nonpathogenic; 129, type 4, nonpathogenic; 2, type 2, moderately pathogenic; 20, type 4, moderately pathogenic; 135, type 4, strongly pathogenic; 36, type 4, strongly pathogenic.

Virulence tests of B. welchii must be made with young cultures; pathogenic cultures lose virulence rapidly after the first 24 hours incubation. When guinea-pigs are given a sublethal dose they frequently suffer a profound intoxication during the first 24-48 hours, associated with the usual gaseous edema. After the subsidence of the acute infection the skin sloughs from the site leaving an open, phlegmonous ulcer that soon becomes foul through secondary aerobic infections. Such ulcers seem to cause little or no general disturbance in guinea-pigs and ultimately heal completely leaving a clean red, later white, scar. Of many guinea-pigs so infected only one died during the chronic course of the infection and this was due to a hernia caused by a perforation of the abdominal wall, i. e., an accident. Frequently the eschar may cover the whole of the belly and thorax and yet the animal recover.

Recovered animals have only a slight but imperfect immunity to reinfection either by the same strain or other strains of the same type. I have repeated a severe but nonfatal Welch infection in a single guinea-pig as many as 3 times. Protection experiments with vaccinated guinea-pigs have therefore little or no diagnostic value for B. welchii.

Robertson[24] concluded that previous vaccination with killed or attenuated cultures of B. perfringens does not cause any appreciable increase of resistance in guinea-pigs against a subsequent lethal dose of living bacilli, "and that recovery from a previous infection with the organism does not prevent a repetition of the illness upon reinoculation with living bacilli, nor does it apparently in any way alter the symptoms or influence the course of the disease."

My experiments (details omitted) support the second statement but not the first and last, although it must be admitted that the advantage of a previous infection in our guinea-pigs, while distinct, was rather slight. (See table 1.)

TABLE 1
PROTECTIVE IMMUNIZATION BY B. WELCHII

Guinea-Pig	Immunized Against B. welchii Culture No.	Number of Injections	Total Cc Injected	Period Covered in Days	Result
39	2—Type 2	4	7	40	Completely recovered
28	20—Type 4	4	7	40	Completely recovered
30	20—Type 4	3	6	20	Died in 23 hours
44	36—Type 4	2	0.7	20	Partially recovered; died in 34 days from complications
66	....	0	0	..	Died in less than 21 hours

Possession of a protective immunity was tested one week after the last immunizing dose by subcutaneous injection of 1 c c 24 hour glucose broth culture of B. welchii 36.

The completeness of the immunity set up by a Welch bacillus infection depends probably on the size and virulence represented in the test dose. A protective immunity induced by one type of B. welchii may be equally protective for another; therefore the protective mechanism of immunity to Welch bacillus is neither strain specific, as in the agglutination reaction, nor even specific as for B. botulinus, but is species specific. This conclusion is in accord with that of Bull and Pritchett who found quantitative but not qualitative differences in the toxins from 27 strains of B. welchii.

I was unsuccessful in completely immunizing guinea-pigs to B. welchii 36, i. e., so that no lesion would develop on inoculation as illustrated by the following record, in which guinea-pig 923 was injected with increasing doses of 24-hour glucose broth culture as follows:

March 12, 1921, 1 c c 1-30
March 15, 1921, 1 c c 1-20
March 18, 1921, 1 c c 1-15
March 20, 1921, 1 c c 1-10
March 23, 1921, 1 c c 1-9
March 25, 1921, 1 c c 1-8
March 26, 1921, 1 c c 1-5
March 28, 1921, 1 c c 1-2
March 29, 1921, 1 c c 1-1

Up to March 29 there had been no lesions. March 30 there was a typical Welch bacillus eschar that healed slowly during the following week. April 10 the scab was removed; the wound which was bleeding was treated with iodine. April 12 the animal died of peritonitis following abdominal perforation.

[24] Lancet, 1916, 191, p. 516.

I was unable to ascribe the striking virulence of glucose-broth cultures of this strain to a filtrable toxin. Ground meat cultures are said to be more favorable for the formation of Welch toxin.

Guinea-pig 3, weight 200 gm., was injected subcutaneously May 19, 1920, with 1 c c of a sterile (tested) Berkefeld filtrate of a 16-hour glucose-broth culture of B. welchii 36. The next day there was a barely perceptible local necrosis, but no edema, emphysema, or toxemia. June 1 this animal weighed 250 gm. and was perfectly well and healthy.

Guinea-pig 76, weight 220 gm., was injected at 10 a. m. May 19, 1920, with 1 c c of a 1-5 dilution of the same 16-hour glucose broth culture 36 previous to filtration used for guinea-pig 3. It was dead at 5 p. m. the same day with the usual findings at necropsy, subcutaneous emphysema, the connective tissue digested away, the skin loosened, pale and not congested or hyperemic.

The characteristic organisms were seen in impression smears.

There was nothing unusual in the pathology of animals killed by Culture 135. They showed the usual symptoms before death and lesions after death.

Impression smears and cultures from the localized lesions both gave positive results. Heart blood cultures in brain medium or glucose broth constricted tubes were always negative.

B. welchii is somewhat less pathogenic in equal doses for rabbits than for guinea-pigs as shown in the animals used in the preparation of agglutinating serums for none died though several showed severe lesions and symptoms.

Bacillus egens

B. egens was described by Stoddard[25] in 1919, but none of the strains encountered in the writer's experience could be so classified.

B. egens is placed tentatively in the centrally spored group not only because of the apparent morphologic resemblance of the vegetative forms to those of B. welchii, and the similarity of the pathology of the gaseous gangrene ascribed to it, but particularly because sparse sporulation is one of the outstanding characteristics of the nonproteolytic members (i. e., B. welchii and B. butyricus) of the central spored group. Stoddard failed to find any spores. The differences recorded in vegetative forms are not significant since the same variation may occur in pure cultures of undoubted B. welchii. The record is clear as to lack of proteolytic action on coagulated albumins but is deficient in not considering gelatin. The failure to ferment lactose and milk is important and appears to have been carefully controlled with B. welchii.

A careful watch should be kept for this species, since, as Stoddard mentions, it might readily escape detection as a contaminant in cultures of B. welchii.

Bacillus centrosporogenes n.sp.

Cultures 76, 116 and 145 were first grouped under the heading of B. bifermentans because of their proteolytic metabolism, their centrally

[25] Jour. Exper. Med., 1919, 29, p. 187.

located spores, and their apparent nonmotility in 24-hour cultures. These properties seemed at first to testify to the true identity of 145 as represented in its label. Culture 82 was later similarly labeled on the basis of its morphology and cultural reactions.

B. centrosporogenes 76.—This culture was recovered from a sterility test of a certain lot of tuberculin about 1914. There was no evidence that the culture was impure.

Repurification started April 18, 1918, and occupied 18 days, during which time single colonies were picked and repicked from the surface of blood-agar slants under alkaline pyrogallol 5 successive times. These colonies were like dew-drops when young, with a tendency to opacity when older and especially when only a few were present on the slant. In two instances when there were only 2-3 colonies they were 3 mm. across and resembled colonies of Bact. coli.

B. centrosporogenes 82.—This was recovered in Oct., 1918, from a tin of canned spinach brought into the laboratory by Dr. Albert Schneider. Several c c of the juice, as well as an initial glucose broth culture, were fed without harm to a guinea-pig, thus disproving B. botulinus. The initial deep brain culture was contaminated with a hay bacillus which was excluded by selective bacteriostasis. In contrast with the culture from the other tin (later identified as B. welchii 36) the present culture blackened the brain medium. It was repurified 3 times by the blood-agar surface colony method, requiring about 8 days.

B. centrosporogenes 116.—This was isolated from a glucose-broth culture of garden soil implanted Sept. 9, 1920. Various aerobic bacteria were inhibited in the subculture by the selective bacteriostasis of crystal violet so that a culture free from aerobes was first secured before starting isolation. Purification consisted in thrice repeated picking of the well separated compact colonies secured in meat infusion 1% agar.

B. centrosporogenes 145.—This was received March 29, 1921, from the Lister Institute, London, to which it had been sent by Miss Muriel Robertson, as B. bifermentans 506, strain 1.

The morphologic, cultural and nonpathogenic properties of the original culture were carefully determined, and while there was no evidence of anaerobic contamination, the culture was repurified 3 times by the deep-agar method, occupying 21 days. The foregoing properties were then confirmed, with the exception of nonmotility; the culture is always motile in the first few hours of growth but not after 24 hours. It fails therefore to conform to the classic description of B. bifermentans.

The first evidence of error in the grouping of these cultures under the specific name B. bifermentans came from the serologic data. Cultures 76 and 116 had already failed to agglutinate in a dilution of 1 : 20 with a specific serum prepared against B. bifermentans 50 active in a dilution of 1 : 2,000. Also a serum prepared against culture 116 with a titer of 1 : 160 for that strain gave negative results on all other cultures tested, including 3 serologically identical strains of B. bifermentans and cultures 76 and 145. I was tempted to conclude that here was another case of sub-species typing or of strain specificity. B. bifermentans happens to be the only species of which all my strains respond to an agglutinating serum produced for a single strain, but this observation is limited to 3 strains.

The second evidence appeared in distinct differences in the form of deep colonies in 1% meat infusion agar when all 6 cultures were compared. Those of cultures 76, 116 and 145 were markedly fluffier and more diffuse than those of B. bifermentans 50, 70 and 102. The form of such colonies is subject to considerable variation in different lots of medium even when they are prepared as far as possible alike. The consistency of the agar has very much to do with colony form; during the isolation of strains 76, 116 and 145, a distinctly more compact opaque type of colony was observed than appeared in the foregoing test. However, a comparative test of this sort ought to have some differential value.

The climax came when all 6 cultures were examined for motility after 8 hours' growth, an examination that was prompted by a single old record of active motility for culture 76. In this test cultures 76, 116 and 145 were shown to be actively motile at 8 hours, but, along with the B. bifermentans strains, nonmotile at 24 hours. Repeated tests have confirmed this finding, both for these 3 strains and for No. 82.

I have searched the literature in vain for a suitable specific name to fit these organisms. They are closely related physiologically to B. sporogenes, from which they differ by their centrally located spores, and by their fermentation of glycerol, and to B. bifermentans from which they differ in possessing motility.

Lüdernitz [26] described such a species in 1889, under the name B. liquefaciens magnus, which, however, being a trinomial, is not in accord with the International Rules for Botanical Nomenclature.[27] Klein's description [28] of "B. enteritidis sporogenes" indicates that the same organism was present, probably in impure culture. Metchnikoff's [29] B. sporogenes, type B., fits quite well, especially in the formation of crystals resembling tyrosin and leucine from certain protein mediums as pointed out by Berthelot [30] and as observed by ourselves in the 3 cultures herewith described. Choukevitch [31] isolated the same forms from the large intestine of horses on 2 occasions. The "central spore bacillus" type 12 of MacIntosh [32] and of Adamson [33] may be identical also.

There is no doubt in the writer's mind that this form should be clearly differentiated from B. sporogenes as a separate species in spite of the willingness of the Medical Research Committee [1] to group the less frequent central spored motile putrefactive anaerobes with B. sporogenes under a single specific name. The specific name "Bacillus centrosporogenes" is herewith proposed for this species.

Morphology.—B. centrosporogenes is a large gram-positive rod occurring singly, in twos, in short chains or even in long filaments. Spores are formed early in nearly all mediums, particularly in those devoid of sugar. They are central in position and do not swell the rod. Oval free spores are present in great abundance in old cultures. The vegetative rods are highly motile in very young cultures, nonmotile in old cultures.

Colony Form.—Surface colonies on blood agar are at first minute hemolytic transparent dew drops that rapidly become more opaque

[26] Ztschr. f. Hyg. u. Infektionskr., 1889, 5 p. 141.
[27] Jour. Bacteriol., 1917, 2, p. 505.
[28] Centralbl. f. Bakteriol., 1895, 18, p. 737.
[29] Ann. de l'Inst. Past., 1908, 22, p. 929.
[30] Ibid., 1909, 23, p. 85.
[31] Ibid., 1911, 25, p. 247.
[32] Med. Research Com., Special Report Series 12, 1917.
[33] Jour. Path. & Bacteriol., 1919, 22, p. 345.

and yellowish in color, spreading where well separated to a diameter of 1-2 mm. and then appearing almost coliform.

Deep agar colonies vary with water content and consistency of the colloid. In 1% agar they are large globular fluffs with a central nucleus when young and with several when older. They resemble the colonies of B. sporogenes.

Physiology.—B. centrosporogenes is actively proteolytic. Coagulated egg albumin, brain and meat mediums with less than an excess of fermentable sugar are digested and blackened. Gelatin is liquefied and blackened. The action on milk consists in slow coagulation followed by liquefaction and slight gas production. Glucose broth cultures of Nos. 76 and 116 were mucoid, as are some Welch cultures; Nos. 82 and 145 were not mucoid.

Old deep brain cultures show round balls of white crystals that are thought to be leucine or tyrosine or possibly a mixture of both. This feature was pointed out by Bertholet [30] in connection with B. sporogenes "B" of Metchnikoff.

Glucose was fermented by all strains; lactose, saccharose, salicin, glycerol, inulin, and sugar-free mediums were not fermented.

Pathogenicity.—Pure cultures are nonpathogenic for guinea-pigs and rabbits. B. centrosporogenes may possibly have a symbiotic effect similar to that of B. sporogenes in wound infections as described by Weinberg and Sequin.[2]

BACILLUS BUTYRICUS

It is a curious anomaly that the species selected as the type of the genus Clostridium in the recent report of the Committee of the Society of American Bacteriologists on Characterization and Classification of Bacterial types [34] should be one of the less common micro-organisms, as well as one whose status until recently had been quite problematic.

Pasteur,[35] the discoverer of anaerobic bacteria in 1861, described a "motile Vibrion butyrique." This organism was probably the prototype of Prazmowski's "Clostridium butyricum," of Gruber's "Bacillus amylobacter," and of Grassberger and Schattenfroh's [36] motile "Buttersäure bacillus." According to Adamson [33] and the Medical Research Committee,[1] B. butyricus is a central spored, motile, nonputrefactive, lactolytic anaerobe that does not liquefy gelatin.

The two following strains meet the requirements of this species except that the second sometimes liquefies gelatin. The identity of culture 125 can be considered tentative only.

[34] Jour. of Bacteriol., 1920, 5, p. 191.
[35] Compt. rend. Acad. des Sc., 1861, 52, pp. 344 and 1260.
[36] Arch. f. Hyg., 1902, 42, p. 219; 1907, 60, p. 40.

B. butyricus 24.—This was recovered April 19, 1917, from water not containing B. coli but giving a spurious presumptive test with lactose broth. The initial brain subculture contained no aerobes, but the blackening and digestion of this medium as well as the liquefaction of the casein that occurred in the later stages of a stormy fermentation of milk pointed clearly to putrefactive anaerobes. These must have been lost during a period of about 8 months, during which the brain culture was stored, for subsequent cultures failed to show any putrefactive tendency. Purification started first in April, 1918, and consisted in 3 repeated isolations of colonies from blood-agar slants under alkaline pyrogallol, and the culture was identified on the basis of its morphologic and cultural characters.

B. butyricus 125.—Oct. 11, 1920, a sterility test in a constricted tube of glucose broth inoculated with the Berkefeld (defective) filtrate of a soil culture in glucose broth developed an anaerobic growth with no evidence of impurity. It was, however, at once repurified 3 times during a period of 14 days by the deep agar method, and the morphologic and cultural properties of the original were reaffirmed in the purified strain.

Morphology.—B. butyricus is a slender gram-positive rod forming centrally located spores sparsely. Cultures older than 3 days are frequently gram-negative, but motility persists for at least this time in some mediums. Both the thickness of the rods and its active motility differentiate B. butyricus from B. welchii. As in B. welchii, spores are difficult to demonstrate.

Colony Form.—Blood-agar surface colonies were minute irregular moist appearing drops with a mild hemolytic activity in culture 125, nonhemolytic in culture 24.

Deep colonies in 1% agar were globular and fluffy and very diffuse. At times it was almost impossible to detect the growth in deep tubes except by the abundant gas production. The Medical Research Committee describes isolated colonies as "small irregular lenticular masses." No doubt the consistency of the agar greatly affects the form of the colonies.

Physiology.—The physiology is remarkably like that of B. welchii, but its proteolytic activities are less. Coagulated albumins are neither liquefied nor blackened; even free iron, which causes most strains of B. welchii to blacken brain mediums, has no such effect with B. butyricus.

The published records regard this species as nongelatinolytic. All of the tests with No. 24 and most of those with No. 125 have proved so. From my experience in the use of gelatin mediums for anaerobes, the failure to liquefy gelatin might be ascribed to poor growth, but this difficulty was not encountered with these cultures. Growth in gelatin mediums, with and without added glucose, always occurred at 37 C. within 24 hours, as shown by turbidity, abundant gas production and the discoloration. Owing to long periods of incubation, paraffine was used as a seal in some of the tests to minimize evaporation. In one such test the medium still hardened on ice after 30 days at 37 C. But in 2 other tests (culture 125), carefully controlled for aerobic and anaerobic contamination, one with added glucose, one without, the gelatin hardened daily up to 7 days, but on the ninth day refused to harden; on another occasion, liquefaction occurred after 4 days.

A possible interpretation is that liquefaction is due to changes in H+ ion concentration rather than to the production of gelantinolytic enzymes.

Glucose, lactose, saccharose and salicin were fermented by both these strains; glycerol and inulin were not fermented. Milk cultures gave rise to considerable gas with a tardy coagulation without subsequent digestion of clot.

Pathogenicity.—Neither culture was pathogenic for small guinea-pigs in 1 c c doses of 24-hour glucose-broth culture inoculated subcutaneously.

Anaerobes with Subterminal Spores

This group comprises B. aerofetidus, B. botulinus, B. histolyticus, B. sporogenes, B. chauvœi, Vibrion septique, B. novyi, B. multifermentanstenalbus, and B. fallax.

B. AEROFETIDUS

B. aerofetidus was named by Weinberg and Sequin [2] in 1916. Five strains were recovered by Henry,[37] and it was described also by the Medical Research Committee.[1] Spores were not discoverable by the French observers, but Bullock [1] states that "they are subterminal." B. aerofetidus would seem from the description to be the only putrefactive anaerobe that ferments lactose. This should differentiate it from other species irrespective of its paucity of sporulation. I have had no opportunity to examine a strain of this species. The only highly putrefactive species in which I have encountered strains that sporulate poorly is B. botulinus and that does not ferment lactose.

BACILLUS BOTULINUS

The central interest in anaerobic bacteriology was suddenly shifted by the cessation of major hostilities in the world war and the growing frequency of food poisoning in the United States, from war wounds to botulism.

With the interesting phases of the problem touching questions of distribution of this species in nature, conditions under which it grows and produces its deadly toxin, its epidemiology, the action of its poison and its sanitary control, this paper has nothing to do except in so far as some of these may relate to the recognition of the types comprising this species as biologic entities.

[37] Jour. of Path. & Bacteriol., 1916, 21, p. 344.

The historical background is in Dickson's excellent monograph.[38] Especial emphasis is laid here on the undoubted fact that many of the cultures circulating in this country, at least until recently, have been contaminated or indeed replaced by other anaerobes, notably by B. sporogenes, and evidence is lacking in some papers to show that the strains studied were either purified or properly identified. Reddish and Rettger [39] found that 18 out of 19 strains contained nontoxic forms resembling B. sporogenes.

I have studied 5 strains as follows:

B. botulinus No. 8, Type A.—This was received Nov. 1, 1916, from Dr. E. C. Dickson of Leland Stanford Junior University School of Medicine, as B. botulinus "Zinsser." It is supposed to have come many years ago from the Kral collection. The culture was free from aerobes and blackened brain medium. Purification began Sept. 20, 1917. There were 2 types of colony on the initial blood-agar slant, and while both were isolated 3 times repeatedly, one of the purified cultures was lost previous to identification. It is uncertain, therefore, whether this culture was actually impure at the start. Nineteen days were occupied in purification. The colonies on blood agar were minute hemolytic, usually rhizoid, but occasionally in certain lots of medium, round in form.

Identity was established by the toxicity of cultures fed to rabbits and guinea-pigs.

B. botulinus 78, Type B.—April 19, 1918, Prof. W. V. Cruess of the Dep. of Agric., Univ. of Calif., brought me a tin can of beans that he had inoculated from a can of spoiled beans found on the shelf of Mrs. M. after an outbreak of limber neck in her chickens fed the contents of another can from the same lot. Dickson [40] has described this outbreak in detail.

There was no swelling of the can due to gas pressure, nor was there any olfactory or visual evidence of spoilage. A Gram stain of the clear fluid failed repeatedly to show any recognizable bacteria. But 1 c c of the fluid injected subcutaneously into a 570 gm. guinea-pig killed the animal within 13 hours, and 4 c c diluted in 10 c c of water and drunk by another pig weighing 500 gm. killed in less than 20 hours, with characteristic pulmonary hyperemia at necropsy and sterile heart blood culture in both cases.

Culture was secured in glucose broth at 37 C. under marble seal in a constricted tube. No aerobes were present. Brain cultures were blackened and digested. Clostridial spores were observed, which, considering that the purified culture has never formed spores that could be recognized visually, suggests but does not prove that the original was impure.

A pure culture was secured during the interval May 1 to July 3, 1918, by the surface colony method. In the first blood-agar surface culture there appeared dew-drop-like colonies that superficially appeared well separated, but careful examination showed an extremely thin confluent growth between them that consisted of gram-positive rods. A culture of putrefactive anaerobes giving this type of growth regularly was isolated but lost before it could be identified. The dew-drop-like colonies were isolated 4 times repeatedly, and while they did not maintain their dew drop form, being flat and leaf-like in some tubes and ameboid in others, the confluent growth was not encountered after the initial isolation culture. There was some difficulty, however, in securing well separated colonies, which accounts for the long time required.

The evidence as to the purity or impurity of the original culture must be admitted as inadequate. It is clear that the form of colonies on blood agar varies considerably.

Identity was established by the toxicity of cultures fed to guinea-pigs.

B. botulinus 80, Type B.—This was received, marked "B_2H," from Dr. Robert Graham of the University of Illinois, June 20, 1918. The accompanying letter stated that several people died from eating beans, and that they were canned by the cold pack method. No aerobes were present.

Isolation required 15 days for 4 repeated pickings. The colonies were always well separated, flat, minute, round plaques, and the original gave no evidence of impurity. Identity was established by feeding.

In April, 1920, this culture was again repurified 3 times by the deep agar method due to an unjustified suspicion based on its abundant formation of spores (see morphology). An unsuccessful attempt was made to utilize Burke's [41] criterion of colony form. All of the deep agar colonies of this culture were alike in similar mediums; none showed a mosaic structure. Nine cultures in brain medium picked from separate colonies showed abundant subterminal spores, and guinea-pigs fed with cultures from 5 separate colonies all died of botulism.

[38] Monograph 8, Rockefeller Institute for Medical Research, 1918.

[39] Abstracts of Bacteriol., 1921, 5, p. 14; Jour. Infect. Dis., 1921, 29, p. 120.

[40] Arch. of Int. Med., 1918. 22, p. 483.

[41] Jour. of Bacteriol., 1919, 4, p. 555.

B. botulinus 119, Type B.—This was labeled "B. botulinus, Type B, Stanford." Its exact origin could not be ascertained. It came into my hands Sept. 21, 1920, free from aerobes and showing the typical morphologic, cultural and pathogenic properties of the species.

Repurification by the deep agar method occupied 11 days. The well separated colonies in 2% agar were opaque disks without mosaic structure. There was no evidence of initial impurity. One c c of a 24-hour glucose broth culture (37 C.) killed a 350 gm. guinea-pig by feeding in less than 24 hours with characteristic symptoms of botulism.

B. botulinus 120, Type A.—This was a mate to B. botulinus 119 B and had a similar history, the brain culture placed in my hands Sept. 23, 1920, being marked "B. botulinus, Type A Stanford."

Brain medium subcultures were contaminated with a gram-positive aerobic coccus that was easily eliminated by selective heating. The initial culture was fatal for a guinea-pig fed with 1 c c.

Deep agar isolation occupied 15 days and comprised thrice picking of the well separated opaque colonies. The purified culture is characteristic in morphology, physiology and toxigenicity.

In addition, 6 cultures were received from other laboratories under the label of "B. botulinus," in which no trace of the indicated species could be detected. It is only fair to say that toxicity tests were not made in the case of the second culture listed until after it had been in the laboratory for some time and had been purified; if this culture contained B. botulinus, it was at least contaminated. In the case of the others, B. botulinus was ruled out before isolation was begun. All were apparently pure (see B. sporogenes 44, 46, 48, 92, 115 and 118).

Morphology.—B. botulinus is a large pleomorphic gram-positive, sluggishly motile rod occurring singly, in pairs and in chains. The spores are clostridial, subterminal and oval in shape. They are formed by some cultures abundantly; by others sparsely, if at all. The most persistent search for spores in brain medium, alkaline egg broth, and blood-agar slants failed to demonstrate them visually in strain 78 B, and only somewhat doubtfully in No. 8 A. Whether some strains produce spores that do not distend the rods should be investigated. The contrast in sporulating activity between these cultures and No. 80 B was so striking that the latter was strongly suspected of a contamination, but this could not be proved; every colony picked from dilutions of B. botulinus 80 B gave rise to actively sporulating cultures that were as highly toxic as those of the apparently nonsporulating Nos. 8 A and 78 B.

Culture 119B also forms subterminal spores readily in brain medium; 120A, on the contrary, has so far failed to reveal any spores.

Heat Resistance of Spores.—Experiments with Professor Chas. A. Hunter of Pennsylvania State College at the University of Chicago, in 1920, showed that the failure to demonstrate spores visually in certain cultures was correlated with a lesser heat resistance; however, it would be impossible to say that these strains are strictly asporogenous.

Forty-eight-hour brain medium cultures were diluted 1:10 in sterile distilled water and heated for the times indicated in the following: Subcultures were made in glucose broth under paraffine and in deep agar. These were incubated at 37 C. The data are tabulated in table 2.

TABLE 2

HEAT RESISTANCE OF THREE STRAINS OF B. BOTULINUS INCLUDING TWO SUPPOSEDLY ASPOROGENOUS STRAINS

Strain	Temper-ature	Time in Minutes							
		Unheated Controls 0	5	10	20	35	45	60	120
8 A	80 C	+1	...	...	...	...	...	+2	+2*
	100 C	+3* +1*	—90	... —90	...	—90			
78 B	80 C	+2*	...	...	...	...	...	—90	—90
	100 C	+3 +2*	+3	... —90	+4* —90	—90			
80 B	80 C	+1	...	...	...	...	...	+2	+2*
	100 C	+2	...	+2	+2	...	—2 +4	—2 +4*	
		+3	+3		+4	+5	—8 +10	—8 +10*	

+3 indicates that the cultures were positive on the 3d day.
—90 means that the cultures were still sterile after 90 days at 37 C.
* = 1 c c fed to a guinea-pig killed with symptoms and lesions of botulism.

In 2 separate tests, B. botulinus 8A failed to resist boiling for 5 and 10 minutes, respectively, and for all greater periods. The subcultures were still sterile after 90 days. Control cultures from the suspensions previous to heating were heavily grown in 24 hours. B. botulinus 8A was a resistant to 80 C. for 2 hours; the subcultures were positive in 48 hours as against 24 hours in the unheated controls.

In one test, B. botulinus 78B failed to resist boiling for 10 minutes. In another the suspension was still alive after 20 minutes' boiling but not after 35 minutes. Both agar- and glucose-broth cultures from the 20 minute suspension appeared on the third day as against the second day for the unheated controls. A few spores must have been present. One c c of the glucose-broth culture fed to a large guinea-pig (845 gm.) killed in about 15 hours with characteristic symptoms and necropsy findings, proving the surviving spores those of B. botulinus. This culture failed to resist 80 C. for 1 hour.

B. botulinus 80B resisted boiling in the first test for 1 hour. The subcultures were still negative after 8 days' incubation but positive on the tenth day. One c c of the glucose broth culture fed to a 290 gm. guinea-pig killed in less than 15 hours, proving the surviving spores those of B. botulinus. The 45 minute cultures were also delayed in growth to the tenth day; the 15, 20 and 35 minute cultures appeared on the third day as contrasted with the second day for the 5 minute cultures and the unheated controls. This experiment was repeated with identical results except that the delay in growth of the cultures from the suspension boiled for 1 hour was not so marked; growth appeared on the fourth day as against the second day in the controls.

It is apparent that considerable differences in spore formation and heat tolerance exist in different strains of B. botulinus. The limit for culture 80B was not reached in these experiments. Emphasis should be placed on the necessity of careful toxin tests in order to exclude results attributable to highly resistant contaminants like B. sporogenes. The work of Weiss [42] on the heat resistance of B. botulinus would have been greatly enhanced by such tests.

Colony Form.—Blood-agar surface colonies are minute round or irregular semi-transparent hemolytic drops.

The form of deep agar colonies varies with the consistency of the agar. The diagnostic value of colony form as emphasized by Burke [41] is questionable, indeed the majority of colonies produced by pure cultures failed to show the reticulate structure when a special search was made for them in 1, 2 and 3% agar. In 1% agar the proportion of disk shaped colonies was low (43%) and none was reticulate; in 2% agar, all the colonies were disk shaped with a nucleus as described by Burke, but only part of them showed the described microscopic structure. It was difficult to secure growth in 3% agar.

Physiology.—While Van Ermengem [43] considered growth to occur only at room temperature, and spoke of B. botulinus as a pathogenic saprophyte, it is now clear that both growth and toxin production occur at 37 C. Orr [44] found that 22 C. was less favorable for growth and sporulation of 16 strains than 37 C. My own repeated observations show that growth is more rapid at 37 C., and that there is no known reason why every routine test for B. botulinus should not be carried out at 37 C. Growth is readily obtained with all the usual mediums for anaerobes.

B. botulinus is predominantly proteolytic. The grouping of this species among organisms with "saccharolytic properties predominating" by the Medical Research Committee [1] certainly is an error. Brain, ground beef mediums, coagulated serum, egg albumin and gelatin are darkened and digested. Milk is slowly coagulated, then digested with gas production.

Sulphuretted hydrogen is produced in the absence of fermentable sugars. No indol production could be proved in controlled tests. All the strains fermented glucose, glycerol and salicin; lactose, saccharose, inulin and sugar-free broth were not fermented.

[42] Jour. Infect. Dis., 1921, 28, p. 70.
[43] Ztschr. f. Hyg. u. Infektionskr., 1897, 26, p. 1.
[44] Proc. Soc. Exper. Biol. and Med., 1919, 17, p. 47.

Pathogenicity.—The animal test constitutes so far the only single certain method of recognition of B. botulinus, in view of the morphology and cultural similarity of B. sporogenes and B. histolyticus. The pathogenicity of B. botulinus is due mainly to its powerful toxin which is produced normally outside the body. The growth of pure cultures appears always to be accompanied by the formation of toxin irrespective of the presence or absence of fermentable sugar, but certain aerobes in mixed culture with B. botulinus inhibit toxin production.

No other bacterial toxin is fatal orally, and no other anaerobe is known that is pathogenic when fed. One may test unknown anaerobes for pathogenicity first by subcutaneous injection of 1 c c of glucose broth culture; in the event of a fatal issue graded doses of culture or filtrate are fed on chopped carrots or better still by pipet. I have no evidence of "nontoxic" strains of B. botulinus. Finally, the protection of control animals by botulinus antitoxin completes the circle of required data for absolute identification.

The symptoms of botulism are highly characteristic, consisting mainly in loss of muscular power. Salivation is frequent but not constant.

At necropsy there may be slight subcutaneous congestion at the site of inoculation; pulmonary congestion is almost invariable in both injected and fed animals, but no other visceral lesions.

With the interesting mooted questions of whether B. botulinus has invasive properties, and whether toxin may be formed in the body, that have arisen recently through the discovery that the organism will grow at 37 C., this discussion has little to do, although this problem was encountered in producing agglutinating serums. That Van Ermengen [43] should have recovered the causative agent from the spleen of a victim seemed to imply some invasive power. Orr [44] recovered cultures "quite frequently from the liver and also occasionally from the heart's blood, the kidneys and the pancreas," and found "toxin-free spores" still pathogenic.

The minimum fatal dose of culture or toxin has not been determined systematically for any of the foregoing 5 strains; 1 c c of a 1: 100 dilution of glucose broth culture has never failed to kill guinea-pigs, either by feeding or by subcutaneous injection; 1 c c of a 1:10,000 dilution of culture 8A has frequently proved fatal on injection.

Heart blood cultures were taken from every animal dying of botulism without, as yet, obtaining a positive result. Spleen, liver and lung cultures were frequently made also with negative results except that lung cultures often developed aerobes that might be interpreted as secondary invaders drawn into the lungs owing to loss of control of the glottis through the action of the botulism toxin. In several cases in which sublethal doses were given, sufficient to cause severe symptoms but from which the animals appeared to be recovering slowly, a fatal aspiration pneumonia intervened. Lung sections in such cases showed marked congestion and beginning consolidation.

Typing Bacillus Botulinus.—(*a*) Protection with Monovalent Antitoxin: That there are two distinct antigenic types of botulinus toxin produced by separate races of B. botulinus, was shown first by Leuchs [45] and confirmed by Burke,[41] Dickson, Burke and Ward,[46] Dickson and Howitt,[47] Hart and Hayes [48] and others.

My 5 strains were typed by means of antitoxic serums kindly provided by Dr. George Hart of the Dept. of Vet. Sc., Univ. of Calif. The cultures employed in the production of the type serums had come from Dr. E. C. Dickson of Leland Stanford Junior University. The serums were preserved with 0.5% phenol and were sterile when received. They had not been standardized.

Three animals were required for each culture, one for each of the 2 serums and one (the heaviest) for a control without serum. A 5-day glucose-broth (37 C.) culture of each organism to be tested was diluted in sterile salt solution 1:100, and 1 c c of each dilution was mixed with 1 c c of the indicated serum, or, in the case of the controls, of salt solution. The mixtures stood 1 hour at room temperature and were then injected subcutaneously. The results are shown in table 3.

TABLE 3

TYPING B. BOTULINUS CULTURES BY THE INJECTION METHOD

Culture Injected 1 c c 1:100	Antitoxin 1 c c		
	Type A	Type B	None
8	Guinea-pig 10 Weight, 205 gm. Lived	Guinea-pig 41 Weight, 205 gm. Dead 18 hours	Guinea-pig 66 Weight, 310 gm. Dead 26 hours
78	Guinea-pig 6 Weight, 206 gm. Dead 40 hours	Guinea-pig 58 Weight, 205 gm. Lived	Guinea-pig 84 Weight, 315 gm. Dead 21 hours
80	Guinea-pig 45 Weight, 250 gm. Dead 18 hours	Guinea-pig 56 Weight, 210 gm. Lived	Guinea-pig 69 Weight, 390 gm. Dead 21 hours

The test was started June 1, 1920. The animals that died presented the usual symptoms previous to death and necropsy findings afterward. The animals that lived all gained weight and were apparently still well when last observed June 14. The living animals indicate the toxic type.

[45] Ztschr. f. Hyg. u. Infektionskr., 1910, 65, p. 55.
[46] Arch. Int. Med., 1919, 24, p. 581.
[47] Jour. Am. Med. Assn., 1920, 74, p. 718.
[48] Am. Vet. Med. Assn., 1920, 10, p. 638.

Cultures 119 and 120 were typed Nov. 3, 1920, by feeding guinea-pigs 1 c c of 1:10 dilution of sterile Berkefeld filtrates on chopped carrots shortly after the subcutaneous injection of the serums. Since the test was to be a confirmation of the labels borne by the cultures, it was possible to pick the lightest animal in each series for protection. The animals were starved for 24 hours and fed separately under observation. The results are shown in table 4.

TABLE 4

Typing B. botulinus Cultures by the Feeding Method

Toxic Filtrate Fed 1 c c 1:10	Antitoxin 1 c c		
	Type A	Type B	None
119	Guinea-pig 138 Weight, 550 gm. Dead 42 hours	Guinea-pig 139 Weight, 490 gm. Lived	Guinea-pig 172 Weight, 600 gm. Dead 42 hours
120	Guinea-pig 145 Weight, 370 gm. Lived	Guinea-pig 142 Weight, 430 gm. Dead 18 hours	Guinea-pig 180 Weight, 540 gm. Dead 26 hours

The symptoms and lesions of the animals that died were typical. The living animals were last observed 3 weeks after the beginning of the test. Both had gained weight.

(*b*) Typing B. botulinus by Means of Chickens: Graham and Schwartz [49] showed that the 2 types of B. botulinus may be distinguished in their toxicity for chickens. This was confirmed for my strains June 9, 1921. Each of 5 chicks, weighing 200 gm. apiece, was fed by pipet 1 c c of a 24-hour glucose-broth culture diluted 1:1,000 as indicated in table 5.

TABLE 5

Typing B. botulinus Cultures by Feeding Chickens

Chicken	Culture and Type	Result
1	8 A	Survived 1 c c 1:100 48-hour glucose-broth culture; died after swallowing 1 c c 1:10 48-hour glucose-broth culture
2	78 B	Survived 5 c c 6-day glucose-broth culture
3	80 B	Survived 5 c c 6-day glucose-broth culture
4	119 B	Survived with slight symptoms 1 c c undiluted 48-hour glucose-broth culture; died after swallowing 5 c c undiluted 6-day glucose-broth culture
5	120 A	Survived 1 c c 1:100 48-hour glucose-broth culture; died after swallowing 1 c c 1:10 48-hour glucose-broth culture

Those receiving the A type strains were separated from those receiving B. type strains in view of a possible cross contamination of the feed by the droppings. There was no result in 6 days, so on June 15 each was fed 1 c c of 1:100 dilution of 48-hour glucose-broth culture (37 C.). Again there was no result. June 20, at 10 a. m., 1 c c 48-hour glucose-broth culture (37 C.) diluted to 1:10 was fed to each chick.

At 4 p. m. chick 5 was weak. While able to stand, it was unable to eat, owing to imperfect coordination of the neck muscles. At 6 p. m. it was prostrate.

All the other chicks at this time were apparently well. At 8 a. m., June 21, chick 5 was dead and chick 1 was prostrate; though still able to sit on the

[49] Jour. Infect. Dis., 1921, 28, p. 317; Jour. Am. Med. Assn., 1921, 76, p. 1743.

perch, its head drooped with the typical symptoms of limberneck. It died about 3 p. m.

The dead chicks showed no macroscopic lesions in the brains, lungs, or abdominal viscera.

The living chicks remained well. June 24, each was fed 1 c c undiluted 48-hour glucose-broth culture of the same strain as before. Chicks 2 and 3 remained well as before; chick 4 showed mild symptoms of botulism on the second and third day, such as reclining while feeding and supporting itself by the wings when forced to stand. On the fourth day chick 4 was distinctly improved.

The 3 were therefore fed, June 28 by pipet, 5 c c of a 6-day glucose-broth culture of the same strain previously administered. On the following day chick 4 was prostrate. It died 46 hours after the last dose. There were no macroscopic lesions in the central nervous system or in the viscera. The two remaining chicks survived and were apparently well and healthy on July 7.

Thus chickens may be utilized as an objective means of distinguishing the 2 antigenic types of B. botulinus. The result with strain 119B shows, however, that sufficiently large doses of certain "B" type cultures may be toxic for chickens.

BACILLUS SPOROGENES

No attempt is made here to trace the early history of B. sporogenes. Weinberg and Sequin [2] and others have indicated the frequent occurrence of this organism among anaerobic cultures studied by the early bacteriologists. The term B. enteritidis-sporogenes was applied by Klein [28] to what seems now to have been a mixed culture, but Metchnikoff's [29] B. sporogenes, type A, is the pure culture prototype.

I have found every culture of "malignant edema bacillus" to be B. sporogenes, but indeed the same has been true of cultures labeled B. welchii, B. botulinus, B. tetani, B. chauvoei, B. novyi and B. feseri. Slightly more than a third (24 out of 73) of my purified strains belong to this species. B. sporogenes is not only one of the commonest anaerobes in nature, but it is also the most frequent contaminator of stock laboratory cultures, owing perhaps to its great resistance to heat.

Of the 24 strains, 21 were received as stock cultures from other laboratories; 2 were isolated by the writer from necropsies on a sheep and rabbit, respectively, and 1 from a sample of spoiled home canned corn. Of the 21 stock cultures, 16 were misnamed, assuming in 3 instances that the now obsolete "bacillus of malignant edema" is a misnomer for B. sporogenes. Of these 16 misnamed cultures, 14 were apparently pure B. sporogenes when received; 1 was questionable but not proved and 1 was certainly impure. Of the five correctly named cultures, 3 were of B. welchii contaminated by B. sporogenes; 1 was pure B. sporogenes and 1 was pure B. tetani which was supplanted in my own laboratory by an accidental contamination by B. sporogenes. I had 1 instance, too, of an incorrectly named culture not containing B. sporogenes when received that became supplanted in my own laboratory by B. sporogenes.

Through the courtesy of Prof. C. E. A. Winslow, I was enabled, during 1920, to study all the cultures of anaerobes then kept in the American Museum of Natural History. Counting those received directly and indirectly from the Museum, 15 in all, every such culture, with but a single exception, contained B. sporogenes, and in 11 out of the 14, only B. sporogenes; in only two instances was the designated species, B. welchii, recovered, while in the remaining instance the designated organism was neither proved nor disproved. The single culture from the Museum that failed to yield B. sporogenes did yield 2 organisms, one of which closely resembles B. sporogenes but differs in its active production of tyrosine. B. tetani as designated on the label was not present. Cultures of known identity have since been placed by the writer in the Museum but one not skilled in anaerobic bacteriology could scarcely be expected to keep them pure and true to name. Nineteen of the 24 B. sporogenes strains proved serologically identical, so that in this species the agglutination reaction has a limited taxonomic value; 5 strains proved heterologous, however, in their agglutination reactions.

B. sporogenes 10.—This was obtained from Dr. Fred Wood of the Cutter Laboratories of Berkeley, March 2, 1916, he in turn having received it from Dr. K. F. Meyer, who published a description of it under the label "malignant edema bacillus Koch" in 1915.[5]

There was no evidence of impurity in this culture, but it was 4 times repeatedly repurified by the blood-agar surface colony method. The purified culture was identical with the original and was renamed B. sporogenes on the basis of Weinberg and Sequin's [2] description. An agglutinating serum was produced with this strain that served to identify 18 other strains of B. sporogenes.

B. sporogenes 42.—This was received May 2, 1916, from the American Museum of Natural History as B. welchii 500. The Museum had obtained it about 1912 from Johns Hopkins University where it was recovered from the soil.

As received, the Welch bacillus was probably present; a stormy fermentation in milk was observed. But brain medium blackened, and the organisms were actively motile. Free from aerobes at first this culture was subsequently contaminated with hay bacillus which was eliminated by selective bacteriostasis.[50]

Purification started March 7, 1918. There were 2 types of colony, one tiny and transparent, the other larger, more spreading and with a dark center, but these were not constant in subcultures, and the separate strains obtained after 4 times repeated isolation proved identical as B. sporogenes by the agglutination test. B. welchii was not recovered.

B. sporogenes 44.—This was received Nov. 9, 1915, from the American Museum of Natural History as B. botulinus 595. The morphologic and cultural properties were those common to both B. sporogenes and B. botulinus. One c c of a brain culture incubated at 37 C. for 48 hours and then at room temperature for 3 days was fed in milk to a cat, without result, Feb. 14, 1916. The same amount was then injected subcutaneously, and followed a few days later by 2 c c intraperitoneally of a glucose-broth culture incubated at 37 C. for 24 hours and then at room temperature for 22 days again without any result. The culture was considered not to contain B. botulinus.

Repurification was started Sept. 29, 1917; three repeated isolations by the blood-agar surface colony method occupied 10 days. There was no evidence that the culture was impure

[50] Hall: Jour. Am. Med. Assn., 1919, 72, p. 274.

in the beginning. The cultural reactions of the purified culture were found to be identical with those of the original, and it was renamed on the basis of these and the specific agglutination reaction.

B. sporogenes 46.—This came Nov. 1, 1916, from Dr. E. C. Dickson of Stanford University as "B. botulinus, Am. Museum of Natural History Strain." It seems probable that this strain was the same as B. sporogenes 44. At any rate, the data of the preliminary tests, of the details of isolation, and of identification, are essentially identical.

B. sporogenes 48.—This came also at the same time from Dr. Dickson as "B. botulinus, San Jose case." Dr. Dickson stated that this strain produced toxin containing 6,000 M L D for guinea-pigs. This culture probably contained B. botulinus originally, but it was lost before our own pathogenicity tests started, April 9, 1917, when the culture was repeatedly found avirulent in large doses.

Purification started Sept. 20, 1917, and occupied 8 days; 3 repeated isolations were made. The morphologic and cultural properties and the lack of virulence pointed to B. sporogenes, and this was confirmed by the agglutination test.

B. sporogenes 52.—This came from the subcutaneous tissues of a rabbit found dead May 15, 1916. It is regarded as an agonal or postmortem invader.

Deep brain cultures showed the presence of an actively motile, subterminally sporulating bacillus that blackened and digested the medium.

As soon after the recovery of this culture as possible 1 c c of an 8-day brain culture was injected intravenously into a 3150 gm. rabbit but without effect. The morphologic and cultural properties of the original culture failed to suggest that it was impure; however, it was purified 4 times by the blood-agar surface method, during the interval between Nov. 8, and Nov. 22, 1917. The purified culture was identified by the agglutination reaction and by its morphologic and cultural features.

B. sporogenes 54.—Dec. 13, 1916, the Laboratory of the California State Board of Health received a small vial of home canned corn accompanied by a letter saying that the corn had caused the severe illness of a woman who had tasted it and the death from eating the discarded corn of an entire flock of chickens. A few grains of the corn fed to a hen in the laboratory produced the typical symptoms of botulism followed by death in about 36 hours. While the presence of botulism toxin in the corn is regarded as certain, it was impossible to recover any obligate anaerobes from crop or gizzard. Heart blood cultures were sterile.

The corn had a sour odor and showed gram-positive rods without spores. The anaerobe culture was free from aerobes and gave the morphologic and cultural reactions of B. sporogenes. Several pathogenicity tests failed to support the assumption of B. botulinus and the latter may be supposed to have been overgrown or lost. The culture was repurified twice by the blood-agar surface method during a period of 8 days and identified by its morphologic and cultural reactions.

B. sporogenes 58.—This was received Sept. 19, 1914, from Prof. K. F. Meyer, of the Univ. of Calif., as "B. oedematis Pasteur." It failed to blacken brain medium, and milk was slowly coagulated with gas production without subsequent liquefaction. Prof. Meyer stated recently that the correct diagnosis of this strain was Vibrion septique (see also Vibrion septique 32). The culture was apparently free from putrefactive contaminants Jan. 18, 1916, but when next examined Dec. 28, 1916, a brain culture was distinctly blackened and digested. Sugar tests made shortly thereafter indicated the undoubted presence of the original strain in the fermentation of lactose and salicin, but not saccharose.

Purification started March 6, 1918, by the surface slant method using at first plain agar. Several types of colony were present but 2 other purified cultures secured from variants, in addition to the one here described, proved identical. Vibrion septique was unquestionably lost during repurification which was repeated on blood agar, 3 more times in each case. The purified cultures were identified as B. sporogenes by the agglutination reaction and by their morphology, cultural reactions and lack of pathogenicity.

B. sporgenes 66.—Jan. 4, 1917, Mr. Frank Bachman of the Bureau of Sanit. Eng. of Calif. State Board of Health submitted an anaerobic culture derived from tap water with a tentative diagnosis of B. welchii.

The fermentation of milk, lactose, saccharose, glycerol and dextrin indicated that B. welchii was present. Blackening of brain cultures, however, showed that the culture was impure.

Purification was not started until Nov. 12, 1917, and consisted of thrice repeated picking of well separated colonies from the surface of blood-agar slants.

B. welchii was not isolated. The purified culture was identified by the agglutination reaction and by its morphologic and cultural properties.

B. sporogenes 72.—This was recovered from stools about 1912 by Prof. J. P. Simonds and sent to the writer by the American Museum of Natural History as "B. welchii No. 521," May 2, 1916. Immediate tests in milk, lactose, saccharose, glycerol, inulin, dextrine and starch, indicated by "stormy fermentation" that B. welchii was present, but blackening of brain cultures showed that a putrefactive organism was present. Also there were motile rods with clostridial subterminal spores.

Purification started March 7, 1918, on plain agar slants under alkaline pyrogallol. Two types of colony were present, one more transparent, the other more opaque. The latter was isolated as B. welchii 2. The former was reisolated 4 times on plain and blood agar with the usual type of sporogenes colony after the primary culture and with the usual morphology and cultural reactions in the purified strain, which was finally identified by the agglutination reaction.

B. sporogenes 74.—This was received Feb. 17, 1916, from the Cutter Laboratories as "B. tetani." It was morphologically characteristic of B. tetani The morphologic data coupled with failure to affect milk or blacken brain medium during 18 days' incubation suggest that the culture was pure B. tetani when received; unfortunately tests for pathogenicity were not made immediately. This record illustrates how anaerobic cultures lose or change their identity in the vicissitudes of the laboratory. March 30, 1917, brain cultures were distinctly blackened, but an inoculated guinea-pig failed to develop tetanus.

Purification started April 17, 1918, and required until May 1 for 3 successful isolations of surface colonies from blood agar. The colonies picked were ameboid drops. The purified culture was first shown to be nonpathogenic for guinea-pigs and rabbits and was later identified as B. sporogenes by the agglutination test. B. tetani was lost during purification.

B. *sporogenes No. 84.*—This was recovered from water in 1910 at the Mt. Prospect Laboratory and sent from the American Museum of Natural History May 2, 1916, as "B. sporogenes No. 120." This culture was apparently pure and correctly named.

The culture subsequently became contaminated on 3 separate occasions with hay bacillus which was eliminated each time by the use of gentian violet.[50] Anaerobic repurification was started April 18, 1918, and continued for about 5 weeks. Four repeated isolations from blood-agar slants were made. It was identified by the agglutination reaction and by its morphology, cultural characteristics, and nonpathogenicity.

B. sporogenes 88.—This was found in the stock collection of the Depart. of Hyg. and Bacteriol. of the Univ. of Chicago, having been received from the American Museum of Natural History, Nov. 20, 1919, as "B. tetani No. 274." According to Miss Ada Bancroft of the Museum, this culture had been isolated from a case of lockjaw in Oct., 1908, and was sent to the Museum by Parke, Davis & Co. of Detroit in April, 1911.

When it came into my hands, Jan. 29, 1921, a deep meat medium culture was blackened and digested, indicating at least an impurity. One c c of a 6-day glucose broth culture injected subcutaneously into a guinea-pig (1.005 gm.) had no effect, indicating the absence of B. tetani and other pathogens.

Purification was started Feb. 9, 1920, using the deep agar method. There were 2 types of colony, one large and fluffy, the other small and compact. The latter was repeatedly isolated until certainly pure. It has not yet been identified and will not be described at this time. The fluffy colony was reisolated 3 more times from deep agar dilutions in none of which more than one type ever occurred. It was identified as B. sporogenes by the agglutination test and by its morphology and cultural reactions.

B. sporogenes 90.—This was received at the Univ. of Chicago Nov. 20, 1919, from the American Museum of Natural History under the label of "B. oedematis-maligni No. 485," having come from Kral.

Deep meat cultures were blackened, but no other differential tests were made previous to purification.

Purification began Feb. 13, 1921, and occupied 26 days for 4 repeated isolations by the deep agar method. The colonies were homogeneous, diffuse and fluffy in appearance. The purified culture presented all the morphologic and cultural features of B. sporogenes and was identified by the agglutination reaction.

B. sporogenes 92.—This was received at the Univ. of Chicago, Nov. 20, 1919, from the American Museum of Natural History as "B. botulinus No. 331," having been isolated by Dr. Dickson and Miss Burke at Leland Stanford University and received at the Museum in Jan., 1919.

Feb. 5, 1921, the writer inoculated a large guinea-pig (weight, 1,150 gm.) subcutaneously with 1 c c of a 6-day (37 C.) glucose-broth culture without effect, showing the absence of B. botulinus. Deep meat cultures were blackened and showed motile rods that stained by Gram's method and bore subterminal spores.

Several failures to secure well separated blood-agar surface colonies were recorded. Although there was no evidence of impurity, the culture was repurified 4 times from deep agar. The morphology and cultural reactions of the repurified culture were as usual for B. sporogenes which was confined by the agglutination test.

B. sporogenes 94.—This was found in the collection at the Univ. of Chicago under the label "B. chauvœi." Its origin was unknown. The blackening and digestion of a deep meat culture inoculated Jan. 30, 1920, indicated an organism more highly putrefactive than B. chauvœi, and the innocuousness of 1 c c of the supernatant fluid from the brain culture incubated 3 days at 37 C. injected subcutaneously into a 230 gm. guinea-pig proved the absence of pathogenic bacteria.

The culture was apparently pure as judged from the similarity of colonies in deep agar but it was repurified four times by repeated isolation from deep agar.

It was identified morphologically, culturally and serologically.

B. sporogenes 113.—This came from the American Museum of Natural History Sept. 1, 1920, as "B. welchii No. 113," having been sent by Dr. Welch to the Mt. Prospect Laboratory and from the latter to the Museum in 1911.

Primary culture in milk gave a result typical of B. sporogenes, not of B. welchii. Primary glucose-broth cultures contained motile clostridial subterminal spores, and deep brain cultures were digested. There was no evidence of the persistence of B. welchii. It was evidently pure B. sporogenes when I received it. Repurification 3 times by the deep agar method required 8 days. It was identified by the agglutination test and corresponds morphologically and culturally.

B. sporogenes 114.—This was an American Museum of Natural History culture marked "B. welchii No. 20," having been obtained from Dr. Ernst at Harvard by the Mt. Prospect Laboratory of Brooklyn and sent to the Museum in 1911. It came into my hands Sept. 1, 1920.

The primary culture in milk failed to confirm the label, but coupled with the motility and morphology of the organism and the digestive action in brain medium pointed to B. sporogenes which was identified by specific agglutination of the repurified culture secured after thrice repeated isolation from deep agar.

B. sporogenes 115.—This was received Sept. 1, 1920, from the American Museum of Natural History as B. botulinus 333, having come to the Museum from Leland Stanford Junior University, Jan. 20, 1919, as the "strain of B. botulinus B. isolated by Dickson and Burke."

The primary subculture in glucose broth was nontoxic at 48 hours for a 200 gm. guinea-pig in a dose of 0.5 c c injected subcutaneously; there was thus no evidence of B. botulinus It showed the morphology and physiology of B. sporogenes, which of course are not distinctive. While the culture was evidently pure, it was repurified 3 times by the deep agar method, requiring 8 days.

B. sporogenes 118.—This was received at the University of California some time during 1919 from the American Museum of Natural History as B. botulinus 575. Its origin was traced only as far back as Kral's Museum from which it was sent several years ago. It came into my hands Sept. 21, 1920, and was then nonpathogenic for guinea-pigs inoculated with 1 c c of glucose-broth cultures. It appeared to be a pure culture of B. sporogenes but was repurified 3 successive times during a period about 9 days by the deep agar method.

B. sporogenes 121.—This was an American Museum of Natural History culture marked "malignant oedema bacillus No. 421." This culture was received by the University of California sometime during my absence in 1919-20. The Museum stated that this culture was isolated in Sept., 1910, at the Bellevue Hospital from a case of malignant edema and was received by the Museum in September, 1911.

It was a brain culture dated April 27, 1920, that came into my hands Sept. 23, 1920. Subcultures in brain medium were free from aerobes and blackened quickly; an 18-hour glucose broth culture was nonpathogenic by subcutaneous inoculation of 1 c c into a 350 gm. guinea-pig; milk cultures gave the usual sporogenes type of reaction.

On dilution in deep agar the identity of colonies suggested the original purity of the cultures, but it was repurified three times. The putrefactive properties in milk and brain medium and the morphology of the purified cultures were again shown to be those of B. sporogenes, which was confirmed by the agglutination test.

B. sporogenes 122.—This was obtained in the same manner as No. 121 from the American Museum of Natural History as "B. Feseri N. 48." A letter from the Museum stated that it came to the Museum in February, 1911, marked "No. 011" from Parke, Davis & Co.

The details of this culture are almost identical with those recorded for B. sporogenes 121. The original was apparently pure as judged by the morphologic and cultural identity with the repurified strain, which was proved serologically to be B. sporogenes.

B. sporogenes 133.—Dec. 4, 1920, a laboratory sheep was found dead, 2 days following a bleeding from the jugular vein. On an admittedly tardy postmortem, the muscular tissue was emphysematous and the lung cavity contained a thick, putrid bloody fluid, which showed thick, gram-positive rods with subterminal spores and slender gram-positive rods. Some of this fluid was injected into a guinea-pig which died, and from it were recovered B. spermoides (see No. 137) and another culture of B. sporogenes. Primary cultures from the pleural fluid contained both gram-positive sporulating anaerobes and gram-negative nonsporulating aerobes, of which the latter were eliminated by heating. The remaining anaerobic culture appeared to be pure B. sporogenes but was repurified 3 times, twice by the deep agar method, and once by the blood-agar surface colony method, before final identification.

B. sporogenes 150.—This was received May 20, 1921, from an assistant in Prof. F. G. Novy's laboratory at Ann Arbor, as B. novyi. The obviously putrefactive action of this culture on milk and brain mediums showed that the culture, if of B. novyi, was at least contaminated anaerobically. The lack of pathogenicity in this culture could not be taken as evidence of the absence of B. novyi, since, while the species is typically quite virulent and the organism recovered by Prof. Novy was so originally, it has almost completely lost its virulence, as shown in a true culture subsequently sent by Prof. Novy himself (see No. 153). It was, at any rate, impossible to find any but B. sporogenes in this culture, but the purity of the strain was insured in thrice repeated isolation by the deep agar colony method.

Morphology.—B. sporogenes is a large, gram-positive, highly motile rod of variable length, occurring singly, in pairs or in chains. In brain cultures chains are less common, but culture 84 was unusually prone to the production of long chains and filaments. Spores are formed abundantly in mediums free from fermentable sugars and to some extent even in mediums containing them.

Colony Form.—Blood-agar surface colonies are variable in form according to the consistency of the agar. With stiffer medium they tend to be round and dew-drop-like; with softer agar they become rhizoid, stellate, ameboid, or even confluent. They are always hemolytic.

Deep 1% agar colonies are fluffy, transparent balls, and if well separated may reach a diameter of 1 cm.; colonies in 2% agar tend to be more restricted, opaque, and even discoid in form.

Physiology.—B. sporogenes is actively proteolytic. It digests rapidly coagulated albumins, such as egg white, minced meat and brain. These mediums are also blackened owing to the liberation of considerable sulphuretted hydrogen and the precipitation of iron sulphide. Salmon flesh is not blackened normally although it is digested and sulphuretted hydrogen is produced, as can be shown by lead acetate, but if an iron nail or certain iron salts be added to this medium, it becomes blackened as do brain and meat mediums. The addition of iron also intensifies the blackening in the latter mediums.

Repeated tests for indol were made with B. sporogenes cultures numbered 10 to 94, inclusive, without results.

Gelatin is liquified and darkened by all cultures.

The action on milk depends on the strain and on the degree of anaerobiosis provided, but the changes always follow a certain order—first, slow coagulation and then liquefaction accompanied by slight gas production. The titratable acidity of the milk always increases greatly during the phase of liquefaction, but the H^+ ion concentration decreases slightly in spite of the increased titer. Further studies are required on the metabolism in milk of B. sporogenes and other putrefactive anaerobes.

B. sporogenes ferments monosaccharides but not higher carbohydrates. Both a change in the direction of higher H^+ ion concentration and gas formation in simple peptone mediums may serve as criteria of fermentation.[15] All of the foregoing cultures formed acid and gas in glucose broth and only traces of gas and no acid in lactose, saccharose, salicin, glycerol and inulin peptone broth.

Pathogenicity.—B. sporogenes in pure culture is practically nonpathogenic. I tested every culture on guinea-pigs and many on rabbits, the former by subcutaneous, the latter by both subcutaneous and intravenous injection. No effect was ever observed from intravenous injection. Subcutaneous injection of 1 c c of glucose broth or brain medium culture, particularly in guinea-pigs, usually produces a slight local tumefaction during the first 24 hours, which then dries up and disappears in a few days.

Barger and Dale[51] and others have noted that larger doses of old putrefactive cultures of B. sporogenes may cause symptoms resembling those of anaphylaxis, shortly after inoculation. These are not to be ascribed either to a pathogenic action of the micro-organism, or to a specific toxin, as Weinberg and Sequin[2] have done, but rather to the effect of ptomaine-like substances produced during growth in mediums rich in protein.[52]

The importance of mixed cultures of B. sporogenes in the problem of pathogenicity is just becoming recognized since the work of Weinberg and Sequin.[2,53] This point is mentioned here only incidentally as it does not bear directly on the problem of identification.

BACILLUS HISTOLYTICUS

Weinberg and Sequin,[54] in 1916, recovered from a case of gaseous gangrene a mildly putrefactive pathogenic anaerobe that they called B. histolyticus because of its marked ability to liquefy living tissues.[55] I am indebted to Dr. Weinberg for a strain of this novel species, which has enabled me to verify the claim regarding its remarkable pathogenic action.

B. histolyticus 141.—This was received from Dr. M. Weinberg of the Pasteur Institute of Paris, March 17, 1921. A stain showed many gram-positive rods, some containing subterminal oval clostridial spores; there were also numerous free oval spores. A brain medium subculture developed Staphy. albus as an aerobic contaminant which was eliminated by 5 minutes' boiling.

A careful study of the morphology, physiology and pathogenicity of the aerobe-free subculture was then made.

Repurification started March 29, 1921, and occupied 13 days for 2 isolations by the deep agar method and one by the blood-agar surface colony method. There was no evidence of anaerobic impurity. The colonies were all alike in 1% agar, compact opaque irregular globules.

Blood-agar surface colonies were hemolytic dew drops.

The morphologic, cultural and pathogenic properties were retested with the purified culture and found identical with those of the original.

Morphology.—B. histolyticus is a gram-positive, motile anaerobic rod that forms subterminal clostridial spores similar to those of B. sporogenes and B. botulinus from which there is no morphologic distinction.

Colony Form.—The form of colony varies according to the medium. Deep agar colonies may be compact lobulate globules or fluffy semitransparent or even cottony balls. On blood-agar slants under alkaline pyrogallol my culture always produced a dew drop type of colony.

Physiology.—Biochemically B. histolyticus is similar to B. sporogenes, but as Blanc and Pozerske[56] found, less actively proteolytic for albumins coagulated by heat. These investigators observed no action of their strain on coagulated egg white, but the one sent by Dr. Weinberg digested this protein in tests slowly. The proteolytic activity

[51] Brit. Med. Jour., 1915, 2, p. 808.
[52] Compt. rend. Acad. des Sc., 1918, 166, p. 1.
[53] Copt. rend. Soc. biol., 1916, 79, p. 1028.
[54] Compt. rend. Acad. de Sc., 1916, 163, p. 449.
[55] Compt. rend. Soc. de Biol., 1917, 80, p. 157.
[56] Compt. rend. Soc. Biol., 1920, 83, pp. 1315, 1343, and 1369.

of B. histolyticus is mild in vitro as compared with its tremendous digestive action in vivo.

A brain medium culture digested slowly, darkened slightly and developed white crystals similar to those pictured for this species as tyrosin by the Medical Research Committee.[1] Gelatin was liquefied on the second day. The action in milk was slow, none at all for 7 days, then coagulation followed by liquefaction without gas production.

Like B. sporogenes, this species ferments only monosaccharides and the easily hydrolyzed disaccharide maltose. I found acid and gas formed in glucose broth, not in lactose, saccharose, salicin, glycerol or inulin.

Pathogenicity.—The pathogenic action of B. histolyticus is unique and consists in a progressive localized liquefaction of living tissues. The following examples confirm the observations of Weinberg and Sequin.[2]

Guinea-pig 945, weighing 470 gm., was inoculated March 26, 1921, with 1 c c of a 24-hour glucose-broth culture of B. histolyticus 141 in the left gluteus muscle. This was with the original culture after the staphylococcus had been eliminated but before the culture had been repurified.

March 27 the skin was gone over an area of 3-4 sq. cm. of the limb at the site of inoculation. The muscles were eroded, and the exposed portion was covered with a bloody slime. Microscopic examination of this showed débris of tissue disintegration, red blood cells, fibrin, a few polymorphonuclear leukocytes and many gram-positive single and double rods mostly without spores. The few spores were subterminal and clostridial. The animal appeared not tc be intoxicated and ate well although suffering pain when handled.

March 28 it was found dead. The flesh of the leg, from hip to knee, was gone completely; the naked joint parted easily at the knee. The abdominal muscles and skin were necrotic and digested away, the intestines extending. There were no macroscopically recognizable lesions of the thoracic or abdominal viscera except that those intestines in contact with the abdominal peritoneum were hyperemic and the kidneys were grayish and friable. The renal lesions attracted our special attention; sections were made by Prof. T. D. Beckwith, to whom the writer is grateful for the following description:

"The kidney tissue on the outer portion of the organ showed an active lytic effect with destruction of tissue complete. Degeneration had spread throughout the mass. The tubular epithelium was undergoing destruction as evidenced by widespread karolysis. In the glomeruli karyolysis was general. Occasionally crescents were noticeable. There was no evidence of infiltration."

I failed to recover a culture from the heart blood.

Guinea-pig 987, weighing 690 gm., was inoculated April 12, 1921, with 1 c c of a 1:10 dilution of a 24-hour glucose broth culture 141 after repurification, in the left gluteus muscle. April 13 the leg was swollen and not used, but the animal appeared to be well otherwise.

April 14 the skin was sloughing off of the external surface of the thigh muscles.

April 15, the animal appeared sick for the first time. The muscles of the injected leg were fluid and dripping. Slides showed a mixed infection of cocci and bacilli with different types of spores, but mostly subterminal clostridia. No leukocytes could be found.

April 16, the guinea-pig was found dead with a peritoneal perforation reaching from sternum to pubis and the intestines hanging out. The leg muscles were gone, but the tendons were intact. The testicles were soft and "mushy." The abdominal muscles were digested away to the pectoral girdle. The lungs were hyperemic. There were no other macroscopic lesions of the viscera except of the kidneys which both macro- and micro-scopically were as before.

An apparently pure culture of B. histolyticus was secured from the heart blood.

The essentials of these results have been repeated several times since.

BACILLUS CHAUVŒI

Until very recently, blackleg in cattle, like gaseous gangrene in human beings, was regarded as a monomicrobic infection, but the work of Heller[57] confirmed the view suggested by the findings of Kerry[58] and others that this disease may be due now to one, again to another, or even at times, to mixtures of B. chauvœi, B. novyi and Vibrion septique. The last 2 have been found in human gaseous gangrene, the first never with certainty. Furthermore, the commonest cause of human gas infections, B. welchii, has not yet with certainty been proved the cause of a natural gas infection in animals.

The writer has been privileged to study only a single strain of B. chauvœi as follows:

B. Chauvœi No. 6.—This was obtained from Dr. F. W. Wood of the Cutter Laboratories, March 2, 1916. It was labeled "Blackleg, Calif.," and had come from Professor K. F. Meyer. This strain was described by Meyer[5] in 1915. The culture was evidently pure, but was repurified 5 times during the interval from March 30 to May 14, 1918. It corresponds with the recent definitions of Meyer,[5] Heller,[57] and Robertson.[60]

Morphology.—B. chauvœi is a gram-positive, motile rod that forms subterminal clostridial spores freely and under certain conditions solidly staining swollen forms that Heller[57] has designated "orgonts." Emphasis was placed by Leclainche and Vallee,[59] Meyer,[5] Robertson[60] and others on a morphologic distinction between B. chauvœi and Vibrion septique in liver smears from experimental animals dead of infection by these organisms; the first never forms chains or filaments, but the latter usually does though not invariably (see Vibrion septique 4).

Colony Form.—Blood-agar surface colonies are flat, leaf-like or round according to the consistency of the medium, and actively hemolytic.

[57] Jour. Infect. Dis., 1920, 27, p. 385.
[58] Centralbl. f. Bakteriol., I, 1894, 16, p. 372.
[59] Ann. de l'Inst. Pasteur, 1900, 14, p. 596.
[60] Brit. Med. Jour., 1918, 1, p. 583.

Deep colonies are semitransparent to opaque spheres with or without raylike growths.

Physiology.—B. chauvœi is easily grown in highly buffered mediums containing a modicum of fermentable carbohydrate. It seemingly requires a more carefully adjusted H^+ ion concentration than some other anaerobic bacteria so that failure to secure growth is not infrequent in poorly buffered mediums, such as broth, agar and gelatin.

B. chauvœi is practically nonproteolytic; chopped brain and meat mediums are neither digested nor blackened. These mediums become acid in reaction and may reach a H^+ ion reaction of $P_H = 5.6$. Even the addition of an iron nail to brain medium gives only a yellowish discoloration (due possibly to iron oxide) after long continued incubation. Sulphuretted hydrogen was not produced in 9 days. Gelatin is liquefied.

The fermentative activities of B. chauvœi are not so vigorous as those of either Vibrion septique or B. welchii. Milk frequently shows no change at all; in the presence of sterile blood there may be gas production and coagulation of the casein. The casein clot is never digested. Glucose, levulose, maltose, saccharose, and lactose were fermented, with acid and gas production; mannite, glycerol, inulin, dextrin and salicin were not fermented, corresponding with Robertson's [60] results. Saccharose fermentation and nonfermentation of salicin are of differential value, as shown in chart 1, in distinguishing Vibrion septique.

Pathogenicity.—My strain is still virulent for guinea-pigs after 5 years' artificial cultivation without animal passage although stock cultures in brain medium were transplanted only at infrequent intervals. In collaboration with Mr. Lee Wah Pond, about 56 guinea-pigs and several rabbits have been inoculated. It is not possible for us to add anything to the elaborate description of acute lesions given by Heller.[57] On several occasions sublethal doses caused severe subcutaneous gaseous edema followed by a sloughing phlegmon and slow but complete healing, as already described for B. welchii.

B. chauvœi is generally regarded as nonpathogenic for rabbits, although Heller [57] noted exceptions in 2 strains. Culture 6 has always proved nonpathogenic for rabbits in doses up to 2 c c of glucose-broth culture inoculated intravenously or subcutaneously.

VIBRION SEPTIQUE

The long standing confusion of the terms Vibrion septique and "bacillus of malignant edema" took a step toward clarification in the work of Ghon and Sachs [61] in 1903 when they pointed out the discrepancies between the Vibrion septique culture of Pasteur, fortunately preserved in the Pasteur Institute in Paris, and the then available descriptions of the "bacillus of malignant edema," a highly putrefactive organism. This point of view was perpetuated in the work of Von Hibler,[62] Werdt [63] and Meyer.[5] We know now that many of the supposedly "authentic" cultures of "malignant edema bacillus" were in reality B. sporogenes. What it was that Koch actually saw in the tissues of his experimental animals but failed to isolate, we can only surmise. But Weinberg and Sequin [2] have elucidated the historical aspects of the question in a highly satisfactory manner. Nor can we overlook Heller's [57] suggestive interpretation of the tangle.

While the essential features of the situation respecting Vibrion septique and "bacillus of malignant edema" may now be regarded as settled, we are far from a unanimity of opinion regarding the nomenclature of Vibrion septique in particular, and of anaerobes in general. No satisfactory excuse can be offered for using a separate generic designation for such closely related organisms as Vibrion septique and Bacillus chauvœi, and indeed Arloing and Mace (quoted by Weinberg and Sequin [2]) have independently suggested the use of Bacillus septicus to replace the former. The writer is unconvinced of the validity of "Clostridium" as adopted by the Society of American Bacteriologists for a generic designation for the sporulating anaerobes and prefers to continue the use of the historic terms until a real unanimity of opinion prevails. For the present, therefore, none will misunderstand what we mean by "Vibrion septique."

I am indebted to Professor K. F. Meyer for all but one of the following 7 cultures. To his great credit, not one gave any evidence of impurity. Some of these strains were misnamed at the time of my receipt of them, Prof. Meyer having passed them on realizing that in some cases they would have to be relabeled. We are now in accord regarding the classification of these cultures.

Vibrion septique 4.—This was received March 2, 1916, from Dr. F. W. Wood of the Cutter Laboratories, he in turn having obtained it from Dr. K. F. Meyer as "Vibrion septique, Pasteur." Purity and identity were confirmed in the morphologic and cultural properties, including the action in brain medium, fermentation of salicin and nonfermentation of saccharose.

The culture was repurified twice by the surface colony method starting March 7, 1918, once from plain agar and again from blood-agar slants under alkaline pyrogallol. The colonies were all alike in each isolation culture—delicate, flat, hemolytic colonies resembling tiny maple leaves. Several further attempts to secure well separated surface colonies failed owing to excessive moisture in the agar.

[61] Centralbl. f. Bakteriol., I, O., 1903, 34, pp. 289, 398, 481, 609.

[62] Unters. über path. Anaëroben, 1908.

[63] Malignes oedem, Kolle u. Wassermann, Handbuch d. path. Mikro-org., 1912, 4, p. 837.

The identity of the repurified culture was confirmed on the basis of its morphology, cultural reactions, and pathogenicity. It alone, of all the Vibrion septique cultures, failed repeatedly to produce filamentous forms on the liver surface of injected guinea-pigs. Precedence is given to the diagnostic value of the fermentative reactions in this case.

Vibrion septique 12.—This was received from Prof. K. F. Meyer Sept. 19, 1914, as Ghon-Sach's "bacillus No. 1." Brain medium cultures failed to blacken, gelatin was liquefied, and blood milk fermented. Sugar reactions were not tested at this time.

Purification by the blood-agar surface colony method started April 8, 1918, and required 25 days for 6 repeated isolations. The colonies were always lobulate, ameboid, and hemolytic.

Vibrion septique 14.—This was received, March 2, 1916, from Dr. F. W. Wood. It came originally from Prof. Meyer as "Ghon-Sach's bacillus." It is doubtful whether this culture is the same as No. 12; it is serologically distinct. Morphologically and culturally it was identical.

Repurification started April 17, 1918, and required 18 days for 4 repated isolations of well separated colonies from blood-agar slants. The colonies were always dew drop like in form.

The culture was relabeled Vibrion septique on the basis of its morphology, cultural reactions and pathogenicity.

Vibrion septique 16.—This was recovered by Dr. F. W. Wood from the tissues of a cow dead of blackleg and sent to the writer with a tentative designation "B. chauvœi," Feb. 1. 1915. No proteolytic anaerobes were present, but looking backward, the fermentation of both saccharose and salicin seems to indicate that both B. chauvœi and Vibrion septique were originally present in this culture. It was pathogenic for guinea-pigs.

Purification started April 17, 1918, and was readily repeated 3 times in 8 days; using the blood-agar surface colony method. B. chauvœi, if actually present at first, was probably lost in this process since the purified culture has never fermented saccharose, but only salicin. It was identified by its morphology, cultural reactions and pathognicity.

Vibrion septique 18.—This was received Sept. 19, 1914, from Prof. Meyer as "B. chauvœi, Kitt, Munich." This latter could be ruled out on the nonfermentation of saccharose and the fermentation of salicin.

Repurification started April 17, 1918, but owing to difficulty in securing well separated surface colonies about 40 days were required for 5 successful repeated isolations out of 12 trials. The colonies, when not confluent, were always flat and somewhat ameboid in form.

Identification was established on the basis of morphology, cultural reaction and pathogenicity.

Vibrion septique 28.—This was Prof. Meyer's "B. chauvœi Pasteur." It came into my hands Sept. 19, 1914. There is nothing in the record of my early tests to indicate impurity; unfortunately the fermentative reactions were not determined prior to repurification.

Repurification started April 19, 1918, and was repeated by the blood-agar surface colony method 3 times. The colonies were of the dew drop type.

The predominance of filaments in a young glucose-broth culture and on the impression smear made from the liver of a guinea-pig dead after inoculation with this culture suggested the new identification of Vibrion septique which was confirmed by the fermentation reactions.

Vibrion septique 32.—This was Prof. Meyer's "B. oedematis Pasteur." It was given to the writer Sept. 19, 1914, along with several others including our B. sporogenes 58. The records fail to distinguish these cultures by their original labels, but they were recorded separately and have been studied separately. I have already mentioned that No. 58 became contaminated in my hands with B. sporogenes which was isolated, whereas the original Vibrion septique was lost. The present culture has never shown any evidence of impurity either when received or since. It was tested carefully and the records of its early morphology, cultural reactions and pathogenicity agree with those of the repurified culture in the designation of Vibrion septique.

Repurification occupied the interval from April 17, 1918, to April 25, 1918, and comprised 3 repeated isolations from blood-agar surface colonies, which were hemolytic ameboid, round, or irregular flat disks in the different tubes.

Morphology.—Vibrion septique is a gram-positive rod. Its gram-staining properties are, however, less intense than those of some other anaerobes. Sporulation occurs abundantly in brain medium. The spores are generally subterminal as to location and swell the rods to form clostridiums. Barrel shaped "orgonts" are formed by the immature spores. On peritoneal surfaces of infected animals long filaments are usually formed which show tremendous variations in the individuals of different or even single cultures.

Vibrion septique is motile in very young cultures but cultures of 24 hours' or more incubation are frequently nonmotile.

Colony Form.—Surface colonies on blood agar are subject to considerable variations as noted in our descriptions of the various strains under isolation.

Deep agar colonies also vary. They tend to be semitransparent, with filamentous or woolly outgrowths.

Physiology.—Vibrion septique is nonputrefactive. It never liquefies or digests coagulated egg white, brain or meat mediums, nor are any of these blackened, even in the presence of metallic iron. Sulphuretted hydrogen is not produced in 0.1% lead acetate. Brain and meat mediums are slightly acidified by the growth of Vibrion septique, owing to fermentation of the natural sugar. Robertson's [6] alkaline egg broth is rendered slightly opaque, never milky as by B. welchii. There is usually no action in milk, except in the presence of blood, when it resembles that of B. chauvœi.

Glucose, levulose, galactose, maltose, lactose, and salicin are actively attacked with acid and gas production; saccharose, inulin, mannite and glycerol are not fermented, in agreement with Robertson's [6] records. Fermentation of salicin and nonfermentation of saccharose distinguish Vibrion septique from the otherwise similar B. chauvœi.

Pathogenicity.—All of the strains described were found pathogenic for guinea-pigs in doses of 1 c c 24-48-hour glucose-broth cultures. Virulence persisted throughout their maintenance in the laboratory without animal passage and indeed with only infrequent transfers in brain medium. I have made no effort to determine the minimal fatal dose. One c c injected subcutaneously produces an emphysematous edema externally similar to that produced by B. welchii and B. chauvœi. The affected area becomes hot, moist, crepitant, and tender to the touch. The hair slips easily. The animals appear to be profoundly intoxicated. They almost invariably die within 48 hours.

At necropsy the subcutaneous tissues are found to be hemorrhagic, emphysematous, and edematous. The differences between animals killed by B. welchii on the one hand and by Vibrion septique and B. chauvœi on the other in our laboratory, accord in general with those described by the English Committee,[1] Weinberg and Sequin [2] and Robertson.[60] They are of corroborative rather than of diagnostic value. Congestion of the intestines is common and gastric hemorrhages have been observed at times. The suprarenals are usually hyperemic, but the kidneys and liver do not as a rule show macroscopic changes.

Impression smears from the peritoneal surfaces usually, but not invariably (see culture 4) show elongated granular filaments. As LeClainche and Vallee,[59] Meyer,[5] Robertson,[60] Heller [57] and others have pointed out, B. chauvœi never forms such filaments; they have therefore considerable diagnostic value.

Heart blood cultures were positive in about 70% of our Vibrion septique necropsies on guinea-pigs.

In rabbits I have made only a few observations incidental to the production of agglutinating serums. Of strains 12, 14 and 18, 1 c c of glucose-broth culture injected subcutaneously failed to cause any inconvenience. An initial injection of 2 c c of Vibrion septique 18 caused a severe but temporary induration in one rabbit. Another, weighing 1,655 gm., after surviving an initial subcutaneous injection of 1 c c of Vibrion septique 18 followed by 2 more of 5 c c each after 4-day intervals without serious illness, succumbed within 24 hours after the third 5 c c dose which was given following an interval of 6 days.

At necropsy there was a bloody and purulent subcutaneous emphysema. The large intestine was hemorrhagic; the kidneys were soft, with the cortex lighter than medulla; the liver was friable; the lungs were normal. Impression smears from the subcutaneous tissues showed single rods with clostridial spores. Impression smears from the liver were negative and heart blood cultures remained sterile on incubation.

It thus seems probable that occasionally strains pathogenic for rabbits may be encountered.

BACILLUS NOVYI

Novy,[64] in 1894, recovered a new pathogenic anaerobe from 3 guinea-pigs that died after injections of nonsterile nuclein prepared from casein, which he named "Bacillus oedematis II." Kerry [65] is thought to have recovered the same organism from the dried flesh of a cow supposedly dead of blackleg, following which, according to Weinberg and Sequin,[2] the 2 descriptions were united by Kruse under the name of "B. oedematis thermophilus" and later given a valid binomial designation, "B. novyi" by Migula. Von Hibler [11] studied 4 strains, including the original (?) and 3 others, recovered respectively from a rabbit inoculated with earth, from a wild boar presumably dead of symptomatic anthrax, and from the lips of a woman supposed to have died of a septicemic disease. Weinberg and Sequin [2] concluded that the organism described by themselves in 1915 [66] as B. oedematiens is identical with "B. novyi." This being true, the earlier name has priority.

I have found 3 strains of B. novyi, including Novy's original culture, one of Weinberg's so-called B. oedematiens, and one recovered in California from a horse essentially identical.

B. novyi 139.—This was received Dec. 10, 1920. It came from a fatal wound infection in a horse, appeared to be pure, and presented all the morphologic, cultural and pathogenic characters that distinguish B. oedematiens in the descriptions of Weinberg and Sequin.[2]

[64] Ztschr. f. Hyg. u. Infektionskr., 1894, 17, p. 209.
[65] Centralbl. f. Bakteriol., 1, 1894, 16, p. 372.
[66] Compt. rend. Soc. de Biol., 1915, 78, p. 507.

It was repurified twice by the deep agar method and twice by the blood-agar surface colony method during the interval from Dec. 15, 1920, to Jan. 4, 1921. The properties of the original were confirmed in the repurified strain.

B. novyi 140.—This was received March 17, 1921, as B. oedematiens 128 from Dr. Weinberg of the Pasteur Institute at Paris. In morphology, cultural reactions and pathogenicity it was identical with the preceding culture.

In the primary deep agar dilution for repurification 2 types of colony suggested impurity. One was more compact, but when the fluffier type was picked into deep brain and further dilutions made in deep agar only compact colonies resulted. Furthermore, when repeated dilutions were made from the original culture only compact colonies appeared. This is cited to show how little reliance can be placed on judgments based on colony differences. We have actually no evidence that the original culture was impure. Four repeated isolations were made from the compact deep agar colonies (none other appeared after those in the initial repurification culture) and a fifth from the well separated minute, dew-drop-like, hemolytic colonies on a blood-agar slant under alkaline pyrogallol. The repurified strain had the same morphologic, cultural and pathogenic properties as the original.

B. novyi 153.—This was received from Prof. F. G. Novy of the University of Michigan, Sept. 13, 1921. The culture was apparently pure and unlike the first culture sent as B. novyi by one of Prof. Novy's assistants (see B. sporogenes 150), was morphologically and culturally identical with strains 139 and 140. It was much less pathogenic for guinea-pigs but not wholly devoid of virulence, for while we have as yet failed to cause the death of guinea-pigs with 1-2 c c doses of glucose-broth culture injected subcutaneously, the characteristic nonemphysematous edema was produced repeatedly.

A single repurification by the deep agar method, although unnecessary, was given this culture; the characteristic morphology, cultural reactions and pathogenicity were reaffirmed for the picked strain.

Morphology.—B. novyi is a gram-positive rod of variable length, sluggishly motile in very young cultures only. Persistent examination is required to prove motility in this species, but the flagella can be stained. Rather large subterminal spores are formed.

Colony Form.—Deep agar colonies are generally compact opaque points when young; as they age they may tend to break up or become surrounded by a delicate corona of short filaments. Later the colonies clear, the center becomes cloudy and surrounded with a corona of tangled filaments.

On blood agar young colonies were like those of B. welchii. Older colonies were flat, transparent, bluish gray with irregular contours.

Little reliance should be placed on colony form for identification.

Physiology.—B. novyi is nonputrefactive, neither blackening nor digesting coagulated albumins, such as meat, brain or egg white. It resembles Vibrion septique and B. chauvœi closely in its protein metabolism, forming little or no sulphuretted hydrogen. An iron nail in brain medium causes only the slightest discoloration on prolonged incubation. There is no visible action in milk. Gelatin is liquefied and blackened.

Fermentable carbohydrates are necessary for vigorous growth. Henry [37] found glucose, levulose, maltose, xylose and starch fermented. The records of McIntosh,[32] Wolf [67] and Weinberg and Sequin [2] disagree as to the fermentation reactions, but a recent report states [1] that glycerol galactose, saccharose, lactose, mannite, dulcite, inulin and salicin are

[67] Jour. Path. & Bacteriol., 1920, 23, p. 254.

not fermented. My cultures fermented glucose and glycerol but not lactose, saccharose, salicin or inulin.

Pathogenicity.—Natural infections have been recorded for guinea-pigs by Novy,[64] for cattle by Kerry,[65] for hogs by von Hibler,[11] for horses by Heller [57] and for man by Weinberg and Sequin,[66,2,68] and by Henry and Lacey.[69] The findings of Novy,[64] Kerry [65] and Weinberg and Sequin [2] in laboratory animals inoculated with pure cultures are in substantial agreement. A massive edema with little emphysema is produced by subcutaneous inoculation of guinea-pigs. Some strains are said to produce a moderately strong filtrable toxin. Weinberg and Sequin [2] described strains whose pathogenicity was due mainly to virulency.

My work confirms the high pathogenicity of strains 139 and 140, the lesser pathogenicity of strain 153, and the character of the lesions described, with the repurified cultures as well as with subcultures of the original received. The data presented concern only the repurified cultures, however.

Culture 139 was tested first on rabbits in an effort to produce an agglutinating serum.

Rabbit 935, weighing 1,900 gm., was inoculated subcutaneously Feb. 21, 1921, with 1 c c of a 24-hour glucose-broth culture. Next day the abdominal tissues were thickened and edematous; the rabbit was visibly intoxicated, and died during the succeeding night. At necropsy the subcutaneous tissues were edematous, slightly emphysematous and not notably congested. Gram-positive rods were present in smears made from the subcutaneous tissues. There were no macroscopic lesions of the viscera. A nonputrefactive anaerobe was recovered from the heart blood.

This result was practically duplicated with doses of 0.1 c c and 0.01 c c of culture.

This culture is also pathogenic for guinea-pigs in which the findings were identical with those in rabbits. B. novyi infections seem always to be characterized by extensive edema with only slight gas production and little congestion—in these respects contrasting both with Welch infection and Vibrion septique infections.

Culture 140 has also been tested both on guinea-pigs and on rabbits, with similar results. Culture 153 is nonpathogenic for rabbits and slightly pathogenic for guinea-pigs in doses of 1-2 c c 48-hour glucose-broth cultures.

[68] Compt. rend. acad. d. S., 1915, 161, p. 744; Compt. rend. Soc. de Biol., 1918, 81, p. 184.
[69] Jour. Path. & Bacteriol., 1920, 23, p. 281.

Guinea-pig 943, weighing 200 gm., was given subcutaneously April 5, 1921, 1 c c of a 1:10 dilution of 24-hour brain medium culture B. novyi 140. Next day the animal was anorectic and in pain from a massive edema that covered the abdomen. The animal died during the following night.

There was extensive subcutaneous edema with necrosis and emphysema covering the abdomen and edema without necrosis over the chest. The abdominal area was very full of gram-positive rods; there were fewer in the pectoral region. The lungs were normal, and the stomach was empty with a slight gastric hemorrhage. The intestines were somewhat hyperemic. A nonproteolytic anaerobe assumed to be B. novyi was recovered from the heart blood.

BACILLUS MULTIFERMENTANS TENALBUS

This species was described by Stoddard [70] in 1919 as an infrequent nonpathogenic anaerobe. According to the description, it should be differentiated from B. chauvœi, Vibrion septique and B. novyi by its failure to liquefy gelatin and from B. fallax by its fermentation of lactose and glycerol. I have encountered no such organism and so far as I am aware, Stoddard's work has not been confirmed; the Medical Research Committee [1] summarizes the details of Stoddard's report.

BACILLUS FALLAX

This is another species that the writer has not yet seen. A culture sent from Paris was lost en route through breakage of the container, and the species has not been encountered otherwise. B. fallax was described as a new species first by Weinberg and Sequin [71] in 1915. Recently isolated strains were said to be pathogenic for guinea-pigs but the property was lost on artificial cultivation.[72] Five strains of B. fallax were studied by Henry.[37] It should be differentiated from B. chauvœi, Vibrion septique, and B. novyi, which it closely resembles, by its nonliquefaction of gelatin and from B. multifermentans tenalbus by its failure to ferment lactose and glycerol.

Details are to be found in Weinberg and Sequin's "La Gangrene gazeuse,"[2] in Henry's paper,[37] and in the Report of the Medical Research Committee.[1]

ANAEROBES WITH TERMINAL SPORES

This group comprises: B. tetani, B. putrificus, B. tetanomorphus, B. tertius, and B. sphenoides, as clearly recognized forms. It is curious that while none of the terminally spored anaerobes is more than mildly proteolytic, the first two species are unable to derive their

[70] Lancet, 1919, 196, p. 12.
[71] Compt. rend. Soc. de Biol., 1915, 78, p. 686.
[72] Ibid., 1916, 79, p. 581.

carbon from carbohydrates and must be regarded as obligately putrefactive. This is the only group in which nonfermentative sporulating anaerobes are known.

B. TETANI

Considering the time elapsed since Nicolaier [73] in 1884 first described and Kitasato [74] in 1889 first isolated the tetanus bacillus, and the peculiar interest that has always attended the study of both natural and experimental tetanus, it is surprising that so much should remain for recent investigators to unravel concerning the bacteriology and serology. Few species have been subjected to such inaccuracy of conception regarding their cultural properties through the presence of anaerobic contaminants. I am able, first, to confirm fully the contention of recent English writers that pure cultures of B. tetani ferment no sugars, and, second, make some contribution to the discussion regarding the proteolytic activities of B. tetani. Some special observations on differences in the form of tetanus colonies are recorded.

Seven strains have been studied, as follows:

B. tetani 1 was received Aug. 26, 1916, from the Cutter Laboratories, they in turn having received it from the Hygiene Laboratory at Washington for the manufacture of tetanus antitoxin. Typical spores were present; 0.0001 c c of a week old broth culture caused fatal tetanus in a guinea-pig, and there was no evidence of aerobic or anaerobic impurity. The culture was nevertheless repurified 6 times during the interval betwen May 16 and June 28, 1918, by the surface colony method, using both plain and blood agar. The well separated colonies varied in size and to some extent in form. They were always flat and when minute were crenate, rhizoid or ameboid; when large (3-5 mm. diameter), feathery. The largest colonies appeared on blood agar which was hemolyzed. Two subsequent purifications by the deep method have shown that in different tubes of medium the size and form of colonies may vary from minute, more or less compact colonies with irregular bodies to larger feathery colonies, such as are generally pictured in the textbooks.

The repurified culture has maintained the morphologic, cultural and pathogenic properties of the original.

B. tetani 130 A.—This was received Nov. 19, 1920, from Dr. Heller of the Hooper Foundation for Medical Research, as a sealed tube of brain medium culture marked "B. tetani U. S. A. 11, Type 1 of Tullock, from Robertson, now impure." A stain showed gram-positive rods with terminal spherical spores. No aerobes were present and 0.001 c c of a glucose-broth culture killed a guinea-pig in 3 days with tetanus, while a control pig inoculated with 1 c c of culture plus 100 units of commercial tetanus antitoxin was fully protected.

Evidence of anaerobic impurity appeared in distinct colony differences in deep meat infusion agar. Certain colonies were diffuse, fuzzy, and larger; these were assumed to be of the tetanus bacillus (see B. tetani 130 B.). Other colonies in the same tube were opaque, compact and smaller; these were assumed to represent the contaminant. Picked into deep brain medium, which was incubated and rediluted in deep agar, they found their counterpart in two successive daughter cultures with none of the fuzzy, diffuse colonies present. The culture was then assumed to be pure. It was surprising to find this culture fulfilling all the requisites of B. tetani. Repeated tests for colony type have since shown the form of colony to be constant for this strain.

B. tetani 130 B.—The diffuse, fuzzy colonies mentioned in the preceding culture were well separated and were picked into deep brain medium, and in 3 repeated serial manipulations for isolated colonies only the fuzzy type was present, but in 3 out of 4 succeeding tests with cultures picked from fuzzy colonies, opaque colonies similar to those of B. tetani 130 A were also present in the deep agar tubes. The proportion of differing colonies in one case was 22 opaque to 5 fuzzy. Efforts to secure a culture by selective picking of fuzzy colonies that would not give also opaque colonies extended almost continuously from Dec. 3, 1920, to June 28, 1921, and involved a total of 14 successive transfers of well separated fuzzy colonies from deep agar dilutions into deep brain, and back again to agar. The last 8 cultures in deep agar have shown only the fuzzy type of colony.

[73] Deutsch. med. Wchnschr., 1884, 10, p. 842.

[74] Ztschr. f. Hyg. u. Infektionskr., 1889, 7, p. 225.

This strain was tested for identity at rather frequent intervals after the first 3 attempts to secure a culture whose colonies would all prove similar in a single tube, and always conformed in morphology of spores, alkalinity of glucose broth cultures, and toxicity, to B. tetani. This experience throws some doubt on the use of colony differences, even in the same tube of medium, as criteria of impurity. It suggests strongly the possibility of a mutating factor in the strain producing the fuzzy type of colony.

B. tetani 131.—This was received Nov. 19, 1920, from Dr. Heller, and this strain too had come from Miss Robertson. It was labeled "B. tetani T67, Type 11 of Tullock, apparently pure." Typical spores were present, there were no aerobes, and 0.001 c c of a 7-day glucose-broth culture killed a 400 gm. guinea-pig with severe tetanus in 3 days, while 100 units of tetanus antitoxin were protective against 1 c c undiluted culture. There was no evidence of impurity. Deep agar colonies observed during 3 successive repurifications were opaque and compact. The repurified culture was re-identified in the usual manner.

B. tetani 132.—This strain also was received Nov. 19, 1920, from Dr. Heller and, like the 3 preceding, had come from Miss Robertson. It was labeled "B. tetani h 22 d, Type III of Tullock, now impure."

It contained gram-positive rods, but no spores that could be demonstrated microscopically. It was free from aerobes and 0.001 c c of a 7-day glucose-broth culture killed a 420 gm. guinea-pig with severe tetanus in 2 days, while 100 units of commercial tetanus antitoxin were protective against 1 c c of undiluted culture. Aside from a colony difference in deep agar shake culture, evidence of impurity was presented in the presence of bizarre forms wholly unlike the classical B. tetani and also in the acid reaction of glucose 1% broth cultures, that persisted even through the fourth successive isolation.

About the time this culture was being studied it seemed reasonable to assume that all pure cultures of B. tetani should be alkaline, irrespective of the presence of carbohydrates, since English investigators had recently found that B. tetani ferments no sugar and my own studies had seemed to show that the best criterion of fermentation is an increase in H^+ ion concentration.[15] It was gratifying, therefore, to find that two further attempts at isolation gave a culture of B. tetani morphologically, culturally and pathogenically characteristic, whose glucose-broth cultures always become more alkaline then when inoculated.

The contaminating organism of this culture, presumably a glucose fermenter, was unfortunately not recovered. The colonies of the purified culture are always alike in the same tube and conform in general to the usual type but vary according to the consistency of different lots of agar. Characteristic pinhead spores were easily demonstrated in the purified culture; their absence in the original culture may be ascribed to the acid reaction produced by the supposed contaminant.

B. tetani 154.—This was received Sept. 16, 1921, from Mr. L. B. Taber, of the Cutter Laboratories as B. tetani 247, having been obtained from the Hygienic Laboratory at Washington under the label "Tetanus O. T. 026580. There was no evidence of impurity or improper labeling. The morphology and cultural reactions in gelatin, glucose broth, milk, and brain mediums were true to our present conceptions. All cultures became alkaline and a dilution of 1:1,000 glucose-broth culture killed a guinea-pig with symptoms of tetanus. The culture was repurified 3 successive times by the deep agar colony method requiring 3 weeks, and the characteristic morphology, cultural reactions, and pathogenicity reaffirmed for the purified culture.

B. tetani 155.—This was also received from Mr. Taber, Sept. 16, 1921, having been obtained only a short time previously from the Hygiene Laboratory under the label "Tetanus-Court Plaster J. P. L." Every statement made for culture No. 154 in the foregoing applies also to No. 155, except that only 10 days were required for 3 repeated reisolations.

In addition to the cultures mentioned in the foregoing, one was received labeled B. tetani that consisted only of B. welchii (see No. 20), one containing B. tetani (not isolated) but contaminated with B.

sporogenes (see No. 74), and 2 others consisting only of organisms other than B. tetani that have not yet been finally identified.

Morphology.—The glass headed pin type of tetanus spores has long been regarded as characteristic; they were present in all our pure cultures. Impure strains frequently failed to reveal spores visually, and the question as to whether the bizarre swollen forms that occur in such cultures are B. tetani or of some other organism requires further study. Kanthack and Connell[75] called attention to the pleomorphism of B. tetani. There is no doubt of the variability of vegetative forms; they range from the ordinary straight single rods to short chains of rods or even long undulating and curled filaments. The rods always seem more slender when attached to spores. Rods both with and without spores are sluggishly motile.

Colony Form.—Five strains (1, 131, 132, 154 and 155) conform in their surface colonies on blood agar to the beautiful illustration shown by Adamson.[76] The same illustration would represent almost equally well a cross section of the deep 1% agar colonies of these strains. Two other strains, separately derived from a single culture diverge from a commoner type; No. 130A forms compact opaque, lenticular colonies with few or no filamentous outgrowths, while 130B forms regularly and exclusively now after some 14 selective isolations, colonies even more diffuse and hazy in outline than usual for B. tetani. The observed differences in colony form seem to be constant and appear both in deep agar cultures and cultures on blood-agar slants under alkaline pyrogallol; the colonies of 130A are minute, discreet, transparent dew drops, those of 130B like Adamson's illustration. Yet all the cultures are apparently identical in morphology, physiology and high toxicity.

Physiology.—Nearly 10 years of almost constant observation of B. tetani have convinced the writer that the claims of Ferran[77] and Rosenthal[78] of its gradual acclimation to oxygen at atmospheric pressure are open to serious question. B. tetani grows only at reduced oxygen tensions.

None of the foregoing strains fermented glucose, lactose, saccharose, inulin, salicin or glycerol. Pure cultures of B. tetani are invariably alkaline, and since the great majority of both aerobic and anaerobic bacteria ferment with acid formation at least monosaccharides, the

[75] Jour. of Path. & Bacteriol., 1897, 4, p. 452.
[76] Jour. Path. & Bacteriol., 1920, 23, p. 241.
[77] Centralbl. f. Bakteriol., I, O., 1898, 24, p. 28.
[78] Compt. rend. Soc., Biol., 1907, pp. 438, 578 & 784.

alkalinity of cultures known to contain B. tetani is to some extent a gage of their purity. A contamination with B. putrificus could not, of course, be detected by this means.

Adamson and Cutler[79] credit Mace[80] as the first to demonstrate the failure of B. tetani to ferment carbohydrates. Mace's findings were confirmed by Dean and Mouat[81] and later by Adamson.[76]

The discovery that pure cultures of B. tetani are always alkaline nullifies the writer's suggestion,[82] made in 1913, concerning the use of magnesium carbonate as an acid buffer in preparing tetanus toxin. No doubt the strain of B. tetani in use at that time was impure since the cultures always became acid without the carbonate.

Tetanus cultures have little or no action on milk, Adamson[76] observed a white flocculent precipitate which is confirmed in my own tests; prolonged incubation sometimes produces a fairly solid coagulum suggesting the operation of a rennet-like enzyme. A slight gas production may occur, but no liquefaction of the casein, although the cultures become slightly alkaline. Some gas is produced by all strains of B tetani in various mediums; it contains some carbon dioxide and is presumably a product of proteolysis. However, the proteolytic activities of B. tetani are feeble as compared with those of B. sporogenes, B. centrosporogenes, B. bifermentans, B. histolyticus and B. botulinus.

Smith[83] recognized the slowness with which it liquefies coagulated egg albumin and its action on brain medium has been a subject of recent controversy. Von Hibler[11] considered B. tetani a brain blackener, and Robertson, who first agreed, later[84] decided with Adamson and Cutler[79] that the discoloration observed by von Hibler and by herself must have been due to a proteolytic contaminant.

The fact is that pure cultures of B. tetani do blacken brain medium, though very slowly and very slightly, so that the reaction is rarely seen except in old cultures. The addition of an iron nail to brain medium greatly accelerates the deposition of iron sulphid to which the discoloration is ascribed, so that cultures only a few days old are distinctly darkened.

Coagulated albumins are also slowly softened and digested but never distinctly liquefied. Gelatin is liquefied and blackened but certain strains (e. g., 130A, 130B, 132), were observed to effect merely a lowering of the solidification point of the gelatin, since after 5 days' incubation at

79 Lancet, 1917, 192, p. 688.
80 Traite pratique de Bacteriologie, 1913.
81 Brit. Med. Jour., 1916, I, p. 77.
82 Univ. of Calif. Pub. in Path., 1913, 2, p. 97.
83 Jour. Am. Med. Assn., 1908, 50, p. 929.
84 Lancet, 1917, I, p. 780.

37 C. with vigorous growth, as shown by gas, turbidity and blackening of the medium, the gelatin would still harden in the ice chest but become liquid again at room temperature, whereas the uninoculated control remained solid.

Indol is produced by all of the strains in mediums containing trytophane, thus confirming Smith.[83] Adamson[76] failed to demonstrate indol, however.

Pathogenicity.—All of the purified cultures were highly toxic; 0.001 c c of the culture or its filtrate almost invariably proved fatal for guinea-pigs, with symptoms of tetanus; 0:0001 c c frequently so. A commercial tetanus antitoxin prepared by the immunization of horses with toxin from culture 1 was equally protective against that from all other strains.

B. PUTRIFICUS

The early history of this species is all but hopelessly confused. Bienstock[85] in 1884 described B. putrificus coli, an obligate anaerobe, as the chief cause of cadaverous putrefaction. Tissier and Martelly[86] referred to B. putrificus coli of Bienstock as the principal agent in the putrefaction of meats, but their description better fits the organism now generally known as B. sporogenes. Klein,[87] in 1901, had described B. cadaveris sporogenes as closely related to B. putrificus and both Bienstock[88] and von Hibler[11] declared the two identical. Bienstock[88] admitted that the earlier descriptions were based on impure cultures; the presence of B. sporogenes may be fairly assumed. In 1906 he clearly defined B. putrificus as a nonpathogenic anaerobe, with oval terminal spores that "ne detruit que les proteines et ne s'attaque pas aux matieres hydrocarbonées," notwithstanding the fact that the proteolytic properties subsequently described sound like those of B. sporogenes.

Bienstock failed to find B. putrificus in the human intestine, but its occurrence there was affirmed by Passini,[89] Metchnikoff,[90] Rettger,[91] and others. Most of these authors agree as to the lack of fermentative power in the species, but there is wide disagreement as to its putrefactive ability. Rettger thought that this property grew weaker under laboratory cultivation, a view that is supported by Weinberg and Seguin.[2]

More recently Sturges and Rettger[92] pointed out that B. putrificus displays marked putrefactive properties only when associated with some other organism, but I was unable to confirm this for any of our strains in brain medium inoculated with B. coli or Staph. aureus.

Certain English writers[1] believe that many of the cultures of B. putrificus, so-called, are really mixtures of B. cochlearius or B. tertius with B. sporogenes."

85 Arch. f. Hyg., 1899, 36, p. 335; 1901, 39, p. 39; Ann. de l'Inst. Pasteur, 1899, 13, p. 854, and 1900, 14, p. 750.

86 Ann. de l'Inst. Pasteur 1902, 16, p. 865.

87 Centralbl. f. Bakteriol., I, O., 1901, 29, p. 991.

88 Ann. de l'Inst. Pasteur, 1906, 20, p. 407.

89 Ztschr. f. Hyg. u. Infektionskr., 1905, 49, p. 135.

90 Ann. de l'Inst. Pasteur, 1908, 22, p. 929.

91 Jour. Biol. Chem., 1908, 4, p. 45.

92 Jour. Bacteriol., 1919, 4, p. 171.

B. cochlearius is the name given by Douglas, Fleming, and Colebrook,[1] in 1919, to an organism that seems to correspond to Bienstock's B. putrificus as defined in the foregoing. But the English view of B. putrificus as a mixed culture fails to account for the lack of fermentative power described by other writers.

My study of 2 strains marked "B. putrificus" from Dr. W. S. Sturges of New Haven, Conn., and of one strain marked "B. cochlearius" from England, proves them identical. The prior use of the former term, not only by Bienstock in 1906, but as well by Sturges and Rettger, in 1919, for cultures of undoubted purity, establishes the validity of "B. putrificus"; "B. cochlearius" should be dropped.

B. putrificus 22 and 38.—These strains were received Feb. 2, 1917, from Dr. W. S. Sturges of Yale University, labeled, respectively, "B. putrificus No. 5" and "B. putrificus M." There was no evidence of aerobic or anaerobic contamination. No acid was formed in glucose, levulose, galactose, mannite, saccharose, salicin, glycerol or starch mediums and only a slight amount of gas. Growth in all mediums was slow. Notwithstanding the apparent purity of the strains, they were repurified during the period between April 15 and July 18, 1918, by five repeated isolations from blood-agar slants. The time involved indicates the patience required in repurifying even an obviously pure culture of B. putrificus.

A third culture that accompanied these two presented identical morphologic and cultural features but was unfortunately lost shortly after these were determined.

B. putrificus 147.—This was received from the Lister Institute, London, March 29, 1921. It was labeled "B. cochlearius No. 535—Strain I. M. I. H. C." There was no evidence of aerobic or anaerobic contamination, but the culture was repurified twice by the deep colony method, requiring 6 weeks of daily effort. This culture is identical morphologically and culturally with the 2 preceding.

Morphology.—B. putrificus is a slender, motile rod with terminal spores that are almost round. Spores are produced in all mediums that support growth, but never, in my experience, abundantly. Blood agar is the most favorable medium for sporulation. Gram's stain is retained imperfectly by the vegetative forms, but, curiously, when the rods stain, so also do the spores.

Colony Form.—In deep agar and on blood-agar slants under alkaline pyrogallol growth rarely appears before the fifth to seventh day when suddenly overnight, particularly in surface cultures, colonies of moderately large size may appear. Surface colonies are at first transparent, round dew drops; later they become opaque. On blood agar they are hemolytic. Deep agar colonies are at first minute opaque points; later, irregular opaque masses. They correspond to the description given by the Medical Research Committee [1] for B. cochlearius rather than to that of Weinberg and Sequin [2] for B. putrificus, as the latter probably studied cultures contaminated with B. sporogenes.

Physiology.—This species is without action on carbohydrates; all of the strains produced a slight alkalinity in sugar peptone medium, glucose, levulose, galactose, mannite, saccharose, lactose, salicin, glycerol, inulin, and starch having been tested. Broth cultures become slightly and slowly turbid and give rise to a little gas.

A definite but mild proteolysis occurs in suitable mediums. Deep meat and brain are softened and slightly blackened after several weeks. An intense blackening occurs in a few days in the presence of metallic iron. Sulphuretted hydrogen is obviously set free in abundance but the feeble proteolytic activity, as of B. tetani and B. welchii, fails to liberate sufficient ionizable iron from the tissues to precipitate the sulphide.

No visible change occurred in milk with my cultures, wherein their record differs from that of Weinberg and Sequin [2] for B. putrificus, but agrees with that of the Medical Research Committee [1] for B. cochlearius.

Gelatin was liquefied by all 3 strains and blackened regularly by No. 22, irregularly by No. 38, but not at all by No. 147. The last 2 cultures grew in gelatin only on heavy inoculation; in some trials no growth at all could be secured with No. 147, judging by the lack of turbidity and production. The Medical Research Committee's statement of nonliquefaction of gelatin by B. cochlearius needs to be qualified by our knowledge of the difficulty of securing growth in gelatin with their strain.

Thus B. putrificus presents an almost complete analogy in its carbohydrate and protein metabolism with that of B. tetani but B. putrificus is a much more difficult micro-organism to cultivate. Deep brain and meat cultures often show no visible evidence of growth on several days' incubation; however, I have repeatedly made the peculiar observation with all of the above strains that if they are then stirred with a sterile platinum rod and reincubated, a moderately vigorous ebullition of gas occurs in a few hours. It seems that growth is so slow that the medium becomes supersaturated.

Pathogenicity.—No claims for pathogenicity have been made for B. putrificus; broth cultures of my strains were nonvirulent for rabbits in doses of 5 c c or less by the intravenous route, and for guinea-pigs in doses of 1 c c by subcutaneous injection. Lack of pathogenicity differentiates B. putrificus from B. tetani.

B. TETANOMORPHUS

Obligately anaerobic, nonpathogenic, "pseudotetanus" bacilli were described by Sanfelice,[93] in 1893, by Tavel,[94] in 1898, and the Latinized "B. pseudotetani

[93] Ztschr. f. Hyg. u. Infektionskr., 1893, 14, p. 339.
[94] Centralbl. f. Bakteriol., 1898, 23, p. 538.

Tavel" and "B. pseudotetanicus Migula" appear in Lehmann and Neumann's "Atlas and Grundriss der Bakteriologie"[95] as synonymous with B. sphaericus. It is impossible to identify the descriptions of any of these with the forms known today.

"B. tetanomorphus" was first described by McIntosh and Fildes as type 9; the published accounts[1] are confirmed in part, and in part not confirmed, in the writer's study of the following strain.

B. tetanomorphus 149.—This strain was received March 29, 1921, as No. 543 strain 259 E. 3 from the Lister Institute. It was said to have been "isolated from a septic wound in 1916." There was no evidence of aerobic or anaerobic impurity; notwithstanding the culture was repurified, twice by the deep agar colony method and lastly by the surface colony method, requiring in all 4 weeks. The morphology, physiology, and nonpathogenicity of the repurified culture proved the same as of the original.

Morphology.—B. tetanomorphus is described as closely resembling B. tetani in the morphology of its spores, hence the name; in the above strain this is true of certain individual rods, but the majority of the spores are slightly oval rather than perfectly round in outline. They are usually located terminally but often subterminally, too, and are formed abundantly in mediums not containing monosaccharides.

Colony Form.—Deep agar colonies are small, opaque, irregular points, not wooly or branched. Surface colonies on blood agar are minute dew-drop-like points, or they may form a spreading, confluent growth according to the consistency of the medium.

Physiology.—Considerable gas is set free in nearly all mediums that support growth. Deep brain and meat medium are not noticeably blackened or digested even on the addition of metallic iron. It is evident that very little H_2S is set free.

My record differs from that of the Medical Research Committee in respect to gelatin. In three separate tests active growth was proved by abundant gas formation within 24 hours, and these cultures hardened again in the ice chest daily for 4 or 5 days, but thereafter remained liquid. The species is therefore mildly gelatinolytic. Unlike most of the anaerobes it fails to blacken gelatin during its growth.

No change occurs in milk, and there is no action on lactose, saccharose, salicin, glycerol or inulin. Glucose is fermented.

Glucose fermentation and failure to blacken brain medium containing metallic iron differentiate B. tetanomorphus from B. putrificus and the fermentation of lactose and salicin differentiates B. sphenoides, which B. tetanomorphus resembles in morphology and in its action on brain medium.

[95] Lehmann, 1912.

Pathogenicity.—B. tetanomorphus has no known significance as a pathogenic micro-organism. Subcutaneous injection of guinea-pigs with 1 c c and repeated intravenous injections of rabbits with 2 c c of 24-48-hour glucose-broth cultures proved quite harmless.

BACILLUS SPHENOIDES

The original discovery and description of this organism is attributed to Douglas, Fleming and Colebrook,[1] in 1919, they having isolated 3 pure cultures from war wounds. The name is derived from the somewhat wedge-like shape of the rods at certain stages in the formation of spores.

I have studied a single culture, presumably one of the foregoing 3.

B. sphenoides 146.—This strain was received March 29, 1921, as a sealed glass tube of meat mash culture from the Lister Institute. It was labeled "B. sphenoides No. 507 Strain 'Tholly.'"

There was no evidence of contamination; notwithstanding, after a preliminary examination for morphology, nonpathogenicity, and cultural reactions in brain, glucose broth, gelatin, and milk mediums, the culture was repurified, 3 times by the deep agar method and once by the blood-agar surface colony method and the correspondence of the reactions in the repurified culture with the initial ones determined.

Morphology.—B. sphenoides is a small, motile, gram-positive rod, fusiform in the vegetative stage, in which the organisms occur in pairs, or even short chains. Spores are formed freely in mediums not containing fermentable carbohydrates in excess, notably in blood-agar surface cultures under alkaline pyrogallol. The spores are at first subterminal but become clearly terminal as they mature and are almost round. The opposite end of the rod maintains its pointed form. The spores are set free in great abundance. The morphology of this organism is believed to be unique among anaerobes.

Colony Form.—In deep 1% agar, isolated colonies are minute opaque disks. On the surface of blood agar they are first like minute dew drops but become whitish and somewhat opaque when older. Hemolysis occurs.

Physiology.—Growth in brain medium is accompanied by turbidity and gas production, but there is little or no change in the consistency of the tissue. No blackening occurs even in the presence of added iron; sulphuretted hydrogen apparently is not set free. Neither is indol produced. Growth in gelatin occurs with blackening and gas production but without liquefaction. Considerable gas is formed from milk but neither coagulation, as observed occasionally by the English workers, nor digestion of the casein, occurred in my culture.

Glucose, lactose, and salicin are fermented with acid and gas production; saccharose, inulin, and glycerol are not fermented by my strain. The English workers reported the fermentation of maltose and galactose by all their strains and of mannite, saccharose, dextrin and starch also by 2 strains.

Pathogenicity.—B. sphenoides is quite nonpathogenic in doses of 1 c c injected subcutaneously into guinea-pigs and 2 c c injected intravenously into rabbits.

BACILLUS TERTIUS

B. tertius was named by Henry[96] as the third most frequent anaerobe encountered in war wounds. It was supposed by him to be identical with an organism found by Rodella[97] in the stools of infants, in 1902, "von Hibler's[11] bacillus"[9] and Fleming's[98] "bacillus y." In addition to the foregoing, good descriptions appear in the work of the Medical Research Committee[1] and Weinberg and Seguin.[2]

I have examined a single strain as follows:

B. tertius 148.—This strain was received March 29, 1921, from the Lister Institute, under the label "B. tertius No. 542—Strain Renard." It was said to have been isolated from a case of gaseous gangrene in 1918. An aerobic coccal contamination was eliminated by boiling a deep brain subculture 2 minutes. After an initial study of the morphology, cultural reactions, and nonpathogenicity, the culture, in spite of its apparent initial freedom from anaerobic impurity, was repurified twice by the deep agar method and once by the blood-agar surface colony method. The properties of the repurified culture were identical with those of the original.

Morphology.—B. Tertius is a slender, gram-positive rod, with elongated oval terminal spores. Blood-agar surface cultures show the morphology most typically. The form of its spores separates B. tertius from all other anaerobes except B. spermoides, from which it may be differentiated by its sluggish motility, failure to blacken iron brain, and to liquefy gelatin.

Colony Form.—Deep agar colonies are minute, compact, opaque, lenticular masses. Surface colonies on blood agar are hemolytic and resemble minute dew drops in their transparency and shape when young. They become more opaque on prolonged incubation.

Physiology.—There is little or no visible action, aside from abundant gas production, on brain medium or other coagulated proteins. Neither brain nor meat is blackened even in the presence of metallic iron. Gelatin is not liquefied, but gas is produced and the precipitate blackened. Milk is fermented with gas and acid formation. In the constricted tube a soft clot forms below the marble seal; the clot never becomes heavily gas blown as with B. welchii, and the fermentation would not be characterized as "stormy." The clot is not subsequently digested. No indol is produced in peptone broth.

[96] Jour. Path. & Bacteriol., 1917, 21, p. 344.
[97] Ztschr. f. Hyg. u. Infektionskr., 1902, 39, p. 201.
[98] Lancet, 1915, 2, p. 376.

B. tertius ferments glucose, lactose, saccharose, and salicin, and not inulin and glycerol, according to my study.

Pathogenicity.—B. tertius is nonpathogenic for guinea-pigs in doses of 1 c c of glucose-broth cultures given subcutaneously and for rabbits in doses of 2 c c given intravenously.

SUMMARY

A critical study of the taxonomy of the obligate anaerobes based on a collection of carefully and repeatedly purified strains, secured from various sources, is presented.

Emphasis is laid on certain purity as an underlying principle in the classification of the anaerobes. Both surface colony and deep colony methods of isolation were practiced successfully, but experience teaches the superiority of the latter for most cultures. The great frequency of misnamed and anaerobically contaminated cultures among those received from various laboratories is pointed out.

Various criteria for identification are discussed in the order of their proper utilization, with respect to their significance, technic and limitations as follows: Morphology, action on proteins, and action on carbohydrates. These points are utilized in setting up a differential key that may be used in the identification of the forms most commonly encountered.

The last section of the article discusses the details of origin, purification, differentiation and identification of these cultures: B. bifermentans, 3 strains; B. welchii, 6 strains; B. centrosporogenes (n.sp.), 4 strains; B. butyricus, 2 strains; B. botulinus, type A, 2 strains; B. botulinus, type B, 3 strains; B. sporogenes, 24 strains; B. histolyticus, 1 strain; B. chauvœi, 1 strain; Vibrion septique, 7 strains; B. novyi, 3 strains; B. tetani, 7 strains; B. putrificus, 3 strains; B. tetanomorphus, 1 strain; B. sphenoides, 1 strain; B. tertius, 1 strain.

PRESENCE OF B. LACTIMORBI IN THE THROATS OF CATS

Roger G. Perkins and James K Shen

From the Department of Hygiene and Bacteriology, Western Reserve School of Medicine

A number of articles and reports have appeared in the last few years dealing with the appearance of diphtheria bacilli in the nose and throat of cats and drawing the inference that these animals are more or less frequent carriers of diphtheria.

In view of the findings in human throats, noted in a previous article,[1] indicating the danger of making an incorrect diagnosis of diphtheria on account of the presence of B. lactimorbi, it occurred to one of us that some of these reports might be due to morphologic appearances of a similarly deceptive nature. To determine the truth or falsity of this theory cultures were made from two series of cats, and all organisms growing out on serum with the formation of metachromatic granules were isolated. It was originally intended to carry out the same technic with other groups of cats, but the results in the first two series made this unnecessary.

One set of cats was examined at the kennels of the Humane Society of Cleveland, and the other in the Department of Pharmacology of Western Reserve Medical School. The first series consisted of 12 and the second of 10 cats.

Swabs were made from the noses and throats and smeared on blood serum, which was incubated for 18 hours at 37 C. Stained preparations were examined for granules. As B. lactimorbi forms spores, all apparently positive cultures were heated in suspension to 80 C. for 10 minutes and inoculated on glycerol agar.

By this method all nonspore-forming organisms were killed, and only the aerobic spore bearers remained. These consisted of 2 groups, one, as might be expected, belonging to the general type usually spoken of as "hay bacillus," though known to represent more than one variety, while the others were typical B. lactimorbi. It is interesting to note, in connection with the hay bacillus group, that many of the forms

Received for publication Dec. 30, 1921.

[1] Perkins, Roger G., and Spreng, D. S.: Jour. Infect. Dis., 1921, 29, p. 513.

contained definite metachromatic granules, though the morphology of course did not suggest diphtheria, and should not cause confusion.

In the first series, 12 animals, B. lactimorbi was isolated in 2 instances, and in the second series, 10 animals, in 5 instances. It seems probable that the larger number in the second series is due to the fact that the cats, which were undergoing a feeding experiment, were in closer contact, and that there was more opportunity for a generalized kennel infection than in the first series in which the animals were separated.

There are, of course, two main possibilities of error: first, that the medium itself was infected with this spore bearer, which then grew out under incubator conditions. Blank tubes incubated under the same conditions and for the same period, remained sterile, and the rest of the batch, which was used in a routine manner did not show any of the organisms. The second possibility is that as this was the organism which had recently been studied in the laboratory there might have been an infection of the tubes in handling. With the exception of the stock cultures in the refrigerator none of these organisms had been available for months and were not under investigation at the time of this special study.

It would appear therefore that in Cleveland there is a widespread distribution of B. lactimorbi, under conditions that make it a frequent contamination accessible to the nose and throat, possibly in dust, or on food. Since it is nonpathogenic, the only importance from the public health standpoint is the danger of false interpretation of the findings, with all the consequences which may follow such error.

In some of the articles referred to there has been described a definite lesion of the throat or nose and the isolation of an organism which was identified as B. diphtheriae and proved to be toxic. It is most interesting that this should be found true, even in a limited number of cases, but the fact of proof that true diphtheria may be found in sickness of animals is likely to lead to more cursory examinations, and the determination of the diagnosis on a morphologic basis alone; the results of our investigations show that this is a distinct danger.

No descriptions of organisms of this type have been published except as found in the Southwest, in the original work of Jordan and Harris, and in Cleveland. It would be of value to learn how wide is the true distribution, and the authors hope that these two articles will stimulate investigations in other parts of the country to determine whether this group is common to all the states or is confined to a limited district.

SUMMARY

The occurrence of B. lactimorbi in the throat of cats is described, and the danger of this bacillus being mistaken for B. diphtheriæ is emphasized.

OBSERVATIONS ON THE PREPARATION OF TOXIN-ANTITOXIN MIXTURE

P. G. Heineman and Charles R. Hixson

From the Research Laboratories, United States Standard Products Company, Woodworth, Wis.

Immunization against diphtheria by toxin-antitoxin has been eminently successful, and this means that another milestone has been passed in the efforts to eradicate the disease. Successful immunization depends on proper balance of toxin and antitoxin. The toxin is the active agent in producing immunity,. while the antitoxin enters into a more or less firm combination with the toxin, thus protecting the system against serious toxic reaction. If the combination between toxin and antitoxin were a firm one, as in many chemical compounds, the excess toxin alone would be of immunizing value. The addition of antitoxin merely enables the system to bear a larger amount of toxin than would be possible without this addition. It is imperative that an effective toxin-antitoxin mixture should be so balanced as to have a slight excess of unneutralized toxin. A completely neutralized mixture has less immunizing value than a slightly toxic one, and a mixture containing an excess of antitoxin is of still smaller value.

Directions for the preparation of the toxin-antitoxin mixture are given by the Hygienic Laboratory, in Washington. According to these directions, the following steps are to be taken:

1. The toxin must be aged for at least three months to insure relative stability.

2. The L+ dose of the toxin is determined against the standard antitoxin issued by the Hygienic Laboratory, and the potency of the lot of serum to be used is determined against the L+ dose of the toxin.

3. A tentative mixture is prepared which is allowed to stand for 24 hours before testing; a toxin is used which contains at least three L + doses for one human dose, and the amount of antitoxin necessary to produce the desired result is calculated and mixed with the toxin.

4. Two tests are made. The first one consists of injecting subcutaneously one human dose into a guinea-pig weighing 250 gm. The second test consists of injecting 5 human doses subcutaneously into a similar guinea-pig. The mixture is properly balanced if the guinea-pig receiving one human dose shows no ill effect, while the one receiving 5 human doses develops paralysis not earlier than the tenth day after

Received for publication Jan. 23, 1922.

injection and dies subsequently within 35 days after injection. A toxin-antitoxin mixture of this quality therefore contains considerably less than one minimum lethal dose of free toxin in 5 human doses. The excess toxicity is distinct, but not large enough to cause serious symptoms.

5. If the guinea-pigs die before the appointed time, the excess of toxin is too large and a further quantity of antitoxin has to be added. The mixture is then tested again. This procedure may have to be repeated several times before a satisfactory mixture is obtained. If by chance the mixture is overneutralized, addition of toxin is not advisable.

6. The toxin-antitoxin mixture is then filled in containers. The contents of several containers are tested for sterility and are injected into guinea-pigs in the same manner as before. After four weeks another pair of guinea-pigs is injected. The first pair is kept under observation for five weeks and the second pair for one week. If the reactions on the guinea-pigs are satisfactory, the mixture is ready for use.[1]

Aging of the toxin is necessary to guard against rapid deterioration with loss of potency. Unfortunately, all toxins do not deteriorate at the same rate. Some lose toxicity more rapidly than others. As a rule, a toxin, when not sufficiently aged, deteriorates more rapidly than does antitoxin, and in this case the toxin-antitoxin mixture soon loses potency. Toxins set aside for preparation of toxin-antitoxin mixture should therefore be tested for L + dose several times until the value remains reasonably constant.

The L + dose of a toxin is tested against the standard antitoxin issued by the Hygienic Laboratory. As a matter of fact, however, a certain antitoxin may give slightly different values when tested against L + doses of different toxins. This is readily understood when Ehrlich's theory of the structure of the toxin molecule is considered. According to this theory the toxin molecule is composed chiefly of the prototoxoid (nontoxic), the toxin (the truly toxic portion) and the toxone (causing postdiphtheritic paralysis). Antitoxin combines more firmly with prototoxoid than with toxin, and more firmly with toxin than with toxone. If, therefore, the prototoxoid fraction in a given toxin is larger than in another one, the former requires more antitoxin to leave one M L D unneutralized than the latter. Although the determination of the value of the antitoxin to be used against the

[1] Since this paper went to press the directions given by the Hygienic Laboratory have been changed and the toxicity of the product is increased thereby.

L + dose of the toxin may not be absolutely necessary, it is advisable and guards against overneutralization.

A test of the tentative mixture of toxin and antitoxin is not made before 24 hours have elapsed in order to allow toxin and antitoxin to combine. A period of 24 hours, however, does not seem to be sufficient. It is possible that a fairly firm combination of antitoxin with prototoxoid may obtain in 24 hours, but the combination between toxin and antitoxin is slower than the former and between toxone and antitoxin still slower. It follows that the death of guinea-pigs injected with five human doses of the mixture must be more and more deferred in proportion to the age of the mixture. After a certain period, which has not been determined and which probably varies in different mixtures, a short-lived stability may obtain. Great caution is necessary in adding antitoxin in small quantity to avoid overneutralization, even though tests, made after the mixture has been prepared, may indicate satisfactory balance. Furthermore, each time an additional quantity of antitoxin is added, the period required for complete combination with toxin is delayed. When finally the reaction of the mixture on guinea-pigs seems satisfactory, disappointment may result in that after a lapse of time the test guinea-pigs fail to die within the required period.

The calculation of the amount of antitoxin required for properly balancing a toxin-antitoxin mixture is accompanied by several complications. If the number of antitoxic units and L + doses of toxin is the same, one M L D for each L + dose should theoretically remain unneutralized and the mixture would be far too toxic. This obviously can but rarely be true for several reasons. The most important one of these reasons is the fact that an exact unitage is usually not determined. The common practice is not to determine the potency of a serum closer than 50 or 25 units apart. This would, for example, mean that an 800 unit serum actually may contain 800 to 849 or 800 to 824 units. A second complication lies in the varying susceptibility of guinea-pigs. While it may be permissible to consider the potency of a serum ascertained when the guinea-pigs barely survive the 96-hour period, as a rule, the value is taken from guinea-pigs surviving a variable period beyond 96 hours. The serum therefore in reality contains a distinct excess of potency over the claimed value. Finally, there is some uncertainty as to the actual value of the antitoxin, since the original standard of Ehrlich has been changed. While Ehrlich's standard called for the control guinea-pig's death in 4 days, the new standard calls for its death in 3 days. The latter standard leaves, therefore, an uncertain excess of potency in the antitoxin, which is a wise measure for safety, but upsets calculations somewhat, because it is not known whether a definite relation exists between the amount of toxin necessary to kill a guinea-pig in three days and the amount necessary to kill in 4 days. As a matter of fact, an exceedingly large amount of toxin rarely kills a guinea-pig in less than 36 to 40 hours. It seems almost unnecessary to add that by using a low potency antitoxin for toxin-antitoxin mixtures the required quantity can be calculated and measured with less chance of overneutralization than by using a high unit antitoxin.

TABLE 1.

RESULTS OF INOCULATION OF GUINEA-PIGS WITH TOXIN-ANTITOXIN MIXTURE

No.	L+ Doses	Units Antitoxin	Results of Inoculation
1	6,876	6,450	After 24 hours; died in 7½ and 9½ days After 30 days; died in 15 and 11 days After 106 days; died in 19 and 19½ days
2	8,700	8,180	After 24 hours; died in 17 and 19 days After 9 days; died in 19 and 25 days After 19 days; died in 20 and 24 days After 30 days; died in 19 and 25 days After 46 days; died in 24 and 25 days
3	8,085	7,550	After 24 hours; died in 18 and 26 days After 28 days; died in 27 and 26 days
4	14,286	14,540	After 24 hours; died in 22 and 19 days After 11 days; died in 16 and 24 days After 24 days; died in 25 and 27 days
5	24,837	22,575	After 24 hours; died in 20 and 25 days After 10 days; died in 25 and 26 days After 20 days; died in 28 and 27 days After 51 days; died in 29 and 28 days
6	21,000	21,395	After 24 hours; died in 15 and 19 days After 11 days; died in 22 and 21 days After 26 days; died in 25 and 27 days

Table 1 gives the amounts of L + doses and antitoxic units of several selected lots of toxin-antitoxin mixture. The results of comprehensive tests of these lots have shown clearly that satisfactory mixtures were obtained. Dead guinea-pigs were always examined for toxin reactions and possible infections.

In some instances the number of L + doses apparently exceeded that of antitoxic units. Sometimes the difference is marked. In other cases the reverse is true. Since the same lot of antitoxin was used in all lots, it seems obvious that the variation must lie in the constitution of the toxin. The variation of quantitative relation between the number of antitoxic units and L + doses may be explained by assuming that the larger the prototoxoid group of the toxin molecule is, the larger is the amount of antitoxin required. In no case, however, is the number of antitoxic units as great as would be necessary were the units accurately determined, because there was an excess of potency in the antitoxin. In other words, the excess toxin, as shown by guinea-pig tests, is actually smaller than the relation of antitoxin to toxin suggests.

In the table appear the records of the guinea-pigs which received five human doses. The deaths of the guinea-pigs were somewhat delayed as the age of the mixture increased. The differences between these periods were not very large, but sufficiently so to suggest a slow combination between toxin and antitoxin. As the combining process proceeds death is deferred, disregarding a similar delay caused by gradual deterioration of both components.

One lot which is not recorded in the table had the effect of shortening the periods between injections and the death of the guinea-pigs. The results were: After 24 hours they died in 6½ and 7 days; after 9 days they died in 8 and 7½ days; after 22 days they died in 5 and 6 days; after 66 days both died in 4 days; after 73 days they died in 2 and 5 days; after 86 days they died in 2 and 3 days. This example is interesting because the second period was greater than the first, but after that the periods grow shorter.

An experiment was made by mixing 4 small lots, one of which did not possess sufficient toxicity to kill a guinea-pig when 5 human doses were injected. There was loss of weight for 10 days followed by increasing weight and recovery. The other 3 lots were fatal to guinea-pigs in 6, 2 and 32 days, respectively. The mixture was tested after 5 days. The guinea-pigs died in 22 and 24 days; 11 days later after 24 and 19 days; 20 days later they died after 18 and 25 days; 25 days later they died in 20 and 22 days; 30 days later they died in 22 and 24 days; 35 days later they died in 21 and 30 days; 60 days later they died in 25 and 29 days. The mixture was fairly stable, but it is doubtful whether such mixtures will always yield dependable results.

After toxin and antitoxin have been mixed there are three possibilities conceivable which may influence the result. These possibilities are:

1. Both toxin and antitoxin deteriorate in approximately the same proportion.
2. The antitoxin deteriorates more rapidly than the toxin.
3. The toxin deteriorates more rapidly than the antitoxin.

Under conditions when antitoxin and toxin deteriorate in the same proportion a simple consideration shows what will happen. The total toxicity and the total antitoxin decrease as time progresses with a corresponding decrease of potency of the mixture. As it is known that both toxin and antitoxin deteriorate in time, a reasonable time limit is placed on the potency of toxin-antitoxin mixtures. The custom at present is to estimate this limit as six months.

The second condition, namely, the more rapid deterioration of antitoxin, is likely to occur rarely, since experience has shown that, as a rule, antitoxin is more stable than toxin. However, such a condition is conceivable and cannot be entirely excluded. The consequence would be an increasing relative toxicity of the mixture.

The third condition probably occurs more frequently than the previous two. When the toxin deteriorates more rapidly than the antitoxin the loss of potency of the mixture is relatively rapid.

Several lots of toxin-antitoxin mixture increased in toxicity as time advanced. An example has been mentioned in which the rate of increasing toxicity may not have been negligible. This puzzling phenomenon is difficult to explain, because the antitoxin used was of considerable age and had been tested several times in order to show its stability. The following explanation is offered as tentative; it may not pass the test of time, but may stimulate further investigation.

Ehrlich assumed that the toxin molecule consists of prototoxoid, toxin and toxone. It is not probable that any two toxins are composed of these portions in the same proportion. But does one lot of toxin always contain only one kind of molecules, or are there sometimes in the same lot molecules whose fractions differ in proportion? When antitoxin is added to toxin, it combines first with the prototoxoid group, next with the toxin group and lastly with the toxone group. This process takes time; how much, it would be venturesome to suggest, but probably the time is not the same in all cases, depending on the constitution of the toxin. Since antitoxin combines first with the prototoxoid group it would seem that the larger this group is the shorter would be the time required for combination.

If it is assumed that some toxins are not homogeneous, antitoxin would combine with the three groups, but on standing it would find some molecules with a larger prototoxoid group than the combined molecules possess. The antitoxin would then go over in part to the newly found molecules, leaving more toxin and toxone free. While this process is going on, the toxicity of the mixture increases. Under varying conditions the increase of toxicity might be relatively slow or rapid. This view is supported by some observations which seemed to show that portions taken from different layers of a mixture gave somewhat different results when tested on guinea-pigs. If the antitoxin combines with molecules of a small prototoxoid group first there is no change in toxicity.

Another possibility is suggested by the fact that toxin deteriorates. During this process the prototoxoid group may increase at the expense of the toxin and toxone fractions, involving a decrease of toxicity. If the enlargement of the prototoxoid group is proportionately greater than the deterioration of the toxin group, the toxicity of the mixture would increase, despite deterioration of the toxin group. In other words, some antitoxin combined with the toxin and toxone groups would pass over to molecules with increased prototoxoid. A condition of this kind becomes more complicated, since probably the rate of deterioration of toxin molecules does not progress at the same rate. However, the increase of toxicity would probably be relatively small.

It has been stated before that toxin should not be added to compensate for overneutralization of a mixture. This might be permissible if the identical toxin were used, although there are no experimental data on this point. If a different toxin is added, the stability of the mixture would be materially injured by gradual movement of antitoxin from molecules with small prototoxoid to those with large ones. This also, as a rule, would involve an increase of toxicity.

The theory suggested is based on the following assumptions: (1) the correctness of Ehrlich's theory of the constitution of the toxin molecule; (2 the greater avidity of antitoxin for prototoxoid than for toxin, and the greater avidity of antitoxin for toxin than for toxone; (3) the relative firmness of the combination between antitoxin and prototoxoid as compared with its combination with toxin and toxone; (4) at best, combination between toxin and antitoxin is a slow process when compared with chemical reactions, and (5) not all toxins are entirely homogeneous.

The theory seems to offer a tentative explanation of some puzzling phenomena observed in the action of toxin-antitoxin mixtures. The necessity of exerting the utmost care in the preparation of toxin-antitoxin mixtures is emphasized by the fact that occasionally a mixture which has given apparently satisfactory tests later increases in toxicity. Toxins should be well ripened, and both toxin and antitoxin should be tested repeatedly until the values obtained are fairly uniform. With care the toxicity probably will never increase to a point at which it becomes really dangerous, but local and systemic reactions may be severe if the excess toxin is too large or becomes so after standing. The greatest aid in obtaining a safe preparation is time. The longer the period of test—within reasonable limits—the more dependable, as a rule, is the product.

AN EPIZOOTIC AMONG GUINEA-PIGS DUE TO A PARATYPHOID B BACILLUS

Katharine M. Howell and Oscar T. Schultz

Morris Institute for Medical Research, Michael Reese Hospital, Chicago

Guinea-pigs are subject to spontaneous infection by a variety of bacteria; such infections have been studied by Holman,[1] who emphasized the bearing that natural infecting agents may have on experimental bacteriologic studies in which the guinea-pig is used. Besides the spontaneous infections which cause the death of single animals, the guinea-pig is subject to infections which may quickly assume epizootic proportions and carry off in a short time a stock which it has taken years to build up. The epizootics, as a rule, are of one of three types: respiratory disease, due usually to B. bronchisepticus (Ferry,[2] Smith [3]), but sometimes to pneumococcus (Smith [4]); a rapidly fatal disease of the hemorrhagic septicemia type; and a disease to which the name pseudotuberculosis frequently has been applied. An epizootic of the last named type of our stock has been studied, and the results are reported because it was found to be due to an organism of the paratyphoid B group.

The bacteria of this group appear to be of constantly increasing importance in animal and human pathology, and the problem of determining relations between the various strains which have been investigated in different parts of the world has become a most bewildering one. So long as we had to limit our consideration to the extremes of the colon-typhoid group, B. coli and B. typhosus, and to the lactose nonfermenting intermediates which ferment dextrose and which do or do not acidify milk, the classification appeared simple. Separation of four main species, B. paratyphosus A, B. paratyphosus B, B. enteritidis, and B. cholerae suis, still appeared clear enough, but with the passage of time there has been isolated an increasing number of strains which can be distinguished only by immunologic methods, and the nomenclature has become so extensive that it is a difficult matter to correlate

Received for publication, Jan. 25, 1922.

1 Jour. Med. Research, 1916, 35, p. 151.
2 Veterinary Jour., 1912, 68, p. 376.
3 Jour. Med. Research, 1913, 29, p. 291.
4 Ibid., 1905, 13, p. 341.

organisms and names. B. cholerae suis, B. suipestifer, B. aertryckii, B. suiseptica, and B. suicida all appear to be the same organism; to paratyphoid A and B has been added paratyphoid C, an unfortunate style of nomenclature; many strains have received nonspecific names derived from the observer or from the locality. The alkali formers in milk, with the exception of paratyphoid B, were supposed to be distributed chiefly among lower animals, and attempts have been made to place those which occur in rodents in a distinct group. Although many members of the intermediate group are identical culturally, they may show quite distinct immunologic differences, and the question arises whether such differences should constitute a valid basis for species differentiation in the face of biologic identities in other respects, or whether such differences are only temporary responses to host environment which tend to disappear with prolonged cultivation. The possible relation of some of the widely distributed and more recently described human pathogens to the strains of animal origin is also a matter of importance.

BACTERIA OF THE INTERMEDIATE GROUP IN GUINEA-PIGS

The earlier literature relating to the occurrence of bacteria of the colon-typhoid intermediate group in guinea-pigs has been reviewed by Holman.[1] They appear to be the chief, if not the sole, cause of so-called pseudotuberculosis in these animals; they have also been encountered in pneumonia and in infectious metritis of guinea-pigs. The older writers place the guinea-pig organisms indiscriminately in the enteritidis or the hog-cholera groups. Ferry[5] isolated 17 organisms which he placed in the B. enteritidis group, no attempt being made to identify them further; some of these were derived from guinea-pigs, but how many is not stated. Krumwiede, Valentine and Kohn[6] studied a number of guinea-pig strains isolated by themselves as well as strains received from other investigators. They found the rodent strains to be distinct from the suipestifer and paratyphoid B groups; from their own animals they isolated also some strains of the enteritidis type. Tenbroeck[7] says that most of the guinea-pig strains which he has encountered belong to the enteritidis group. Busson[8] isolated paratyphoid organisms from two guinea-pig epizootics of the hemorrhagic septicemia type. The character of disease with which organisms of this group are associated is, therefore, quite varied, and the various diseases are world-wide in their distribution. In addition to accounts relating specifically to paratyphoid bacilli and to diseases caused by them in guinea-pigs, there are numerous references in the literature which make casual mention of the interference with other work caused by the presence of these bacteria, and the word "ubiquitous" is frequently applied to them.

[5] Jour. Path. & Bacteriol., 1914, 18, p. 445.
[6] Jour. Med. Research, 1919, 39, p. 449.
[7] Jour. Exper. Med., 1920, 32, p. 19.
[8] Centralbl. f. Bakteriol., 1, O., 1921, 86, p. 101.

RELATIONS WITHIN THE INTERMEDIATE GROUP

The question of the relation of the various paratyphoid B organisms of animal origin to each other and of those of human origin to those derived from animals is an important one, which deserves greater elucidation. From the standpoint of the prevention of disease among lower animals it is essential to know whether the members of the group are readily transmissible from one species to another, or whether there is any limitation of strains to host species in spite of cultural and immunologic similarities. From the standpoint of human disease it is important to know whether infection of human beings by strains of animal origin is possible in the ordinary course of events, or only as food infections; a further possibility exists that a strain which has been derived from a lower animal might gain a foothold in the intestinal tract of a human being, adapt itself to its new surroundings, and, after spread by those channels through which typhoid is disseminated, become pathogenic for other human beings into which it might be introduced. From the purely biologic standpoint the matter of strain relations within the group is of the utmost interest and has a direct bearing on questions relating to mutation and variation among bacterial species.

Of human strains supposedly different from the four type species, Hirschfeld's[9] B. paratyphosus C belongs serologically to the hog-cholera group according to Tenbroeck,[10] although the Hirschfeld organism ferments dulcite and arabinose readily. Bacilli of human origin of the Voldagsen type and several other strains from epidemics of food infection were studied by Manteufel, Zschucke and Berger[11] and were found also to belong to the suipestifer group; they conclude that it is impossible to determine the human or animal origin of a strain from its cultural or serologic characters.

Although B. suipestifer is the group representative most frequently encountered in swine, Spray,[12] Doyle and Spray,[13] Tenbroeck[7] and others have isolated strains like the paratyphoids A and B of human origin.

Krumwiede, Valentine and Kohn,[6] who concluded that the strains of rodent origin form a distinct group, found 13 of their 15 guinea-pig strains, 2 of 4 mouse strains, 1 rabbit strain and 1 cat strain to be identical and different from B. suipestifer and human B. paratyphosus B. The series of organisms studied by them did not, however, include any of the so-called paratyphoid B strains from other animal sources, so that the possibility of affinity with such strains is not excluded. The tendency to consider the bacteria associated with pseudotuberculosis in rodents a distinct group is apparent in the older literature relating to this subject, in which the name B. pseudotuberculosis rodentium is applied to the organism. Klein[14] has recently reported a study in which he

[9] Lancet, 1919, 1, p. 296.

[10] Jour. Exper. Med., 1920, 32, p. 33.

[11] Centralbl. f. Bakteriol., 1, O., 1921, 86, p. 214.

[12] Jour. Infect. Dis., 1920, 26, p. 340.

[13] Ibid., 27, p. 245.

[14] Centralbl. f. Bacteriol., 1, O., 1921, 86, p. 564.

compared a strain, isolated from an epizootic of pseudotuberculosis among guinea-pigs in Cologne, with an original culture of B. pseudotuberculosis rodentium and one of B. paratyphosus B of human origin. His own strain and the original pseudotuberculosis strain did not ferment dextrose. The original strain was not agglutinated by human para B antiserum, whereas his own was agglutinated by this serum. He concludes that the organisms causing pseudotuberculosis in guinea-pigs belong to the paratyphoid B group and that the strain isolated by himself is intermediate between B. pseudotuberculosis rodentium and human B. paratyphosus B. Whether the inability to ferment dextrose, if this is a fixed character, warrants the placing of these organisms in the colon-typhoid intermediate group appears questionable. Litch and Meyer [15] accept the existence of a rodent group, in which they place the organism isolated by them from an epizootic among rabbits. However, their own agglutination results hardly seem to warrant such a definite conclusion, since the relation between their rabbit strain and 1 guinea-pig strain, on the one hand, and 3 avian strains, 2 swine strains and 1 human paratyphoid B strain on the other, appear closer than the relation of 3 other guinea-pig strains, 1 rabbit strain and 1 mouse strain to their rodent group. The organisms causing hemorrhagic septicemia in guinea-pigs have usually been placed, together with the bacteria of hemorrhagic septicemia in other animals species, in the nonmotile pasteurella group of Lignières, but Busson's [8] study indicates that this is not a homogeneous group; furthermore, the organisms isolated by him from 2 epizootics among guinea-pigs separated by a time interval of 5 years and characterized by the anatomic lesions of hemorrhagic septicemia, belonged to the paratyphoid group. His strains from the 2 epizootics gave only slight cross agglutination, and one formed gas in dextrose while the other did not. Plasaj and Pribram [16] have studied the bacteria of the hemorrhagic septicemia group in the Král collection. They also find that this group includes a heterogeneous variety of organisms, some of which are nonmotile, others motile. For some of the latter, like B. cuniculicida, B. cavisepticum, B. suisepticum, B. suicida, the close relation to or identity with members of the colon-typhoid intermediates is admitted, yet they are retained in the hemorrhagic septicemia group under the subheading B. multoseptica. The tendency to name bacterial species according to the diseases of lower animals with which the bacteria may be associated is a regrettable one, and the bewildering confusion to which it may lead is well illustrated by the hemorrhagic septicemia bacteria. An organism which in the beginning of an epizootic causes the more chronic lesions of pseudotuberculosis, may, as the epizootic reaches its height and the bacteria increase their virulence, cause typical hemorrhagic septicemia.

The organisms from rats and mice are usually placed in the enteritidis group, rather than in a possible rodent para B group. In a comparative study, Bahr, Raebiger and Grosso [17] found the ratin bacillus to be distinct from B. enteritidis and B. paratyphosus B. The work of Krumweide, Valentine and Kohn [6] indicates that some, at least, of the mouse strains have a closer relation to the so-called animal paratyhoids than to B. enteritidis. The organism isolated from infectious diarrhea of calves by Meyer, Traum and Roadhouse [18] was considered by them B. enteritidis, and strains from horses were placed by Graham, Reynolds and

[15] Jour. Infect. Dis., 1921, 28, p. 27.
[16] Centralbl. f. Bakteriol., O., 1921, 87, p. 1.
[17] Ztschr. f. Infektionskr. d. Haustiere, 1909, 5, p. 295.
[18] Jour. Am. Vet. Med. Assn., 1916, 49, p. 17.

Hull[19] in the same species. Zeller[20] found that strains isolated by himself from calves had a closer relation to human paratyphoid B than to enteritidis.

Of the avian strains, B. psittacosis is placed by Jordan[21] in the enteritidis group. Litch and Meyer's work, however, indicates closer relations to the guinea-pig strains studied by them. B. pullorum and B. sanguinarum, usually termed avian paratyphoid bacilli, were found by Mulsow[22] to be antigenically related to B. typhosus, B. enteritidis and B. abortus-equinus, but not related to B. paratyphosus A, B. paratyphosus B and B. suipestifer. In spite of relations to species so distinct as B. typhosus and B. enteritidis, the propriety of including these 2 avian species in the colon-typhoid intermediate group appears doubtful, since both are nonmotile. Motility is a fundamental biologic character which should have weight in determining relationships equal to that given to immunologic or cultural reactions. Spray and Doyle[23] found 22 of 23 strains isolated from chicks with white diarrhea and from hens to be B. pullorum, while one strain was like human paratyphoid B culturally, but distinct from the latter agglutinatively.

It is possible that the difficulty in determining relations among the members of the group which diverge from the four main species may be due to instability of biologic characteristics, resulting in altered immunologic properties when strains become transferred from one species of animal to another, or in loss or acquisition of fermentative powers when cultivated. Smith and Reagh[24] have held that a change from one host species to another might possibly change serologic characters. Fletcher[25] and Thjötta and Eide[26] have isolated capsulated paratyphoid variants. Jordan[27] has studied several strains which split off variants whose fermentation reactions differed from the parent strains. Two statements made by Jordan in this study are of fundamental significance: "Agglutinative reactions . . . in the paratyphoid-enteritidis group especially are to be accepted only guardedly as criteria of relationship." "Variations both in nature and in artificial test-tube cultures are exceedingly common throughout the paratyphoid-enteritidis group. These variations affect agglutination and fermentation characters, as well as less fundamental qualities."

To variations which actually occur within species and to the use of unauthentic strains of the four main species of the group in the comparative study of other strains, we believe that much of the present confusion is due.

Description of the Epizootic

The epizootic among our animals began in the spring of 1920 and manifested itself at first simply by a slightly progressively increasing death rate among the animals. By the middle of the summer the death rate had increased to such an extent that study of the disease became imperative if the rearing of guinea-pigs was to be continued. The results of the postmortem examinations at this time were so uniform as to indicate that we had to deal with an epizootic disease.

19 Ibid., 1920, 56, p. 378.
20 Ztschr. f. Infektionskr. d. Haustiere, 1909, 5, p. 361.
21 General Bacteriology, 1914, p. 275.
22 Jour. Infect. Dis., 1919, 25, p. 135.
23 Ibid., 1921, 28, p. 43.
24 Jour. Med. Research, 1903, 9, p. 270.
25 Lancet, 1918, 2, p. 102.
26 Jour. Bacteriol., 1920, 5, p. 501.
27 Jour. Infect. Dis., 1920, 26, p. 427.

Our guinea-pigs are kept on the second floor of a separate, brick animal house which is well lighted and ventilated. The floors are of concrete. The breeding animals are kept in a series of open pens 3 by 4 feet in a room 14 by 24 feet. Inoculated animals are kept in small cages in a separate room. How the infection entered is unknown. No new guinea-pigs had been placed among our stock, which had been bred from carefully selected animals for a period of about 3 years before the epizootic developed, until which time the stock had been exceptionally healthy and strong. The animals are fed on hay and oats stored in the animal house and on fresh vegetables and stale bread received daily from the hospital kitchen. It is probable that the infection was introduced with some of the green food. In the spring of 1920 our stock consisted of about 150 breeding females, from which about 100 young per month were being received. There were, in addition, about 150 young animals of both sexes which had been removed from the mothers and from which the supply of breeding animals was replenished as the animals matured. There were, further, about 100 males, about three-fourths grown, which had been separated from the other animals and which were used for bleeding, inoculation, etc. While an exact census of the number of guinea-pigs on hand previous to the epidemic cannot be given, 500 is a close estimate and this number was being increased by about 100 young per month. When the epidemic was brought under control, at the end of the summer, there were left only about 30 breeding females, and all the young animals on hand at the beginning of the epizootic and those born during its course had died. Our breeder estimates the number of young animals, which did not reach breeding age and which were lost during the epizootic, at about 500. The older males suffered much less severely. Throughout the epizootic the greater susceptibility of the females was striking, and pregnancy and parturition were important predisposing factors. Many of the females gave birth to dead young prematurely; when the young were born alive both the mother and the young frequently died within a few days after delivery. The greater suspectibility of female guinea-pigs in the different kinds of epizootic infections has been repeatedly referred to by others.

Symptoms

Often a peculiar cough was the first thing which called attention to a sick animal. In other cases the attitude and the appearance indicated that the animal was ill; it sat quietly huddled in a corner and the coat was rough. Emaciation was a marked feature. When the epizootic was at its height the animals died without having previously shown any symptoms which called attention to their condition. Diarrhea was absent; although the infection was probably intestinal in origin, the symptoms indicated freedom of intestinal involvement, which was borne out by the postmortem findings. In a small proportion of the animals the hind legs became paralyzed shortly before death.

Pathologic Anatomy

The most striking and constant lesions occurred in the spleen. This organ was enlarged to several times its normal size; the largest encountered measured 5 x 3.5 x 1.5 cm. Beneath the capsule and in the substance of the spleen were multiple, opaque, yellowish round areas which usually measured from 0.5 to 1 mm. in diameter and bore a close resemblance to tubercles. These were usually sharply defined and surrounded by a narrow zone of congestion. The splenic tissue between the nodules had a grayish-red color. In the largest spleen, mentioned in the foregoing, the areas were up to 1 cm. in diameter; as in the smaller lesions, the opaque necrotic material was dry and friable. The liver was usually moderately enlarged, pale and fatty. In addition to these changes, the tissue frequently contained indistinct, poorly defined, opaque areas of necrosis or more sharply defined and more opaque abscesses like those present in the spleen. There was no change in the lungs, except the atelectatic areas which occur so frequently in the lungs of the guinea-pig. The gastro-intestinal tract was uniformly negative, even in animals that died suddenly without spleen or liver lesions. In females that had had young and that died within a period varying from 1 day to 3 weeks following parturition, the uterus at times contained one or more abscesses, or without definite localized abscesses pus might be present in one or both horns. In a few instances the pleura was thickened and the pleural cavity filled with thick friable pus, and in about an equal number of cases the peritoneal cavity was the seat of similar changes. The left pleura was more frequently involved than the right, and both pleural and peritoneal involvement usually appeared to be the result of a spread of the inflammatory process by direct continuity from the spleen. At times the lesions of the pleura, peritoneum and spleen had the appearance of having been present for a relatively long time; other organs, such as the stomach and intestine, might be firmly united to the spleen or the abdominal wall by fibrous adhesions. When the epizootic was at its height, the animals apparently died acutely, without characteristic lesions; the internal organs were congested, but in no case were there any of the lesions characteristic of hemorrhagic septicemia; heart blood cultures from such cases were positive. In some of the animals that became paralyzed shortly before death, the central nervous system was examined, without, however, revealing any gross changes.

In the microscopic examination of the splenic lesions, the similarity to tubercles was almost as striking as in the gross. Each lesion was made up of a relatively large center composed of necrotic material, derived largely from fragmented leukocytes and lymphocytes. About the center was a narrow zone in which the tissue was better preserved; there was slight proliferation of the stroma cells and moderate infiltration by leukocytes and lymphocytes. The spleen pulp between the abscesses was somewhat congested and contained moderate numbers of large oval cells, apparently proliferated endothelium or stroma; this diffuse proliferative reaction was not nearly so marked as in the human spleen in typhoid fever. Some of the liver lesions were sharply defined abscesses like those present in the spleen. More frequent were the poorly defined areas of necrosis; microscopically, the smaller of these had an appearance identical with that of the focal necroses of the human liver in typhoid. The intervening liver tissue was usually markedly fatty. The gross lesions of the other organs had the same necrotic and purulent character as those of the spleen and liver. No changes were seen in the central nervous system which would account for the paralyses.

In animals with definite lesions the anatomic characteristics were those of a disease of rather prolonged duration. In other cases at the height of the epizootic, the absence of definite lesions, the presence of bacteria in the blood, and the clinical manifestations indicated that the disease had run a rapid course.

Bacteriology

Between July 24 and Aug. 15, 1920, necropsies were made on 31 guinea-pigs. Three were males and had been used for inoculation with suspected tuberculous material; the other 28 were females from the breeding stock. A culture was made from the heart blood of each guinea-pig and, in addition, cultures were made from the trachea, spleen, liver, pleura, uterus and tubes, peritoneal and pleural fluids, as indicated by the gross lesions.

A gram-negative bacillus was obtained from 26 of the 31 heart blood cultures and from all of the lesions from which cultures were taken. Two of the negative heart cultures were from guinea-pigs inoculated with tuberculous material. One negative culture was from a female guinea-pig with no definite symptoms or lesions. Another negative culture was from an emaciated, pregnant female guinea-pig that had been sick a year, but which had no typical lesions at necropsy. The fifth negative culture was obtained from the heart blood of an emaciated female guinea-pig that had a typical spleen from which a positive culture of gram-negative bacilli was obtained.

Microscopically, the organism isolated in this epizootic was a gram-negative bacillus, somewhat inclined to be pleomorphic, since there were coccus-like forms and longer, slender bacilli in the same culture. The bacillus was slowly motile. No capsule could be demonstrated by special staining methods.

The first cultures were made in dextrose broth, ascitic dextrose broth, plain agar, and blood agar, and they were grown anaerobically as well as aerobically. However, a good growth was obtained in plain broth and agar under aerobic conditions in 24 hours, so the other cultural methods were not used as a routine. In most instances, the gram-negative bacillus was obtained in pure culture. In two of the heart blood cultures a gram-positive coccus was isolated in addition to the gram-negative bacillus, and in one uterine culture a gram-positive bacillus was also obtained which did not grow in subcultures.

Broth cultures of the gram-negative bacillus were diffusely cloudy. The colonies on agar plates were elevated, moist, 1 to 3 mm. in diameter, rather opalescent, and with a smooth or slightly indented edge. On blood-agar plates the colonies were more moist and larger, but no hemolysis took place. On Endo's medium the colonies were faintly pink. Russell's double sugar medium had acid and gas in the lower part of the tube, and a trace of acid in the upper part of the medium. Growth on potato was not characteristic. Gelatin was not liquefied. Lead acetate medium was darkened in 24 hours. Litmus milk showed a faint trace of acid 24 hours after inoculation, then became increasingly alkaline until the milk was dark blue after 3 or 4 days. The alkalinity persisted for 8 weeks, at which time the cultures were discarded. There was in no instance any peptonization of the milk. There was no production of indol in 2-day, 7-day or 14-day cultures. The sugar reactions of all the strains were as follows: acid and gas were formed in dextrose, levulose, galactose, maltose, mannite, dulcitol, arabinose, and xylose; in lactose, salicin, saccharose, and inulin, there was no production of acid or gas. Cultures were made in the sugars and in litmus milk after 6 months' cultivation of the strains, and again after 1 year. The reactions in the sugars and in litmus milk remained the same.

The more important differential cultural reactions are given in table 1. In this and in the succeeding tables and throughout the rest of this communication, the guinea-pig organism under investigation is referred to as A 5. This was a pure strain isolated from a single colony derived from the heart blood culture of one of the animals that died early in the epizootic.

VIRULENCE

Three half-grown normal guinea-pigs were injected with salt suspensions of living A 5 bacteria. The first guinea-pig was injected intraperitoneally with 1 c c of a suspension which contained one-fourth of a 24-hour growth from a plain agar slant. The next morning, the guinea-pig was found dead. At necropsy, a small amount of cloudy fluid was found in the peritoneal cavity. The blood vessels on the injected side of the peritoneum were very congested, although the point of inoculation could not be determined. The blood vessels of the omentum, intestine and stomach were also very congested. The spleen, liver and kidneys were large and congested. The lungs and pericardium were slightly congested. The bacillus was recovered from the heart blood culture.

The second guinea-pig received less than 0.1 c c of the same suspension intravenously. It died on the second day. At necropsy, there was a slightly increased amount of fluid in the pleural and peritoneal cavities. All the blood vessels were congested. The omentum was very congested. No gross lesions were found. A 5 bacillus was isolated in pure culture from the heart blood.

The third guinea-pig received subcutaneous injections into the lower right quadrant of the abdomen, with 0.5 c c of the same A 5 suspension. This guinea-pig also died on the second day. The blood vessels at the site of inoculation

TABLE 1

CULTURAL REACTIONS

	Lactose	Dextrose	Xylose	Arabinose	Dulcitol	Litmus Milk		Lead Acetate
						24 Hours	6 Weeks	24 Hours
B. paratyphosus A (Army)	0	AG	0	AG	AG	A	A	0
B. paratyphosus A (Jordan)	0	AG	0	AG	AG	A	A	0
B. paratyphosus B (Army)	0	AG	AGs	AGs	AGs	Alk.s	Alk.	Dark
B. paratyphosus B (Jordan)	0	AG	AG	AG	AG	Alk.	Alk.	Dark
B. suipestifer......	0	AG	AG	AGs	AGs	Alk.s	Alk.	0
B. enteritidis......	0	AG	AG	AG	AG	Alk.s	Alk.	Dark
A 5...............	0	AG	AG	AG	AG	Alk.s	Alk.	Dark

A = acid; G = gas; s = slight; Alk. = alkaline.

were very congested. Apparently the infection traveled through the abdominal wall, for there was an acute plastic peritonitis. The pleural cavity was also invaded. There was general congestion of all the organs, but there were no gross lesions. A 5 organisms were recovered from the peritoneal fluid and from the heart blood.

Two guinea-pigs were fed on 3 consecutive days with an A 5 culture. This was done by pouring a 24-hour broth culture of A 5 bacteria over the bread and lettuce leaves fed to the guinea-pigs. On the second day the guinea-pigs were apparently affected by the feedings, since there was a loss of appetite and an appearance of weakness. However, in a few days they appeared normal. On the tenth day after the first feeding, the guinea-pigs coughed considerably. One guinea-pig became emaciated, and on the twenty-fifth day after the first feeding, the hind legs were partially paralyzed, and the animal appeared almost dead. It was killed and necropsy examination performed. The positive findings were a large fatty liver with numerous abscesses from 1 mm. to 2 cm. in diameter, large and congested spleen, and congestion of the upper lobes of the lungs. Films from the abscesses contained gram-negative bacilli. Bacilli typical of the epizootic were isolated from a liver abscess and from the heart blood.

Several c c of blood were taken from the heart for an agglutination test. This serum did not agglutinate A 5 or several other guinea-pig strains. The second guinea-pig which had been fed A 5 bacteria apparently recovered from the infection. After about 6 weeks, it was killed. No lesions were found at necropsy, the blood cultures remained sterile and the serum did not agglutinate A 5 bacteria.

A half-grown rabbit was inoculated subcutaneously with 0.1 c c of a suspension of A 5 bacilli similar to the one used in the guinea-pig virulence tests. The rabbit stopped eating after one day. It was very limp and obviously ill on the second day, and it died that night. A typical A 5 bacillus was recovered from the heart blood. No lesions were found at necropsy.

Necropsy examination was performed on the rabbit that was bled to death for immune A 5 serum. The positive findings were a large and congested spleen and a liver with several abscesses varying from 1 to 5 mm. in diameter. Cultures from the heart blood of this rabbit were sterile, but those of the liver lesions yielded the organism.

While rabbits were quite susceptible to artificial inoculation, they were apparently not very susceptible to spontaneous infection. Our stock of rabbits is kept on the first floor of the building in which the infection occurred among the guinea-pigs; a few rabbits were also kept on the same floor with the guinea-pigs. None of the rabbits developed the infection spontaneously.

White mice were readily susceptible to artificial infection. A mouse, inoculated intraperitoneally with ½ million organisms, died in 18 hours, and one each with 1 million and 1 billion died in 36 hours. A mouse which received ¼ million lived. These inoculations were made after the organism had been under artificial cultivation for 14 months. A half-grown white rat was not killed by an intraperitoneal inoculation of ½ million bacteria; when given a second intraperitoneal injection of the growth on one agar slant, it died in less than 18 hours.

IMMUNOLOGIC REACTIONS

Rabbits were immunized with the following bacterial strains: guinea-pig strain A 5; B. paratyphosus A; B. paratyphosus B; B. suipestifer; B. enteritidis. Guinea-pig strain A 5 was isolated at necropsy from the heart blood of a guinea-pig that had had typical symptoms of the infection and that had the characteristic lesions of the liver and the spleen. The strain was bacteriologically similar to the other gram-negative bacilli isolated in the epizootic. Paratyphoid strains A and B were obtained from the Army Medical School, Washington. The B. suipestifer and B. enteritidis strains were obtained from Prof. E. O. Jordan of the University of Chicago.

Agglutinins.—The macroscopic agglutination method was the one used for these tests. To varying serum dilutions (starting with undiluted serum and stopping with 1:10,000 serum dilution) was added an equal amount of an opalescent suspension of killed bacteria in physiologic salt solution. The tests were incubated in the hot-water bath at 56 C. for one hour, and the readings were made at once. Each immune serum and a normal rabbit serum was tested for agglutinin with each bacterial suspension. In addition to the bacterial suspension of the bacilli used for immunization were 3 suspensions of animal paratyhoid B strains 240, 244 (guinea-pig strains) and 245 (rabbit strain), which were obtained from Professor Jordan after the 5 rabbits had been immunized. The results of the agglutination tests were very clear-cut (table 2). There was no spontaneous clumping of the bacterial suspensions, and even undiluted normal rabbit serum failed to agglutinate any of the bacterial suspensions. A 5 serum in 1:10,240 dilution agglutinated A 5 suspension; in 1:5,120 dilution, No. 240 suspension; in 1:2,560 dilution, No. 244 suspension; in 1:1,280 dilution, No. 245 suspension; in 1:20 dilution, B. enteritidis suspension; and in 1:10 dilution, B. paratyphosus A suspension. Undiluted A 5 serum failed to agglutinate B. suipestifer and B. paratyphosus B suspensions. B. suipestifer serum agglutinated the homologous suspension in 1:5,120 serum dilution and B. enteritidis suspension in 1:1,250 serum dilution. This serum did not agglutinate A 5, B. paratyphosus A, B. paratyphosus B, 240, 244, or 245 suspensions. B. enteritidis immune serum in 1:5,120 dilution agglutinated B. enteritidis suspension, and in 1:1,280 dilution agglutinated B. suipestifer suspensions. This serum failed to agglutinate the other suspensions. B. paratyphosus A serum agglutinated B. paratyphosus A suspension when it was diluted 1:5,120; and B. paratyphosus B and B. enteritidis suspension when

TABLE 2

AGGLUTINATION REACTIONS

Serums	Suspensions							
	B. paratyphosus A (Army)	B. paratyphosus B (Army)	B. suipestifer	B. enteritidis	A 5	No. 240	No. 244	No. 245
B. paratyphosus A (Army)	1:5120	1:10	0	1:10	0	0	0	0
B. paratyphosus B (Army)	1:10	1:2560	0	0	0	0	0	0
B. suipestifer......	0	0	1:5120	1:1280	0	0	0	0
B. enteritidis......	0	0	1:1280	1:5120	0	0	0	0
A 5...............	1:10	0	0	1:20	1:10240	1:5120	1:2560	1:1280
Normal...........	0	0	0	0	0	0	0	0
None.............	0	0	0	0	0	0	0	0

it was diluted 1:20. The other bacterial suspensions were not agglutinated by this serum. B. paratyphosus B serum agglutinated B. paratyphosus B suspension in 1:2,560 serum dilution; and B. paratyphosus A in 1:1,010 dilution. The other organisms were not clumped by this immune serum.

The agglutinin titer of A 5 serum was so high for Nos. 240, 244, and 245 bacterial suspensions that it was considered unnecessary to immunize animals with these strains in order to perform the reverse tests (immune serum with A 5 suspensions), since the relation between the bacterial strains was already clearly established. The agglutination tests also showed the close relation between B. suipestifer and B. enteritidis, and to a lesser degree between the 2 human paratyphoid strains; but they did not place the A 5 strain or the 3 known animal paratyphoid B strains with either group. Agglutination tests were made, using A 5 immune serum with each of the bacteriologically similar strains isolated in the epizootic. With the exception of 2 strains, A 20 and A 22, all agglutinated with this serum. The agglutinin titer varied from 1:160 to 1:5,120.

Absorption Tests.—One c c of undiluted A 5 immune serum and 1 c c of a heavy, killed suspension of A 5 bacteria in normal salt solution were placed in a large bottomed test-tube and incubated in a hot-water bath at 56 C. for one hour. The mixture was centrifugalized and the clear supernatant fluid removed. The supernatant was again incubated with a heavy A 5 suspension, and the process was repeated until A 5 serum had no agglutinin for A 5 bacteria. A 5 immune serum was treated in a similar way with No. 240 bacteria until there was no agglutinin for No. 240. Serum A 5 (table 3), after A 5 agglutinin had been absorbed, clumped No. 240 suspensions in 1 : 30 serum dilution and suspensions of Nos. 244 and 245 in serum dilutions of 1 : 60. Serum A 5 after No. 240 agglutinin had been removed, agglutinated A 5 suspension in 1 : 40 serum dilution, but it did not clump No. 244 or 245 suspensions.

TABLE 3

AGGLUTININ ABSORPTION

Serum A 5 Absorbed with	Suspensions			
	A 5	No. 240	No. 244	No. 245
A 5	0	1:30	1:60	1:60
No. 240	1:40	0	0	0

The absorption tests show that strain A 5, though clearly related to the known paratyphoid B animal strains, is not identical with any one of them.

Opsonins.—The opsonic content of A 5 immune serum to the bacteria A 5, B. suipestifer, B. enteritidis, the human paratyphoids A and B, and the animal paratyphoids 240, 244 and 245 was measured by the opsonic index method. For comparison, the opsonins of B. suipestifer immune serum were determined for the same bacteria.

TABLE 4

OPSONIC INDEX

Immune Serums	A 5	No. 240	No. 244	No. 245	B. paratyphosus A (Army)	B. paratyphosus B (Army)	B. enter-it'dis	B. suipestifer
A 5	7.0	4.1	6.8	6.0	2.0	2.0	1.5	1.7
B. suipestifer	2.5	1.5	1.8	1.3	0.75	2.0	1.9	4.7

The technic was as follows: One part of the serum under examination, one part of a faintly cloudy suspension of killed bacteria, and one part of washed rabbit leukocytes were thoroughly mixed in a capillary pipet and were incubated for 15 minutes at 37 C. Films were made from the mixture and stained, 50 leukocytes were examined, and the number taking part in phagocytosis was noted. The number of phagocytic leukocytes in the immune serum divided by the number of phagocytic leukocytes in the normal serum constituted the opsonic index.

The opsonic index of A 5 immune serum (table 4) to A 5 bacteria was 7; to B. paratyphosus A, 2; to B. paratyphosus B, 2; to B. suipestifer, 1.7; to B. enteritidis, 1.5; to No. 240, 4.1; to No. 244, 6.8, and to No. 245, 6. The opsonic index of B. suipestifer immune serum to A 5 bacteria was 2.5; to B. paratyphosus A, 0.75; to B. paratyphosus B, 2; to B. suipestifer, 4.6; to B. enteritidis, 1.9; to No. 240, 1.5; to No. 244, 1.8; and to No. 245, 1.3.

The results of the opsonic index point to a close relationship between the guinea-pig A 5 strain, and the animal paratyphoid B strains 240, 244 and 245. However, from the opsonic indexes with serum B. suipestifer, A 5 would seem to be closer than the other animal paratyphoid strains to that bacterium.

Complement-Fixation.—Bacterial complement-fixation tests were made, using each immune serum, and a normal serum with all the antigens. Some difficulty was encountered in devising a method of antigen preparation which would prove satisfactory for each bacterium. Simple suspensions of either living or killed bacteria in normal salt solution gave good antigens for all the bacteria except A 5 and B. suipestifer. These two antigens were nonspecific in that they fixed complement to some extent with all the immune serums, and with several normal serums even when the amount of antigen used in the test was only a small fraction (1/264) of its anticomplementary unit. After trying various methods of antigen preparation, a fairly specific A 5 antigen was obtained by boiling a faintly cloudy suspension of bacteria in salt solution for 5 minutes. The resulting antigen was opalescent and of uniform density. Antigens of the other bacteria were similarly prepared, and they proved to be fairly satisfactory. Each antigen was standardized so that 0.1 c c of antigen equaled one-fourth of the anticomplementary unit of that antigen.

The bacterial complement-fixation tests were made according to the original Wassermann test (one-tenth method). The antigen and complement were kept constant, 0.1 c c. of each, and the inactivated serums were used in the following amounts: 0.04 c c, 0.02 c c, 0.01 c c, and 0.005 c c. Serum, antigen, and complement were incubated 45 minutes in a hot-water bath at 37 C., then sheep corpuscles and antisheep amboceptor were added to the contents of each tube, and the whole was incubated for 30 minutes at 37 C., in the hot-water bath.

When there was complete inhibition of hemolysis in the tube containing 0.005 c c serum, the result was considered + + + +. Similarly, when 0.01 c c serum was the least amount which inhibited, + +; and when 0.04 c c inhibited, +. When there was complete hemolysis in all the tubes, the result was regarded as negative.

The results of the complement-fixation tests (table 5) were not as clear-cut as were those in the agglutination tests (table 2). Serum A 5 gave a + + + + fixation with A 5, No. 240 and No. 244 antigens, a + + + fixation with B. suipestifer antigen, a + fixation with B. paratyphosus B, and B. enteritidis antigens and no fixation with B. typhosus A antigen. Antigen A 5 was less specific than the A 5 serum, since it gave a + + + fixation with B. paratyphosus A, B. paratyphosus B, and B. suipestifer serums, and a + + fixation with B. enteritidis serum. However, the close relation between A 5 and the 3 animal paratyphoid B strains was again demonstrated.

PREVENTIVE IMMUNIZATION

Although preventive immunization by means of killed bacteria is generally considered to yield poor results in the diseases of animals due to the paratyphoid group, it was decided to make use of this procedure as a final resort in an endeavor to overcome the infection. A vaccine was prepared, using 12 typical strains of the gram-negative bacillus that had been isolated in the epizootic. Eighteen-hour growths on plain agar sants were washed off with sterile salt solution, heated at 56 C. for 30 minutes, and standardized by Wright's method. On Aug. 6, 1920, a test group of 16 guinea-pigs was vaccinated. Three inoculations of the vaccine were given at 2-day intervals. The first dose contained one-half billion bacteria; the second, one billion; and the third, two billion.

There were no fatalities after the first dose. One guinea-pig died after the second injection. At necropsy, the liver had typical abscesses and the gram-negative bacillus was isolated from the heart blood. Since the death rate was not increased by the vaccination, the entire stock was vaccinated. One guinea-pig from the first vaccinated group died on October 4, and another on October 25. Both had typical liver and spleen lesions, and a bacillus was isolated in each case from the heart blood that was bacteriologically similar to the organisms isolated in the summer. Jan. 3, 1921, a fourth pig in this group died. There were no typical lesions found at necropsy, and the heart blood cultures remained sterile. The death rate became normal within several weeks after the vaccine had been given to the guinea-pig stock.

Agglutinins in Vaccinated Guinea-Pigs.—A group of 4 vaccinated guinea-pigs, including a young animal, 2 half-grown ones, and a full-grown one were bled several times, and their serums tested for agglutinin. Eight days after the

TABLE 5

COMPLEMENT-FIXATION

Serums	Antigens							
	B. paratyphosus A (Army)	B. paratyphosus B (Army)	B. suipestifer	B. enteritidis	A 5	No. 240	No. 244	No. 245
B. paratyphosus A (Army)	++++	+	0	++	+++	+++	+	0
B. paratyphosus B (Army)	+	+++	0	+	+++	++++	++++	++++
B. suipestifer......	0	0	++++	++++	+++	0	0	++
B. enteritidis......	0	0	+++	++++	++	+	0	0
A 5...............	0	+	++	+	++++	++++	++++	+++
Normal...........	0	0	0	0	0	0	0	0

++++ = Inhibition of hemolysis in 4 tubes (0.005 c c serum).
+++ = Inhibition of hemolysis in 3 tubes (0.01 c c serum).
++ = Inhibition of hemolysis in 2 tubes (0.02 c c serum).
+ = Inhibition of hemolysis in 1 tube (0.04 c c serum).
0 = Complete hemolysis.

third dose of vaccine, serum from guinea-pig 1 agglutinated the polyvalent suspension that had been used for vaccination in 1:5 dilution; this serum agglutinated A 5 suspension also in 1:5 dilution. Guinea-pig 2 serum agglutinated A 5 bacteria in 1:20 lilution, and the polyvalent suspension in 1:40 dilution. Guinea-pig 3 serum agglutinated A 5 suspension in 1:5 dilution, and the polyvalent suspension in 1:20 dilution. Guinea-pig 4 agglutinated A 5 in 1:5 dilution and the polyvalent suspension in 1:10 dilution. Fifteen days after vaccination, the results of the agglutination tests with A 5 bacteria were as follows: Guinea-pig 1 serum did not agglutinate; guinea-pig 2 serum agglutinated in 1:160; guinea-pig 3 serum in 1:40; guinea-pig 4 serum in 1:20. The results of the agglutination tests with a polyvalent suspension at this time were agglutination in 1:20, 1:80, 1:40, 1:40 serum dilutions, respectively. Twenty-four days after vaccination, the serums agglutinated A 5 bacteria as follows: With guinea-pig 1 serum there was no agglutination; with guinea-pig 2 serum there was agglutination in 1:40; with guinea-pig 3 serum, in 1:20; and with guinea-pig 4 serum, in 1 : 160. Agglutination experiments with the polyvalent suspension were not performed at the 24-day period. The results of these experiments on the vaccinated animals are given in table 6.

Protection Experiments.—The 4 guinea-pigs used for the agglutination experiments just described were given living, virulent A 5 bacteria in order to test the protective power of the vaccine. Twenty-seven days after the third dose of vaccine, guinea-pig 1, which had no agglutination for A 5, and guinea-pig 2, which had agglutinin for A 5 in 1 : 160 serum dilution were each injected subcutaneously with 250,000 live virulent A 5 bacteria. Guinea-pig 1 developed a red indurated mass about 1 cm. in diameter at the point of the injection, but it was not apparently ill. Guinea-pig 2 showed no ill effects from the inoculation. Five days later guinea-pigs 1 and 2 were inoculated subcutaneously with 0.5 c c of a heavy suspension of living A 5 bacteria. Both guinea-pigs developed red fluctuating masses at the point of the injection, which opened within a week and discharged pus for several days. The abscesses appeared clean and started to heal as soon as the pus was discharged. Guinea-pig 1 lost weight rapidly after the second inoculation of virulent bacteria, and it did not appear well.

TABLE 6

AGGLUTININS OF VACCINATED GUINEA-PIGS

Guinea-Pig	Number of Days After Third Vaccination				
	8		15		24
	A 5 Suspension	Polyvalent Suspension	A 5 Suspension	Polyvalent Suspension	A 5 Suspension
1	1:5	1:5	0	1:20	0
2	1:20	1:40	1:160	1:80	1:160
3	1:5	1:20	1:40	1:40	1:10
4	1:5	1:10	1:20	1:40	1:160

Guinea-pig 2 showed no systemic symptoms. The local ulcerated lesions healed quickly and completely. The smaller animal, which had become emaciated, regained its weight; it was killed 3 months after the inoculation; there were no lesions, and the blood culture was negative. The other animal has remained apparently well since its recovery from the local effects of the inoculation.

Guinea-pig 3, whose serum agglutinated A 5 bacteria in 1 : 10 dilution, and guinea-pig 4, whose serum agglutinated the same organisms in 1 : 160 dilution, were fed on consecutive days 2 large doses of living, virulent A 5 bacteria. Neither animal showed any ill effects from the feedings and both have since remained well.

DISCUSSION

The infection with which we had to deal apparently made headway slowly at first, but increased in severity as it gained momentum. At the beginning of the epizootic the disease ran a more protracted course and was characterized by chronic tubercle-like abscesses of the spleen and liver, together with focal and larger necroses of the liver. At the height of the epizootic the animals died quickly, without lesions and without definite clinical manifestations. The readiness with which the same organism was cultivated from the infected animals and its almost uniform isolation in pure culture was striking. All of the strains isolated were culturally identical. The degree to which they were agglutinated by the monovalent serum made against one of the strains isolated in the beginning of the epizootic varied from 1 : 160 to 1 : 5,120.

Motility, morphology and fermentative reactions place the organism in the colon-typhoid intermediate group. In its reactions on xylose, arabinose, dulcitol, litmus milk, and lead acetate agar it is identical with the Jordan strains of B. paratyphosus B and B. enteritidis used for comparative study (table 1).

The organism is one of that increasingly large group of bacteria which are considered to be paratyphoid B bacilli of animal origin. A relationship close enough to the strain of human B. paratyphosus B used by us in the immunologic studies reported in the foregoing to warrant calling the organism a paratyphoid bacillus is not apparent. Immunologically our organism is no more closely related to the human paratyphoid B strain used than to any of the other members of the group on which table 2 is based; the only relations which appear in that table are between the guinea-pig strain isolated by us and the 2 guinea-pig strains and 1 rabbit strain received from the Jordan collection. The human paratyphoid B strain obtained from the Army Medical School and used by us in our comparative study is not a typical strain, in that it does not ferment xylose, arabinose and dulcitol at all or only slightly and slowly (table 1). The determination of a possible closer relationship to a more typical paratyphoid B strain appeared to be of sufficient importance to warrant further investigation, since we have felt that much of the confusion that exists today in the colon-typhoid intermediate group depends on the use of irregular strains of the 4 fixed species for comparative study. After the work described in the foregoing had been completed and while the manuscript was in preparation, strains of human paratyphoid A and B were received from Professor Jordan and were used for the preparation of immune serums. These strains react typically on the differential mediums (table 1) and conform to the criteria which Jordan and his collaborators [28] have laid down in an important series of investigations. The Jordan paratyphoid B immune serum, which gave marked agglutination of its homologous organism in a serum dilution of 1 : 10,240

[28] Ibid., 1917, 20, p. 456; 1917, 21, p. 554; 1918, 22, p. 511.

(the dilutions were not carried further than this), agglutinated our organism in a dilution of 1:160, and the Jordan animal strains 240, 244 and 245 in dilutions of 1:320, 1:640 and 1:2,560, respectively (table 7). The relations of our organism, and of the other guinea-pig and rabbit strains which we had, to human B. paratyphosus B is now more apparent. Furthermore, the irregularity of the first strain of paratyphoid B used by us is evident; the Jordan antiparatyphoid B serum agglutinated the Army Medical School organism in a dilution of only 1:1,240, and the latter organism was agglutinated by the Jordan antiparatyphoid A serum in a dilution of 1:320 (table 7).

The agglutinin and opsonin experiments indicate a close affinity of our organism with the 2 guinea-pig and the 1 rabbit strain received from another source. Absorption of the agglutinins of the A 5 serum

TABLE 7

Agglutination Reactions with Antiparatyphoid A and B Serums (Jordan Strains)

Serums	Suspensions									
	B. paratyphosus A (Jordan)	B. paratyphosus A (Army)	B. paratyphosus B (Jordan)	B. paratyphosus B (Army)	B. suipestifer	B. enteritidis	A 5	No. 240	No. 244	No. 245
B. paratyphosus A (Jordan)	1:10240+	1:320	0	1:320	0	0	0	0	0	0
B. paratyphosus B (Jordan)	0	1:20	1:10240+	1:1280	0	0	1:160	1:320	1:640	1:2560
Normal...........	0	0	0	0	0	0	0	0	0	0
None..............	0	0	0	0	0	0	0	0	0	0

by the homologous organism did not remove completely the agglutinins for the other 3 strains; for the latter the titer was reduced from 1:5,120, 1:2,560 and 1:1,280 to 1:30, 1:60 and 1:60, respectively. A 5 serum absorbed with strain No. 240, one of the 2 Jordan guinea-pig organisms, lost its agglutinins for the 3 heterologous strains but still agglutinated our organism in 1:40 dilution (table 3). This may be accepted as evidence of slight differences between our strain and the 3 other animal strains; the latter, all derived from the same laboratory, are apparently more closely related to each other than to our strain. Although these 3 strains and our strain are closely related, we are unable to offer any conclusive evidence of the existence of a distinct rodent strain because of the small number of such strains that were available for study; the American Museum of Natural History informed us that they had no strains of rodent origin in their collection. While the small number of such strains that we had for comparison does not permit us to reach any conclusion as to the occurrence of a distinct rodent group of paratyphoid B bacilli, the work of others indicates that members of the intermediate group, other than those which may be supposed to constitute a rodent subgroup, occur frequently in rodents. The rodent origin of a given strain is not, therefore, in itself sufficient proof that the strain belongs to the rodent group. Immunologic study must establish that it has no close affinities with paratyphoid B, suipestifer and enteritidis. And then still further study is required to show that the strains of rodent origin, which are not related by their serologic reactions to the species mentioned, are closely enough related to each other to constitute a homogenous subgroup. If, as appears probable, such a distinct rodent subgroup can be established, it should receive species rank equal to that of the 4 members of the intermediate group at present recognized as distinct species.

In the complement-fixation reactions, our organism yielded some unexpected results. The fresh suspension was markedly anticomplementary and inhibited hemolysis in the presence of normal rabbit serum; our strain of B. suipestifer had this property to a less marked degree. By boiling the suspension and using the supernatant, this anticomplementary action could be overcome. Such a boiled antigen of the guinea-pig organism, however, gave strong fixation, not only with its homologous serum but also with the immune serums against the 4 fixed species (table 5). Used as an antigen for complement-fixation, our organism was, therefore, markedly nonspecific. This nonspecific action did not apply to the immune serum against the organism; the serum fixed complement completely in the presence of its homologous antigen, but did not bind complement at all when B. paratyphosus A was used as antigen, and fixed slightly in the presence of B. paratyphosus B, B. enteritidis and B. suipestifer. It fixed complement strongly with the 3 other rodent strains (table 5). The variability with which certain members of the intermediate group are agglutinated and fix complement before and after boiling has been observed by several investigators.

Immunization of the guinea-pigs by means of a killed polyvalent suspension appeared to bring the epizootic quickly under control. We make this statement with some trepidation, since it is generally held that immunization against the animal paratyphoid B organisms is without demonstrable effect. Previous to vaccination the death rate among our animals had been high and many of the animals were dying with acute rather than with chronic lesions or with no evident lesions.

During the course of the immunization 1 guinea-pig died with typical chronic lesions, and during the second month after the vaccination was completed 2 other animals died with typical abscesses of the spleen and liver. We believe that these animals were infected before the immunization was begun. A fourth animal died still later, but was free of lesions, and cultures were negative. The sudden decrease in the death rate we believe is to be ascribed to the immunization. It is possible, of course, that the infection may have run its course as the result of such sanitary measures as were undertaken and as the result of depletion of the stock. We do not feel, however, that these were the main or even important factors in the decrease in mortality, since they had been in operation for some time without noticeable effects. The loss of animals had been a progressive one and ceased rather sharply with immunization. A small group of guinea-pigs which was especially studied with regard to the results of immunization developed agglutinins in titers varying from 1:20 to 1:80 on the 24th day after completion of the vaccination (table 6). Inoculation and feeding of these animals with living suspensions established that they were protected against infection; even after subcutaneous inoculation of a large dose there developed only local purulent lesions which healed quickly.

The protection afforded by the immunization appears to have persisted. The death rate increased again in May, 1921. A necropsy examination was made of every guinea-pig dying, and a culture was made from the heart blood in each instance, and also from any suspicious lesions. The positive findings were usually gastro-intestinal in nature, and it was thought that this might be an early stage of the previous epizootic disease. The necropsy findings were similar to those of the preceding summer in only one guinea-pig. This was an emaciated female with a few suspicious areas on the spleen. However, cultures from the heart blood and from the spleen were negative, and the blood serum did not agglutinate A 5 bacteria. A large variety of bacteria was isolated during this second summer, i. e., B. coli, staphylococci, diplococci, yeasts, B. proteus and various gram-negative bacilli. Only one of the latter was culturally similar to the strains isolated in 1920. This strain agglutinated with A 5 immune serum in 1:320 dilution. Four other gram-negative bacilli resembled the A 5 strain, but on further investigation did not prove to be the same bacillus.

The organism was highly virulent for nonimmunized guinea-pigs when fed or when inoculated subcutaneously, intraperitoneally or intravenously. It was also virulent for rabbits on inoculation, but rabbits kept in contact with infected guinea-pigs during the epizootic were not spontaneously infected. White mice were susceptible; after more than a year of artificial cultivation the organism was still fatal to a white mouse in 18 hours in a dosage of one-half million bacteria. White rats were more resistant.

SUMMARY

An infectious disease which developed among our guinea-pigs during the summer of 1920 was characterized by the occurrence of multiple tubercle-like lesions of the spleen and of the liver. The disease was of the type to which the name pseudotuberculosis has been applied.

The infection quickly assumed epizootic proportions and led to the death of more than 500 animals before it was brought under control. At the height of the epizootic many of the guinea-pigs died without typical lesions but with positive blood cultures. Females were much more highly susceptible to spontaneous infection than males, and pregnant females were especially susceptible. In the pregnant animals purulent metritis was not infrequent.

From the infected animals there was isolated a gram-negative, motile bacillus which had the cultural characteristics of the colon-typhoid intermediate group. It fermented xylose, arabinose and dulcitol readily, quickly formed alkali in milk, and darkened lead acetate agar within 24 hours. The bacillus was isolated, usually in pure culture, from the lesions and from the heart blood.

Immunologically the organism was distinct from the representatives of the 4 fixed species of the group, namely, B. paratyphosus A, B. paratyphosus B, B. enteritidis and B. suipestifer, which were used for comparative study; it was agglutinated in low dilutions (1:160) of a serum against the Jordan strain of human paratyphoid B. It was closely related to, although not absolutely identical with, 2 guinea-pig and 1 rabbit strain received from another source.

It was virulent, on artificial inoculation, for guinea-pigs, rabbits, white mice, and white rats.

The epizootic was apparently brought under control by immunization of the guinea-pig stock with a killed polyvalent suspension of the organism.

THE EFFECT OF PEPTONE ON THE TOXIGENIC PROPERTY OF B. DIPHTHERIAE NO. 8

HARRIET LESLIE WILCOX

From the Research Laboratories, Department of Health, New York City

It is known to all laboratory workers who are familiar with the production of diphtheria toxin that the strain of B. diphtheriae used in obtaining a potent toxin is called No. 8. This strain was isolated by Dr. Williams in the summer of 1895 and so stable has been its toxigenic property that it is used, not only in the serum laboratories of the United States but in those of England and Europe as well.

The idea that different cultures of this strain should vary in their toxic productions was not entertained up to about 1916. However, from time to time, requests for new transplants of No. 8 had been received at this laboratory from other workers who said that their cultures had lost the ability to produce a potent toxin. Previous to 1914, our strain was still producing a potent toxin, though with some irregularities in strength.

More recently and coincident with the reports from other laboratories, the potency of the toxin produced at the Bureau of Laboratories has shown a marked decline. The average toxicity of the years 1914, 1915 and 1916 was 1:200 (or less) as compared with an average potency of 1:350-1:400 for the years 1911, 1912 and 1913.

In the summer of 1916 I was privileged to work a few weeks at the Pasteur Institute in Paris and to observe the preparation and inoculation of the diphtheria toxin broth. This procedure consisted of seeding Martin peptone broth [1] in Fernbach flasks with fairly large amounts of broth culture of No. 8. This culture had been taken to the Pasteur Institute in 1896 by Dr. Williams. The usual routine for the preparation of diphtheria strain was as follows:

> The stock culture was kept on coagulated ox-serum while the other culture was cultivated entirely on Martin peptone broth and was transferred 3 times weekly. The culture on serum was subcultured every 4 weeks and was not used for toxin production unless the broth culture became contaminated; in such case a fresh culture in Martin peptone broth was made from the serum culture. How often recourse to this culture was made, I do not know, but from the careful technic employed one would say, rarely, if ever.

Received for publication Jan. 27, 1922.

[1] Ann. de l'Institut Pasteur, 1897, 12, p. 26.

On my return several experimental preparations of diphtheria toxin were made. The method of the Pasteur Institute was used as well as their culture of No. 8 which had been brough back to New York. The results were so superior to those obtained by employing Witte peptone broth and our own culture of No. 8 that in January, 1917, Martin peptone broth inoculated with the Pasteur culture of B. diphtheriae No. 8 was adopted as our method of toxin production. Since we were following as closely as possible the Pasteur method, we used the same procedure for the propagation of the culture of B. diphtheriae.

Comparative tests of our culture of No. 8 with that of the Pasteur No. 8 were made at Dr. Williams' request. The first two or three tests showed such marked difference in favor of Pasteur No. 8 that we decided to discover whether, after a cultivation of several months or longer on Martin peptone broth, our No. 8 culture would produce as high a toxin in Martin peptone broth as the Pasteur No. 8.

To differentiate between these two cultures of the same strain of No. 8 we have called the culture which has been propagated exclusively at the Bureau of Laboratories, Research No. 8, whereas the culture obtained from Pasteur Institute is designated as Pasteur No. 8. These two cultures were inoculated in Martin peptone broth Dec. 28, 1916, and transferred three times weekly in this medium.

At about the same time these cultures were inoculated similarly into Witte peptone broth, Research No. 8 being planted Dec. 23, 1916, and Pasteur No. 8 Dec. 28, 1916, and were transferred three times weekly.

In the summer of 1919 a second culture of No. 8 was obtained from the Pasteur Institute and this was planted Aug. 19, 1919, in Martin peptone broth, Berna peptone broth and Witte peptone broth; it was designated as Pasteur 2 No. 8.

The records of these cultures, that is, the date each was planted in a different medium, the number of transfers weekly, together with the date and result of the planting to determine purity, were kept on separate cards.

In order to obviate any possibility of the substitution of one medium for another while making the subcultures, the following procedure was adopted:

The cultures Research No. 8, Pasteur No. 8, and Pasteur 2 No. 8 in the Martin peptone broth were kept in a different container than the same cultures in the other peptone broths. At the time of transferring only one container with its respective broth tubes was on the work table, thus avoiding any possibility of a Witte peptone broth tube being substituted for a Martin peptone broth tube and vice versa.

The dilutions of the filtered cultures for the animal inoculation were made in 0.8% NaCl. In the tables in which the toxicity is given as being below 1:100 or 1:200, etc., it indicates that those were the dilutions inoculated and that they did not kill the test animals, or if they did so, not within the time limits. When a toxin is stated to be of a given strength it means that the given dilution killed a 250 gm. guinea-pig within the 4 days with the classical toxic symptoms. Occasionally it was not possible to obtain pigs weighing 250 gm., but in those tests made with heavier pigs, the surplus weight was always discounted in estimating the toxicity. No guinea-pigs weighing below 230 gm. were inoculated.

MARTIN PEPTONE BROTH

The comparative tests of Research No. 8 and Pasteur No. 8 in Martin peptone broth are given in table 1. It is to be recalled that the cultures were subjected to cultivation in this broth, were transferred three times weekly and were then cultivated under identical conditions. To give the reader the approximate number of generations before the different tests were made, the date of starting the cultures in the different broths is given in the tables.

TABLE 1.

Toxicities Produced in Martin Peptone Broth by Three Different Cultures of B. Diphtheriae No. 8 After Cultivation in the Same Broth; Transfers Made Three Times a Week

Date of Test	Research No. 8 Cultivation Begun Dec. 28, 1916	Pasteur No. 8 Cultivation Begun Dec. 28, 1916	Pasteur 2 No. 8 Cultivation Begun Aug. 19, 1919
Jan. 19, 1917	1:100	1:400	Not tested
May 31, 1917	1:300	1:400	Not tested
June 30, 1917	Below 1:200	1:500	Not tested
Oct. 11, 1917	Below 1:100	1:300	Not tested
Oct. 19, 1917	1:150	1:800	Not tested
Feb. 2, 1918	1:100	1:200	Not tested
Sept. 19, 1919	1:200	1:600	1:600
Oct. 2, 1919	Below 1:100	Below 1:200	Below 1:200

It will be seen that in one test only Research No. 8 approximated Pasteur No. 8 in its toxic production. In the experiment dated May 31, 1917, Research No. 8 gave a toxicity of 1:300 as compared with a toxin of 1:400 produced by Pasteur No. 8. The greatest difference in their toxigenic powers was shown in the test dated Oct. 19, 1917, when the M L D of Research No. 8 was 1:150 in contrast to a potency of 1:800 produced by Pasteur No. 8. Subsequent comparative tests showed a diminution in the toxigenic production by both cultures in Martin peptone broth.

The first test comparing the 3 cultures, Research No. 8, Pasteur No. 8 and Pasteur 2 No. 8, was made Sept. 19, 1919. The results showed that the two Pasteur cultures gave a toxicity of 1:600 whereas the Research No. 8 gave a low M L D of 1:200. The last comparative test in Martin peptone broth was made in October, 1919, but the toxicities in this test were so low that only negative results were obtained.

WITTE PEPTONE BROTH

The number of tests made using Witte peptone broth was limited, due to the scarcity of the peptone. The broth used in these tests was made according to the formula recommended by Theobald Smith [2] for obtaining a potent toxin. As in the test made with Martin peptone, the 3 cultures were transferred in the Witte broth 3 times weekly. The period of cultivation may be judged from the dates in table 2 in which the results are given.

TABLE 2

TOXICITIES PRODUCED IN WITTE PEPTONE BROTH BY THREE DIFFERENT CULTURES OF B. DIPHTHERIAE NO. 8 AFTER CULTIVATION IN THE SAME BROTH; TRANSFERS THREE TIMES A WEEK

Date of Test	Research No. 8* Cultivation Begun Dec. 23, 1916	Pasteur No. 8 Cultivation Begun Dec. 28, 1916	Pasteur 2 No. 8 Cultivation Begun Aug. 19, 1919
Jan. 19, 1917	Below 1:100	1:400	Not tested
Oct. 26, 1917	1:150	1:700	Not tested
Sept. 15, 1919	1:100	1:400	1:250
Mar. 12, 1920	Below 1:100	Below 1:100	Not tested
May 27, 1921	Below 1:100	Below 1:200	1:450

* This culture had been carried on in Witte broth since 1895 and transferred every other day as the routine procedure.

It will be noticed that despite the fact that Research No. 8 had been cultivated in a medium containing Witte peptone practically ever since its isolation in 1895, its toxigenic property was much less in the first three tests than that of Pasteur No. 8. The test made May 27, 1921, was a great surprise for it was the first time that Pasteur 2 No. 8 had given a higher potency than Pasteur No. 8. Whether this difference would have been demonstrable in the March 12, 1920, test it is impossible to say, but it is evident that the toxigenic property of Pasteur No. 8 in Witte broth had deteriorated. Further reference to this will be made in the following pages.

[2] Jour. Exper. Med., 1899, 4, p. 373.

BERNA PEPTONE BROTH

It was stated in the foregoing that Martin peptone broth was used during the year 1917 at the Bureau of Laboratories for the routine production of diphtheria toxin, with satisfactory results. In the early months of 1918, however, the potency of the toxin was irregular, and in the late spring several successive preparations of the broth gave too low a toxin for practical use. At this time we had just begun to use the Berna peptone for the production of tetanus toxin, and the idea occurred to us that this peptone might be satisfactory for obtaining a potent diphtheria toxin. Therefore a small amount of broth was made according to the method of Theobald Smith, but with the Berna peptone instead of Witte. The result of this test was very gratifying as a M L D of 1 : 350 was obtained. No comparative tests of Research No. 8 and Pasteur No. 8 were made at this time as I began a year's leave of absence. During this time all of the cultures in the different mediums were carried on by Miss Alice G. Mann whose cooperation is greatly appreciated. The 2 cultures, Pasteur No. 8 and Research No. 8, were planted in Berna peptone broth and were transferred 3 times weekly.

On my return from France in 1919 the comparative tests in Berna peptone broth of the 2 cultures, Research No. 8 and Pasteur No. 8 were made, together with the second culture of No. 8 that had been obtained from the Pasteur Institute in the summer of 1919 and which is spoken of in the test as Pasteur 2 No. 8. The results are given in table 3.

TABLE 3

TOXICITIES PRODUCED IN BERNA PEPTONE BROTH BY THREE DIFFERENT CULTURES OF B. DIPHTHERIAE NO. 8 AFTER CULTIVATION IN THE SAME BROTH; TRANSFERS THREE TIMES A WEEK

Date of Test	Research No. 8 Cultivation Begun May 4, 1918	Pasteur No. 8 Cultivation Begun May 4, 1918	Pasteur 2 No. 8 Cultivation Begun Aug. 19, 1919
Aug. 22, 1919	Below 1:100	1:100	1:100
Sept. 13, 1919	Below 1:100	1:250	1:250
Sept. 15, 1919	1:100	1:500	1:500
Sept. 19, 1919	Below 1:100	1:500	1:400
Sept. 26, 1919	Below 1:100	1:100	1:100
Oct. 4, 1919	Below 1:100	1:100	1:100
Oct. 10, 1919	Below 1:100	1:250	1:250
Oct. 18, 1919	Below 1:100	1:150	Below 1:100

Four of the 8 tests given in table 3 showed decidedly the greater toxigenic property of the two Pasteur cultures over that of Research No. 8. The toxicities of the other 4 tests were so uniformly low that less definite comparisons were possible.

The toxin made from the Berna peptone broth was so inferior from October, 1919, through to the new year that efforts were made to discover whether there was a domestic peptone on the market which would be more satisfactory for diphtheria toxin production. A comparative test of Parke-Davis peptone and Berna peptone broths was made and inoculated with only Pasteur No. 8. The results were encouraging for the toxin made from Parke-Davis broth had a M L D of 1 : 700 in contrast to a M L D of 1 : 200 obtained with Berna peptone broth. Accordingly, the 3 cultures were cultivated in broth made with Parke-Davis peptone. However, no comparative tests of the toxigenic powers were made until March, 1920. These and subsequent results are given in table 4 in which is also included three tests of the culture "American."

TABLE 4

TOXICITIES PRODUCED IN PARKE, DAVIS PEPTONE BROTH BY THREE DIFFERENT CULTURES B. DIPHTHERIAE NO. 8 AFTER CULTIVATION IN THE SAME BROTH; TRANSFERS THREE TIMES A WEEK

Date of Test	Research No. 8 Cultivation Begun Jan. 1, 1920	Pasteur No. 8 Cultivation Begun Jan. 1, 1920	Pasteur 2 No. 8 Cultivation Begun Jan. 1, 1920	"Americain"*
Mar. 3, 1920........	1:100	1:1000	Not tested	Not tested
Mar. 12, 1920........	1:100	1:800	Not tested	Not tested
Nov. 16, 1920........	1:300	1:900	Not tested	Not tested
Nov. 26, 1920........	1:200	1:1000	1:700	1:1000†
Jan. 21, 1921........	1:200	1:1000	1:300	1:700‡
April 7, 1921........	1:100	1:1500	1:700	1:800

* This culture was obtained from Dr. Durand, Lyons, France, and was the B. diphtheriae No. 8 which had been sent him probably from the Pasteur Institute, Paris.

† This culture had been inoculated into Parke-Davis peptone broth for seven generations before seeding of toxin flasks.

‡ This had been in Parke, Davis broth for five generations before seeding of toxin flasks.

The marked differences in the toxigenic power of these strains were again in evidence. As far as was known, there was no explanation for the low toxicity of Pasteur's 2 No. 8 in the test made Jan. 21, 1921. This was 1 : 300 as against the M L D of 1 : 1,000 produced by Pasteur No. 8. In all the other comparative tests with the different peptones, the toxin made from Pasteur 2 No. 8 had corresponded very closely with the toxins made from Pasteur No. 8 with the exception of the experiment of Sept. 15, 1919, made in Witte peptone broth (table 2). Here Pasteur No. 8 produced a M L D of 1 : 400 as compared with a toxicity of 1 : 250 made from Pasteur 2 No. 8.

It is interesting to note that the "American" culture (table 4, Nov. 26, 1920) gave after only 7 generations in Parke-Davis peptone broth a toxin with as high a potency as the Pasteur No. 8 which had been cultivated 11 months in that medium.

When it was evident that Research No. 8 produced consistently a very much lower toxin than either of the other strains, regardless of the length of cultivation in any particular broth, the thought occurred to us that it would be interesting to see what effect the different peptones may have had on the toxigenic power of Pasteur No. 8 after its cultivation in the different peptone broths. Accordingly, a preparation of Berna peptone broth was inoculated on July 23, 1920, with the Pasteur No. 8 culture which had been cultivated exclusively in Martin, Witte, Parke-Davis and Berna peptone broths. The day before the test was started, seed cultures in Berna peptone broth were planted from these cultures, as fairly large amounts of the seed cultures were used to inoculate the toxin flasks and we wished to obviate carrying over any of the other peptone broths into the Berna broth. The results of this test, together with the dates of first cultivation in the different broths, are given in table 5.

TABLE 5

TOXICITIES PRODUCED IN BERNA PEPTONE BROTH BY PASTEUR NO. 8 AFTER CULTIVATION IN BROTHS MADE WITH DIFFERENT PEPTONES

Transplanted Three Times Weekly		Date of Test	Toxicity
First Transplant of Series	Cultivated in Broth with		
May 4, 1918	Berna peptone broth	July 23, 1920	1:500
Dec. 28, 1916	Witte peptone broth	July 23, 1920	Below 1:100
Dec. 28, 1916	Martin peptone broth	July 23, 1920	1:450
Jan. 1, 1920	Parke-Davis peptone broth	July 23, 1920	1:450

TABLE 6

TOXICITIES PRODUCED IN WITTE PEPTONE BROTH BY PASTEUR NO. 8 AFTER CULTIVATION IN BROTHS MADE WITH DIFFERENT PEPTONES

Transplanted Three Times Weekly		Date of Test	Toxicity
First Transplant of Series	Cultivated in Broth with		
Dec. 28, 1916	Witte peptone broth	Dec. 9, 1920	1:150
Dec. 28, 1916	Martin peptone broth	Dec. 9, 1920	1:300
May 4, 1918	Berna peptone broth	Dec. 9, 1920	1:500

The results of the foregoing test show that the cultures of Pasteur No. 8, which had been cultivated exclusively in Berna, Martin and Parke-Davis peptone broths, gave satisfactory toxins. The culture, however, which had been transferred in Witte broth since Dec. 28, 1916, gave a potency of below 1 : 100.

Another test was made with these same cultures which had been cultivated in broths made with Witte, Berna and Martin peptone, but instead of the Berna peptone broth, Witte peptone broth was used. As in the former test, the seed cultures were planted in Witte peptone broth before the inoculation in the Witte toxin broth.

Here again the culture which had been in Witte broth gave the lowest toxicity. This test was repeated 9 months later, on April 22, 1921 (table 7).

TABLE 7

TOXICITIES PRODUCED IN WITTE PEPTONE BROTH BY PASTEUR NO. 8 AFTER CULTIVATION IN BROTHS MADE WITH DIFFERENT PEPTONES

Transplanted Three Times Weekly		Date of Test	Toxicity
First Transplant of Series	Cultivated in Broth with		
May 4, 1918	Berna peptone broth	April 22, 1921	1:800
Dec. 28, 1916	Witte peptone broth	April 22, 1921	Below 1:100
Dec. 28, 1916	Martin peptone broth	April 22, 1921	1:700
Jan. 1, 1920	Parke-Davis peptone broth	April 22, 1921	1:700

It will be seen that these results confirm the former test in the Witte peptone broth and also that in the Berna broth, in that the culture of Pasteur No. 8 which had been cultivated in the Witte broth gave the lowest toxicity.

Attempts will be made to confirm the results reported in this paper: (1) By subcultivating in Witte broth the culture Pasteur No. 8 which has been propagated continuously in Parke-Davis peptone broth since January, 1920, and which has given regularly a potent toxin in this medium; and by comparing these two cultures from time to time in order to determine whether the toxigenic powers of the culture in Witte broth has been adversely affected while the culture kept in Parke-Davis peptone broth retains its ability to produce strong toxin.

(2) By subcultivating Pasteur No. 8, which has apparently lost its toxigenic power by cultivation in Witte broth, in Parke-Davis peptone broth to determine whether this culture after varying lengths of time in Parke-Davis broth may not regain its power to produce a potent toxin.

(3) By further cultivation of Pasteur 2 No. 8 in Witte broth to determine whether this culture will lose its toxigenic power in Witte peptone broth as Research No. 8 and Pasteur No. 8 have apparently done.

SUMMARY

The culture of Research No. 8 which has been propagated exclusively in Witte broth since 1895 at the Bureau of Laboratories has apparently lost its power to produce a potent toxin in any of the broths tested.

The Pasteur cultures of No. 8 which were planted in Witte broth Dec. 28, 1916, has also apparently lost its ability to produce a potent toxin in both Witte and Berna peptone broths. The same culture kept in Berna, Martin and Parke-Davis peptone broth produces strong toxins in both the Berna and Witte broths.

The cultures of Research No. 8 which have been carried on in Berna, Martin and Parke-Davis peptone broths have not as yet recovered their powers to produce a potent toxin in any of the broths tested.

The toxigenic property of Pasteur 2 No. 8 culture has not as yet been affected deleteriously by the 2 years' cultivation (1919-1921) in Witte peptone broth.

CONCLUSIONS

It would seem in view of the foregoing results:

That Witte peptone broth had an inhibitory or destructive influence on the toxigenic powers of both Research No. 8 and Pasteur No. 8 cultures.

That Pasteur 2 No. 8 may be similarly affected after a still longer cultivation in Witte broth.

That the different preparations of Witte peptone received in this country just prior to 1914 may be responsible for this deleterious effect on the cultures. The fact, that culture Research No. 8 from the time of its isolation in 1895 to 1912-1913 had been cultivated in Witte peptone broth without any signs of the lowering of its toxigenic property, as shown by the production of a potent toxin, tends to confirm this conclusion.

That it is possible that the different preparations of any peptone may vary in their effects on the toxigenic property of B. diphtheriae No. 8.

That the continuous cultivation of a culture of B. diphtheriae No. 8 in the same broth as that used for the toxin production is apparently not necessary for obtaining a potent toxin, is shown by the "American" strain of No. 8, which after only 7 generations in Parke-Davis broth gave as potent a toxin in that medium as Pasteur No. 8 which had been cultivated for 11 months in Parke-Davis broth.

THE ACTION OF NEOARSPHENAMIN AND NEOSALVARSAN ON THE PHAGOCYTIC ACTIVITY OF LEUKOCYTES

Ruth Tunnicliff

From the John McCormick Institute for Infectious Diseases, Chicago

In connection with certain experiments on the action of chemicals on phagocytosis, I found that solutions of neosalvarsan, 1 : 10,000, caused a well marked increase in the activity of leukocytes. I have made similar experiments with neoarsphenamin, to determine whether it would cause an increase in phagocytosis and what its action on the leukocytes might be.

Normal human serum and leukocytes were used in the following experiments. It is necessary that the organisms used do not clump, and strains of Streptococcus viridans from measles and influenza were chosen, which were not spontaneously phagocytable, yet not so virulent as not to be readily engulfed. The cocci were grown 24 hours either on moist goat blood agar and the growth washed off in salt solution, or they were grown in meat infusion broth. The suspensions to be satisfactory can be only slightly cloudy.

To test the action of the arsenic compound on phagocytosis equal parts of the compound in salt solution, serum, suspensions of washed leukocytes and of bacteria are incubated 25 minutes. Salt solution alone is used in the controls. Such mixtures are smeared on slides and stained with carbol thionin. At least 100 polymorphonuclear leukocytes are counted, and the number of cocci per leukocyte as well as the number of cells taking part in phagocytosis noted. The results of such tests are illustrated in table 1.

To determine whether the effects on the degree of phagocytosis shown in table 1 are on the leukocytes themselves, tests may be made as follows: Equal numbers of washed leukocytes are suspended in different dilutions of the arsenical compound for one hour at room temperature; the leukocytes are then washed twice with salt solution by centrifugation, equal parts of serum and bacteria added, and the whole incubated for 25 minutes, when smears are made and the results determined by studying 100 polymorphonuclear leukocytes (table 2).

Received for publication Jan. 27, 1922.

It appears that in vitro solutions of neoarsphenamin, below 1 : 1,000, as a rule, stopped or greatly reduced phagocytosis, while dilutions between 1 : 10,000 and 1 : 100,000 promoted phagocytosis, phagocytosis being increased on an average more than two times. Higher dilutions produced no effect. This increase in phagocytosis was found to be due to the action of the drug on the leukocytes, which were about twice as active in the diluted arsenical solution as in salt solution. These experiments were repeated six times with similar results, two different organisms being used, as a rule, in each experiment.

TABLE 1

PHAGOCYTOSIS IN MIXTURES OF HUMAN SERUM, HUMAN LEUKOCYTES, STREPTOCOCCI AND NEOARSPHENAMIN

Dilution of Neoarsphenamin	Average Number of Streptococci in 100 Leukocytes	Percentage of Leukocytes Taking Part in Phagocytosis
1: 400	0.08	4
1: 1,000	1.6	44
1: 10,000	3.3	44
1: 100,000	4.7	56
1: 1,000,000	2.2	32
Salt solution	2.3	38

TABLE 2

PHAGOCYTOSIS IN MIXTURES OF HUMAN SERUM, STREPTOCOCCI, AND LEUKOCYTES, WHICH HAD BEEN SUSPENDED FOR ONE HOUR IN NEOARSPHENAMIN OR SALT SOLUTION AND THEN WASHED TWICE WITH SALT SOLUTION

Dilution of Neoarsphenamin	Average Number of Streptococci in 100 Leukocytes	Percentage of Leukocytes Taking Part in Phagocytosis
1: 1,000	0.16	8
1: 10,000	0.82	28
1: 100,000	0.76	28
1: 1,000,000	0.33	12
Salt solution	0.34	16

Next 7 rabbits, weighing about 1,800 grams, were injected intravenously with 1 c c of distilled water containing 0.007 gm. of neoarsphenamin, prepared as for human injection. Leukocyte counts were made before and every 15 minutes following the injections, for from 1 to 2 hours, or until the counts became normal. The opsonic and cytophagic (phagocytic activity of the leukocytes) indexes were determined, the opsonic determinations being made in the usual way, equal parts of serum, rabbit leukocytes and bacterial suspension being incubated 25 minutes.

In these experiments the phagocytic activity of the leukocytes was determined as follows: The leukocytes of the rabbits were collected in 2% sodium citrate solution, centrifugated and washed once in normal salt solution to remove all traces of serum. It is, of course, essential to use suspensions containing approximately the same number of polymorphonuclear leukocytes. Such suspensions may be obtained by counting the number of cells in the circulating blood, collecting the same amount of blood from each rabbit, and then equalizing according to count. The same serum was used to provide opsonin in the tests of the leukocytes. Equal parts of serum, equalized leukocytic suspensions and bacterial suspensions were mixed in bent capillary pipets and incubated 25 minutes when the mixtures were smeared on glass slides and stained. The phagocytic activity of the leukocytes, that is cytophagic index, was determined by comparing the number of bacteria taken up by the leukocytes before and after the injection of neoarsphenamin.

Five of the 7 rabbits injected with neoarsphenamin showed a decided increase in the number of leukocytes in from 15 to 30 minutes following the injection. This increase varied from 3,200 to 22,000, the average increase being 10,000. The leukocytosis was transitory rarely lasting 15 minutes. The leukocytes were from 2 to 6 times more actively phagocytic than normal at 15 minutes after the administration of neoarsphenamin. In the other 2 rabbits leukocytosis developed in 45 and 75 minutes, and in these animals an increased phagocytic activity of the leukocytes was present 30 and 45 minutes, respectively, after the injection. No changes in the opsonic index were observed, that is, there was no increase in opsonin. The number and activity of the leukocytes remained normal after the intravenous administration of 1 c c of salt solution and after 1 c c of salt solution containing 0.0002 gm. of mercuric cyanide.

According to Dinnick,[1] the intravenous administration of arsenical compounds is followed by an appreciable leukocytosis. He found that arsenic disappeared from the blood in a few hours and concludes that probably the therapeutic effect is only exerted during the short time the drug is circulating in the blood stream.

The fact that the leukocytes of most of the rabbits were more active during the height of the leukocytosis raised the question whether the presence of young leukocytes or the arsenic directly was responsible for this increased activity. To study this question further, two patients were examined before and after the injection of 0.6 gm. of neo-

[1] Lancet, 1919, 1, p. 1055

salvarsan. In neither case was there a leukocytosis, but in each instance 30 minutes after the injection, there was an increase in the phagocytic activity of the leukocytes, the index being 3.6 in one patient and 4.3 in the other. No increase of phagocytic activity could be made out 15 minutes later, that is 45 minutes after the injection of neosalvarsan. As the activity of the leukocytes and the leukocytosis did not always coincide in the rabbits, and as there was increased leukocytic activity in both patients, but without leukocytosis, the conclusion seems warranted that the neoarsphenamin or neosalvarsan was directly responsible for the increased phagocytic activity.

Various investigators have demonstrated that arsenical compounds increase antibody production. Boehncke [2] and Strubell [3] found that salvarsan stimulates opsonin production, and according to Strubell the increase in opsonin occurs from 2 to 8 hours after intravenous injection. An increase in other antibodies (agglutinins, hemolysins, precipitins) and also in complement, after the administration of arsenical compounds, has been observed by Aggazzi,[4] Friedberger and Maruda,[5] Lippmann,[6] Boehncke,[2] Weisbach [7] and Togama and Kolmer.[8] Kröcher,[9] Brekke,[10] and Reiter,[11] however, were unable to demonstrate any influence on the formation of antibodies by the injection of salvarsan into rabbits.

The results presented in this paper emphasize once more that to analyze thoroughly the effects of certain conditions or substances on phagocytosis, it is necessary to determine their action on the leukocytes as well as on the opsonin. Cross [12] concluded that because there was no reduction of the opsonic power of the serum in certain conditions there was no reduction in the phagocytic activity of the blood; but manifestly this is not a safe conclusion because it is not known that the phagocytic power or activity of the leukocytes, themselves the active agents of phagocytosis, remained unchanged.

[2] Ztschr. f. Chemother., O, 1912, p. 136.
[3] Berl. klin. Wchnschr., 1912, 49, p. 1078.
[4] Ztschr. f. Immunitätsf., O, 1909, 1, p. 736.
[5] Therap. Monatsch., 1911, 25, p. 288.
[6] Deutsch. med. Wchnschr., 1911, 37, p. 1693.
[7] Ztschr. f. Immunitätsf., O, 1914, 21, p. 187.
[8] Jour. Immunol., 1918, 3, p. 301.
[9] Ztschr. f. Hyg. u. Infectionskrankh., 1914, 78, p. 321.
[10] Beretning for Gades, Path. Inst., 1912-3, p. 74.
[11] Ztschr. f. Immunitätsf., O, 1912, 15, p. 116.
[12] Bull. Johns Hopkins Hosp., 1921, 32, p. 350.

SUMMARY

In proper concentrations, neoarsphenamin and neosalvarsan may increase the phagocytic activity of leukocytes, both in vitro and in vivo. In vivo the stimulating effect is rapid and of short duration, occurring, as a rule, within 30 minutes after intravenous injection. Further study is necessary to determine what part, if any, this stimulus of the phagocytic activity of the leukocytes plays in the curative action of neoarsphenamin and allied products.

CONDUCTIVITY OF BACTERIAL CELLS

R. G. GREEN AND W. P. LARSON

From the Department of Bacteriology and Immunology, University of Minnesota, Minneapolis

During late years much has been written concerning electrical conductivity of cells as a method of measuring permeability of cell membranes. While there seems to be doubt as to the validity of this method in the minds of some, most writers on this subject accept the method as measuring permeability and draw conclusions from their results on this basis. Our experiments with conductivity of bacterial cells were begun with the idea of determining whether immunologic reactions could be demonstrated to bring about changes in the permeability of bacterial membranes. The progression of our experimental work on this problem led us to doubt more and more that we were measuring an actual change in permeability of the bacterial membranes to the ions carrying the electric current, and we seem to have found an explanatory analysis of our results much more complex than has been indicated by the conclusions of other investigators.

The fundamental principle that a solution containing cells has a higher resistance than the same solution without cells seems to have been established before 1900, being used by Fischer,[1] Roth,[2] Burgarsky and Tangl,[3] Stewart,[4], and Oker-Blom,[5] working with red blood cells in serums and salt solutions. Stewart [6] demonstrated that the resistance of a suspension of erythrocytes decreased on hemolysis, and McClendon [7] showed a decrease in the resistance of a suspension of echinoderm eggs on fertilization. This and similar experimental work by others has formed the basis for the more elaborate work which has been done in applying the conductivity method to the measurement of functional changes in permeability of cell membranes. The decrease observed in the resistance of a suspension of live cells on injury or death of the cells seems to be accepted by most investigators as a

Received for publication, Jan. 25, 1922.

* Aided by a grant from the National Dental Research Association.

[1] Jahrb. d. Botanik, 1895, 27, p. 1.

[2] Elect. Leitfähigkeit thierischer Flüssigkeiten, 1897.

[3] Ztschr. f. Phys., 1897, 2, p. 297.

[4] Jour. Physiol., 1899, 24, p. 356.

[5] Pflüger's Arch., 1900, 79, p. 111 and 510.

[6] Jour. Pharmacol. & Exper. Therap., 1910, 1, p. 49.

[7] Am. Jour. Physiol., 1910, 27, p. 270.

quantitative measure of an increased conductance by the cells due to a change in the cell membrane. Osterhout [8] definitely subscribes to this view in his work with Laminaria and finds that the resistance of a cylinder of Laminaria disks in sea water drops to the resistance of an equal cylinder of sea water when the cells die. Gray [9] working with echinoderm eggs reports similar findings. Shearer [10] finds that when a suspension of B. coli in Ringer's solution is heated, the resistance drops to that of Ringer's solution alone. He states that the resistance is produced by the living state and that dead cells offer no more resistance than so much agar or gelatin. The idea that the observed changes in resistance are due to an increased permeability of the membrane to the ions carrying the electric current was not held by Stiles and Jorgensen,[11] and they pointed out that the exchange of salts between the cell interior and the liquid surrounding the cell must be taken into consideration. Stiles and Kidd [12] measured the osmosis of salts by measuring the conductivity of the solution surrounding plant tissues and considered this a measurement of permeability. However, experimental work taking into account all factors involved in this complex problem with consideration of the relative effects of each, seems at present to be lacking.

In our work, suspensions of bacteria were used. Results from the use of free cells suspended in a simple solution would seem to be more easily analyzed than those obtained from the use of mass tissue in that there is only one type of cell present and because there is no intercellular substance to complicate the interpretation of measurements. Bacterial cells may be preferred to eggs for this type of experimentation in that we are not sure the membrane of a dormant egg is comparable in properties of permeability to the membrane of a complete individual making use of its membrane by virtue of an active metabolism. Above all, with the use of suspended cells, the liquid may be separated from the cells and studied separately.

Our experiments were made with B. coli and Staphylococcus albus which were grown in Kolle flasks, washed off, centrifuged from the wash water and resuspended in salt solutions, the strength and character of which varied with other experimental conditions. The measurements were made with a modified Wheatstone bridge using an

[8] Science, 1912, 35, p. 112.
[9] Proc. Roy. Soc., B, 1916, 207, p. 481.
[10] Jour. Hygiene, 1919, 18, p. 360.
[11] Ann. Bot., 1915, 29, p. 611.
[12] Proc. Roy. Soc., B, 1919, 90, p. 448.

oscillating current of 4,000 cycles obtained from a Vreeland oscillator. Duplicate readings with radio-frequency from an audion bulb showed that variations in frequency do not produce variations in measured resistance and so introduce no error. Very delicate and accurate readings were obtainable by the use of a variometer in series with the electrolytic cell. The measurements were made in a water bath constant to 1/25 degree Centigrade. The electrolytic cell was an L or boot shaped cell, the horizontal portion, which carried the electrodes, having a capacity of 1.5 mils.

The experiments here reported concern changes in resistance of suspensions of bacteria on death of the bacterial cells as produced by heat and liquor formaldehydi. Experiments were carried out in general according to the following technic:

The suspension of bacteria having been made in a salt solution of the desired strength, its resistance was measured by transferring 2 mils to the electrolytic cell. On replacing this, the suspension was centrifuged and the clear supernatant liquid obtained, the resistance of which was measured. A suspension was formed once more by means of a rotating glass stirrer until constant readings were obtained and the suspension resistance again measured as a check. The suspension was then heated at a definite temperature for a definite time which varied in different experiments. After a thorough mixing the resistance of the heated suspension was determined. Again centrifuging to obtain the supernatant liquid from the killed bacteria, its resistance was measured. After mixing the dead cells with the solution once more, the resistance of the suspension of dead bacteria was again obtained. The measurements of the unheated or live organisms before and after centrifuging showed that the operation did not bring about any change in resistance, so experimental error from that source seems to be eliminated.

For convenience the suspensions are designated as live or dead, the degree of heat applied being above the thermal death point for the bacteria used. The liquid suspending the cells is referred to as the menstruum live, or menstruum dead, depending on whether it was suspending live or dead cells when separated for measurement. The results of several experiments using B. coli are given. They are put in graphic form to show the relation of the different values at a glance. The ordinates represent resistance in ohms, the abscissas merely indicate the operation which brought about a change in the ordinates.

Fig. 1 represents the results obtained with the heating of B. coli in approximately 0.5% NaCl solution at 60 C. for 90 minutes.

Fig. 2 shows the changes in resistance which occurred when B. coli was heated in approximately 0.3% NaCl at 92 C. for 6 minutes. The menstruum in these experiments was mainly an NaCl solution as specified, but the solution contained some calcium and other ions carried over from the nutrient medium.

From these data the following points are to be noted for subsequent discussion.

1. Coincident with a drop in resistance of the bacterial suspension, there is a marked drop in the resistance of the menstruum.

2. The dead bacterial cells act to raise the resistance of the solution in which they are suspended similar to live cells, but it would appear, on superficial consideration at least, to a lesser extent.

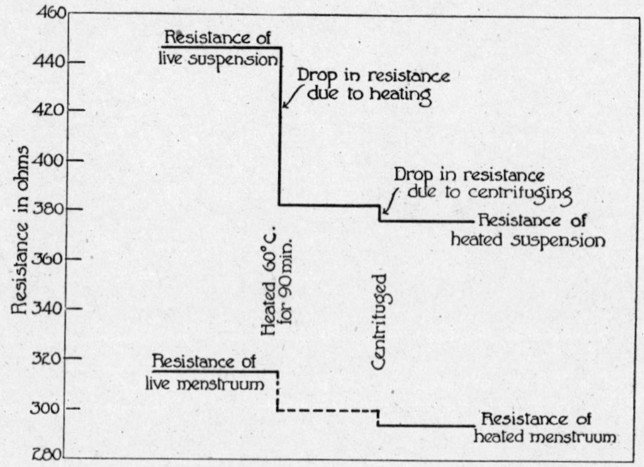

Fig. 1.—B. coli suspended in 0.5% NaCl solution and heated to 60 C. for 9 minutes.

3. After the cells are heated and the resistance of the suspension determined, a further drop in resistance is found to occur on centrifuging and remixing.

The first of these points has its explanation in the exosmosis of salts from the cells into the surrounding medium. This decrease in resistance of the menstruum is always included in the measurement of the cells plus the menstruum, and of course becomes an error when the drop in suspension resistance is interpreted as measuring increased penetration of the plasmic membrane to mobile ions. To eliminate this error it is evident that the concentration of salts inside and outside the cell must be balanced in such a manner that when the membrane of the cell is made completely permeable there will be no increase in the number of current carriers in the liquid between the cells. These experimental conditions are probably never fulfilled. In our experiments we have found that bacteria growing on ordinary media store up salts to a greater concentration than is found in the media on which they are grown. On killing Spirogyra in the pond water in which they were rapidly growing, we likewise found a great exosmosis of the salts from the cells into their natural habitat. We have termed these diffusible salts the physiologic, in contradistinction to the structural salts which are bound up in body structure and demonstrated only by ash analysis. It is our ignorance of the conditions controlling or determining the concentration of these physiologic salts that makes this factor so difficult to estimate or eliminate in conductivity measurements.

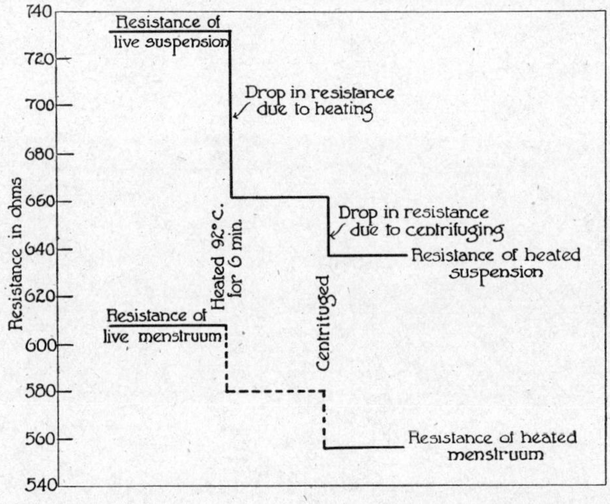

Fig. 2.—B. coli suspended in 0.3% NaCl solution and heated at 92 C. for 6 minutes.

The second point noted, that dead cells increase the resistance of a solution in which they are placed, is a constant finding in all of our experiments. A comparison with live cells made on the basis of solutions of equal resistance shows that the dead cells raise the resistance of the solution 75% or more of the amount observed when the same cells were alive. While this finding is contrary to the results of other investigators, we call attention to the simplicity of the technic used in our experiments. The suspension of bacteria was broken up by centrifuging and remixing repeatedly, the resistance of the solution alone and then the solution suspending the cells being measured each time. The result was not affected by the degree of heat used, and findings were similar when the cells were killed by liquor formaldehydi.

We also noted that the heated suspension was different from the unheated in that a drop in resistance took place on centrifuging and remixing. A further drop did not take place on repeating the manipulation. It does not seem possible to say definitely whether this is due to a change in the menstruum or in the bacteria themselves. There are several possibilities. A change in permeability of the membrane due to centrifuging seems unlikely. It might be due to a decrease in the size of the bacteria, a possibility given in detail below. A

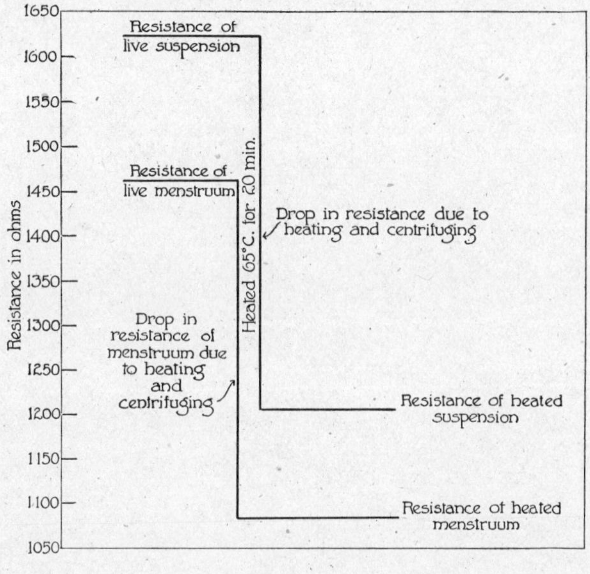

Fig. 3.—B. coli suspended in 0.7% NaCl solution and heated at 65 C. for 20 minutes.

third possibility is that there is a further exosmosis of salts from the bacteria into the surrounding menstruum due to the mechanical action of centrifuging. It is seen from the graphic representation of our results that we subscribe to the latter view as the explanation.

The quantitative effect of exosmosis must depend on the relation between the concentration of electrolytes within and around the cells. Figures 3, 4 and 5 are graphic representations of an experiment in which the same number of bacteria, grown under identical conditions, were killed by heat when suspended in equal quantities of NaCl solution varying in NaCl content.

A suspension of B. coli was divided into equal parts by weight and after centrifuging, NaCl solutions were substituted for the original menstruum in weighed amounts. This experiment again demonstrates the results previously discussed and illustrates the relation of the electrolyte concentration of the menstruum surrounding the cells to the results obtained by conductivity measurements. Fig. 4 is an example of experimental conditions being right to make the resistance of the menstruum plus the dead bacteria equal to the live menstruum alone, from which it might be erroneously assumed that dead cells offer little or no resistance if the heated menstruum were not separated and measured.

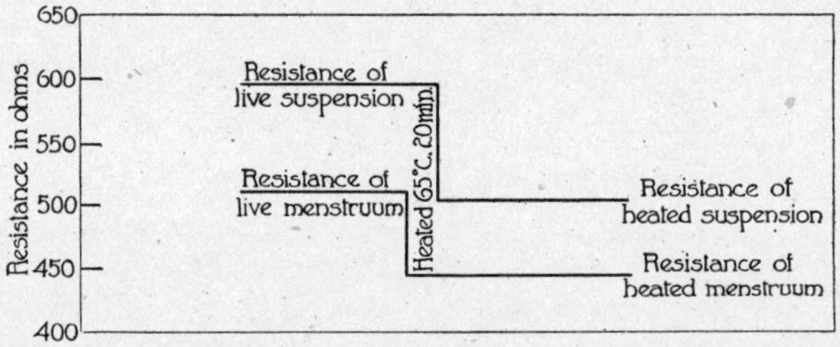

Fig. 4.—B. coli suspended in 0.3% NaCl solution and heated at 65 C. for 20 minutes.

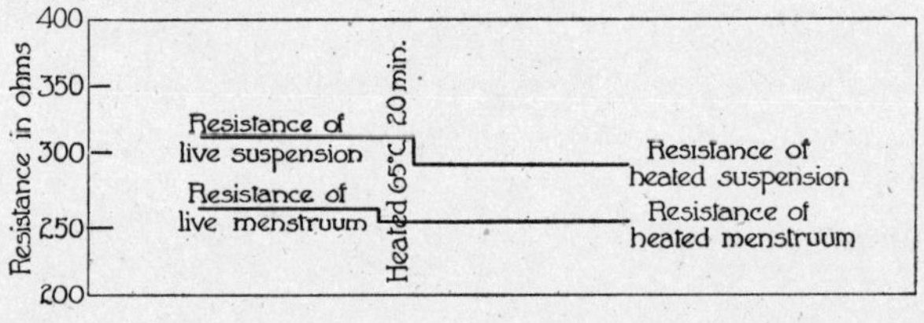

Fig. 5.—B. coli suspended in 0.1% NaCl solution and heated at 65 C. for 20 minutes.

Another important factor that must be considered in the interpretation of conductivity measurements is the variation in volume of cells if there is any. If it is true that cells store up salts to a greater concentration than is found in their liquid habitat, the resulting turgor must keep the cell expanded to a maximum volume. It might be expected that an exosmosis of salts might allow a shrinking of the volume of the cell and that this might be increased by the packing of the cells in centrifuging. Some support for this view is gained from the common observation that the centrifuged volume of bacterial cells is much decreased after the cells are heated.

Direct measurements made on live and dead bacterial cells when prepared by both positive and negative stains show considerable decrease in the size of individual cells on death. The effect of a decrease in the size of the bacterial cells on death is that less space will be taken up between the electrodes by the dead bacterial bodies which we have found to have a higher resistance than the suspending solution, and there will be a corresponding decrease in total resistance due to this factor.

It appears that if the resistance of a suspension of bacteria decreases, such a decrease may be due to at least three factors. exosmosis of salts; decrease in the size of the cells, and the passage of ions through the bacterial membrane owing to increased permeability.

In our experiments exosmosis seems to be the factor of greatest moment. Our findings that at death there is only a slight decrease in the ability of the bacterial cells suspended in a solution to offer resistance to an electric current makes it appear that any change in permeability of the cell membrane must be of minor value. This is further emphasized by the finding that the dead cells have a lessened ability to obstruct an electric current in that they displace less conducting solution.

In this discussion no values for the resistance of bacterial cells have been assigned, as in such a system the resistances are not in series and the total resistance does not indicate the value of the individual resistances concerned.

SUMMARY

Dead bacterial cells offer resistance to an electric current almost if not equal in amount to that exhibited by live bacterial cells.

Bacterial cells growing in ordinary mediums store up diffusible salts within their bodies to a greater concentration than is found in their habitat.

On the death of bacterial cells by heat or liquor formaldehydi there is an exchange of salts between the cells and the surrounding medium.

In our series of experiments the drop in resistance on cell death could be shown to be due in greatest part to an exosmosis of salts into the surrounding solution.

On death of bacteria there is a definite decrease in the size of the cell.

From our findings it appears that conductivity measurements do not measure a change in permeability of bacterial membranes, but that permeability is only indicated by the exosmosis of salts from the cells killed by heat and by liquor formaldehydi.

THE OCCURRENCE OF ENTAMOEBA HISTOLYTICA WITH TISSUE LESIONS IN THE TESTIS AND EPIDIDYMIS IN CHRONIC DYSENTERY *

Aldred Scott Warthin

From the Pathological Laboratory of the University of Michigan, Ann Arbor

Amebas associated with pathologic processes have been reported as occurring in nearly every organ of the body, with the exception of the parts named in the title of this paper. As Dobell has pointed out, a large number of these reports on pathogenic ameboid organisms observed in man are either mistaken identifications of nonpathogenic forms, or misinterpretations. This is particularly true of the ameboid organisms reported as having been found in the urinary tract, lungs, pleural and peritoneal cavities, skin, and in pus from abscesses in various portions of the body. Many of these reports are probably misinterpretations of epithelial, mesothelial or endothelial cells, atypical cell-forms derived from granulation tissue, or of degenerating flagellates or other organisms. The vague and imperfect descriptions of most of these reports give additional grounds for their rejection.

No positive proof exists at the present time that there is any species of ameba pathogenic to man other than Entamoeba histolytica (Loeschia histolytica). This organism is widely distributed throughout the world; and, with the evidence at hand, this is the only species responsible for any amebic pathologic condition in man. It is generally recognized now as the sole etiologic agent in amebic dysentery and the secondary complications of this infection, such as hepatic, hepatopulmonic, splenic and cerebral abscess. In all of these secondary conditions amebas have been repeatedly demonstrated that cannot be distinuished from those in the primary intestinal lesions. The same thing has also been claimed by various observers for the skin, blood and urine; but the evidence given in these cases is too incomplete to be convincing.

There is no literature more confused and perplexing from the zoological standpoint than that on the ameba. To Dobell we are much indebted for his attempts to unravel this synonymic tangle. He shows that the species pathogenic to man is preferably called Entamoeba histolytica and this appellation is accepted by most writers. On the

Received for publication, Feb. 1, 1922.

other hand, Castellani prefers Schaudinn's term, Loeschia histolytica. Without going further into this discussion the writer accepts for this report the views of Dobell and his criteria for the recognition of this organism.

The case reported here is a product of the routine microscopic study of all the organs and tissues from the necropsies made in this laboratory.

Case History.—A Russian Hebrew, aged 33, a boilermaker, was admitted to the Medical Clinic (Dr. Hewlett) April 20, 1916. He had acquired syphilis at the age of 17, and had been treated by injections over a period of five years; he has had no symptoms of the disease since. Eleven years previously (1904-5) he was in China during the Russo-Japanese War, and contracted dysentery. He had at that time from 20 to 40 bloody stools daily, but without pain. Food did not affect the condition. After three months he went back to Russia, where

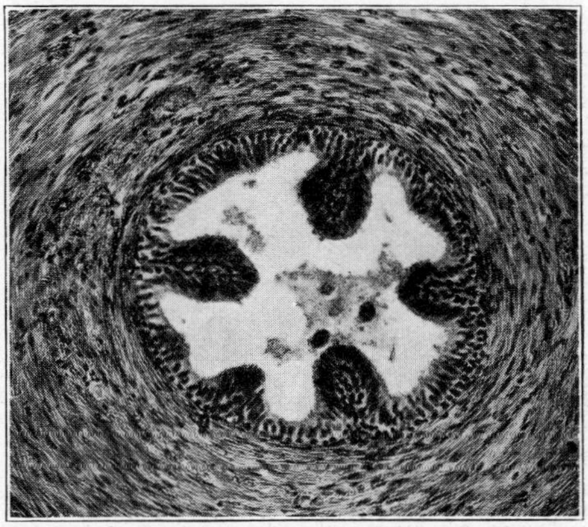

Fig. 1.—Section of upper portion of vas deferens, with small fibrin clot containing several amebas.

he apparently recovered. He came to the United States in 1910, going first to Chicago, and then to Detroit. Eighteen months before admission his intestinal trouble had returned. He had about ten stools daily, small in amount and bloody; they were painless, but he has always had a feeling of soreness in the right lower quadrant. His appetite remained good; he never vomited; food had no effect on his diarrhea. He was treated for about five weeks in Harper Hospital without any improvement. Six months before admission the blood disappeared from the stools, and after that time he continued to have from 8 to 9 watery stools a day. He took treatment all the time without results. He had lost 32 pounds during the last six months. He had had night sweats during the last 3 weeks. He did not cough; he was never jaundiced. He was always thirsty, and he had to get up four times nightly to pass water. There were no other symptoms.

Physical examination revealed an anemic, underweight and undersized man, with numerous scars over the face and upper thorax, slight scarring at the angles of the lips, a brown, slightly indurated scar on the penis. There were tattoo marks on both arms. The cervical glands only were enlarged. The lower border of the liver was three finger breadths below the edge of the ribs in the nipple line. There was some tenderness on pressure over the liver. The spleen was not palpable. There was soreness in the right shoulder without limitation of movements or swelling. Examination of lungs was negative. The heart was over-active. The pulse rate was 120, regular and easily compressed. The temperature was 99.6 F.; respiration, 24. Roentgenologic report showed pleural thickening on the left side, with early tuberculosis of the right apex. A sclerosing glossitis (Dr. Wile). The blood contained 2,400,000 red blood

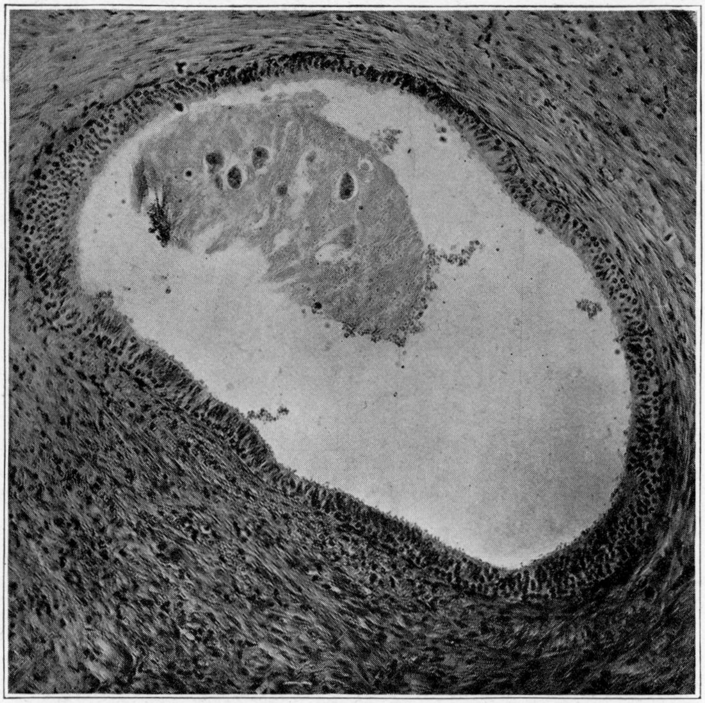

Fig. 2.—Section of tail of epididymis with fibrin clot containing a number of Entamoeba histolytica. The form of the amebas is made elliptical through contraction of the fibrin during fixation.

cells, 16,000 white cells and 65% of hemoglobin. Urine examination was negative. The stools were soft and yellow, containing fat and meat fibers, occult blood, and many amebas of the type of *Entamoeba histolytica.*

Clinical Diagnosis: Amebic dysentery; syphilis.

He was placed on emetin hydrochloride, bismuth, saline rectal irrigations, dilute hydrochloric acid and forced special milk diet. By May 8 the amebas had entirely disappeared from the stools, but his general condition was not improved. He ran a septic temperature, and the lower border of the liver descended, easily palpable and tender. He was, therefore, thought to have an amebic abscess of the liver and was referred to the Surgical Clinic (Dr. Darling) for operation. An exploratory laparotomy was performed May 9. No abscess was found at operation. Following the operation he developed pneumonia and died May 14. The stools remained free of amebas during the last 6 days.

Necropsy (Dr. Warthin) 2½ hours after death: The most important points of the protocol were:

Small, slender build; general nutrition poor; anemic; general edema; numerous scars over the face and trunk; pigmented scar on the penis; scars in angles of the lips; recent laparotomy wound in right hypochondrium, to the right of the

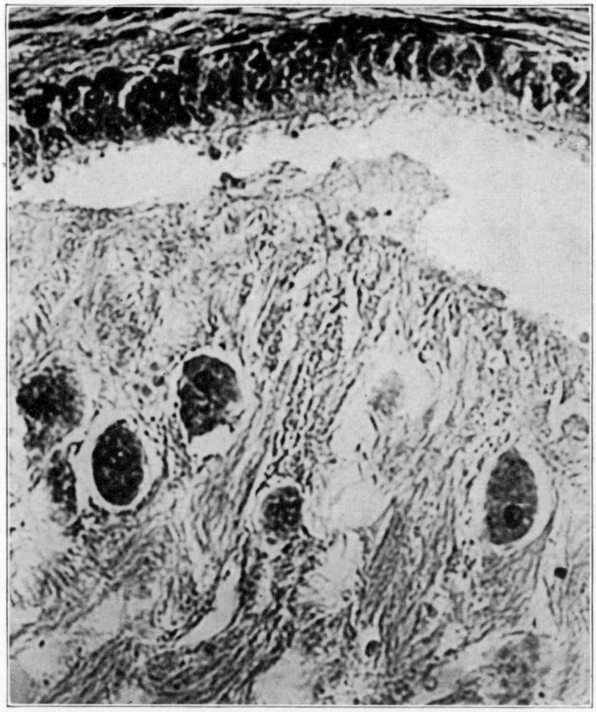

Fig. 3.—Higher power view of portion of clot containing Entamoeba histolytica, from tail of epididymis.

median line, extending vertically, 10 cm. in length; abdomen below level of ribs; right arm tattooed with Russian characters; testicles small and firm; left epididymis enlarged; hydrocele and spermatocele on left side.

Upper portion of peritoneal cavity filled with a fibrinopurulent exudate; peritoneum cloudy and covered with exudate; surface of liver adherent to abdominal wall and to colon by fresh adhesions; heart small, "droplet heart"; large patch of sclerosis; orifices and valves negative; fatty change in muscle; lungs adherent by firm adhesions; left lower lobe airless, firm, on section presenting numerous small encapsulated abscesses; pressure forces many fibrinopurulent plugs from bronchioles and alveoli; unresolved croupous pneumonia;

spleen slightly larger than normal, firmer, purplish-red; on section, purplish-red, marked congestion, trabeculae not prominent, follicles small. No abscess.

Intestinal coils free throughout, with the exception of adhesions of colon to liver; peritoneum of small intestine cloudy and covered with thin layer of exudate; on section, mucosa congested, thickened, covered with mucus, appearance of a chronic catarrhal enteritis; no ulcers; the wall of the colon thickened throughout its entire length, showed many congested points but no ulcers, mucosa covered with thick layer of mucus; no pigmentation of mucosa; irregular patches of thinning in the mucosa, apparently wholly covered by mucous

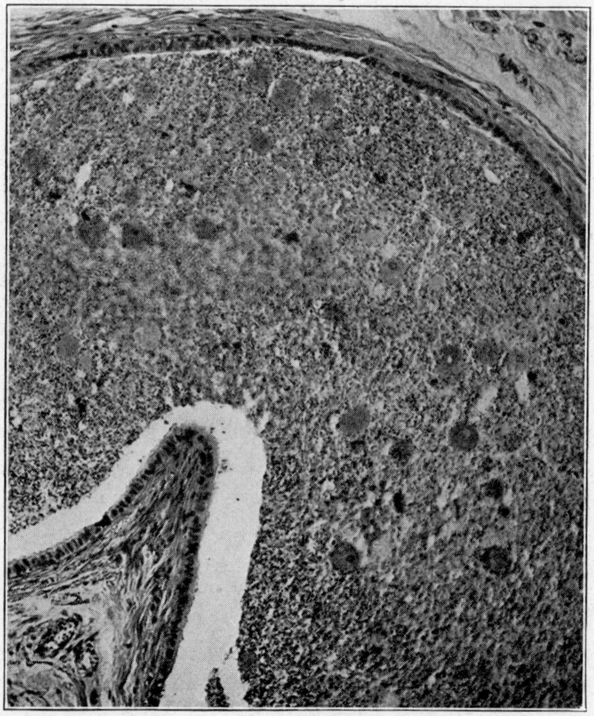

Fig. 4.—Section of body of epididymis showing duct filled with spermatozoa, through which are scattered many amebas. In the semen the amebas are more round and the characteristic annular nucleus and karyosome are clearly seen.

membrane, probably healed ulcers; appendix plump, wall thickened, lumen patent; peritoneal surface of stomach covered with fresh fibrinopurulent exudate; wall edematous.

Surface of liver covered with fresh adhesions uniting it to abdominal wall and to incision; liver somewhat enlarged, of firmer consistency, capsule thickened and opaque, particularly on under side, where it shows shallow stellate contractions over the surface; on section, liver is firm, light yellow-brown, lobules small, stroma between lobules increased—early atrophic hepatitis; no abscess; gallbladder dilated, filled with clear pale yellow bile; bile passages patent;

pancreas negative; peripancreatic lymph nodes much enlarged, grayish, translucent, edematous; mesenteric nodes moderately enlarged and edematous.

The suprarenals showed atrophy and excessive lipoidosis; fatty capsules of both kidneys poor in fat; right kidney somewhat larger than left; fibrous capsules slightly adherent, surfaces smooth; small calculus in pelvis of left kidney; both kidneys pale.

Aorta showed numerous patches of fatty change in its intima.

Retroperitoneal lymph nodes and hemal nodes enlarged.

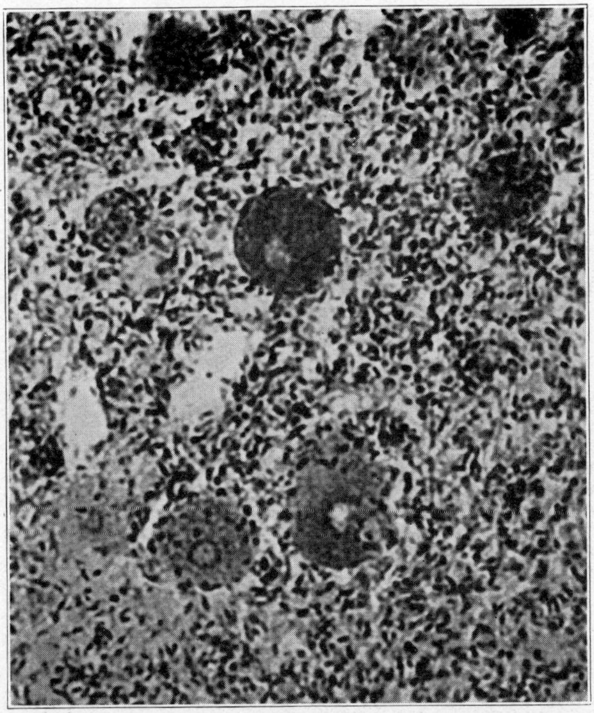

Fig. 5.—Higher power view of portion of field shown in preceding figure; entamoeba histolytica in mass of sperm in epididymis. The characteristics of the nucleus are well shown, as is also the phagocytosis of spermatozoa by them.

Epididymis dilated; spermatocele on left; left testis large, on section showed fibroid patch; right testis smaller and firmer, stroma increased; prostate slightly enlarged; seminal vesicles dilated, full of semen; seminal ducts dilated. The bladder contained purulent urine, mucosa negative.

The microscopic examination of the different organs and tissues revealed:

Heart: Sclerosis of epicardium; fatty infiltration of subepicardial tissue with beginning serous atrophy; simple atrophy, cloudy swelling and fatty degenerative infiltration of heart muscle; early coronary sclerosis; a few small active areas of syphilitic myocarditis; sclerosis of endocardium.

Lungs: Croupous pneumonia, delayed resolution, multiple abscesses and beginning organization; purulent bronchitis; no amebas in abscesses; marked anthracosis.

Tongue: Marked fibroid hypeprplasia of the papillae with atrophy of the lymphoid tissue; chronic syphilitic glossitis.

Aorta: Slight sclerosis of the intima; a few small plasma cell infiltrations around the vasa vasorum; early syphilitic mesaortitis.

Spleen: Marked chronic passive congestion with marked increase of stroma; diffuse fibrosis with atrophy of the lymphoid tissue; sclerosis of artioles; acute fibrinous perisplenitis.

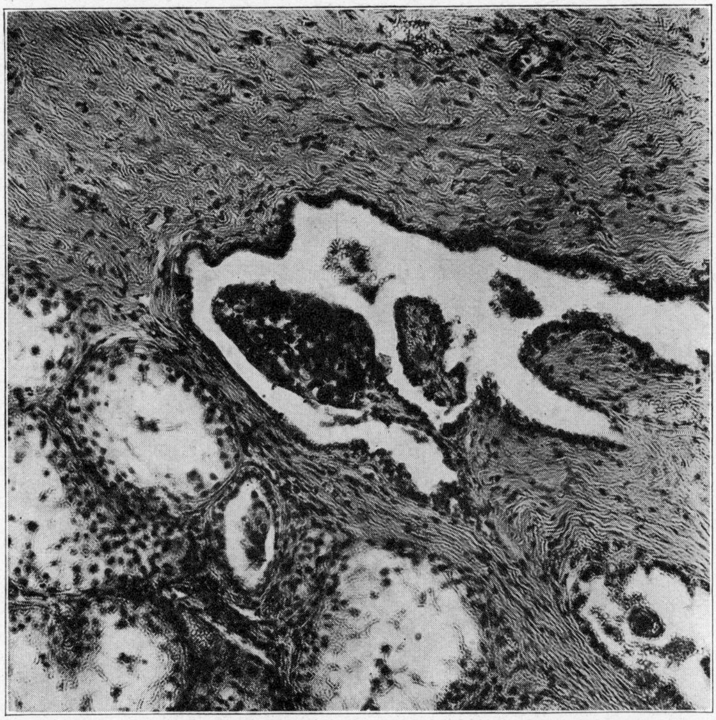

Fig. 6.—Mass of ameba cysts attached in clot to small ulcer or erosion in duct of rete testis.

Liver: Well advanced atrophic cirrhosis; areas of plasma-cell infiltration and proliferation of blood vessels and stroma (syphilitic hepatitis), most marked at periphery of lobules; new formation of bile ducts; acute fibrinopurulent perihepatitis; no abscesses in liver.

Pancreas: Slight fatty atrophy; areas of interstitial pancreatitis (syphilitic); fibrosis of some of the islands; marked dilatation of pancreatic ducts.

Suprarenals: Capsules thickened; atrophy with lipoidosis of the parenchyma; small plasma-cell infiltrations in the medulla.

Kidneys: Slight atrophy and cloudy swelling; marked passive congestion; few casts; many of the tubules dilated; early sclerosis.

Ureters: Dilated; otherwise negative.

Bladder: Negative.

Stomach: Chronic catarrhal gastritis; mucosa atrophic in areas, in others showing a polypoid hypertrophy; no normal gastric glands; acute fibrinopurulent peritonitis.

Small Intestine: Marked chronic catarrhal enteritis; no ulcers; subacute peritonitis.

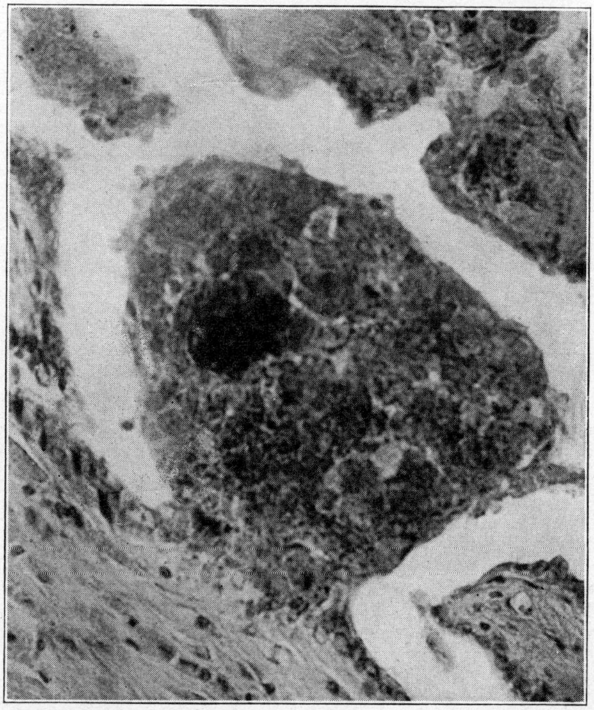

Fig. 7.—Higher power view of blood clot attached to small ulcer in tubule of rete testis, containing Entamoeba histolytica in various stages of development, many adult forms filled with red blood cells. Precystic and cyst forms. The faint granulation of the stroma cells in the lower right hand corner is hemosiderin.

Colon: Severe chronic catarrhal colitis; mucosa atrophic in areas, hypertrophic in others; numerous small healing and healed ulcers with regeneration of epithelium and hyperplastic margins; no amebas found; nearly healed dysentery; fibrosis of all coats.

Appendix: Chronic catarrh.

Mesenteric Lymph Nodes: Chronic lymphadenitis with marked sinus catarrh.

Prostate: Slight glandular hyperplasia and cystic dilatation; no inflammatory changes; no amebas found in any of the gland spaces or ducts.

Seminal Vesicles: Dilated with albuminous fluid containing many spermatozoa; no amebas found.

Vas Deferens: Both seminal ducts were moderately dilated above, more markedly so below. In the lower dilated portions there were pink-staining fibrinous clots of loose texture containing numerous typical amebas of the histolytica type. These clots only partly filled the lumen of the duct and were not attached to the wall; they increased in size toward the epididymis, giving the appearance of floating up into the tube from below.

Epididymes: Both, but particularly the left, showed marked dilatation of the ducts. These were filled in part with masses of spermatozoa through which great numbers of amebas were scattered. In the sperm-filled ducts there was little fibrin, and the amebas were rounder than in the fibrin clots in the vasa. No blood cells were found in the amebas in the semen; but there was marked phagocytosis of spermatozoa by the amebas. On the left side a number of the large dilated ducts in the head of the epididymis contained a heavy albuminous, almost hyaline, precipitate, without spermatozoa or amebas, apparently blind tubules. About the ducts the connective tissue was thickened and the blood vessels were sclerotic, but there was slight active inflammatory reaction. The ductuli efferentes of the lobules of the epididymis and of the mediastinum testis and extending into the rete testis were all dilated but were free of sperm. They contained, however, numerous small fibrin clots, in the meshes of which amebas in various stages of development were present. These clots were either attached at some point to the wall of the duct, or extended into the ducts of the rete where they were attached. At the point of attachment of the clot the epithelium was absent, and the duct wall showed a superficial ulceration. Small hemorrhages in the tissues of the wall of the duct occurred beneath the attachment of the clot and in its neighborhood. The stroma cells were increased in number and size, and contained fine yellowish-brown granules of a pigment giving the iron reaction (hemosiderin). In the clot attached to the lining of the duct amebas in all stages of development were present, many precystic and cystic forms. The adult types showed marked phagocytosis of red blood cells, especially those in the portion of the clot next to the denuded tissue. In many of the clots a layer of amebas lay in direct contact with the connective tissue, and in a few places some of the amebas had penetrated a slight distance into the tissue-spaces. The appearances were those of an actual active erosion of the duct wall by the parasites. Fresh hemorrhages of minute size accompanied this invasion, and the invading amebas showed active phagocytosis of the red blood cells. No phagocytosis of seprmatozoa was seen in the amebas in the rete testis.

Testes: Many seminiferous tubules showed aspermatogenesis with vacuolation of germ cells; other tubules showed active spermatogenesis. The stroma was increased and edematous. Small patches of fibroid atrophy (syphilitic) occurred, more marked in the left testis than in the right. A few seminiferous tubules near the rete were dilated, filled with sperm, and contained amebas mixed with spermatozoa. These amebas showed phagocytosis of the sperm, as in the epididymis. No red cells were distinguishable in these amebas. There was no reaction, and no pigmentation around these tubules.

The amebas found in the testes corresponded in every way to those previously found in the stools of the patient when first seen, and were identified as Entamoeba histolytica. The size of the organisms, the character of the nucleus, its annular appearance, the characteristic central karyosome with halo, eccentric position of the nucleus, the marked phagocytosis of spermatozoa and red blood cells, the production of slight but definite tissue lesions, and the character of the precystic and cystic forms—all of these points establish the diagnosis beyond doubt. In the dilated duct of the epididymis many degenerating forms were present, as well as precystic and cystic forms. In the clots the contraction of the fibrin reticulum caused more or less distortion during fixation, the organisms being slightly compressed or contracted into a more elliptical form.

The complete pathologic diagnosis was: Unresolved croupous pneumonia, with early abscess-formation and organization; purulent bronchitis; early atrophic cirrhosis; chronic passive congestion of spleen with fibrosis; healed chronic dysentery (amebic); metastasis of Entamoeba histolytica to epididymes and testes with local lesions; latent syphilis (leptomeningitis, myocarditis, hepatitis, pancreatitis, mesaortitis, orchitis, etc.); early sclerosis; atrophy, parenchymatous degeneration and passive congestion of all organs; recent laparotomy; tattoo.

This case, therefore, presents the unique occurrence of the metastasis of Entamoeba histolytica to the epididymes and testes with definite, though slight, local lesions in these organs, in a patient affected for many years with amebic dysentery, at the time of death nearly completely healed, with disappearance of amebas from the stools. It is the first recorded instance of such a localization of Entamoeba histolytica, and presents additional evidence of the mildly pathogenic character of this parasite, in the slight tissue destruction caused by it and its phagocytosis of red blood cells and spermatozoa. A point of some interest is the localization of the small lesions in the rete testes and tubuli efferentes, with long streaming clots extending upward into the epididymis, the amebas being held within these clots. In the dilated semen-filled portions of the epididymis the organisms were found in greater numbers and free in the semen. Their commensal character is shown by the phagocytosis of red blood cells in the clots, and by that of spermatozoa in the semen particularly; that is, they show the same tendency in the semen to feed on substances contained in it as they do on the substances in the intestinal contents.

THE EXCRETION OF SPIROCHAETA PALLIDA THROUGH THE KIDNEYS

Aldred Scott Warthin

From the Pathological Laboratory of the University of Michigan, Ann Arbor

That spirocheturia is a striking phenomenon in Weil's disease was first demonstrated by Inado and Ito,[1] who, in February, 1915, announced the discovery of Spirochaeta icterohaemorrhagica as the cause of this infection. The excretion of the spirochetes in the urine was shown by successful transmission of the disease through inoculations of urine from infected animals and patients. Dark-field examinations of the urine in the early stages of infectious jaundice reveal the presence of the spirochetes in small numbers; from the tenth to the twenty-fifth days they are usually found in enormous numbers. After this time they degenerate and finally disappear by the fortieth day. Their appearance in the urine in numbers is usually coincident with the beginning formation of immune bodies. Pathologic studies showed that the spirochetes are present in the kidneys in great numbers, even more so than in the liver. They are massed in the intertubular interstitial tissues especially, but are found also in the wall and lumen of the tubules. The kidneys present the appearance of acute degenerative nephritis. In November of the same year Uhlenhuth and Fromme,[2] independently working on Weil's disease in Germany, reported also the discovery of the presence of a spirochete in the blood, liver, kidneys and urine of human cases and inoculated guinea-pigs which they regarded as the cause of infectious jaundice. The occurrence of icterogenic spirochetosis was recognized in the British and French armies during 1916-17; and the importance of spirocheturia as an early diagnostic factor was insisted on by a number of writers, particularly in France. Recognition of the spirocheturia was one of the chief points leading to the establishment of the identity of "trench" or "war jaundice" with Weil's disease. The value of this sign became questioned by a number of observers because

Received for publication Feb. 1, 1922.

This investigation was carried out under a grant from the Interdepartmental Social Hygiene Board, Washington, D. C.

[1] Jour. Exper. Med., 1916, *23*, p. 377.

[2] Med. Klin., 1915, 11, pp. 1202 and 1264; Ztschr. f. Immunitätsf., 1916, *25*, p. 317.

of the possible contamination of urine with the spirochetes present in the meatus or on the glans. Other workers showed that with proper precautions such urethral contaminations could be avoided; and the demonstration of a renal spirocheturia remains one of the most important phenomena of Weil's disease of diagnostic value.

In 1917, Garnier and Reilly[3] studied especially the renal lesions of infectious jaundice and their relation to the excretion of the spirochetes. They found that the elimination of the spirochetes takes place chiefly through the convoluted tubules. The degenerative lesions are confined to the epithelium of these tubules, while the glomeruli remain unaffected. Accompanying the epithelial degeneration there is an interstitial reaction which in cases running a long course may approach sclerosis In cases in which death occurs early there is an arrest of the renal function with or without cytolysis of the tubular epithelium. In patients dying later the lesions are more marked and extensive, with homogenization of the cytoplasm. Fatty degeneration does not occur. The spirochetes at first are massed in the intertubular spaces, and later pass through the epithelium toward the lumen of the tubule. At the inner pole of the cells they begin to show fragmentation and attenuation, finally breaking up in part into granules, while others pass apparently unchanged into the lumen of the tubule and out with the urine. Throughout the tubules desquamated epithelial cells and casts containing spirochetes also occur.

Other observers have confirmed the importance of the renal lesions and the spirocheturia occurring in infectious jaundice during the septicemic stage of the disease. Spirochetes regarded as identical with the parasite of infectious jaundice have been found in the kidneys and urine of wild rats in Japan, Belgium, France and America. We possess, however, little knowledge concerning the excretion of other forms of spirochetes through the kidneys. Futaki found spirochetes in the kidney in typhus fever, but his observations have not been confirmed. This stimulated a group of Japanese workers to an intensive research on the occurrence of spirochetes in the kidneys. Kou, Watabiki and their associates[4] found by the Levaditi method what they took to be spirochetes in 26 of 50 kidneys from cadavers and in 15 of 26 kidneys removed surgically. The spirochete-like bodies were found only in casts or detritus in the lumen of the tubules, and were not present in the interstitial tissue, epithelial cells or blood vessels with the exception of an occasional occurrence in the glomeruli. There was no reason to believe that they were associated with any definite disease or that they were being eliminated by the kidneys. It was thought that they might represent an ascending saprophytic infection from the smegma. Three types were described, always mixed together. They were not all sharply differentiated from Spirochaeta pallida, but were considered different morphologically. Other evidence of syphilis was not present in these cases. There can be little doubt that the bodies found were not true spirochetes, but represent the same silver-impregnation forms somewhat resembling them seen by a number of European observers in the tubules of kidneys showing lesions of acute nephritis.

Ido, Ito and Waji[5] state that in seven-day fever a condition of spirocheturia closely resembling that of infectious jaundice is found. The spirochetes (Sp.

[3] Compt. rend. Soc. de biol., 1917, 80, p. 38; Arch. de méd. et d'Anat. path., 1918, 28, p. 375; Presse méd., 1918, 26, p. 505.

[4] Tokyo Med. News, 1917, p. 2375.

[5] Tokyo Med. News, 1917, No. 2053.

hebdomadis) appear in the urine after the eighth day, the organisms occasionally occurring in great numbers. From the eighteenth to the twenty-fifth day they are found constantly, and may persist to the thirty-ninth day. The disease resembles very much an atypical Weil's disease. According to Kusama, Koboyashi and Kuzunshi,[6] the spirochete of rat-bite fever (Sp. morsusmuris) is rarely excreted in the urine of infected guinea-pigs. The spirochetes of relapsing fever (Sp. recurrentis) have been demonstrated in sections of the kidney taken from patients and infected animals, but no study seems to have been made of the occurrence of spirocheturia in this infection. It is of great

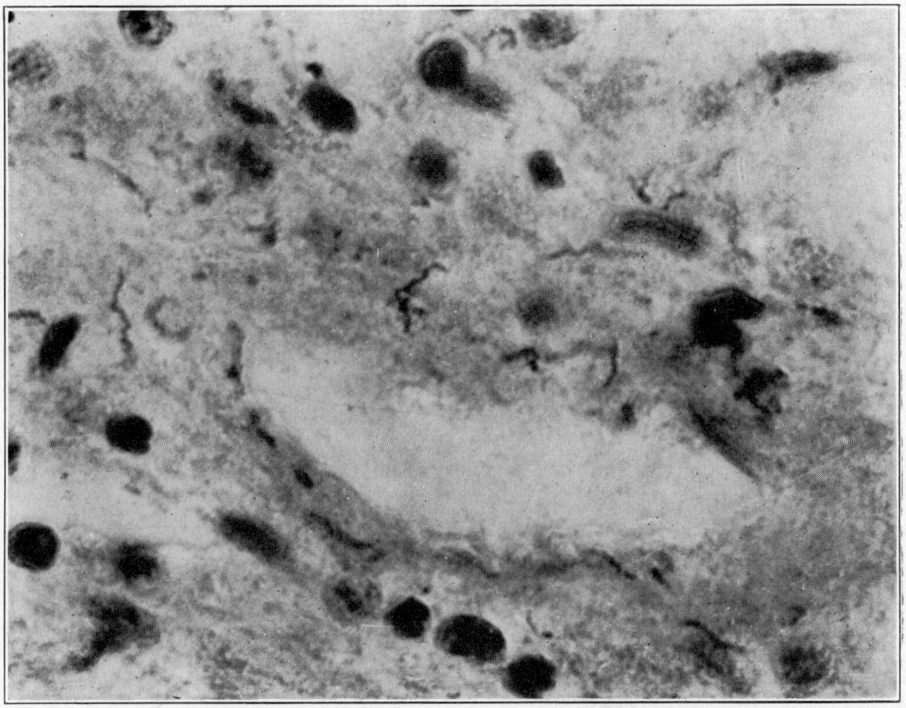

Fig. 1.—Low power view of small kidney arteriole showing numerous Spirochaetae pallidae in wall of vessel and perivascular interstitial tissue. Warthin-Starry silver-agar method. Photomicrograph, Zeiss objective F, compensating ocular, No. 4, bellows length 85 cm.

Note on illustrations. All material used in the photomicrographs was fixed in formol, imbedded in paraffin, sections mounted on coverglasses and stained according to the Warthin-Starry silver-agar method with the additional treatment with hydrogen peroxide to clear the background.

interest that the first observation of the occurrence of spirochetes in yellow fever was that made by Stimson,[7] in 1907. In Levaditi preparations of kidney from a case of yellow fever occurring during the epidemic in New Orleans in 1905, Stimson found a spirochete in the renal tubules, both in the epithelial cells

[6] Saikingaku Zasshi, 1918, p. 1.
[7] U. S. Public Health Reports, 1907, 22, p. 541.

and in the lumen (Sp. interrogans). According to Noguchi,[8] the morphologic characteristics of this organism appear to be identical with those of Leptospira icteroides, which he regards as the possible cause of yellow fever, and which he finds in the kidneys of guinea-pigs inoculated with this organism. No study of the excretion of this organism through the kidneys has yet been made.

In the case of Spirochaeta pallida few observations exist of the demonstration of this organism in the urine. In 1912, Vorpahl[9] reported the case of a woman, 38 years of age, who had had, 12 years before, an ulcer on the genitalia, and had taken a "Schmierkur" with apparent success. There was no history of

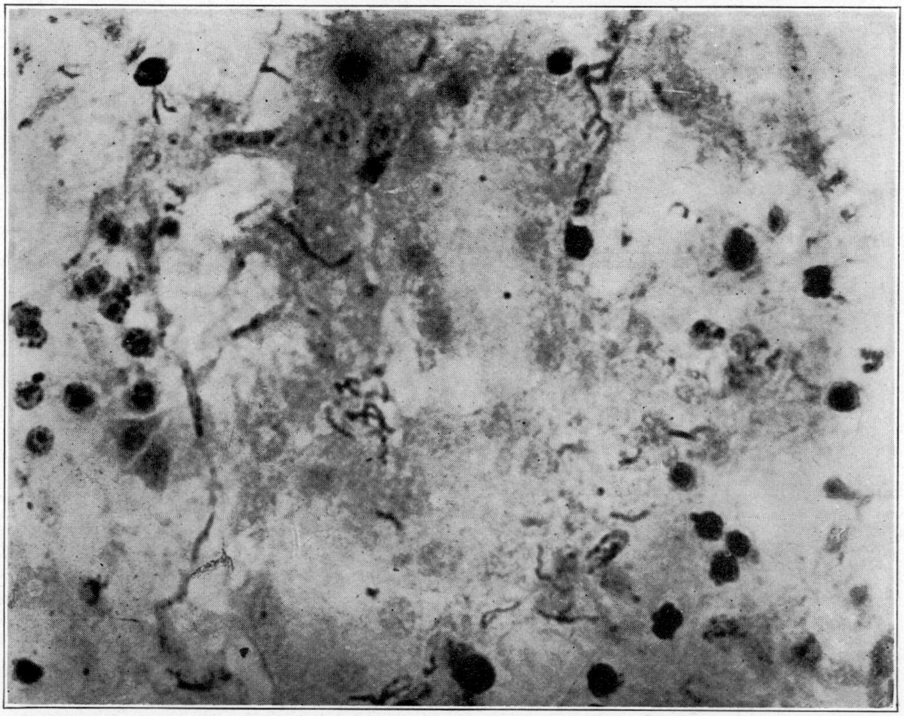

Fig. 2.—Low power view of convoluted tubule showing arrangement of Spirochaeta pallida in wall of tubule and in renal epithelium. Warthin-Starry silver-agar method. Photomicrograph, Zeiss objective F, compensating ocular, No. 4, bellows length 85 cm.

a new infection. For 3½ months she had had symptoms of nephritis. The Wassermann reaction was strongly positive, and gummatous ulcers were found in the throat. In the urine obtained by catheterization, centrifugated and examined by the India-ink method, 3 spirochetes, said to be morphologically like pallida, were found. Antisyphilitic treatment gave good results as far as the symptoms of nephritis were concerned. In the same year, Hoffmann[10] reported two cases of

[8] Am. Jour. Hyg., 1921, 1, p. 118.

[9] München. med. Wchnschr., 1912, 59, p. 2811.

[10] Deut. med. Wchnschr., 1913, 39, p. 353.

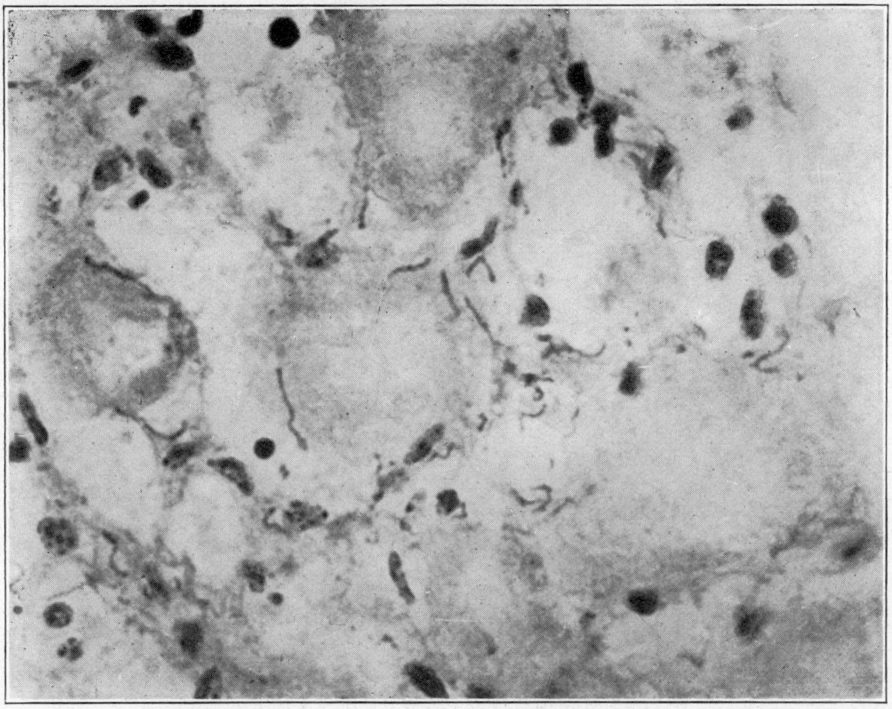

Fig. 3.—Low power view of renal tubules showing great numbers of spirochetes in walls of various portions of convoluted tubules. Warthin-Starry silver-agar method. Photomicrograph, Zeiss objective F, compensating ocular, No. 4, bellows length 85 cm.

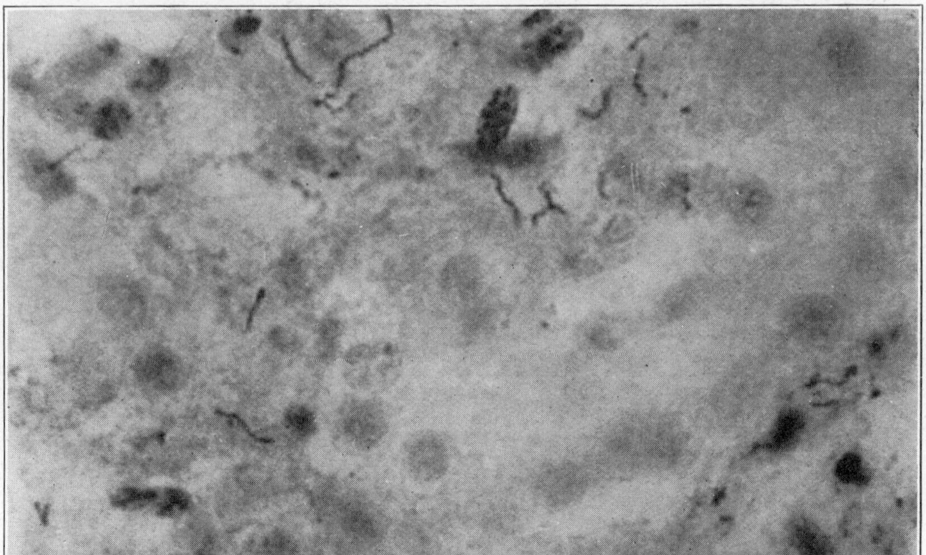

Fig. 4.—Slightly higher power view showing massing of Spirochaeta pallida between and in the walls of tubules. Warthin-Starry silver-agar method. Photomicrograph, Zeiss objective F, compensating ocular, No. 4, bellows length 85 cm.

early acute syphilitic nephritis. In one of these the patient showed a roseolar eruption with nephritic edema, massive albuminuria and granular casts. The urine obtained under precautions to avoid contamination showed numerous living Spirochaetae pallidae in dark-field examinations.

In 1919, Lévy and Guilé[11] conducted researches to ascertain the presence of Spirochaeta pallida in the urine of syphilitic patients. They concluded that the demonstration of syphilitic spirochetes in the urine of patients with untreated syphilis is difficult and rarely successful. They found 2 spirochetes of the

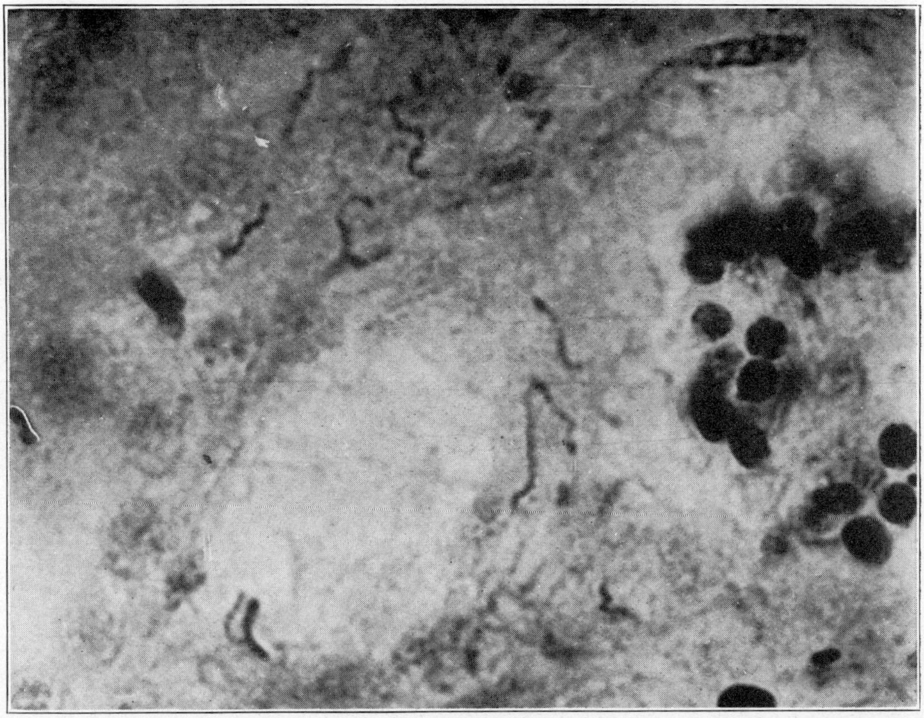

Fig. 5.—Medium power view of Spirochaeta pallida in wall of tubule and in interstititial tissue near a glomerulus, a portion of which is seen at the right. Warthin-Starry silver-agar method. Photomicrograph, Zeiss objective 5, compensating ocular, No. 4, bellows length 150 cm.

syphilitic type in one case at the beginning of the roseolar stage. They were not certain whether they were of renal or of local origin. They believe that the most favorable time for the demonstration of syphilitic spirocheturia is at the end of the first month after the appearance of the chancre, at the appearance of the roseola. Such an elimination of spirochetes, they believe, would be of fleeting duration, but its demonstration at this time, when the diagnosis is often in doubt, might be of great value in fixing with certainty a diagnosis of syphilis.

[11] Compt. rend. Soc. de biol., 1918, 82, p. 65. Bull. et mem. Soc. méd. d'hôp. d. Paris, 1919, 43, p. 48.

The same writers also studied the action of urine on Spirochaeta pallida. They found some organisms still recognizable after 17 hours' standing in urine; others showed elongated, straightened or effaced spirals, while great numbers showed contraction and degeneration. In 1921, Fiessinger and Huber [12] found Spirochaeta pallida in the urine of a young man with a roseolar syphilid, about one month after the development of the primary lesion. In 12 other cases of secondary syphilis seen during 3 years, and given especial examination with reference to the occurrence of spirocheturia, no spirochetes could be found in the urine.

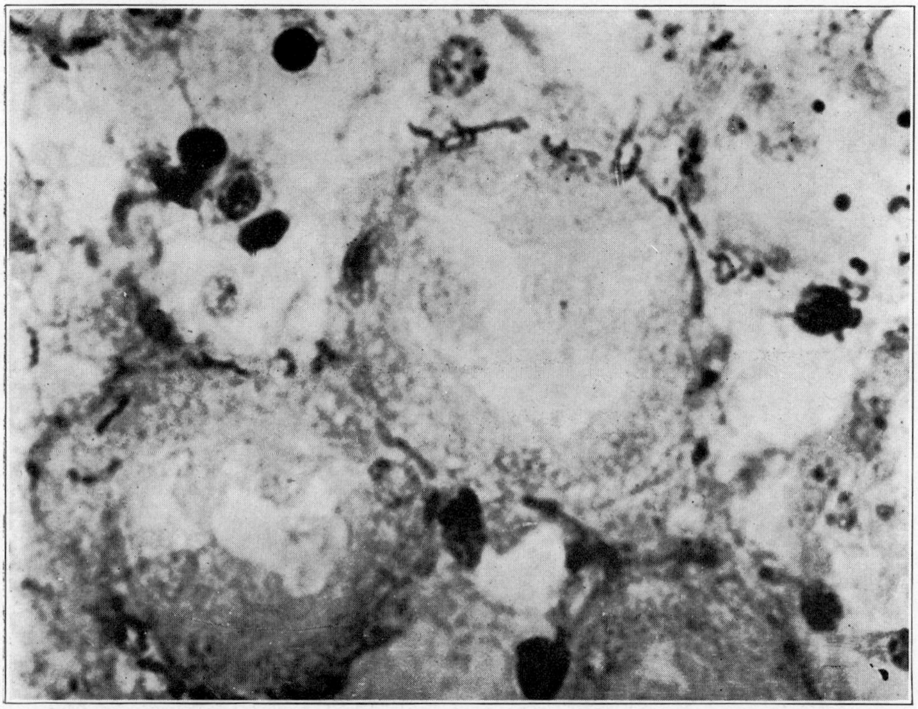

Fig. 6.—Medium power view of constricted portion of convoluted tubules showing massing of spirochetes in basement membrane. Warthin-Starry silver-agar method. Photomicrograph; same magnification as fig. 5.

On the other hand, Le Play, Sèzary and Pasteur Vallery-Radot [12] insist that in certain nonsyphilitic forms of nephritis there may be found in sections of the kidney impregnated with silver according to the methods of Bertarelli and Volpino certain spiral structures which are not true spirochetes although they resemble spirochetes and might, therefore, be mistaken for them. It is probable that the spirochete-

[12] Bull. et mém. Soc. méd. d'hôp. de Paris, 1921, 45, p. 146.
[13] Comp. rend. Soc. Biol., 1912, 73, p. 635.

like forms seen in Levaditi preparations of kidney by the Japanese workers mentioned may be identical with these. Such gross errors of identification of spirochetes in silver-impregnated tissues are due entirely to inexperience in spirochete morphology, and should not occur today. With the improved methods of silver staining applied to single sections, spirochete-like artefarcts are never produced.

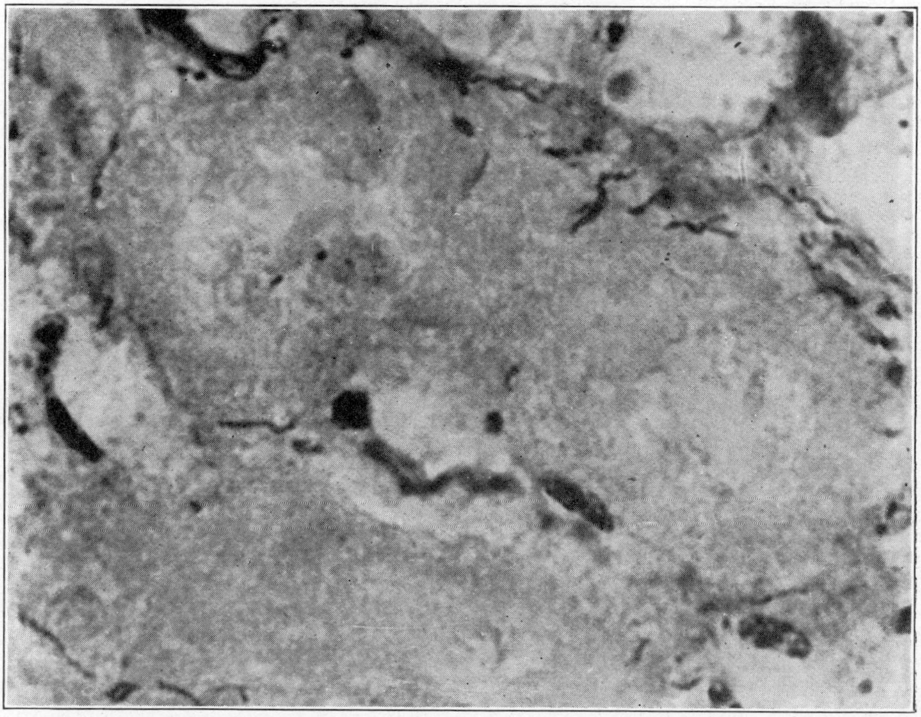

Fig. 7.—Medium power view of convoluted tubule showing spirochetes in basement membrane and epithelium of the tubules. Warthin-Starry silver-agar method. Photomicrograph; same magnification as fig. 5.

Excluding all palpable errors of this kind with reference to the demonstration of spirochetes in the urine and in the renal tubules, the observations cited are the only ones in which the excretion of Spirochaeta pallida in the urine has been demonstrated. It is true that in some of the studies on the distribution of the spirochetes in the organs and tissues of congenital syphilis Spirochaeta pallida has been seen in sections of kidney tissue in great numbers without apparent coincident

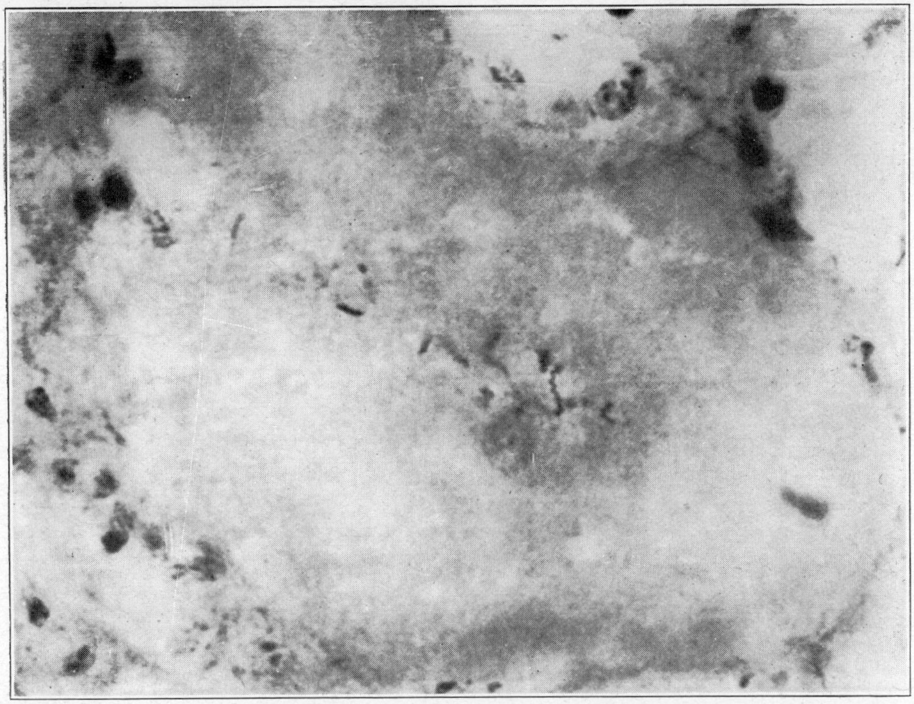

Fig. 8.—Medium power view of convoluted tubule showing degenerating spirochetes in renal epithelium. Warthin-Starry silver-agar method. Photomicrograph; same magnification as fig. 5.

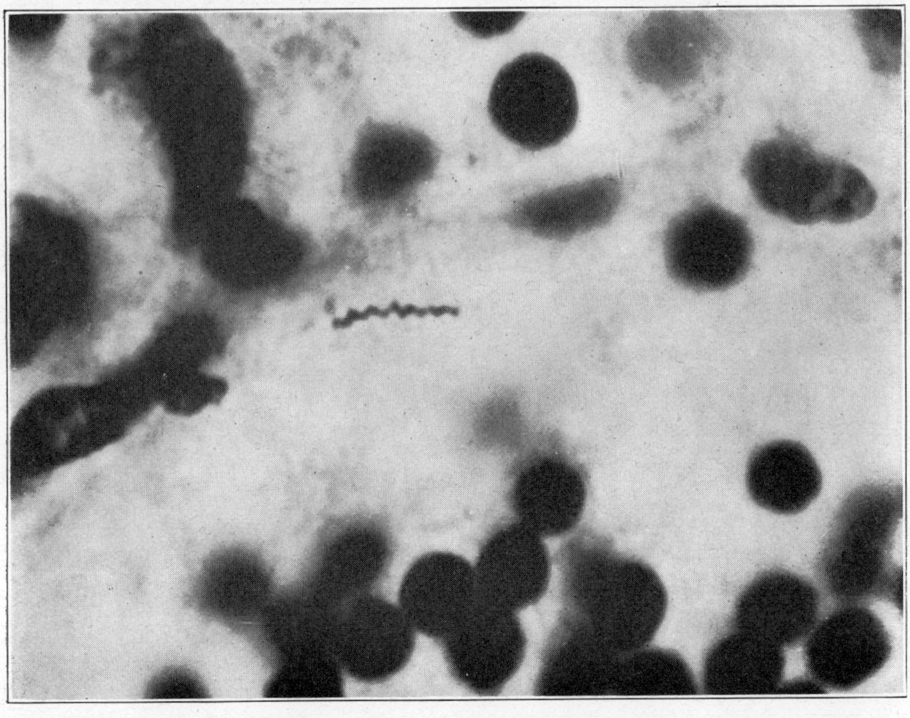

Fig. 9.—High power view of single Spirochaeta pallida in subcapsular glomerular space. Warthin-Starry method. Photomicrograph, B. L. oil-immersion, 2 mm.; compensating ocular No. 4, bellows length 85 cm.

tissue lesions, but no note has been made of the excretion of the organism through the renal tubules. In my own experience, in the study of spirochete distribution throughout the tissues in congenital syphilis, I have found the organisms in varying numbers in the kidneys in all cases in which there was a marked spirochetosis of other organs. With the exception of the three cases to be mentioned, this renal localization seemed to be unassociated with any lesion of the renal epithelium, and no especial attention was paid to the demonstration of an excretion of

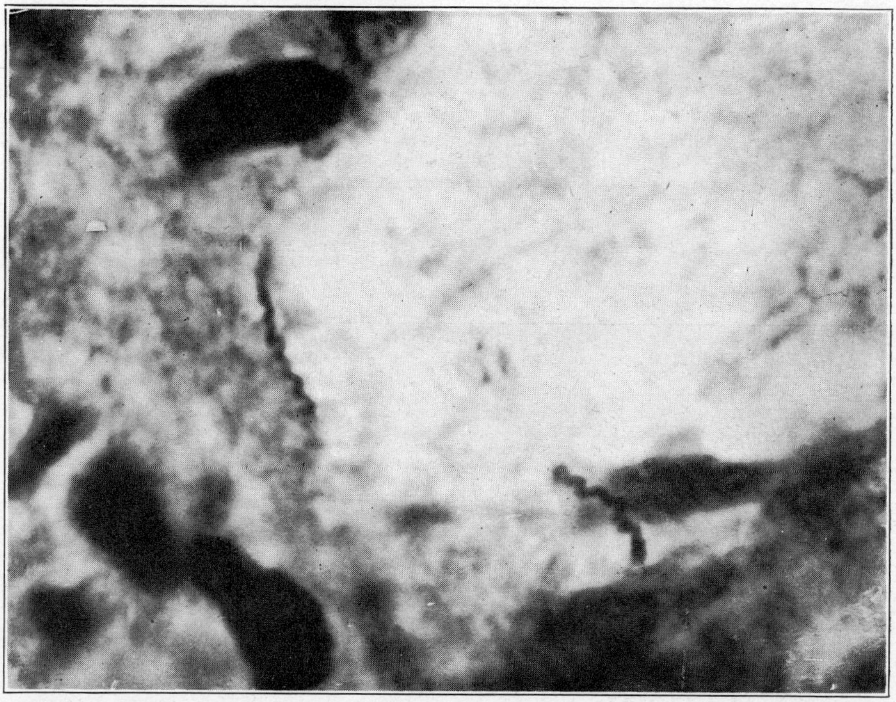

Fig. 10.—Spirochaeta pallida in endothelium of small intertubular vessel. The straightened appearance of one of the spirochetes on the endothelial surface is characteristic. The lower spirochete is passing through an endothelial cell. Warthin-Starry method. Photomicrograph; same magnification as fig. 9.

the spirochetes by way of the urine, although this was regarded as a possibility and has often been mentioned in my teaching.

In 3 cases of congenital syphilis studied, one of a child dying at birth, another dying 8 days after birth, and the third at $3\frac{1}{2}$ years of age, the kidneys presented an unusual degree of spirochete localization with definite lesions. In 2 cases of acquired syphilis, those of a young man with a roseolar eruption and a young woman with maculopapular eruption, both dying from arsphenamin poisoning, a similar localization of spirochetes in the kidneys with positive evidences of excretion through the renal epithelium into the tubules was observed. The material from these 5 cases constitutes the basis of this study. Identical conditions and changes were present in all 5 of these cases. No arsphenamin treatment had been administered to the patient with the

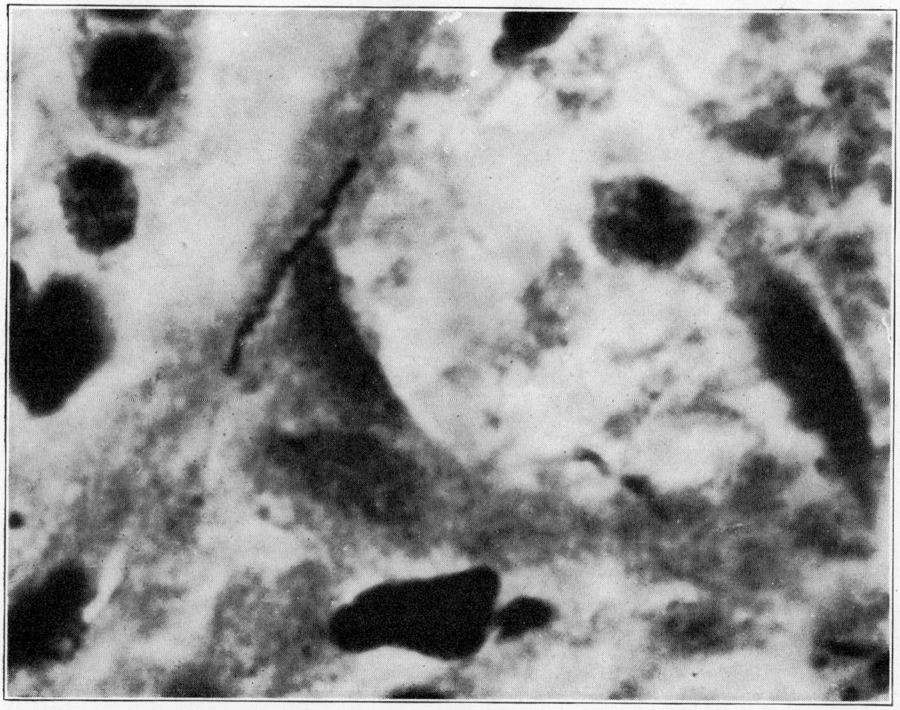

Fig. 11.—Wall of small intertubular capillary. Straightened-out Spirochaeta pallida in endothelial cell. Warthin-Starry method. Photomicrograph; same magnification as fig. 9.

congenital case dying soon after birth or to the child of 3½ years; but it had been given to the child dying at 8 days of age, and the death was supposed to have been due to the treatment, although the details are unknown to me. The child of 3½ years of age had albuminuria and symptoms suggesting poliomyelitis, the young woman of 23 years had casts and albuminuria; the urine of the young man had not been examined. He was supposedly in good condition except for the chancre and roseolar eruption.

The tissues from these 5 cases were well fixed in 10% formalin, and had been preserved in formol for some time. Blocks from the kidneys were embedded in paraffin and the sections cut and mounted on cover glasses, and stained according to Warthin and Starry's silver-agar cover-glass method, with the additional use of hydrogen-peroxide as

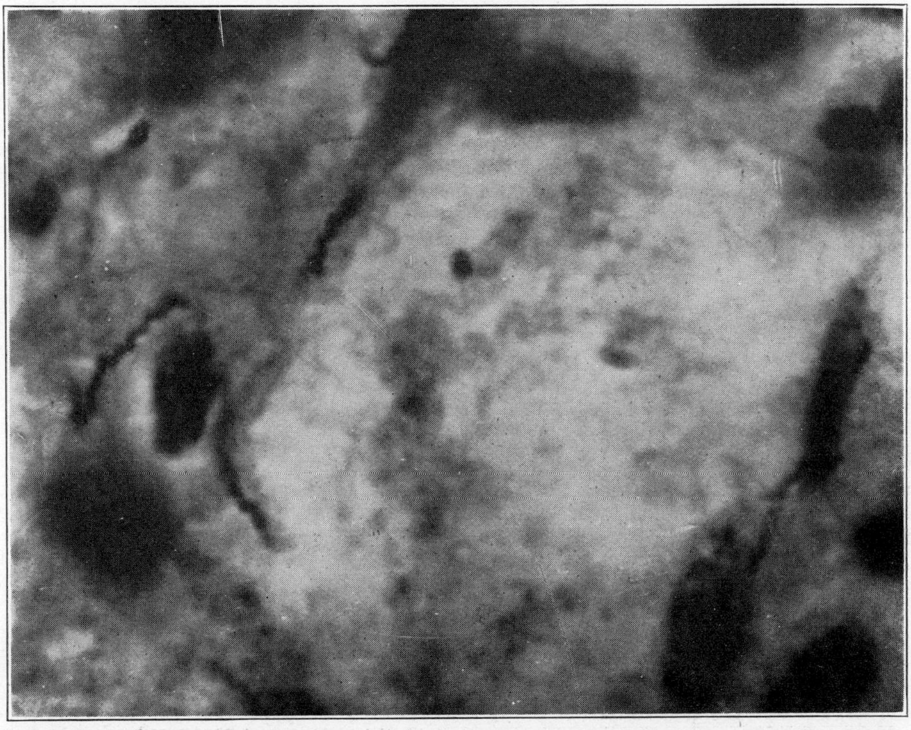

Fig. 12.—Small intertubular vessel. Two straightened-out spirochetes are seen on the left in the endothelium, several in the interstititial tissue to the left of the vessel; in the capillary wall on the right another straight organism in the endothelium out of focus. Warthin-Starry silver-agar method. Photomicrograph; same magnification as fig. 9.

an agent to clear out the tissue background and throw the individual spirochetes into greater relief. The Levaditi method and its variations have also been applied to the study of these tissues, but we have found our own method to be more constant, to show a greater number of spirochetes, and with greater contrast and detail of the organisms.

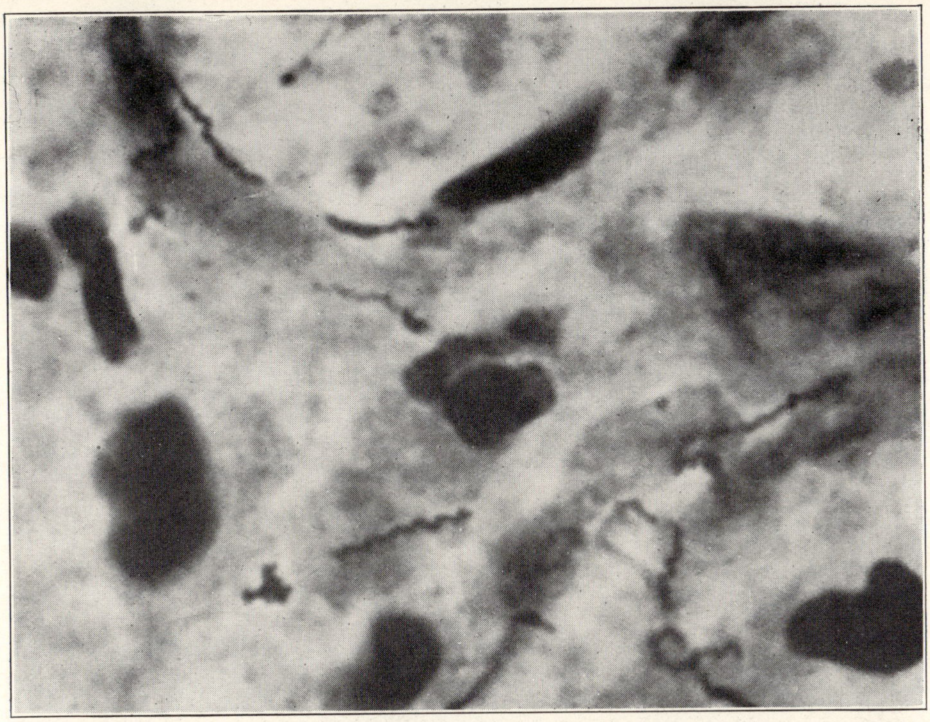

Fig. 13.—High-power view with intertubular capillary at top showing straightened spirochetes in the wall; below it numerous spirochetes massed in the intertubular interstitial tissue. Warthin-Starry silver-agar method. Photomicrograph; same magnification as fig. 9.

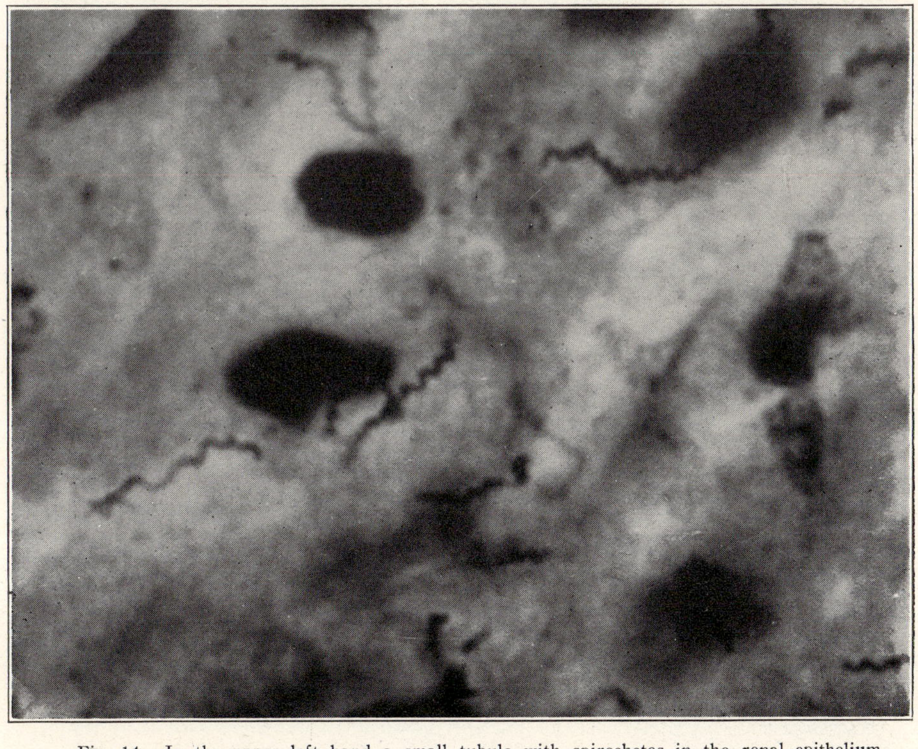

Fig. 14.—In the upper left hand a small tubule with spirochetes in the renal epithelium and spirochetal fragments in the lumen of the tubule. In the interstitial tissue numerous spirochetes in varying focus to show their massing between the tubules. Warthin-Starry silver-agar method. Photomicrograph; same magnification as fig. 9.

General Pathology of Kidney.—All 5 kidneys showed a general passive congestion and a parenchymatous degeneration most marked in the renal epithelium of the convoluted tubules, but involving the loops and straight tubules to some degree in the 2 adult cases. The intertubular interstitial tissue showed edema and an increase in the number of small cells, the majority of these being of the lymphocyte or plasma-cell

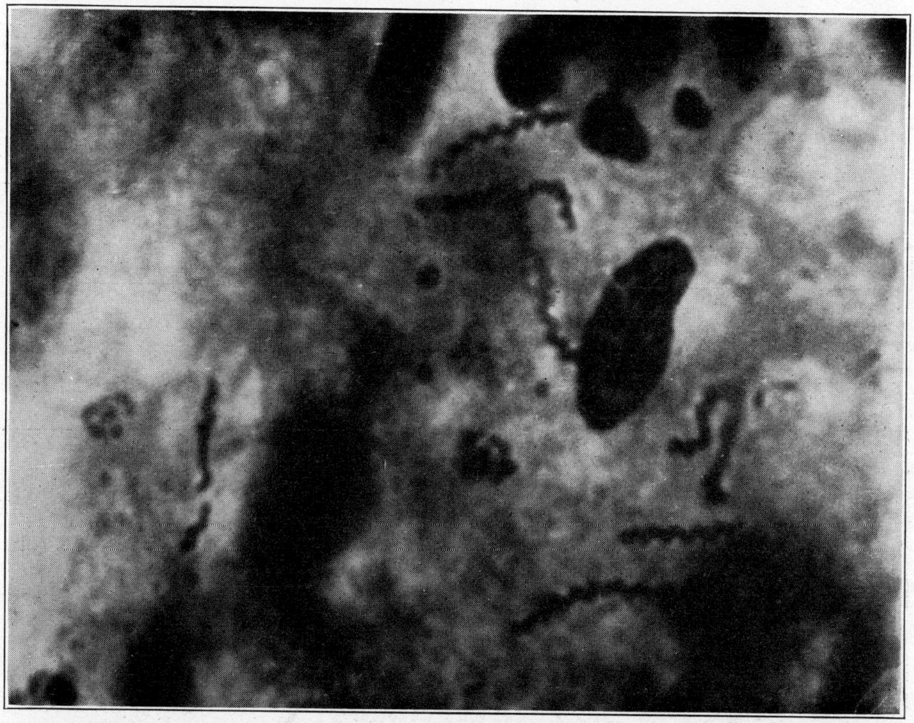

Fig. 15.—High power view of Spirochaeta pallida massed in intertubular interstitial tissue. Tubule at left with two degenerating spirochetes in renal epithelium. Warthin-Starry silver-agar method. Photomicrograph; objective B. & L., oil-immersion 2 mm., compensating ocular No. 4, bellows length 155 cm.

type. In one case only, that of the child of 3½ years with congenital syphilis were there any definite interstitial inflammatory areas. These were found between the tubules, particularly in the neighborhood of the larger blood vessels. They showed the same plasma-cell infiltrations with slight fibroblastic proliferation that characterize the localization of spirochetes elsewhere in the body. In these areas the silver stains showed the presence of great numbers of Spirochaeta pallida.

Glomeruli.—No degenerative or inflammatory lesions were found in the glomeruli. The capillaries were dilated. In these, occasional spirochetes were found, usually one to two in a glomerulus, never in greater numbers; and in many glomeruli no organisms were found. Occasionally they were seen in the subcapsular space or in the capsule itself. No degenerated forms of the organisms were found in the glomeruli.

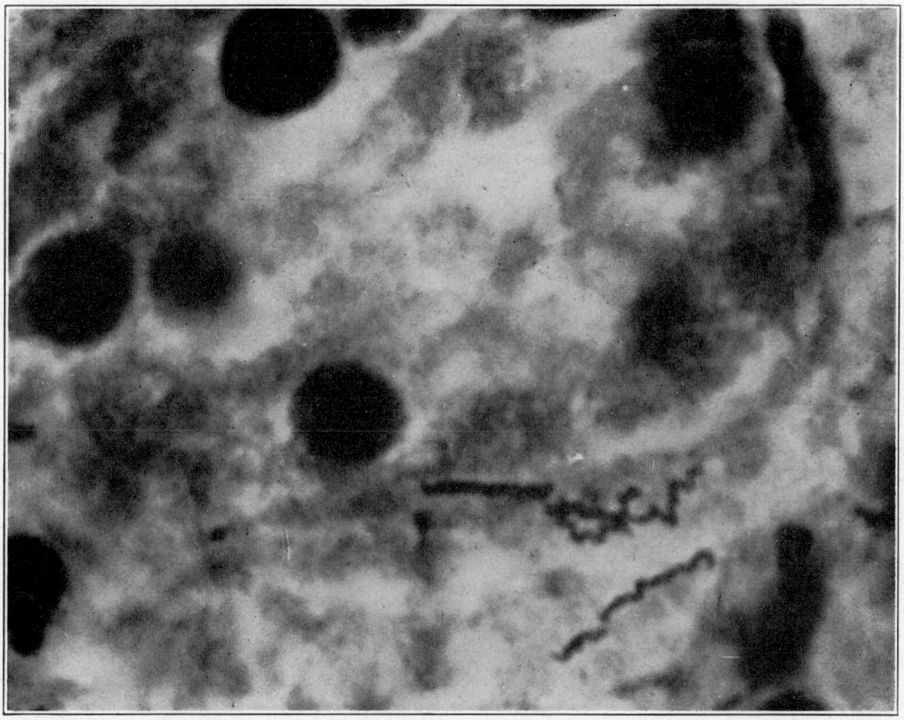

Fig. 16.—High power view of degenerating spirochetes in wall of tubule. Lumen of tubule contained many degenerating forms out of focus in this picture. Warthin-Starry silver-agar method. Photomicrograph, B. & L., 2 mm. oil-immersion, compensating ocular, No. 4, bellows length 85 cm.

Convoluted Tubules.—The spirochetes were massed in greatest numbers in the intertubular capillaries and lymph spaces of the edematous interstitial substance between and around the convoluted tubules. In the capillaries and small arteries they were present in great numbers in the lumen, but were often straightened out on the endothelium as if agglutinated to the endothelial cells. Some vessels seemed to be lined with an internal layer of spirochetes. Passage of the organisms into and through the endothelium was seen in all stages. No degenerative changes were seen in the endothelial cells and no degenerative forms of the organisms were found in the vessel walls. In the interstitial tissue between the capillaries and the tubules the spirochetes were collected in great numbers, apparently free and unchanged. Around the basement membrane of the convoluted tubules they were heaped up, often entangled, sometimes attenuated, or straightened out, or coiled up into bizarre forms. They were often collected at certain portions of the

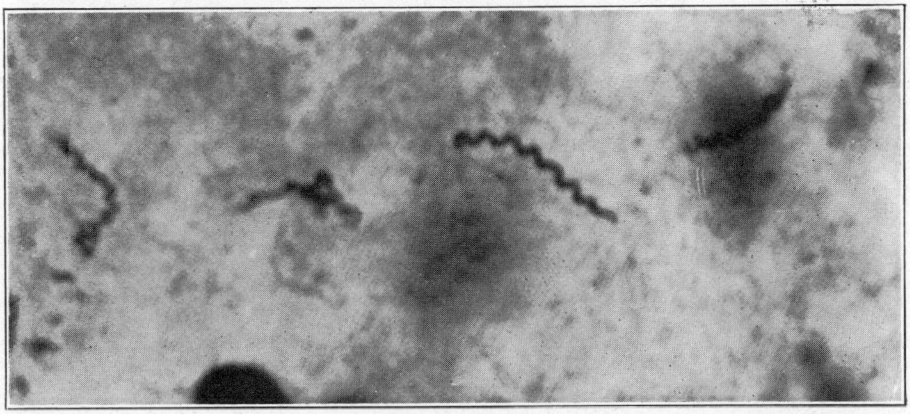

Fig. 17.—High power view of segment of convoluted tubule showing spirochetes in degenerated epithelium. Some of the organisms show degeneration. Spirochetes are toward the lumen, one nucleus showing below. Warthin-Starry silver-agar method. Photomicrograph, B. & L. oil-immersion 2 mm., compensating ocular, No. 4, bellows length 155 cm.

basement membrane as if drawn to that point. In other tubules the organisms formed a tight barricade entirely around the basement membrane of the tubule. Passage through the basement membrane into and between the renal epithelium was seen in all tubules. Phagocytosis of the organisms by the renal epithelum and by polymorphonuclear leukocytes was evident in the tubules. In the renal cells the spirochetes were well preserved until they approached the inner pole of the cells. Toward the lumen there was seen a marked fragmentation of the organisms, the spirochetes breaking up into fragments of all sizes, ultimately becoming granules which still become impregnated with silver. Other spirochetes reached the lumen apparently unchanged, and were found free in the lumen. As the spirochetes approach the lumen and begin to fragment they are often found arranged in a radiating position about the lumen.

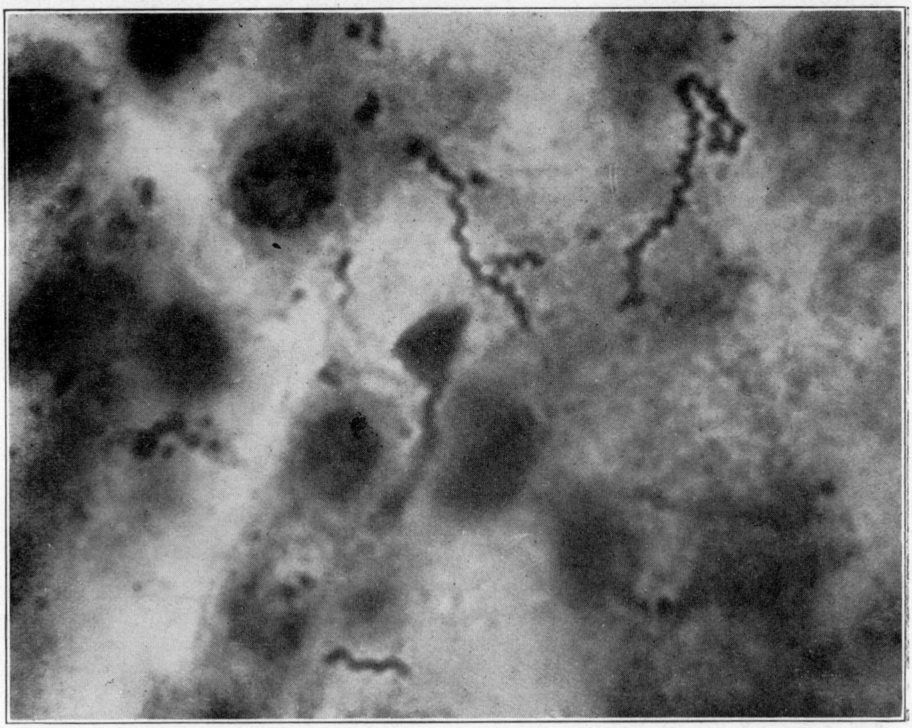

Fig. 18.—High power view of Spirochaeta pallida in walls of tubules; in the upper field the large organisms are in the renal epithelium. Warthin-Starry silver-agar method. Photomicrograph; same magnification as fig. 17.

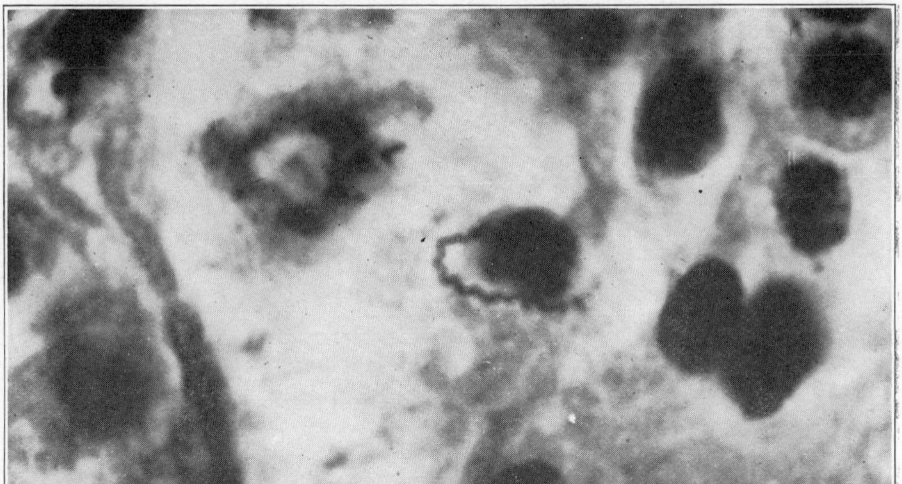

Fig. 19.—Phagocytosis of Spirochaeta pallida by renal epithelium; in the tubule a desquamated degenerating renal epithelial cell contains numerous fragments of degenerating spirochetes. Warthin-Starry silver-agar method. Photomicrograph; same magnification as fig. 17.

The tubular epithelium through which this process of elimination is taking place shows varying degrees of cloudy swelling, hyaline change or complete cytolysis. Fat droplets are not present in the degenerating cells. The lumina of the tubules are narrowed, often completely blocked by the swollen cells, or are filled with a granular detritus from exudate or broken-down cells. In such granular casts spirochetes, either unchanged, or presenting various stages of disintegration are

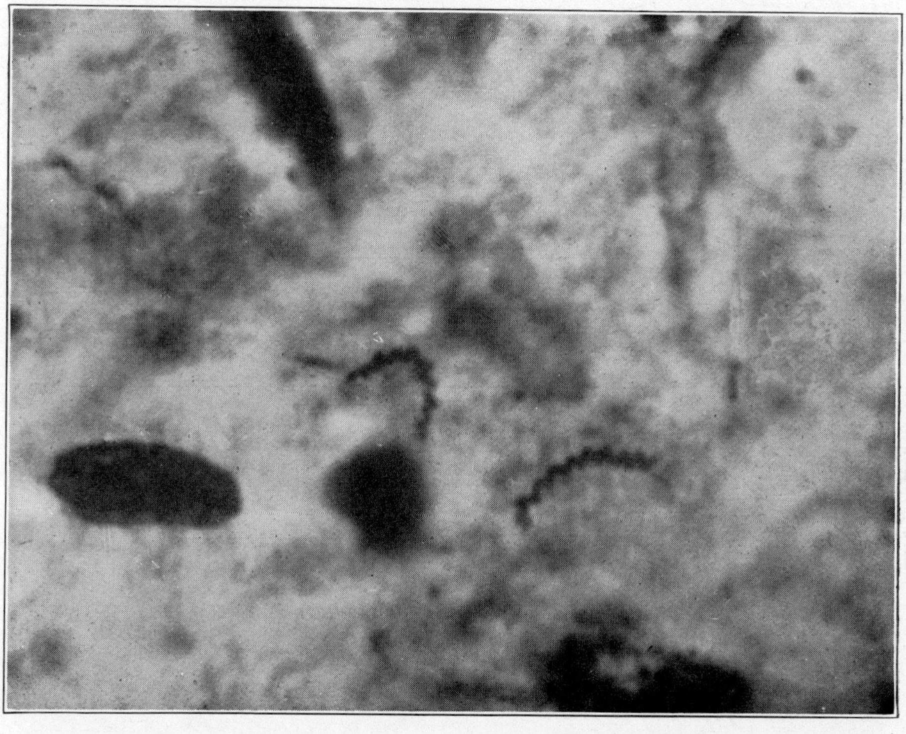

Fig. 20.—Tubule with lumen blocked by detritus and swollen epithelium; in the latter two spirochetes showing beginning coiling. Warthin-Starry silver-agar method. Photomicrograph; same magnification as fig. 17.

present in great numbers. Desquamated cells containing single or numerous organisms are common in the lumina. In the phagocytes the spirochetes often become coiled into a loop or circle, which gradually contracts and condenses until it forms a round granule still taking the silver impregnation. All stages of this phagocytosis and destruction of the organism are shown. The great majority of the organisms reaching the lumina show signs of disintegration. In the loops of Henle the passage of the organisms through the walls of the tubules occurs at a greatly reduced rate, although the intertubular tissue is often closely packed with them. In the straight tubules the organisms within the lumen of the tubules diminish in number until in the medullary pyramids they almost entirely disappear from the tubules, only occasional ones being found free within the tubule or in casts. Granular

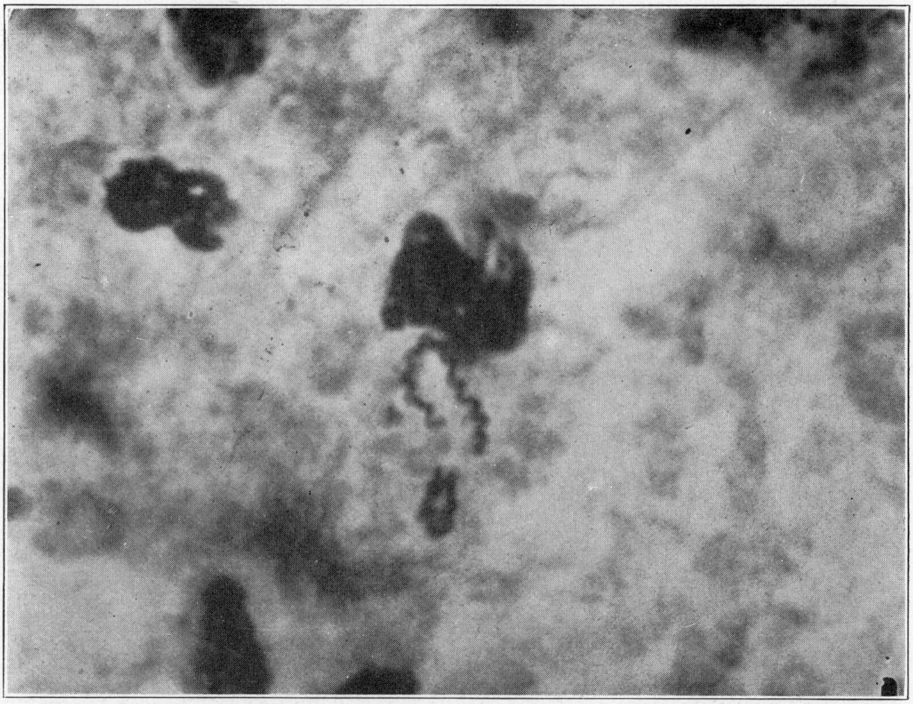

Fig. 21.—Lumen of tubule with swollen epithelial cell showing two enclosed spirochetes in different stages of coil formation, the lower one contracting and condensing, the final stage of phagocytosis. Warthin-Starry silver-agar method. Photomicrograph; same magnification as fig. 17.

and beaded spirochetes were numerous in the lumina. The fragments of the disintegrated organisms apparently lose their affinity for silver impregnation in the straight tubules as these become fewer and fewer in the collecting tubules. The intertubular vessels in the medullary pyramids, however, contain great numbers of spirochetes, as does also the intertubular interstitial tissue, decreasing however toward the papilla.

From the appearances presented by the sections of these kidneys the excretion of Spirochaeta pallida takes place chiefly through the convoluted tubules. The majority of the organisms appear to pass directly through the renal epithelium. These cells show a marked degeneration, cloudy swelling or a hyaline parenchymatous degeneration, both leading ultimately to complete cytolysis. The cytoplasm shows more change than the nuclei, although with cytolysis the latter lose their staining

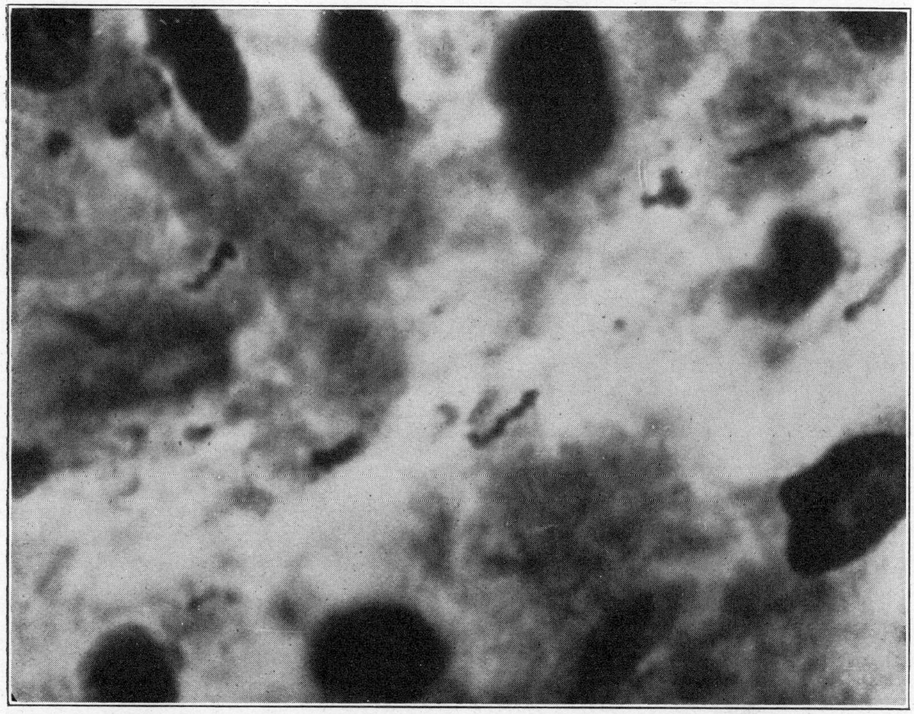

Fig. 22.—Fragments of spirochetes in the detritus in lumen of tubule. In the epithelium at top spirochetes radiating toward the lumen can be seen. Warthin-Starry method. Photomicrograph; same magnification as fig. 17.

power. A definite relation seems to exist between the degree of degeneration of the cells and the disintegration of the spirochetes. The destruction of the organisms appears to take place chiefly toward the lumen and in the latter. In the urine the great majority of them must disappear completely; and only a small number of them, presumably the viable ones, may reach the bladder and appear in the excreted urine.

The search in the urine for such evidence of syphilitic infection cannot, therefore, be expected to be of any great value as a diagnostic method. If in all cases the destruction of the excreted spirochetes is as great as it is in these kidneys, the demonstration of spirocheturia in syphilis must be a rare and largely accidental observation.

The excretion through the kidneys of Spirochaeta pallida takes place under the same conditions and apparently with the same mechanism as

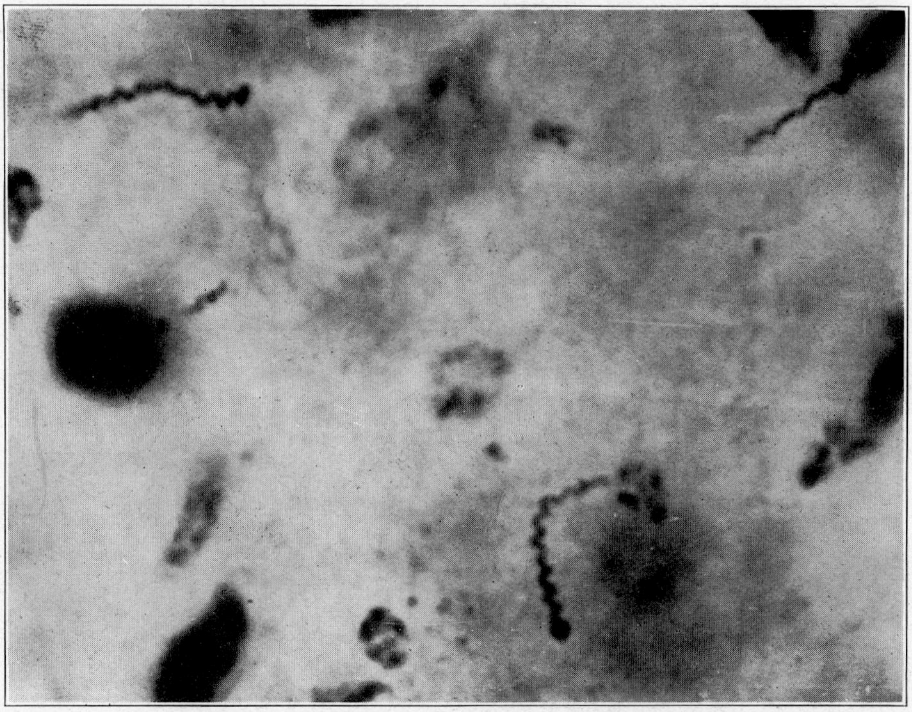

Fig. 23.—Tubule showing radial arrangement of spirochetes toward the lumen; in the latter numerous degenerating fragments of spirochetes were present, only a few in focus. Warthin-Starry silver-agar method. Photomicrograph; same magnification as fig. 17.

described for the spirocheturia of infectious jaundice. There is a more or less generalized spirochetosis in the body, with spirochetemia. In the kidney there occurs a massing of the spirochetes about the convoluted tubules and a passage of the organisms from the vessels and interstitial tissues into the tubules where they undergo disintegration for the greater part. This destruction of the organisms in the kidneys is more marked in the case of syphilis than in infectious jaundice. The spirocheturia of the latter disease is a more marked and constant feature of the infection than it would appear to be in syphilis. This point can be settled only by future examinations of urine on a more extensive scale during the stage of spirochetemia following the development of the chancre and the early cutaneous manifestations. It does not seem likely, however, that spirocheturia in acquired syphilis will become a diagnostic factor of importance as it is in Weil's disease. In the case of septicemic congenital syphilis such spirocheturia is more likely to be found.

In the icterigenic spirocheturia and that of syphilis definite renal lesions are present. In Weil's disease the renal injury is much greater than in these five cases of syphilis, and in proportion to this greater degeneration of the epithelium of the convoluted tubules there is a much greater excretion of Spirochaeta icterohaemorrhagica. The occurrence of spirocheturia in syphilis has, nevertheless, an important bearing on the much discussed question of a precocious syphilitic nephritis. From these cases it would appear that such a syphilitic injury of the kidneys does occur during the septicemic stage of the infection. In suspected cases of early syphilitic nephritis the examination of the urine for the presence of renal spirochetes, by using proper precautions to prevent urethral contamination, might become an important diagnostic procedure in determining the nature of the renal lesion.

The fact that three of these patients had been given arsphenamin treatment may be of importance in determining the degree of primary or secondary injury to the kidneys, as well as the degree of spirocheturia. As spirocheturia does not take place to any marked degree in Weil's disease until after the tenth day when immune bodies are forming, it is possible that the same is true of syphilitic spirocheturia. Further, any spirocheticidal treatment may in itself be a factor in rendering the spirochetes of syphilis more susceptible to passage through the renal epithelium, or the injury to the latter resulting from the therapeutic measures may make the kidneys more pervious to their passage.

CONCLUSION

Spirocheturia appears to be a striking phenomenon of the entire group of spirochetal infections. The elimination of the spirochetes through the kidneys with the production of associated renal lesions appears to constitute a family characteristic in so far as the known types of the organisms have been studied thoroughly. It is best known in the case of infectious jaundice, and in this disease is a factor of considerable diagnostic value.

Syphilitic spirocheturia occurs in the stage of septicemic syphilis, in both the congenital and acquired infections. Spirochaeta pallida, as is Spirochaeta icterohaemorrhagica, may be excreted in enormous numbers through the convoluted tubules. During such excretion through the kidneys the spirochete of syphilis suffers greater destruction than does the icterogenic parasite, so that fewer spirochetes may reach the urine in syphilis than in infectious jaundice. The demonstration of the occurrence of syphilitic spirocheturia, is, therefore, not likely to possess such diagnostic value as that of icterogenic spirocheturia.

It seems probable that spirocheturia is more likely to occur when the spirochetes in the blood stream are exposed to the action of antibodies or spirocheticidal drugs. Further, spirocheturia in any degree, both in the case of syphilis and infectious jaundice, appears to be associated with definite degenerative lesions of the epithelium of the convoluted tubules. Such lesions may make the tubules more pervious to the passage of the spirochetes.

THE STAINING OF SPIROCHETES IN COVER-GLASS SMEARS BY THE SILVER-AGAR METHOD *

A. S. Warthin and A. C. Starry

From the Pathological Laboratory of the University of Michigan, Ann Arbor, Mich.

The methods in practical use at the present time for the immediate clinical and laboratory demonstration of spirochetes are the dark-field and the India-ink methods. Both of these methods are dangerous for the inexperienced laboratory worker of the type common today in the smaller hospitals scattered throughout the country. Within the last year we have been consulted with reference to three cases of carcinoma of the lip and mouth and one of the genitalia in which mouth and smegma spirochetes were mistaken in the dark-field for Spirochaeta pallida. In one of these cases the patient was treated for syphilis until hopeless generalized metastases developed, and in this case the mistaken diagnosis was made by an expert in the use of the dark-field and the clinical recognition of syphilis. We have reason to believe that such mistakes are not uncommon. Certain forms of spirochetes of the mouth so approach the pallida in appearance in the dark field that morphologic differentiation by this method is sometimes impossible. We believe that fine morphologic differences are more easily recognizable in the stained smear, and regard the use of the latter as the safest procedure in the clinical diagnosis of syphilis. There has, however, not yet been devised any simple staining method for the demonstration of spirochetes in cover-glass smears. No stain or dye has yet been discovered that will stain spirochetes sufficiently well for diagnostic purposes. The silver-impregnation methods are the only ones that will. We offer here a method of application of silver-impregnation to the study of spirochetes in smears.

Method for Silver-Impregnation of Spirochetes in Smears on Cover-Glasses

1. Prepare smears on No. 1 cover-glasses.
2. Dry thoroughly in the air.
3. Place in absolute alcohol 3 - 5 minutes.
4. Wash in distilled water.

Received for publication Feb. 1, 1922.

* Aided by a grant from the Interdepartmental Social Hygiene Board, Washington. D. C.

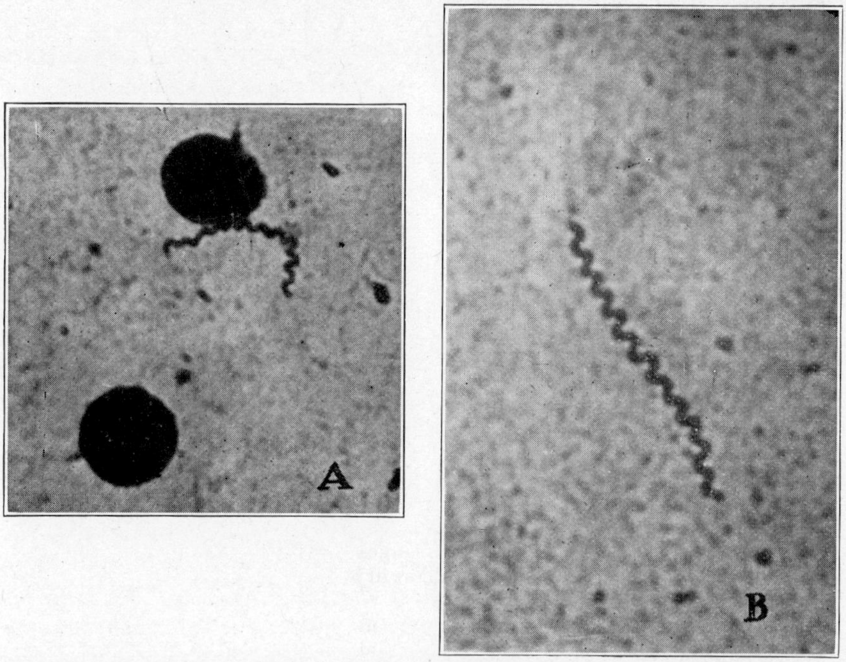

Fig. 1.—Smear from chancre, stained by Warthin-Starry silver-agar method. A, Spirochaeta pallida with two red blood cells, photomicrograph, B. & L., oil-immersion 2 mm., compensating ocular No. 4, bellows length 85 cm. B, another organism from same smear with bellows length of 155 cm.

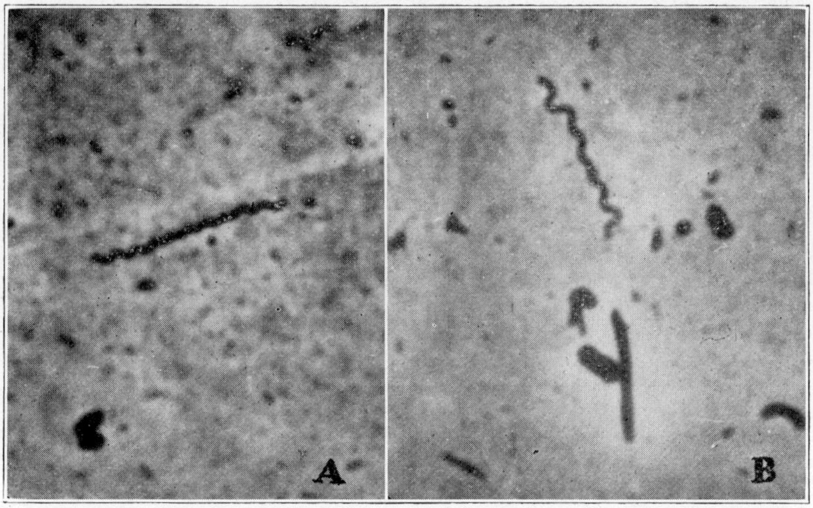

Fig. 2.—Smear from gums. A and B, two types of mouth spirochetes, the ones most commonly mistaken in the dark-field for pallida. Photomicrograph, B. & L., oil-immersion 2 mm., compensatory ocular No. 4, bellows length 155 cm. Smear stained by Warthin-Starry silver-agar method.

(If hydrogen peroxide is used to clear background, the smear is placed in concentrated hydrogen peroxide for 5 - 20 minutes, and then washed thoroughly in distilled water.)

5. Rinse cover-glass with smear in 2% silver nitrate. Cover the smear side with another perfectly clean cover-glass also rinsed in the silver nitrate solution. Place the adherent pair of cover-glasses carefully, so as not to separate them, in a bottle of 2% silver nitrate, and place in an incubator for 1 -2 hours; then remove the cover-glasses from the silver nitrate solution and separate them.

6. Place the cover-glass with the smeared side up in the following mixture:

2% silver nitrate solution....................	3 c c
Warm 10% aqueous gelatin solution........	5 c c
Warm glycerol	5 c c
Warm 1.5% agar suspension................	5 c c
5% aqueous hydroquinone solution..........	2 c c

7. After the solution is reduced remove and rinse in 5% sodium thiosulphate solution.

8. Rinse in distilled water.

9. Absolute alcohol, xylol, balsam.

Discussion of the Method.—Clean cover-glasses are essential. The cover-glass smears are prepared in the usual way. It is important that they be thoroughly dried in the air before attempting to stain them. Long exposure to air does not affect the staining quality if they are protected from dust and dirt. Dried smears containing Leptospira icteroides stained readily after standing 4 weeks. After drying, the smears are placed in absolute alcohol for 3-5 minutes, and are then washed with 2 changes of distilled water. It is essential that no other method of fixation than drying in air followed by absolute alcohol be used.

The silver-impregnation is carried out in wide-mouthed dark bottles fitted with tightly fitting corks. The smear is taken from the distilled water, and rinsed in 2% silver nitrate solution; the smeared side is then covered with another perfectly clean cover-glass also rinsed in the silver nitrate solution, so that the wet cover-glasses adhere. The silver nitrate solution should be fresh, not over 6 - 7 days old. During this time the silver nitrate solution can be used over and over if kept in the dark bottle and free from contamination. The adhering pair of cover-glasses are put into the bottle so that they stand on edge against the side of the bottle, and enough silver nitrate is poured into the bottle to come about half way up the cover-glasses. If round bottles are used a small meniscus is formed between the cover-glasses and the side of the bottle, thus holding them in place. It is a good routine measure always to place the smeared cover-glass next to the wall of the bottle, so that there will be no danger of getting the cover-glasses mixed and placing the wrong one in the reducing mixture.

The reducing mixture is prepared by mixing the silver nitrate solution, gelatin and glycerol in order. This mixture is thoroughly stirred, and the agar suspension stirred in last. The hydroquinone solution is added just before using. About 2 c c give the best results. If the reduction takes place too rapidly add less, if too slowly, add more. The agar suspension should be carefully made as follows: One and a half gm. of agar are broken up fine, and placed in 20 - 30 c c of distilled water, and allowed to soak for a few minutes until the agar is saturated with water. The excess is then poured off and the agar washed with

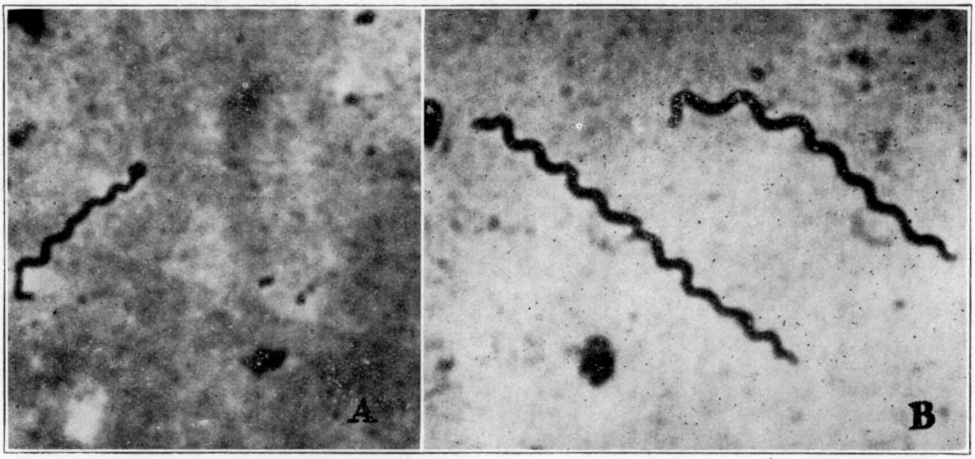

Fig. 3.—Smear of rat's blood, stained by Warthin-Starry hydrogen-peroxide, silver-agar method. A, Sp. obermeieri. Photomicrograph, B. & L., oil-immersion 2 mm., compensatory ocular No 4, bellows length 85 cm. B, two Sp. obermeieri from same smear, same stain, with bellows length of 155 cm

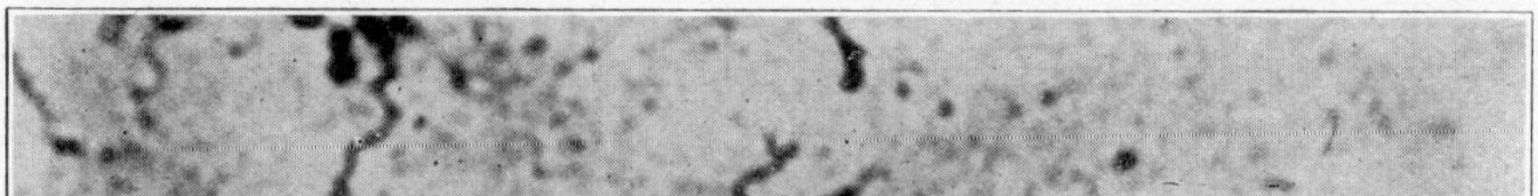

Fig. 4.—Smear from old culture of Sp. icterohaemorrhagica, stained by Warthin-Starry hydrogen-peroxide, silver-agar method. Photomicrograph, B. & L., oil-immersion 2 mm., compensatory ocular No. 4, bellows length 85 cm. Organisms show some involution.

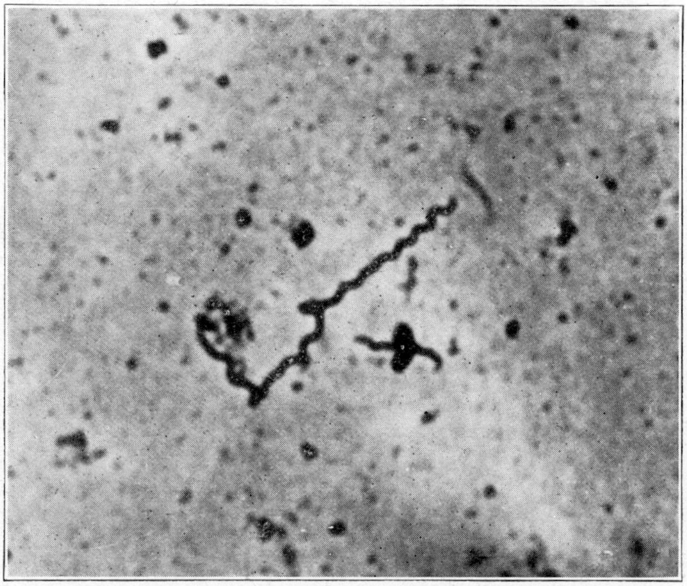

Fig. 5.—Spirochaeta icterohaemorrhagica from same stained smear as preceding, taken with a bellows length of 155 cm.

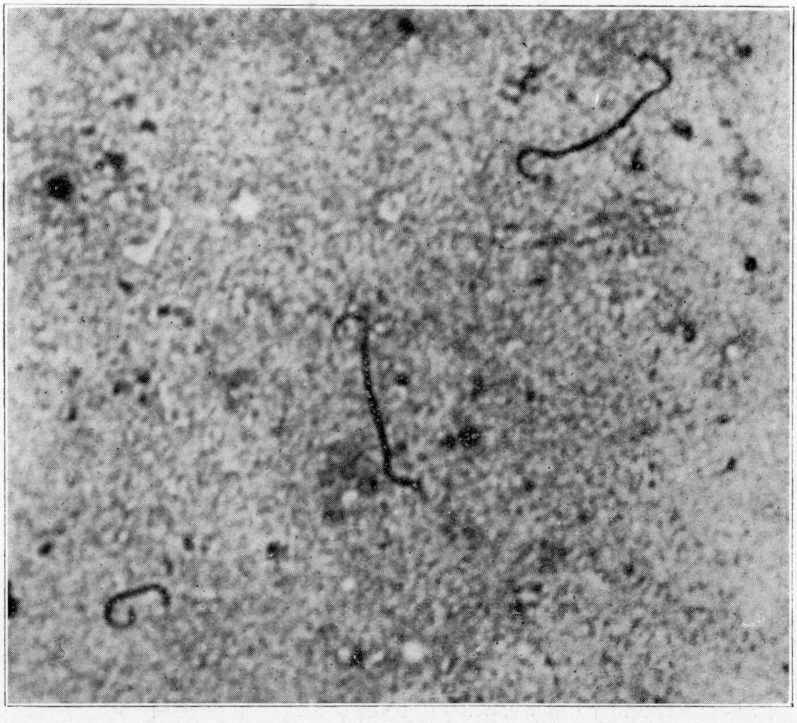

Fig. 6.—Leptospira icteroides in smear from guinea-pig's liver, stained with Warthin-Starry hydrogen-peroxide silver-agar method. Photomicrograph, B. & L., oil-immersion 2 mm., compensatory ocular No. 4, bellows length 100 cm. Organisms show typical "shepherd's crook ends." "Granule" near motile segment also indicated.

several changes of distilled water; 100 c c of distilled water is then added, and it is carefully brought to the boiling point with constant stirring. When the agar has gone into fine suspension the mixture is poured into a clean bottle, corked and allowed to cool. As the agar thickens it is occasionally shaken, and when it begins to set it is thoroughly broken up by violent shaking. It is then placed on top of the paraffin oven, after which it will remain a thick heavy mixture just fluid enough barely to run. All of the solutions used should be made up in clean porcelain or glass ware, and not in metal containers.

The hydroquinone is added just before using. After it has been added the mixture is stirred vigorously for a short time, when it is poured into staining

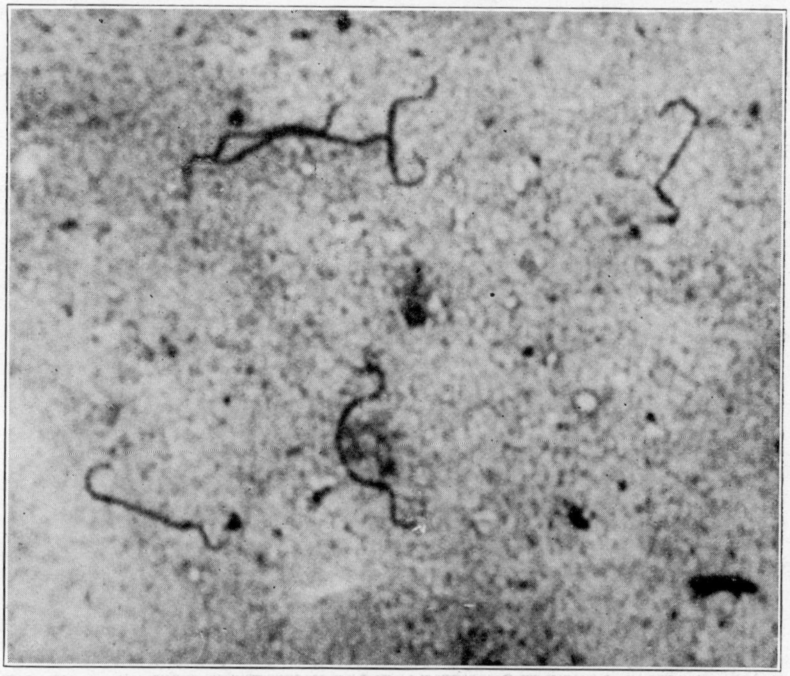

Fig. 7.—Leptospira icteroides in smear from macerated guinea-pig's liver, stained by Warthin-Starry hydrogen peroxide, silver-agar method. Photomicrograph with B. & L. oil-immersion 2 mm., compensatory ocular No. 4, bellows length 100 cm.

dishes, and the smears removed from the silver nitrate solution, the cover-glasses separated, and the one having the smear is immersed in the reducing mixture for a number of seconds (30 seconds to 2 minutes) until the reduction is complete. The smears turn a light brown; if very thin they may scarcely change color. When reduced, the smears are removed and placed in a 5% sodium thiosulphate solution for a few seconds. They are then rinsed in water, dehydrated in absolute alcohol, cleared in xylol and mounted in balsam. The longer the smears are in the reducing fluid the darker they are; it is, therefore, advisable to leave them in it until the reduction is nearly or wholly completed.

The use of the extra cover-glass in the silver solution seems to be essential. Good results are rarely obtained if the smear is left uncovered, as the serum and cellular elements of the smear take a deep brown stain and the spirochetes are usually indistinguishable.

It is essential that all reagents used be chemically pure and free from all contamination. The alcohol must be pure; if it contains phenol, mercuric chlorides, etc., the smears are easily mordanted, and the staining of the spirochetes becomes difficult.

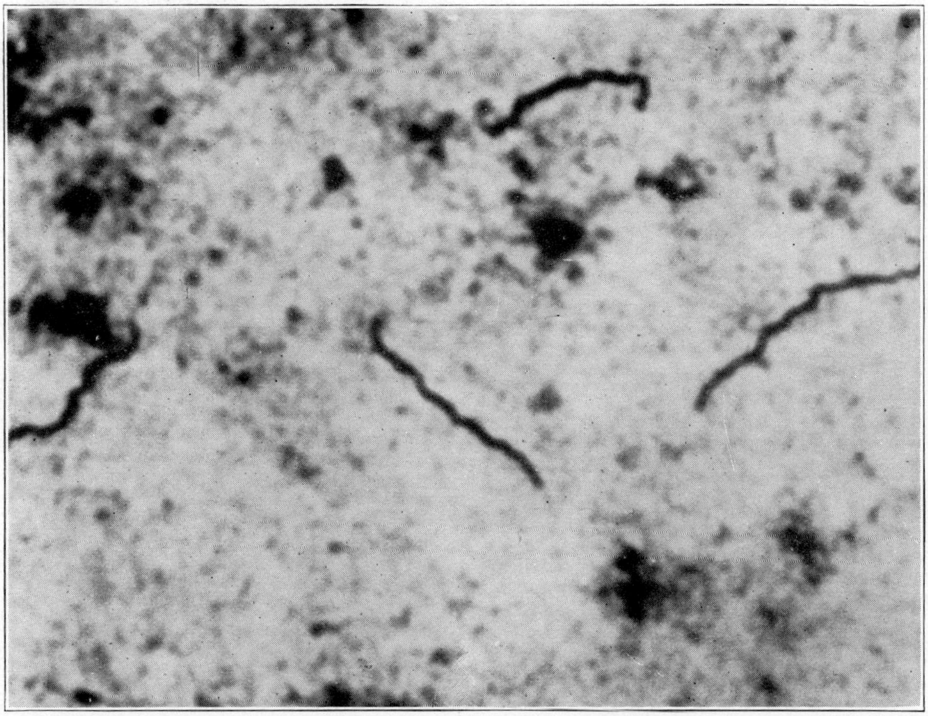

Fig. 8.—Leptospira icteroides in smear of macerated guinea-pig's liver. Same preparation. Taken with bellows length of 155 cm.

The spirochetes in the stained smears should appear black against a light background. In heavy smears with much serum or cell material we have found it of great advantage to use hydrogen peroxide to clear up the background. Between steps 4 and 5 of the method the cover-glass is placed in concentrated hydrogen peroxide for 5 - 20 minutes. It is then washed in 2 changes of distilled water before proceeding with the silver-impregnation in No. 5. In smears made from macerated liver we have found it possible to secure nearly colorless backgrounds for the spirochetes. The hydrogen peroxide must be pure and free from such impurities as barium chloride and other substances commonly found in commercial hydrogen peroxide. We have found that put up in pure form in slightly acidulated water, made by Parke, Davis & Co., to be satisfactory. With care the same solution can be used over and over for several weeks.

The spirochetes are increased in apparent size by this method, particularly in so far as their thickness is concerned. The precipitation of silver is chiefly a surface reaction on the spirochete. There is apparently some difference between different forms of spirochetes with relation to the intensity of this precipitation. The spirochetes of syphilis, relapsing fever, mouth and smegma precipitate silver much more intensely than Spirochaeta icterohaemorrhagica and Leptospira icteroides, and the thickness of the first-named group is increased proportionately, that of Sp. obermeieri about three times. This magnification of the size of the organisms is of the greatest advantage in diagnostic work, as every morphologic detail of the organism is proportionately increased in size and intensity and differential morphological characteristics are accentuated. The number, size and character of the turns of the organisms are easily determined, more so than by any other method.

The stained smears are not always permanent. After 4-6 weeks some of them fade, while others have retained their original intensity for a year and longer. We have found this fading particularly marked in the case of Leptospira icteroides. When for purposes of record it is desirable to make permanent preparations we have found that the smears made according to our method can be stabilized and, so far as our present experience goes, made permanent by toning with gold chloride. We have found Perrin's[1] method very satisfactory. After the smears are stained they are washed in a solution of sodium hyposulphite, then with distilled water and then toned in the following solution:

Ammonium sulphocyanide	6.25 gm.
Tartaric or citric acid	.50 gm.
Sodium chloride	1.25 gm.
Distilled water	250 c c
Solution of gold chloride (1:100)	6.25 c c

After a short time in this solution (5-15 minutes) the stain turns to a blue-black color. The smears are then washed in distilled water, dehydrated and cleared, and mounted in balsam.

We believe that our method of demonstrating spirochetes in cover-glass smears by silver-agar silver impregnation is the surest and safest diagnostic method yet devised. It should replace the use of the dark-field and the India-ink method in the diagnosis of syphilis. The morphologic details of Spirochaeta pallida and the mouth and smegma organisms so often mistaken for it by workers using the dark-field or India-ink method are so accentuated that differential diagnosis is made much easier. The India-ink method is especially dangerous for inexperienced workers. If spirochetes are present in the smear they will be stained by our method if directions are followed. The method is not formidable as it may seem because of the full directions given. It is easily acquired by laboratory workers. Aside from the time

[1] Arch. f. Dermat. u. Syphilis, 1920, 21, p. 354.

required for silver-impregnation in the incubator, it is a relatively short method, and a large number of smears can be kept going in different bottles at the same time. For bacteriologists and laboratory workers engaged in spirochete studies this method is of the greatest advantage in recovering organisms from the organs of inoculated animals, or from the blood or urine. It lends itself particularly well to the laboratory study of Sp. icterohaemorrhagica and Leptospira icteroides. Nevertheless, it is in its application to the clinical diagnosis of syphilis that it possesses its greatest value.

AN UNUSUAL CASE OF NOCARDIOSIS

G. R. Callender and J. F. Coupal

From the Division of Laboratories, Army Medical School, Washington, D. C.

This case is considered worthy of record for several reasons: 1. The patient was a physician and, as in this case, physicians often fail to receive as good attention as other patients. Too much is taken for granted by the physician himself, while the view of the rest of the world is: "Physician, heal Thyself." 2. The diagnosis was completely missed during life. 3. Necropsy with bacteriologic and pathologic study cleared up the whole condition. 4. The infection is a rare one.

The physician was 53 years of age and owned and managed a sanatorium for mental and nervous diseases near a large Eastern city. He had always enjoyed unusually good health up to two years ago. He was a tall, thin man of English type. His family history and previous history are uninstructive except that one sister had a mild attack of tuberculosis several years ago from which she has recovered.

Present Illness.—In October, 1919, the patient, while eating soup inhaled what he thought was a small piece of bone. It seemed to lodge in the right side of the chest. A nurse who was present said, after the death of the patient, that he nearly suffocated at the time of the accident. The patient, however, minimized the accident and cautioned the nurse to say nothing about it to his family. Shortly afterward, a physician on a nonprofessional visit observed that he apparently had a "bad cold" and was coughing considerably. He made light of the trouble, and though it was suggested that he have a bronchoscopic examination, he did not consider it necessary, saying that he thought that if he had inhaled the bone it was only a small splinter. During the following months he complained of pain in the right side and coughed a good deal. In February, 1920, he had a severe attack of influenza, with high temperature and some pneumonia. The trouble was especially marked on the right side and was accompanied by pain on breathing and a good deal of expectoration. Cultures of sputum at this time showed Staphylococcus aureus and Micrococcus catarrhalis; the leukocyte count was 15,900. After partial recovery he was given a thorough examination. Roentgen-ray plates were negative, especial search being made for the bone; examination of the sputum proved negative for tubercle bacilli; guinea-pig inoculations were inconclusive because of the early death of three animals from complicating infections. Another specimen of sputum was requested but was not received. The Wassermann reaction was negative; blood sugar 0.11%; urea nitrogen 13.7 mg. It was concluded at this time that the case was one of postinfluenzal bronchitis or bronchiectasis. The teeth were examined with the roentgen ray, and several teeth with apical abscesses were extracted. The patient improved a great deal during the summer and the following fall of 1920 seemed to be active and well. In February, 1921 he had another attack—influenzal in character—and became considerably run down in weight and vitality. In May, 1921, he went to Atlantic City for recuperation, but felt so bad that he returned

Received for publication Feb. 23, 1922.

after about two weeks. He had a slight fever at this time, shortness of breath, pain in the right side and coughed a good deal. He was seen at this time by a nose and throat specialist and a lung specialist, and they found evidences of what was thought to be a latent tuberculosis in both apexes with a somewhat more active lesion in the lower part of the right lung. A roentgenogram showed a slight lesion in the latter location. It was recommended that the patient go to a northern sanatorium for rest and treatment for tuberculosis. Sputum examinations at this time were negative for tubercle bacilli; some nonacid-fast rods were seen but no importance was attached to them. During July and September, 1921, the patient was in the north, where physicians thought he showed slight tuberculous lesions of both apexes, especially the right. The sputum was negative for tubercle bacilli. He improved considerably in weight, walked and drove about a good deal and was preparing to return when, on Sept. 7, he had an attack of mental confusion and developed a slight general paralysis. This passed off in a day or two, but he had a red nodule on one wrist, and an old buckshot wound on the right leg became somewhat inflamed. He was making further plans to return home when, on Sept. 9, he had a convulsive attack accompanied by unconsciousness, a wrist drop of the right hand appearing after the first convulsion. The blood examination showed: leukocytes 25,200; polymorphonuclears 78%. The next day he was mentally clear but weak. A spinal puncture on the 11th showed an increase in globulin, cells 4, polymorphonuclears 13%, lymphocytes 84%. On that day there was another attack of confusion followed by convulsion, after which the entire right side was paralyzed. The urine showed a trace of albumin, a few casts and some red blood cells. Blood cultures were made which were sterile at the end of a week. Blood count: leukocytes 24,000; polymorphonuclears 85%. The temperature was elevated very little. A probable diagnosis of cerebral hemorrhage or embolism was made. The patient was taken home barely alive on Sept. 11 and died on the 15th. A consultant at his home made a probable diagnosis of thrombosis. Another leukocyte count was requested, but the patient died before it could be made. He never became fully conscious. During the last few days his left side also showed some paralysis.

Extracts from the Necropsy Report

The body was that of a well developed, somewhat emaciated white man. Panniculus moderate in amount but contains little fat.

Brain.—The dura is adherent to the brain along the superior longitudinal sinus where the pacchionian bodies seem to be increased in size. All vessels are markedly injected, and there is some exudate about the vessels in the posterior portion of the left cerebrum which bulges posteriorly. There is considerable edema of the membranes. On section, two abscesses were found, the larger in the left cerebrum being 9 cm. in length from before backward, and about 5 cm. in diameter, occupying the greater part of the middle of this lobe. In the right lobe was a similar abscess about 5 cm. in diameter, more or less spherical in shape. The abscesses have a ragged wall, not clearly outlined, and the centers contain fluid pus. The right ventricle contains a cloudy fluid, while the left is clear. The abscesses compress the periphery and both involve the internal capsule.

Thorax.—Left pleural cavity is moist, and there is one fibrous adhesion at the apex. Elsewhere the lung is free, the visceral pleura being somewhat duller than the parietal.

Right pleura shows a few firm adhesions at the apex and a free portion from about the lower margin of the second rib to the upper margin of the fourth rib in the midaxillary line. From there, to and including the base, the lung is adherent by large delicate fibrous adhesions, the interstices between the adhesions being filled with a gelatinous exudate.

Lung.—The left lung shows the pleura at the apex markedly thickened by elevated opaque, yellowish white, firm, coalescing nodules, the area covered by this thickening being approximately 2.5 cm. anteroposteriorly and 5 cm. from within outward. The thickening extends only a few millimeters into the lung-parenchyma, and while there are a few small points of yellowish opacity between these raised nodules, there is no marked activity. The rest of the upper lobe is air-containing, and, although somewhat congested, appears relatively normal. The lower lobe shows scattered areas of thickening, the centers of which are apparently about smaller bronchi and therefore occupy the centers of the lobules. The color of the lung is a deep red with a lighter, brighter red with a yellowish tint as the color of these consolidated areas.

The right lung shows a similar condition at the apex except that its extent is 3.5 to 4 cm., maximum anteroposterior measurement, and 12 cm. maximum measurement from within outward. The area, therefore, forms a cap over the apical portion of the lung. The maximum extension of the thickening into the parenchyma of the lung is 1 cm., and there is a yellowish caseous looking area where the thickening joins the air-containing tissue. Below this area the tissue for a distance of 2 to 3 cm. appears relatively normal. It then becomes a darker red and indurated. In about the mid-portion of this lobe is a yellowish white opaque area approximately 2 cm. in diameter, the center of which, about 1.3 cm. in diameter, is soft and composed of a cheesy-like material, of a granular consistency. From this area to the hilus of the lung the nearest bronchus is surrounded by an indurated thickened area, and the wall of the bronchus itself is markedly thickened and lined by a dirty brownish red membrane covered with an exudate of similar color. The interlobar fissure has been obliterated by adhesions. At about the midaxillary line, the tissue of the upper lobe just above the interlobar separation presents an indurated mass about 3 cm. in diameter, in the center of which is a cavity about 1.5 cm. in greatest diameter lined by a dark brownish red membrane. The cavity appears to be vacant except for a small amount of dirty reddish exudate on the surface of the lining. In the upper portion of the lower lobe extending outward from the main bronchus of this lobe about 4 cm. from its origin, is an indurated mass which extends into the lung for a distance of about 5 cm. This consists of indurated dark red tissue in the periphery with a slaty reddish zone of connective tissue forming a center with soft, small abscesses averaging 3 mm. scattered through it. This right inferior bronchus shows a markedly thickened wall which is irregularly dilated surrounding a cervical vertebra of a chicken which had lodged 2.5 cm. from the origin of the right inferior bronchus. It was situated with its inferior or ventral aspect posteriorly and had lost its two inferior prolongations. The rest of the lower lobe shows an occasional bronchopneumonic patch like those described in the left lung, while the pleura over the entire lung is thickened, particularly where covered by adhesions, as described in the foregoing.

The tracheobronchial glands are relatively small in the upper areas. The large gland below the primary bronchus of the right lung has enlarged to a size of 1.5 cm. in thickness and 3 cm. in length. On section it is mottled a rather deep red and an opaque yellowish red. The upper series of glands show a few hardened foci but no evidence of tuberculous activity.

Kidneys.—These show cloudy swellings and are rather opaque, but the capsule strips normally. In one section near the lower pole of the right kidney is an opaque yellowish area about 2.5 mm. in diameter.

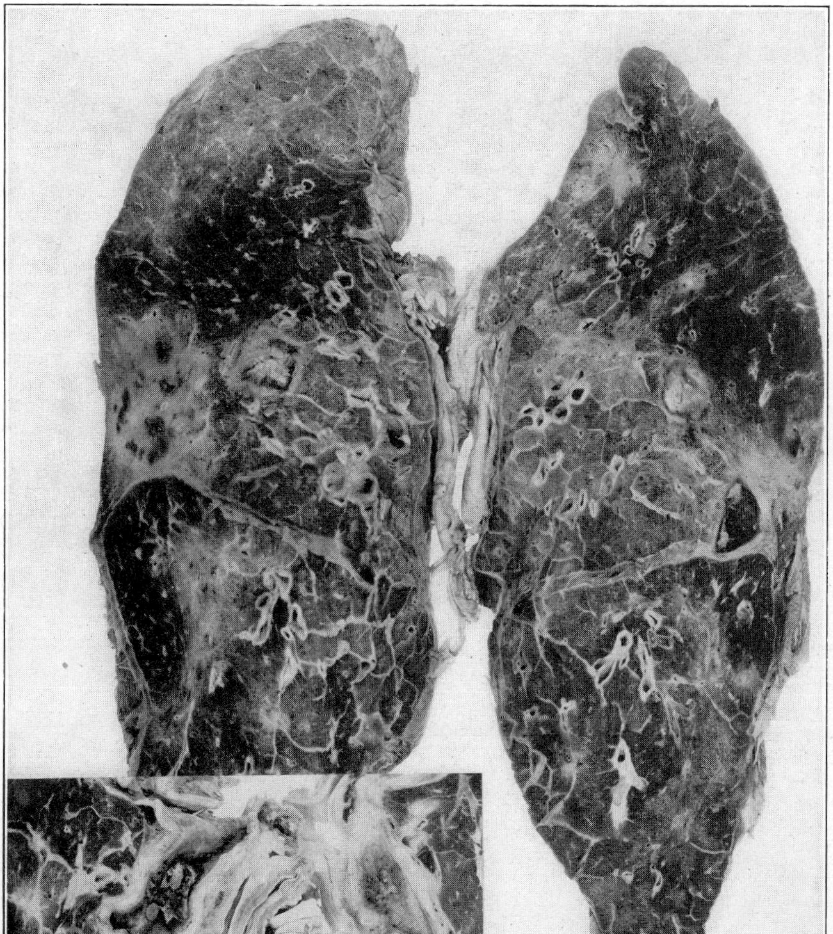

Fig. 1.—Sections of right lung showing lesions caused by Nocardia. Insert: Chicken vertebra in right bronchus.

BACTERIOLOGIC FINDINGS

Bacteriologic studies were made by Major H. J. Nichols, M. C., U. S. A. At necropsy, smears were made from the pus of the largest abscess of the brain. These showed no tubercle bacilli, but a number of clusters of short, threadlike gram-positive organisms, which were diagnosed as Streptothrix (Nocardia). Several slants of infusion agar were inoculated with the pus at the time of necropsy. These remained sterile except for a slight growth of Streptothrix in one tube which could not be transferred to other slants. Pus from the abscess was collected in a sterile tube, and on return to the laboratory was inoculated into several deep glucose agar tubes. After a week's incubation one tube showed three distinct colonies made up of threadlike organisms similar to those found in the abscesses. These colonies have a characteristic trilobular appearance (fig. 2). The organism was in pure culture and has been transferred a number of times in deep agar, and grows freely after several days' incubation. It is a strictly anerobic, gram-positive, pleomorphic bacillus. It stains unevenly both by Gram stain and with Loeffler's methylene blue. Branching forms are seen in the tissues; in culture no definite branching forms were seen. It was evidently in pure culture in the abscess.

Animal Inoculations.—A guinea-pig, inoculated subcutaneously with the pus, developed a small abscess lasting for two weeks, which showed a mixed growth of numerous threadlike organisms and staphylococci. A guinea-pig inoculated subcutaneously with the culture developed a small nodule which disappeared after about a week without breaking down. Further inoculations were made as follows: One guinea-pig was inoculated intraperitoneally with culture, one rabbit intravenously, one monkey intratracheally, and one monkey intracerebrally with culture. None of these animals showed any evidence of infection in two months. Necropsies were performed on all, and none was infected.

The organism which appears to have been the cause of the disease belongs to the anaerobic group of Streptothrix but is a somewhat unusual type. When injected in the pus from human lesions, it was only slightly pathogenic for guinea-pigs and lost its virulence rapidly in culture. A guinea-pig which was inoculated intraperitoneally with the pus, showed two weeks later, after a subcutaneous inoculation, an anaphylactic reaction of redness and induration about the inoculation site.

HISTOLOGIC EXAMINATION

Brain.—Sections from the brain show an abscess, the contents of which are composed of polymorphonuclear leukocytes with numerous colonies of Streptothrix (Nocardia) scattered throughout the pus. The wall is composed of brain tissue over a considerable area, though in places there is thickening of the glia forming a delicate margin of gliosis. The leukocytes have infiltrated the tissue to a greater extent where this protective wall has not been formed. Blood vessels in the vicinity of the abscess show escape of leukocytes, both polymorphonuclear and lymphocytes, and brain tissue for considerable distance around these abscesses shows similar leukocytic infiltration, lymphocytes gradually predominating at a distance from the abscess wall. The meninges show some thickening in the sulci, and deep between the convolutions or lobules there is considerable exudation, particularly where the abscess approaches the surface. This exudate is composed of fibrin with rather numerous leukocytes largely of the polymorphonuclear variety. The pia is somewhat thickened over the surface of the brain which overlies the abscess. The process has destroyed brain tissue and surrounding it ganglion cells show advanced degenerative changes and there is considerable edema throughout.

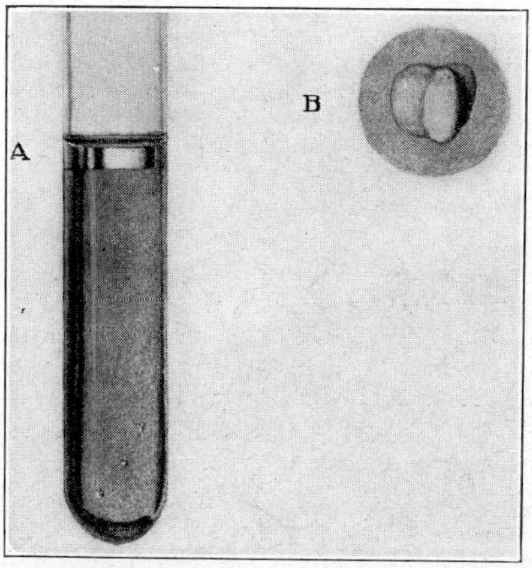

Fig. 2.—*A*, anaerobic culture from brain abscess; *B*, enlarged colony.

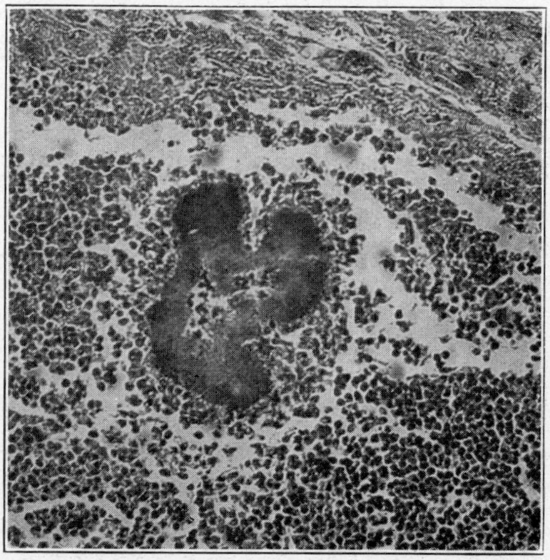

Fig. 3.—Nocardia in brain abscess; × 100.

Right Lung.—Sections taken from the bronchus in the vicinity of the chicken bone show an intense hyperemia and denudation of the bronchial mucosa with formation of granulation tissue from the submucosa. The bronchial glands are swollen and dilated with secretion, their walls infiltrated with leukocytes, and there is an increase in connective tissue extending down from the granulating layer on the surface to the cartilages and involving to a considerable degree connective tissue between the cartilages and beneath them. Lymph nodes are hyperactive as indicated by marked increase of epithelioid cells in the nodal centers. Bacterial stains show various types of organisms, both cocci and bacilli. There are no colonies of Streptothrix in these areas.

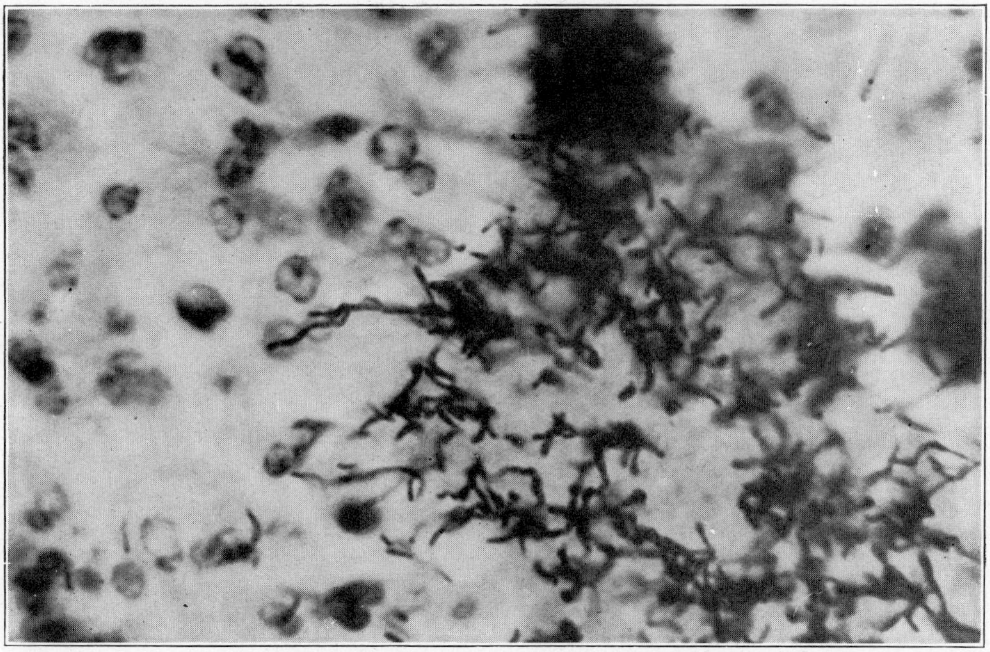

Fig. 4.—Nocardia in tissue; × 1,000.

Sections from the pearly masses of the apexes show fibrosis and connective tissue which in places has become hyaline. Scattered here and there are small lymph nodes containing anthracotic pigment surrounded by a smaller zone of some younger fibroblasts than are present in the rest of the tissue. The lymph nodes are more abundant just beneath the endothelial surface. This fibrosis appears to extend only a short distance into the lung.

A section taken from one firm nodule surrounding the bronchus of the right upper lobe shows bronchial mucosa partially desquamated; the walls are thickened and the surrounding blood vessels are engorged. The surrounding air cells show a marked thickening of the alveolar walls and an atelectatic condition. The epithelium of the alveoli have for the most part become cuboidal in character. This probably represents a blocking off of this small section of the lung by reason of inflammatory changes in the bronchus.

Sections from the bluish area at the junction of the upper and lower lobes of the right lung show an advanced fibrosis of the alveolar walls resulting in an organizing process compressing the alveoli which contain desquamated epithelial cells. There is no tendency in this area for the alveolar epithelium to become cuboidal but rather to degenerate. In the outer layers there is considerable hyalin change where alveolar structure has been eradicated by the overgrowth of connective tissue. In sections nearer the abscesses in the indurated tissue the early stages of these processes are seen and vary from thickening of the alveolar wall by edema and lymphocytic infiltration to the fibrosis of the older areas. All of this tissue contains numerous lymphocytes and quite a few polymorphonuclears.

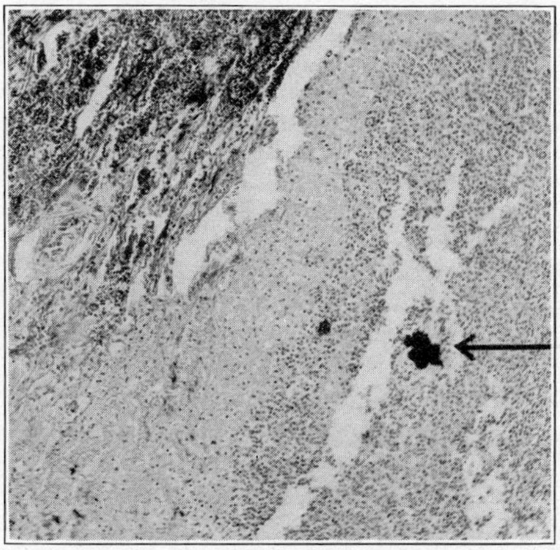

Fig. 5.—Nocardia in lung abscess.

Sections from the bronchus of the upper lobe of the right lung taken about 4 cm. from its origin show a marked thickening of the wall due to connective tissue increase in the submucosa which has surrounded and partially obliterated the glands. Gram-positive organisms, both cocci and bacilli and gram-negative bacilli, are found in the bronchi and to some extent in occasional alveoli where the exudate consists largely of leukocytes. The abscesses of the lung where filled with leukocytes show numerous colonies of Streptothrix or Nocardia (fig. 5).

Left Lung.—Sections taken from the bronchopneumonic areas show numerous small patches 3 or 4 mm. in diameter where the alveoli are partially filled with polymorphonuclear leukocytes. The bronchial epithelium is desquamated. The bronchi contain considerable pus. The walls of the alveoli are not markedly thickened though the blood vessels are filled with blood. There is some tendency in portions to proliferation of connective tissue cells. In addition to the leukocytes, the alveoli contain blood cells and a moderate amount of fibrin. The organisms present are a mixture of gram-positive and negative cocci and bacilli. There are no colonies of Streptothrix in this lung.

Kidney.—Glomeruli show some proliferation of the capillary endothelium and a slight degree of hydropic change. The cells of the convoluted tubules are swollen and granular. One section of the right kidney shows two small abscesses surrounded by connective tissue thickening of considerable extent with leukocytic infiltration and vascular hyperemia throughout the thickened tissue. The abscesses contain colonies of Streptothrix.

Skin.—A section from the skin shows an infiltrating abscess in the deeper layers of the subcutaneous tissue with a slight degree of fibrosis. The abscess contains colonies of Streptothrix.

Anatomic Diagnosis.—Nocardiosis of the right lung with metastatic abscess in the brain, kidney and skin; tuberculosis of apical pleura, both lungs; bilateral bronchopneumonia; degeneration (toxic) of kidneys and liver; foreign body (chicken neck vertebra) in right inferior bronchus with secondary bronchitis and bronchiectasis.

GENERAL SUMMARY

The patient, two years before death, inhaled into his right bronchus a chicken vertebra. He minimized the importance of the size of the bone and repeated roentgen-ray examinations failed to reveal it. A few months after the accident the patient had a severe attack of "influenza" with pneumonia, which was especially localized on the right side. A year later there was a train of symptoms of the same character. During the interim the patient was in comparatively good health. Following this second attack until his death (a period of seven months) the patient gradually failed. He had a cough, high temperature, pain in the right side and shortness of breath. Bacteriologic examinations were negative but physical examination and roentgenograms indicated a tuberculous process. Two weeks before death there was evidence of embolic processes as indicated by the cerebral attack and the abscess on the leg. Signs were found of old tuberculosis of the apexes.

It is impossible to determine accurately the exact onset of the infection with Nocardia. From the clinical history it would appear that if this infection occurred prior to the second influenzal attack in February, 1921, it must at least have remained well localized, as no generalized symptoms occurred. It seems not unreasonable to suppose that the focus of diminished resistance produced by the bone in the bronchus gave a satisfactory lodging place for this organism, which probably came from the mouth and that it slowly developed during the last seven months of the patient's life, then by its formation of abscesses it gained access to the blood stream and produced a nocardial pyemia during the last two weeks. The general age of the lesions in the lung and brain indicates that this is the probable story.

The organism belongs to the Streptothrix group and is a rather unusual type in that it is apparently an absolute anaerobe. Such organisms have been described, but no attempt is made at this time to review the literature on infections with this type of organism.

A PECULIAR FAILURE OF HEMOLYTIC ACTION IN A STRAIN OF HEMOLYTIC STREPTOCOCCUS

EUGENIA VALENTINE

From the Bureau of Laboratories, Department of Health, City of New York.

While titrating by the tube method the hemolytic capacity of a series of streptococcus cultures of the beta hemolytic type, a peculiar absence of hemolysis was observed with one culture.

This strain, W 12, isolated from a case of pleurisy has been described by Williams,[1] Valentine and Mishulow,[2] and Mishulow.[3] It is unusual in many respects. In blood-agar pour plates, it forms a rosette or complex colony unlike most beta hemolytic streptococci. It has the characteristics of the beta type in that microscopic examination shows that the red cells about the colony are completely dissolved, although the hemolyzed zone develops slowly, being very narrow after 24 hours' incubation and increasing in diameter to 3 mm. after 48 hours. The relatively feeble hemolytic capacity of this strain was also shown by the general absence of demonstrable hemolysin in the supernatant broth of centrifuged broth cultures. After 68 hours' growth in glucose broth, it reaches a H-ion concentration of P_H 4.7, which is more acid than the reaction produced by the majority of strains of human origin.

With the strain W 12, 0.5 c c of an 18-hour broth culture failed to give hemolysis when mixed with 1 c c of 5% washed red cell (horse), while 0.4 c c of the culture plus 0.1 c c of sterile broth resulted in

TABLE 1

THE FAILURE OF HEMOLYTIC ACTION BY STRAIN W 12

Broth culture, 18 hours....	0.5 c c	0.4 c c	0.3 c c	0.2 c c	0.1 c c	0
Sterile broth..............	0	0.1 c c	0.2 c c	0.3 c c	0.4 c c	0.5 c c
Red cells, 5% suspension...	1 c c	1 c c	1 c c	1 c c	1 c c	1 c c
Strain 60..................	Complete lysis	Complete lysis	Complete lysis	Complete lysis	Complete lysis	No lysis
Strain W 12................	No lysis	Lysis	Lysis	Lysis	Slight lysis	No lysis

Horse, sheep and rabbit cells gave the same results.

almost complete hemolysis of the red cells (table 1). Twenty-five other strains did not show this phenomenon; the result with strain 60 is representative of the hemolytic activity of these other strains and is

Received for publication, Feb. 18, 1922.

[1] Jour. Immunol., 1921, 6, p. 62.
[2] Ibid., 1921, 6, p. 301.
[3] Ibid., 1921, 6, p. 329.

given in table 1 for comparison. Another strain having the same characteristics as W 12, but differing from it agglutinatively, also showed hemolysis in all the tubes.

The failure of the whole culture of strain W 12 to lake red cells until the addition of sterile broth is of interest from the practical standpoint, for it may be a source of error in testing the hemolytic activity by the tube method usually employed. From the theoretical standpoint it seemed of interest to explain, if possible, the mechanism of this phenomenon.

In most of the further experiments, 0.5 c c and 0.2 c c of culture were used. The phenomenon was observed with marked constancy without regard to the kind of broth employed, that is, whether made of veal or of beef, the mode of sterilization, the period of storage and the variation of reaction within the limits suitable for growth.

It was found, however, that 0.5 c c of a broth culture of W 12, which had been incubated for only 6 hours, caused hemolysis, without the addition of fresh broth, but that the same culture incubated for 15 or 18 hours did not (table 2). The failure of hemolysis by the 18-hour culture was always prevented by the addition of 0.1 c c of sterile broth, and the addition of as little as 0.03 c c of broth resulted in the development of some hemolysis.

TABLE 2

THE HEMOLYTIC ACTION OF CULTURES OF STRAIN W 12 INCUBATED ONLY SIX HOURS; ABSENCE OF HEMOLYSIS AFTER LONGER INCUBATION

Broth culture, 6 or 18 hours	0.5 c c	0.5 c c	0.2 c c	0.2 c c
Sterile broth	0	0.1 c c	0	0.1 c c
Salt solution	1.0 c c	0.9 c c	1.3 c c	1.3 c c
Red cells, 5% suspension	1.0 c c	1.0 c c	1.0 c c	1.0 c c
Results, 6 hours culture	Complete lysis	Complete lysis	Lysis	Lysis
Results, 18 hours culture	No lysis	Complete lysis	No lysis	Lysis

When the clarified supernatant broth of an 18-hour culture of W 12 was used in place of sterile broth in an experiment parallel to that shown in table 2, no hemolysis took place. Heating this supernatant broth to 56 C. and 100 C. for 15 minutes, gave no different results. The supernatant broth from an 18-hour culture when added to a 6-hour culture did not prevent hemolysis. Adding peptone water to 18-hour broth cultures was as effectual in renewing hemolytic activity as the addition of sterile broth. Sterile horse serum, however, did not serve so well. Acid production was evidently not a factor, for neutralization of the small amount of acid produced did not result in hemolysis.

The outstanding points were therefore: the active hemolysis after 6 hours' incubation, the absence of hemolysis after longer incubation, the renewal of hemolytic action by the addition of broth or peptone water, that is, a fresh food supply. This raised the question: Was the failure of hemolysis due to the cessation of growth and was the resumption of hemolytic action, after the addition of fresh broth, due to renewed multiplication?

This point was investigated by making poured plates. After 2 hours' incubation of the tube to which no fresh broth had been added, plate counts showed at most a slight increase in the number of cocci. The tube, however, to which fresh broth had been added, showed after 2 hours' incubation an increase of 30 to 60% in the number of colonies developing in the plates.

SUMMARY

It would seem that the failure of hemolysis of the strain of hemolytic streptococcus studied was due to cessation of growth which was renewed by the addition of a small amount of fresh broth. The reason, however, why this culture should present this peculiarity remains obscure.

BACTERIOLOGIC STUDIES OF GASTRIC FRACTIONS OBTAINED BY THE REHFUSS METHOD

Nicholas Kopeloff

From the Department of Bacteriology, Psychiatric Institute, Ward's Island, New York City

The fractional method of gastric analysis makes possible a study of the stomach contents at the different stages in the process of digestion and in the resting or "interdigestive" phase as well. Until recently this method has been employed almost exclusively for obtaining chemical data which would be of assistance to the clinician. However, this method can likewise be used for the determination of the bacterial content of the stomach. So far as could be ascertained, no quantitative studies concerning numbers of bacteria present in various gastric fractions have hitherto been reported. In fact little is known with regard to the types of bacteria to be found in these fractions beyond the work of Cotton [1] who claims that, "The stomach and duodenum are very frequently the seat of secondary foci. . . . The bacteria invade the stomach wall and appear to interfere with the secretion of hydrochloric acid, so necessary to digestion. Cultures of the stomach contents will reveal the presence of various types of streptococci and frequently of various types of colon bacilli. The chemical examination of the stomach contents will show either a very low secretion of hydrochloric acid, or in many cases, its entire absence during the test meal." On the administration of autogenous vaccines the acidity of the stomach is said to be increased and the bacteria to disappear.

The first criticism which can be advanced against such a position is that these conclusions are based on single determinations by the Rehfuss method of fractional analysis. I have shown [2] that repeated analyses carried out on the same person within a short period of time yield different acidity curves. In other words, the same subject may show a low, high and intermediate acidity on three separate analyses carried out within a single week. Obviously, therefore, it is not valid to base any conclusions on a single determination.

The Rehfuss method of fractional gastric analysis was carried out in the usual way on a number of healthy and psychotic persons. The

Received for publication Jan. 28, 1922.

[1] New York Med. Jour., 1920, 111, pp. 672, 721 and 770. The Defective Delinquent and Insane, p. 201.

[2] Nicholas Kopeloff: Jour. Am. Med. Assn., 122, 78, p. 404.

modifications introduced were as follows: Sterilization of the Rehfuss tubes and syringes; rinsing of the mouth with chlorazene solution (1 teaspoonful of powdered aromatic chlorazene to a cup of sterile water) followed by several thorough rinsings with sterile distilled water. The conditions for bacteriologic study, consequently, were somewhat more aseptic than those generally employed. Broth tubes were inoculated with the gastric fractions during analysis and incubated for 24 hours at 37½ C. Gram stains were made of all fractions. From these broth cultures streaks were made on lactose meat infusion agar having brom cresol purple as an indicator, and pure colonies were fished therefrom. Holman [3] was followed for the classification of streptococci, and Chester [4] for all other organisms. In all, a qualitative study was made of about 1,000 gastric fractions.

TABLE 1

BACTERIAL SPECIES FOUND BY THE FRACTIONAL METHOD OF GASTRIC ANALYSIS

Staphylococcus albus	Bacterium bossonis
Staphylococcus aureus	Bacterium acidiformans
Staphylococcus citreus	Bacterium ambiguum
Streptococcus viridans	Bacterium aerogenes
Streptococcus pyogenes	Bacterium mycoides
Streptococcus fecalis	Bacterium I
Streptococcus equinus	Bacterium II
Streptococcus salivarius	Bacillus vulgatus
Streptococcus mitis	Bacillus dendriticus
Streptococcus ignavus	Bacillus vulgaris
Streptococcus subacidus	Bacillus cloacae
Enterococcus	Bacillus coli
Bacterium lacticum	Bacillus I
Bacterium acidi-lacti	Bacillus II
Bacterium viscosum	Yeasts, nonchromogenic
Bacterium desidiosum	Yeasts, chromogenic

However important such a qualitative bacteriologic investigation may be, it soon becomes apparent that quantitative results are of equal, if not greater, significance. Invariably, infection connotes numbers of bacteria. Therefore, in addition to classifying the bacteria found in the various gastric fractions, an attempt was made to determine the actual number of bacteria present at each stage of the analysis. The procedure was as follows: One c c of each gastric fraction on withdrawal was at once plated out in duplicate (at the bedside) on lactose meat infusion agar. The plates were incubated in the usual way and counted in 24 hours, and again in 3 days.

Another factor of considerable importance in the proper interpretation of analyses by means of the Rehfuss method is the saliva. Varying

[3] Jour. Med. Res., 1916, 29, p. 377.

[4] A Manual of Determinative Bacteriology, 1902, p. 401.

quantities of saliva are swallowed by different persons, and it is of importance to determine the bacterial flora of the saliva in question, as well as to note the amount swallowed. Careful record, therefore, has been kept of the numbers of bacteria occurring in composite samples of saliva obtained during the analysis, as well as of the types found, and the chemical reaction.

In table 1 will be found a list of the species of bacteria isolated from the various gastric fractions. The streptococci and staphylococci are well represented, as are the lactobacilli. Many of the listed names represent approximations due to atypical characters of the organisms, rather than constituting exact species. Thus it has been necessary to call several atypical strains of nonhemolytic streptococci: Streptococcus viridans. It will be noted, however, that the great majority of these organisms are generally regarded as nonpathogenic. Many of them are, to be sure, facultatively pathogenic and merely await a favorable opportunity to become true pathogens. The species found are in close agreement with some unpublished data, very kindly placed at our disposal by Dr. L. W. Famulener.

The occurrence of these organisms in the various gastric fractions is shown in table 2, which gives a summary of data to be given in detail elsewhere.[5] The high acidity average is an average of the 3 highest total acidity values obtained during the analysis of that date; the average number of bacteria is the average found concomitantly with the acidities just mentioned; the low acidity average is the average of the 3 lowest total acidity values obtained in the same analysis; the average number of bacteria found concomitantly with those acidities; and the last column gives the names of these types of bacteria. The table itself is divided into 2 parts, the first half being the results obtained with healthy normal persons and the second half being devoted to psychotic patients. These results have been greatly condensed and these subjects may be considered representative of the larger group studied.

Certain rather broad features can be clearly distinguished. In the first place, if one glances down the column of types of bacteria found for the three highest total acidities and compares them with the types found for the lowest total acidities during the same analysis, a marked similarity will be discerned between the parallel columns at almost every point. This holds true for psychotic as well as for normal persons. For example, in the very first subject, C.Te., on August 31, when the

[5] Nicholas Kopeloff: State Hosp. Quart. (N. Y.), May, 1922.

TABLE 2

Bacteria in Gastric Fractions of High and Low Acidity

Name	Date	Average Three High Acid	Average No. Bacteria	Types	Average Three Low Acid	Average No. Bacteria	Types
				Normal			
C. Te.	8/31	64	47	Yeasts.................	24	46	Yeasts, S. fecalis
	9/ 2	68	25	S. viridans, Bact. ambiguum	30	14	S. viridans, Bact. ambiguum
	9/ 6	81	3	Yeasts, Bact. ambiguum	45	2	Yeasts
S. Mc y.	8/31	43	943	Yeasts, Bact. lacticum, S. viridans, Bact. ambiguum	9	30,000	B. coli, S. viridans
	9/ 2	72	1,166	Bact. ambiguum, S. viridans, yeasts	23	720	Bact. ambiguum, S. viridans, yeasts
	9/ 6	84	428	Bact. ambiguum, S. viridans, yeasts	30	405	Bact. ambiguum, S. viridans, yeasts
M. Mc a.	8/31	52	0	S. viridans, yeasts.....	25	27,000	S. viridans, yeasts
	9/ 2	64	0	Nil......................	40	1	Bact. mycoides
	9/ 6	64	0	Enterococcus..........	46	1	Enterococcus
				Psychotic			
E. Zn.	7/ 7	28	22	Bact. lacticum, Bact. mycoides, B. vulgaris	9	15,434	Bact. mycoides
	7/21	23	8	B. cloacae, yeasts......	7	78,000	B. cloacae
M. Sl.	3/14	44	68	S. viridans, S. albus, yeasts, Bact. lacticum	18	5,000	S. albus, S. viridans, yeasts
	3/16	39	2	Bact. aquatilis, S. albus, yeasts, Bact. lacticum	8	4,500	S. albus, S. fecalis, Bact. acidi-lacti, yeasts
	6/28	38	64	B. vulgatus, yeasts, S. mitis	8	21,518	B. vulgatus, S. mitis
	11/16	43	18	S. mitis................	13	5,533	S. mitis
I. Sn.	7/29	48	....	S. aureus, S. fecalis, yeasts	16	......	S. aureus, S. fecalis, yeasts
	8/14	40	285	S. aureus..............	21	436	S. aureus
M. Hr.	6/30	56	39	Bact. lacticum, yeasts	31	16	Bact. lacticum, yeasts
	7/ 7	63	31	Bact. lacticum, yeasts	24	49	Bact. lacticum, yeasts
	7/14	51	12	S. aureus, yeasts......	22	6,335	S. aureus, yeasts
E. Kg.	4/19	57	11	S. albus, Bac. I, yeasts	43	3	S. albus, Bac. I, yeasts, S. salivarius
	6/30	67	1,517	Bact. lacticum.........	34	623	Bact. lacticum
E. Mc y.	7/ 7	24	618	Bact. lacticum.........	9	15,000	Bact. mycoides, Bact. lacticum
	7/14	22	32	S. aureus, Bac. I.......	11	4,133	S. aureus, yeasts
	11/ 4	22	203	Bact.	10	4,650	Bact.
M. Dn.	7/ 7	25	17	S. aureus, Bact. lacticum, yeasts	16	8,513	Bact. lacticum, yeasts
	7/21	67	308	S. aureus, Bact. lacticum, yeasts	23	591	Bact. lacticum, S. aureus
	7/26	55	693	Yeasts.................	15	320	Yeasts
I. Be.	4/19	78	2,966	Bact. lacticum, yeasts	21	20,430	Bact. lacticum, yeasts, Bact. I
	4/26	72	118	Bac. I, yeasts..........	41	87	S. albus, B. vulgatus, Bact. I
	6/28	62	113	S. ignavus, Bact. lacticum, yeasts	39	885	S. albus, Bact. lacticum, yeasts
B. Cy.	3/16	50	19	Bacterium acidi-lacti, yeasts, Bact. ambiguum, S. ignavus	26	43	Bact. I, yeasts, S. ignavus
	4/19	55	2	Yeasts.................	19	2,420	S. albus, yeasts
	4/26	54	58	Bac. I, yeasts..........	10	3,176	S. albus, B. vulgatus
M. By.	7/14	64	450	S. aureus, yeasts......	24	53	S. aureus, yeasts
	8/14	95	61	Yeasts.................	21	1,064	S. aureus, yeasts, S. mitis
T. Cd.	6/30	51	3	Bact. lacticum, S. mitis	27	4	Bact. lacticum, S. mitis
	7/21	46	1	Bact. lacticum, yeasts	19	6,040	Bact. lacticum, S. aureus, yeasts
	7/26	63	3	Bact. mycoides, S. viridans, yeasts	31	175	Bact. mycoides, S. viridans

average high total acidity was 64, and 47 bacteria per c c were found, yeasts were present. The average low total acidity was 24, and the number of bacteria 46. Again yeasts were found, together with S. fecalis. On September 2, with an acidity of 68, 25 bacteria were found, the types being S. viridans and Bact. ambiguum. With the low acidity of 30 there were only 14 bacteria comprising identically the same types as those just mentioned. Such close parallelism occurs with great frequency throughout both series.

This observation is of considerable significance, for it shows rather convincingly, that acidity is not of prime importance with regard to bacterial species found. In other words, instead of finding a great many more delicate organisms at the lower acidities, we find virtually the same flora as occurs at higher acidities. This is further emphasized by the fact that the flora remains the same, irrespective of the numbers of bacteria present at the differing acidities. It will be noted that there is great inconsistency in the bacterial numbers at different acidities. In some instances, notably C.Te., one actually finds fewer bacteria with lower acidity, which is contrary to expectation. Again this would indicate that acidity is not the limiting factor as far as the bacterial content of the stomach is concerned. This will warrant further discussion in connection with other quantitative results still to be considered. It is interesting to observe that the more common organisms appear in the same person at different times, but this occurrence is scarcely any more regular than the occurrence of the same species in different persons on the same day—indicating that external factors are fully as important as the internal factors. However, the fact that the more uncommon organisms are not found with any degree of regularity, either in the same subject or on the same day, makes it inadvisable to draw any inferences, but rather to consider these phenomena as being instances of the law of probabilities.

Concerning the occurrence of streptococci, it will readily be seen that in general gastric acidity does not appear to be of much concern to them. Thus in the subject showing the lowest gastric acidity, namely, E.Zn. (the first of the psychotic patients)—in whom the highest average acidity is below 30—no streptococci were found. On the other hand, in the first two normal subjects, C.Te., and M.Mca., Streptococci viridans occurs in conjunction with high gastric acidity. Thus there is little to be said for the close association of streptococci with low gastric acidity, and still less for its importance as an etiologic factor in the psychoses, considering its cosmopolitan appearance in normal persons. The same may be said for B. coli, which occurred, not in the subject with the lowest acidity, but in the one showing the highest acidity. Incidentally, it may be mentioned that this subject was a healthy young nurse rather notorious for her good digestion. Finally, it must be stated that almost invariably the same organisms found in the stomach were isolated from the saliva and the test meal. The former supplied the members of the streptococcus and staphylococcus groups, and the toast accounted for the remaining yeasts and bacteria.

All the considerations, therefore, point to the conclusion that bacterial species found by the Rehfuss method occur independently of the acidity present, and that there is no correlation in psychotic patients between low acidity and a development of streptococci or B. coli. Consequently, under such conditions it cannot validly be asserted that the stomach (without lesions) is a focus of infection.

Turning now to a consideration of bacterial numbers, it has been stated that in only one half of the number of instances has there been found a correlation between high acidity and low bacterial numbers or vice versa. This, together with the observations on the bacterial species found in the saliva and test meal, indicated that the latter relatively external factors were of greater importance in determining the bacterial content of the stomach than was the gastric acidity. In this connection it may be mentioned that the only subject who showed an absence of bacteria in the stomach on repeated analysis was a patient with profound depression. Her mouth was exceedingly dry, and therefore the absence of saliva was regarded as the limiting factor.

A method was finally devised for conducting a fractional gastric analysis in such a manner as to isolate the saliva as a factor for special study. A dental suction tube attached to a running water pump was inserted in the patient's mouth throughout the analysis. This reduced the swallowing of saliva to a minimum. An attempt was made to have all conditions as aseptic as the circumstances would permit. In this way, counts made on the bacteria would be a true approximation of the numbers and kinds actually present in the stomach and could be satisfactorily compared with previous results obtained when saliva was present in greater amount.

In table 3, are presented the bacteriologic and chemical results obtained with a psychotic patient (diagnosed manic-depressive: manic). The first two main headings "Saliva Not Removed" are for the fractional gastric analyses carried out at two different times with the technic employed in previous work. Under the final heading "Saliva Removed" appear the data obtained with the modified technic described. In the first column of figures giving bacteria per c c, when saliva was not removed, we see that the fasting contents contained 15,500 bacteria per c c. During the process of digestion the numbers are considerably lower until 2¼ hours have elapsed, when there is a tremendous increase. This occurs despite the fact that the acidity in the stomach is generally sufficient to decimate a large proportion of the original number of bacteria ingested. Contrast the first two columns of bacterial numbers when saliva was not removed with the column of bacterial figures when saliva was removed. In the latter column, the first number is 2, and the last, which is the highest, is 32. The results speak for themselves. Such a striking reduction makes the conclusion irresistible: namely, that bacterial numbers in the stomach depend almost entirely on the saliva

TABLE 3

INFLUENCE OF SALIVA

M. Sl.	Saliva Not Removed			Saliva Not Removed			Saliva Removed		
	Bacteria per 1 C c	T A	PH	Bacteria per 1 C c	T A	PH	Bacteria per 1 C c	T A	PH
F. C.	15,500	5	2.8	.....	..	...	2	12	2.8
¼ hour	380	11	2.7	310	35	2.9	5	23	2.5
½ hour	78	41	2.2	5,100	37	3.0	8	52	1.7
¾ hour	5	46	1.8	925	41	2.8	2	70	1.4
1 hour	60	25	2.5	2,800	28	3.0	0	71	1.3
1¼ hours	800	18	2.7	110	36	2.2	1	42	1.5
1½ hours	215	25	2.3	95	43	1.9	1	29	1.7
1¾ hours	55	6	2.7	12	45	1.8	32	12	2.0
2 hours	110	28	2.7	5,400	10	3.7	*	2	3.0
2¼ hours	48,000	9	2.7	3,200	9	4.3	*		
2½ hours	46,000	10	2.7	6,800	16	3.5	*		

* Empty.

swallowed—when the bacterial content of the food may be disregarded. It would naturally be expected that the greatest multiplication of bacterial and maximum numbers would be attained in the "inter-digestive" phase, when the stomach is relatively at rest and the secretion of acid is at a minimum. Accordingly, therefore, the fasting contents should show the highest bacterial count. But such is not the case. As a matter of fact, the last fractions, whether saliva be removed or not, contain a far greater number of bacteria. Unquestionably the secretion of acid during the actual process of digestion together with the natural motility of the stomach would be expected to reduce the numbers of viable bacteria present at the beginning of the analysis. Contrary to this inference, the numbers are actually increased, and this is additional evidence that the continual swallowing of saliva (which contains millions of bacteria per c c) is in reality the factor which determines the bacterial content of the stomach. Again, the fact that the bacterial numbers when saliva was removed were so small as to be negligible is significant when it is noted that the secretion of acid is without much influence, i. e., only 2 bacteria appear when the total acidity is as low as 12 and as high as 70. All the facts mentioned indicate that the saliva is the most important single factor in influencing the bacterial content of the stomach under the conditions employed. Similar results were obtained when these tests were made on a healthy normal person and on other manic patients having very low gastric acidity. The most important consideration, however, is that these patients having a very low acidity would be precisely the type of subjects in whom bacteria might gain a foothold and make the stomach a focus of infection. Judging from the results when saliva is removed, this is far from being the case.

Therefore, Cotton's [1] contention that the stomach is a focus of infection finds no substantiation after a critical inspection of the fundamental facts. His conclusions are based on results obtained by the Rehfuss method, and therefore are open to the following objections: 1. Repeated analyses by the Rehfuss method on the same person yield different curves and little constancy in bacterial species. 2. No correlation can be established between low acidity and high bacterial numbers or species since it has been shown that acidity is not the limiting factor in determining the bacterial content of the stomach during a fractional analysis by the Rehfuss method. 3. Saliva is the most important factor in influencing the bacterial content of the stomach (without gastric lesions) although the bacterial content of the food ingested must be considered.

Should the objection be raised that the bacterial content of the stomach is an academic one, the burden of proof falls on him who asserts that it is possible to determine infection in the lining of the stomach wall. Removal of the stomach is the only positive method yet known of proving whether or not such infection exists. The advantage of obtaining the knowledge in such a manner could scarcely be considered worth while from the standpoint of treatment. Therefore, infection in the stomach (without lesions) has been diagnosed by Cotton from results obtained by the Rehfuss method. Two possibilities are open. The first is that the infection is secondary and has been brought by means of the blood stream and lymph channels; the second is that it results from the swallowing of infected material. In either event if the infection is "hidden" in the living stomach wall, the gastric contents on withdrawal will not show the bacteria in question. On the other hand, if the bacteria from the focus are being actively discharged into the stomach contents, if the infection has come by way of the blood or lymph stream, the number of bacteria found in the gastric contents should not be decreased by cutting off the flow of saliva. However, such is not the case, and it has been shown that the removal of saliva reduces the bacterial content. Consequently, it must be inferred that the bacteria in the gastric contents are introduced by the swallowing of saliva. It naturally follows, then, that there should be a multiplication of microorganisms when the stomach is at rest. However, it has been previously shown [2] that no such multiplication exists, even in stomachs having a low acidity.

It may be of interest in this connection to cite several cases of functional psychoses in which the patients showed approximately the same bacterial content, quantitatively as well as qualitatively, in the fasting contents and during analysis a considerable time after the primary foci were removed. Furthermore, the curves of acidity did not show any material improvement. The limitations imposed on any of the foregoing generalizations by virtue of the comparatively small number of persons under observation are fully realized, and only an intensive study of a great many cases can actually decide the points at issue. For the present the chain of evidence seems reasonably definite and points clearly to the conviction that the stomach (without lesions) cannot be considered a focus of infection on the basis of results obtained by the Rehfuss method of gastric analysis.

SUMMARY

The following results were obtained by the Rehfuss fractional method of gastric analysis carried out on normal and psychotic persons. Subject to limitations and to the material under observation it was found that:

The organisms most frequently found in the stomachs of normal and psychotic persons were members of the staphylococcus, streptococcus, lactobacillus and yeast groups.

During an analysis, approximately the same types and numbers of bacteria were found in the stomach irrespective of high or low acidity fluctuations. This indicates that the gastric acidity is not the most important factor limiting the bacterial content of the stomach during a fractional analysis.

Streptococci were found associated with high, as often as with low, gastric acidity; consequently there seems to be no reason to attach undue importance to their presence or therefore to consider the stomach a focus of infection.

A method was devised for studying the influence of saliva on the bacterial content of the stomach. A striking reduction in numbers of bacteria occurred when the swallowing of saliva was thus reduced, indicating that saliva was a factor of considerable importance. This was even observed in subjects having a low gastric acidity contrary to expectation, if the stomach was to be considered a focus of infection.

The removal of primary foci of infection has not caused any material change in the gastric acidity, types or numbers of bacteria found in the patients examined.

THE PRECIPITIN REACTION IN THE DETERMINATION OF THE INFECTIVITY OF GONORRHEAL DISCHARGES

MARGARET F. KELLEY

From the Department of Bacteriology, New York University and Bellevue Hospital Medical College *

After the subsidence of the acute symptoms of gonorrheal infection, a condition of chronic inflammation commonly results. This may persist over a long period of time. The demonstration of gonococci by either the culture or the smear method may be difficult or impossible. The complement-fixation test of the blood of treated or untreated patients may be negative. Such negative findings do not necessarily exclude continued infectiousness. There is need, therefore, of a method which could be easily carried out and which would be a better index as to the persistence of infectiousness than are the methods now available.

The work of Robinson and Meader,[1] who reported encouraging results with the application of the precipitin reaction to discharges of gonorrheal origin, seemed to offer a step in this direction. They state that extracts of discharges from gonorrheal inflammations give precipitin reactions with antigonococcus serum, even when examinations of smears of such discharges fail to reveal gonococci. We are indebted to them for an actual demonstration of their original methods which we used as follows:

Production of Immune or Precipitin Serum.—Rabbits whose serum diluted 1:2 did not give ring reactions with the control antigen (see below) were used for inoculation. They received intravenous injections of 1 c c of a suspension containing 500 million per c c of "live" gonococci for the first injection and increasingly larger doses 3 to 5 days apart; later, they were injected at weekly intervals to keep up the antibody content. Trial bleedings, tested against the specific control antigen (see below) showed that the animals varied in their ability to produce precipitins; about 10 injections were necessary before the immune serum could be used. The animals were bled whenever a new supply of serum was needed. Robinson and Meader used the Brady strains 1, 2 and 3 for immunization; we used the 10 Torrey strains.

Received for publication Feb. 18, 1922.

* This work was carried on under a grant from the United States Interdepartmental Social Hygiene Board.

[1] Jour. Urol., 1920, 4, p. 551.

We are indebted to Robinson and Meader for a sample of the immune serum which they were using. This gave us the means of determining that the serums we prepared were at least equally as potent as theirs as determined with our gonococcus antigens. With antigens prepared from the Torrey strains both their serum and ours always gave clearly visible reactions when diluted to 1 : 80. Dilutions to 1 : 160 gave faint reactions which appeared irregularly in successive tests.

Antigen for Control Tests.—The 48-hour growth of the gonococcus on North medium was scraped with a platinum loop into 5 c c of salt solution, autolyzed from 3 to 7 days, centrifugalized and the clear supernatant fluid used. The term antigen, unless otherwise specified, is used throughout to signify this specific gonococcus autolysate or precipitinogen.

We avoided the use of blood or serum mediums in the preparation of the gonococcus antigen in order first, to exclude a possible effect on the cultures; second, to avoid the possible transfer of serum or blood to the suspension to be used in the preparation of the antigen. Robinson and Meader used blood agar. The question of the possible influence of the medium on the antigen is noted later.

Material from the Cases to be Tested.—Secretion from the vagina or cervix was obtained on a cotton swab. This was rubbed in 2 c c of salt solution and the mixture incubated over night. In some instances, which are noted, we used salt solution containing 0.3% phenol (carbolic acid). The purpose of incubation was to autolyze the gonococci if they were present. On the following morning, the mixture was centrifugalized. This clear supernatant fluid might or might not contain gonococcus precipitinogen, as the term antigen or even extract is not really applicable, unless one may be justified in using this term for a reagent to be tested. Because of the difficulty of finding a suitable term, "discharge extract" is used throughout to signify the clarified test material. This term is also used for specimens not of gonorrheal origin.

The Reaction to Determine the Presence of Gonococcus Substance.—Two-tenths c c of the "discharge extract" was layered or floated over 0.2 c c of a 1 : 2 dilution of immune serum. A control of the "discharge extract" with a 1 : 2 dilution of normal rabbit serum was also made. The specific antigen as well as salt solution was employed with a 1 : 2 dilution of both immune and normal serums to serve as further controls.

All were placed in the water bath for one hour at 40 C. and then in the icebox for one hour. Observations were then made. The tests were returned to the refrigerator and observed again the following morning. The development of a contact ring of varying opacity and thickness at the line of contact between serum and superimposed clear fluid was recorded as a positive precipitin reaction.

In applying these methods we found that in some instances a ring reaction was not apparent until the tests had been kept in the icebox over night. In other instances, the ring observed after one hour's incubation and one hour in the refrigerator had disappeared when the test was again observed on the following morning. With few exceptions, the disappearance of the ring was accompanied by the development of a precipitate, the few exceptions being almost entirely with normal serum. In other instances a ring reaction was never observed,

TABLE 1

DISCHARGES, GONORRHEAL, SMEARS POSITIVE

Number of Specimens	Precipitin Reaction			
	Normal Serum		Immune Serum	
	Percentage Positive	Percentage Negative	Percentage Positive	Percentage Negative
92	21.7	78.3	82.6	17.4

The specimens from male cases (52) were extracted in salt solution containing 0.3% phenol. The proportion of nonspecific reactions with these and with normal serum was practically the same as with the specimens from females when no phenol was added.

but a precipitate was visible after holding the tests over night. For these reasons the later tests were observed only after refrigeration over night. All other factors excluded, there was another reason for this procedure: Only after this longer period was the percentage of positive reactions with the immune serum sufficiently high from the practical standpoint. Further discussion of this point is given later. The following tables include both ring and precipitate reaction readings as positive, although precipitate readings were not taken at the very beginning of our study.

The first step in our investigations was to apply the test to the discharges of male and female patients; 92 were tested. The smears from these discharges were all positive.

The results in this series of tests (table 1) were disappointing. In spite of the fact that all of the smears were positive and that the majority showed abundant gonococci, only 82.6% gave positive reactions with the specific serum; 17.4% gave negative reactions. With normal serum, 78.3% gave no reaction but 21.7% gave reactions. These reactions were unexpected and disconcerting. If the reactions obtained with normal serum (21.7%) were deducted from those obtained with immune serum (82.6%), the reactions presumably specific would be about 60%.

The results with the "smear negative" patients, the type in which a successful application of the method would be more important, are likewise disappointing. As seen in table 2, the positive results with the immune serum fall to 61%, and the positive reactions with the normal serum rise to 51%. This leaves us with only about 10% of positive reactions which might presumably be considered as specific in character.

Even the reactions which appear superficially to be specific in character and the percentage of which seems to correlate with the smear findings cannot be accepted as such without further analysis.

TABLE 2

DISCHARGES, CLINICALLY GONORRHEAL, SMEARS NEGATIVE

Number of Specimens	Precipitin Reaction			
	Normal Serum		Immune Serum	
	Percentage Positive	Percentage Negative	Percentage Positive	Percentage Negative
49	51	49	61	39

One observation shows this clearly, namely, that of several normal rabbit serums one or more may give a positive reaction, the others not. In other words, the results of the tests are dependent to a considerable extent on the sample of normal rabbit serum used as a control.

Evidently even if specific reactions are present, the results are obscured by a nonspecific factor. The following tests were made in the attempt to determine what this factor was and whether it could be eliminated: Vaginal secretions were obtained from supposedly nongonorrheal children; at the same time, nasal secretions were collected from the same children for further controls. Nasopharyngeal secretions from adults were also obtained. A miscellaneous group of specimens was also tested; one pleuritic fluid; 6 sputums; 6 samples of pus, 2 each from tuberculous, streptococcal and staphylococcal abscesses. Other specimens not of human origin were also included; they were the washings from the peritoneum of one normal and 5 inoculated mice.

The results with these specimens of nongonorrheal origin are contrasted in table 3 with the total number of specimens obtained from presumably gonorrheal sources. The striking point in this table is the high percentage of positive reactions with nongonorrheal material. These reactions occurred with both the normal and the immune serum. If the former are deducted from the latter, it gives the untenable conclusion that from 5 to 20% of these specimens were gonorrheal. This shows at once that the subtraction method is not justified as a criterion of the significance of the reactions. The nonspecific reactions obtained with nongonorrheal material indicate that the method as employed did not yield reliable results.

TABLE 3

COMPARISON OF REACTIONS WITH MATERIAL FROM GONORRHEAL AND NONGONORRHEAL SOURCES

Extracts of Secretions	Number of Specimens	Precipitin Reaction			
		Normal Serum		Immune Serum	
		Percentage Positive	Percentage Negative	Percentage Positive	Percentage Negative
Suspected gonorrheal..........	174*	24.3	75.7	69.2	30.8
Nongonorrheal vaginal.........	17	94.1	5.9	100.0	0
Nose and throat................	21	66.7	33.3	81.0	19.0
Miscellaneous..................	19	73.7	26.3	94.7	5.3

* Includes cases on which no smear examinations were made.

The nonspecific reactions with material of other than gonorrheal origin were shown to Robinson and Meader. They had not observed such a percentage of nonspecific reactions and suggested that this factor might be eliminated by greater dilution of the serum or the extract, or of both.

The results of tests made with a higher dilution (1:4) of serum and diluted "discharge extracts" are given in table 4. Although the tests with specimens from gonorrhea are at first glance favorable, the results with the other specimens indicate how little reliance can be placed on the dilution method. The results with the two nasal specimens are especially noteworthy.

In all the preceding work no attempt was made to have the mixture of secretion and of salt solution uniform in turbidity prior to centrifuging. The question arose whether the contradictory results obtained might not be influenced by this factor of irregularity. A turbidity control was prepared which consisted of a suspension of gonococci containing 2,000 million organisms per c c. The control gonococcus antigen originally of the same turbidity reacted in a dilution of 1 : 5 with a 1 : 5 and with a 1 : 10 dilution of the immune serum, not in higher serum dilutions. The standardized specimens were tested, therefore, in these dilutions, as it was unbelievable that the gonorrheal specimens could contain more gonorrheal substance than was contained in the suspension from which the gonococcus antigen was made. Two immune serums and 2 normal serums were used.

TABLE 4

REACTIONS WITH NORMAL AND IMMUNE SERUM DILUTED 1: 4 AND GONORRHEAL AND NON-GONORRHEAL MATERIAL

Specimen from	Normal Serum		Immune Serum	
	Extract Dilution	Result*	Extract Dilution	Result*
Nose	1-8	+	1-8	+
Nose	1-2	—	1-8	+
Vagina, nongonorrheal child	1-64	+	1-16	—
Cervix, gonorrheal smear positive	1-8	+	1-32	+
Cervix, gonorrheal smear positive	1-8	+	1-32	+
Cervix, gonorrheal smear negative	1-8	+	1-32	+
Cervix, gonorrheal smear negative	1-8	+	1-32	+

* Highest dilution of extract in which a positive result was obtained or lowest dilution in which a negative result was obtained is recorded.

Symbols used in this and the following tables: ++ = marked reaction; + = moderate reaction; ± = slight reaction; ± = very slight reaction; — = no reaction.

TABLE 5

REACTIONS WITH EXTRACTS STANDARDIZED BY TURBIDITY*

Specimens from	Normal Serum		Immune Serum	
	Rabbit a	Rabbit b	Rabbit c	Rabbit d
Tuberculous abscess, pus	+	+	+	+
Tuberculous abscess, pus	+	—	+	—
Urethra, male, gonorrhea†	—	—	(1:5)+	—
Urethra, male, gonorrhea‡	—	—	+	+
Cervix, chronic, gonorrhea†	—	—	+	+
Cervix, chronic, gonorrhea‡	—	—	+	+
Cervix, chronic, gonorrhea‡	—	—	—	—
Cervix, chronic, gonorrhea‡	+	+	+	+
Cervix, subacute, gonorrhea‡	+	+	+	+
Vaginal, normal‡	+	+	+	+

* Results refer to a dilution of serum of 1 : 10, except where otherwise noted, and a dilution of extract of 1 : 5.

† Smear positive.

‡ Smear negative.

The comparison between the results obtained with the gonorrheal cases showing negative smears and those showing positive smears, and of both these types of gonorrheal cases with the nongonorrheal cases, demonstrated that the standardization by opacity was of no value in excluding the nonspecific factor.

The next point studied was whether the nonspecific reaction was due to bacterial substance other than that of the gonococcus.

Suspensions of various bacteria were made in distilled water and the number of bacteria in the suspensions estimated by comparison of the turbidity of each with counted vaccines of the same bacterium. After a few drops of chloroform had been added to prevent multiplication of bacteria, these suspensions were placed in the incubator for 48 hours to autolyze. A concentrated salt phenol solution was then added to bring the salt content to 0.9%, and the phenol content to 0.3%. The equivalent content per c c after this dilution is given in table 6. The suspensions were then centrifuged and the clear supernatant fluid used for test. The results with 3 normal and 2 immune (gonococcus) serums are also shown in table 6.

TABLE 6

REACTIONS WITH GONOCOCCUS AND OTHER BACTERIAL ANTIGENS

Bacterial Antigens	Immune Serum								Normal Serum											
	Rabbit 344				Rabbit 354				Rabbit 321				Rabbit 369				Rabbit 371			
	1:5		1:10		1:5		1:10		1:5		1:10		1:5		1:10		1:5		1:10	
	R*	P†	R	P	R	P	R	P	R	P	R	P	R	P	R	P	R	P	R	P
Torrey, 2,000 million	—	+	—	++	—	++	+	++	—	—	—	—	—	—	—	—	—	±	—	±
Brady, 2,000 million	—	+	—	±	—	±	—	+	—	—	—	—	—	—	—	—	—	±	—	±
Staphylococcus, 2,000 million	—	±	+	—	—	±	—	+	—	+	+	±	—	±	+	±	—	±	—	±
Streptococcus, 300 million	—	±	—	±	—	—	—	±	—	—	—	—	—	±	—	±	—	—	—	—
Pertussis,‡ 1,000 million	—	±	—	±	—	±	—	±	—	—	—	—	—	±	+	—	—	—	—	±
Pneumococcus, 100 million	—	±	—	+	—	—	±	—	—	—	—	—	—	—	—	—	—	±	—	±
Colon, 500 million	—	—	—	±	—	—	—	±	—	±	—	±	—	—	—	—	—	—	±	—
Catarrhalis,‡ 2,000 million	—	—	—	±	—	—	—	±	—	—	—	±	—	—	—	—	—	±	—	±
0.9% salt solution with 0.3% phenol	—	—	—	—	—	—	—	—	—	—	—	—	—	—	—	—	—	—	—	—

* Ring.

† Precipitate.

‡ Grown on "chocolate" agar. Formula: Glycerol veal agar, neutral to phenolsulphonephthalein before autoclaving. About 5% normal citrated horse blood added while veal agar is about 85 C.

A considerable number of nonspecific reactions were obtained. They were relatively more frequent with the two immune serums. The reactions obtained with normal serums varied considerably. The staphylococcus gave the greatest number of nonspecific reactions. The amount of reaction obtained with the different antigens is recorded in this table in quantitative terms. The degree of reaction obtained with the heterologous antigens is approximately equal to that obtained in the majority of tests with "discharge extracts." The lack of difference between the reactions obtained with the gonococcus serum with the gonococcus antigens and the reactions with the heterologous antigens is probably due to the fact that the time element was not considered. These tests were made not to determine the optimum conditions under which specific differences could be elicited with bacterial antigens but to determine to what degree nonspecific reactions would develop with the method as adopted for testing the "discharge extracts."

As noted, practical considerations led us to adopt the method of observing reactions only after the tests had been refrigerated over night. The results with the bacterial antigens would seem to indicate that the nonspecific factor was exaggerated by this method.

The overnight method was continued, however, because although the total number of reactions between normal serum and gonorrheal material or between immune serum and nongonorrheal material was increased, this increase was accompanied by a proportionate increase (doubled) in the positive results with the immune serums, and gonorrheal extracts. It seemed, therefore, better to use the method which would give the highest level of positive reactions between immune serum and gonorrheal material and then try to find a means of eliminating the nonspecific factor.

In connection with the results obtained with bacterial antigens it is of interest that extracts of the Brady strains, of relatively recent isolation, were somewhat less sensitive to precipitin action than were the Torrey strains which had been in cultivation for a long time. This naturally raised the question whether the gonococci obtained directly from man might not yield an autolysate which would be still more resistant to precipitin action. Possibly this might be a factor in the failure to obtain with a vaginal discharge, containing numerous gonococci, a reaction which in rapidity and quantity was decidedly greater than with nonspecific material.

The question then arose whether the nonspecific factor might not be limited by heating the extracts. That the reaction between precipitin and its specific precipitinogen (bacterial) is not influenced by heating the precipitinogen is generally accepted. We found no difference in precipitability with the gonococcic antigen whether heated or not heated, when tested with serum dilutions up to the point of extinction of reaction.

Heating of the heterologous bacterial antigens did not reduce appreciably the degree of nonspecific reactions (table 7).

The results obtained with heated and unheated "discharge extracts" are given in table 8. Included in this is the use of both distilled water and salt solution as extractives. Where the former was used the extracts were made isotonic before use by addition of an appropriate amount of concentrated salt solution. The suspensions were all of a uniform capacity before subsequent treatment.

As seen from table 8, there was no constancy in the results before and after heating the extracts, whether the original material showed gonococci in smears or not.

TABLE 7

EFFECT OF HEAT ON REACTIONS WITH BACTERIAL ANTIGENS

Bacterial Antigens	Immune Serum								Normal Serum			
	Rabbit 344				Rabbit 354				Rabbit 316			
	1:5		1:10		1:5		1:10		1:5		1:10	
	N*	H†	N	H	N	H	N	H	N	H	N	H
Torrey, 2,000 million	++	++	+	+	++	++	+	+	—	—	—	—
Brady, 2,000 million	+	+	+	0	+	+	+	0	—	—	—	0
Streptococcus, 300 million	—	—	$\underline{\pm}$	$\underline{\pm}$	—	—	$\underline{\pm}$	$\underline{\pm}$	—	—	$\underline{\pm}$	—
Pertussis, 1,000 million	±	±	—	—	—	—	±	±	—	—	$\underline{\pm}$	—
Colon, 500 million	±	±	$\underline{\pm}$	$\underline{\pm}$	—	—	±	±	—	—	—	—
Pneumococcus, 100 million	—	—	$\underline{\pm}$	$\underline{\pm}$	—	—	$\underline{\pm}$	$\underline{\pm}$	—	—	—	—
Catarrhalis, 2,000 million	±	±	—	—	—	—	—	—	—	—	—	—
0.9% salt solution with 0.3% phenol	—	—	—	—	—	—	—	—	—	—	—	—

* Not heated. † Heated to 100 C. for 10 minutes. 0, No test, insufficient material.

Three factors—dilution of the extract, dilution of the serum and heating of the extract—were of no aid in excluding the nonspecific factor.

The persistence of reactions after the bacterial antigens or the "discharge extracts" had been heated to 100 C. for 10 minutes, seemingly answers the possible criticism that a precipitate due to bacterial growth during the time of extraction and test, might have simulated positive reactions, especially those which were obviously nonspecific.

Naturally, if the reactions were due to bacterial growth a reaction should always appear with both the immune and with the normal serum when both of the salt serum controls showed no evident reaction, thus demonstrating the absence of bacterial growth originating from the serums. It is difficult to understand how a ring reaction, developing after one hour's incubation, or how a later ring reaction or sediment after 24 hours could be due to bacterial growth when the remaining fluid was nearly always clear. The appearance of reactions with extracts of pus aspirated from unopened cold abscesses is significant. It should also be noted (table 1) that "discharge extracts," containing 0.3% phenol, gave reactions.

TABLE 8

EFFECT OF HEAT ON REACTIONS WITH "DISCHARGE EXTRACTS"

Specimens from	Smear	Extracted With	Extract Diluted	Serum Diluted	Normal Serum Plus Extract		Immune Serum Plus Extract	
					Extract Not Heated	Extract Heated to 100 C. for 10 Min.	Extract Not Heated	Extract Heated to 100 C. for 10 Min.
Cervix, gonorrhea	..	Salt solution	—	1:5	+	—	+	±
		Distilled water	—	1:10	—	±	—	±
Cervix, gonorrhea	—	Salt solution	—	1:5	±	+	±	+
		Distilled water	—	1:10	—	+	—	+
Urethra, male, gonorrhea	—	Salt solution	—	1:5	±	±	±	—
		Distilled water	—	1:10	—	—	—	+
Urethra, male, gonorrhea	..	Salt solution	—	1:5	±	—	—	—
		Distilled water	—	1:10	—	—	±	±
Vagina, nongonorrheal	—	Salt solution	—	1:5	—	—	±	—
		Distilled water	—	1:10	—	—	—	—
Cervix, gonorrhea	..	Distilled water	1:5	1:5	±	—	—	±
		Distilled water	1:5	1:10	—	—	±	—
Cervix, gonorrhea	—	Distilled water	1:5	1:5	—	—	+	—
		Distilled water	1:5	1:10	—	+	±	—
Cervix, gonorrhea	—	Distilled water	1:5	1:5	+	—	+	—
		Distilled water	1:5	1:10	+	—	±	—
Urethra, male, gonorrhea	..	Distilled water	1:5	1:5	—	±	—	±
		Distilled water	1:5	1:10	—	—	—	—
Urethra, male, gonorrhea	—	Distilled water	1:5	1:5	—	±	—	±
		Distilled water	1:5	1:10	—	±	±	±
Vagina, nongonorrheal	—	Distilled water	1:5	1:5	+	—	+	—
		Distilled water	1:5	1:10	+	—	+	—

Distilled water extracts made isotonic with salt before use.

For the direct demonstration that bacterial growth was not a factor in the reactions and especially in the reactions with nonspecific material, extracts clarified by prolonged centrifuging were tested with immune and with normal serum and then tested culturally. The materials extracted were obtained from tuberculous abscess, 3 specimens; urethral discharge (male), 4 specimens; and nasal discharge, 2 specimens.

The reactions with the immune and with the normal serums were the same as those previously obtained with similar material. After the tests were completed the contents of each tube were added to melted serum agar and the mixture poured into a petri dish. The majority of the tests yielded no growth. Some showed the development of from 1 to 5 colonies, obviously an insufficient bacterial content to simulate a reaction.

Robinson and Meader have recently attempted to eliminate the nonspecific factor by absorbing gonococcus immune serum with a mixed antigen of Sarcina lutea and Staphylococcus aureus. They have found that these two organisms gave nonspecific reactions.

We have absorbed three samples of our gonococcus immune serum with suspensions of gonococci, meningococci and staphylococci, respectively. When the antigonococcus serum was absorbed by the heterologous types, the precipitin content for the gonococcus was reduced either very slightly or not at all, whereas the precipitin content for the absorbing type was completely or nearly completely removed. When the serum was absorbed by the gonococcus to the point where the precipitins for this organism were removed, the degree of reaction with antigens of the staphylococcus and of the meningococcus was reduced either very slightly—or not at all. This indicates that the reactions obtained with these antigens had no relation to the specific immunization by the gonococcus.

The absorbed serums were also tested with extracts of material from (1) urethra, gonorrheal, smear positive, male; (2) cervix, gonorrheal, smear positive; (3) cervix, gonorrheal, smear negative; (4) vagina, nongonorrheal; (5) tuberculous abscess.

With only one of the extracts, and that from a gonorrheal case (3), did the absorption of the gonococcus immune serum by the staphylococcus or by the meningococcus, result in a diminution of the reaction. As stated, the serums thus absorbed no longer reacted with the staphylococcus or the meningococcus antigen, or at most reacted only slightly.

With the immune serum absorbed by the gonococcus, only one specimen, that from case 3, failed to give a reaction. The extracts from the other two gonorrheal cases still gave undiminished reactions. We have, therefore, the striking result that a gonococcus serum absorbed to the point where it no longer reacts with a specific gonococcus antigen still reacts with the "discharge extracts" from two gonorrheal cases showing positive smears.

These results indicate that some reacting substance in the extracts, other than of bacterial origin, is most frequently responsible for the nonspecific reactions.

Some observations on the reactions obtained with antigens prepared in different ways are suggestive in this connection. Robinson and Meader prepared their antigens by growing the gonococcus on blood agar. They obtained reactions with immune serums in extraordinary high dilutions. On the other hand, with gonococcus antigens prepared from North medium cultures, we obtained reactions with our immune serums and even with their immune serum in dilutions of only 1:80 or slightly higher. These observations indicated that the blood in the medium might influence the results. We prepared two antigens, therefore, with the same medium, using rabbit blood in one case and not in the other. With the medium containing no blood, the resultant antigens reacted slightly with one [2] immune serum as high as 1:100, with 3 others diluted 1:50. With the medium containing blood, the resultant antigens reacted when these 4 serums were diluted 1:500 to 1:1,000 and with 2 of these serums even in dilutions of 1:2,000. One of these rabbits was immunized with vaccine grown on blood medium, the other with vaccine grown on medium without blood. Diluted normal rabbit serum likewise gave a reaction when added instead of the gonococcus antigens to the gonococcus immune serums used in the foregoing tests. Normal rabbit serum diluted 1:10 gave a reaction with one immune serum obtained from Robinson and Meader diluted 1:250.

These observations indicated that the addition of blood to the medium might be a factor in the reaction. The importance of this factor varied apparently with the serums of the individual immune rabbits.

Because of the variation noted with the gonococcus antigens, the experiment was repeated with the serums from 4 rabbits immunized with a vaccine grown on blood-free medium and from one rabbit immunized with vaccine grown on blood mediums. The results with the serums from all 5 rabbits have shown an average lower reaction (1:40) with blood-medium grown antigens as compared with the reaction (1:60) with antigens grown on blood-free medium, these results differing very much from those obtained in the experiment outlined in the foregoing.

As has been previously noted, the serums from normal rabbits vary considerably as regards reactions with bacterial antigens, including gonococcal, or with "discharge extracts." The two series of experi-

[2] Sample of serum used by Robinson and Meader in most of their tests.

ments with animals immunized by the injection of gonococci show, a still more marked variation. The fact that certain rabbits after immunization give materially higher reactions with blood grown antigens than with antigens prepared with blood-free mediums indicates that the nonspecific reactions obtained with "discharge extracts" are due to some substance present in the extracts which give such reactions.

The fact that the sample of serum received from Robinson and Meader, which they employed for most of their tests, gave very high reactions with the blood-grown antigen seems significant in view of their high incidence of positive results with "discharge extracts."

The heating of blood-grown antigens reduced the reactivity of these antigens slightly, if at all. This was true even when the blood-grown antigen reacted with the immune serum in dilutions as high as 1 : 1,000.

SUMMARY

Although reactions are obtained when extracts of discharges from gonorrheal patients are added to the serum of a rabbit immunized with gonococci, similar reactions are frequently encountered with the serums of normal rabbits. Likewise, extracts of material from the genital organs, known not to be infected with the gonococcus, as well as extracts of exudates due to infection by other organisms, give reactions with both antigonococcus serum and normal serum.

Attempts to exclude the nonspecific factor and thus obtain a specific reaction have failed. Dilution of serum of extract or of both, has not served to differentiate between a specific and a nonspecific reaction. Likewise, absorption of the antigonococcus serum by heterologous bacteria has failed to eliminate the nonspecific factor.

This nonspecific factor has obscured any reaction which might have occurred between the gonococcus serum and any gonococcus precipitinogen which might have been present in the known gonorrheal specimen.

Comparison between the probable amount of gonococcus substance present in the specimens as indicated by smear examination with the number of organisms necessary in a suspension to give a satisfactory precipitating antigen, raises a strong presumption that a specific precipitate development infrequently if at all.

When the gonococcus precipitins were absorbed from the serum, there was no uniform diminution in the reaction obtained with extracts from gonorrheal cases.

The precipitin reaction as recommended by Robinson and Meader is not applicable for the determination of the presence of the gonococcus in discharges from the cervix, urethra, etc.

AN AMEBA-LIKE ORGANISM IN THE KIDNEYS OF A CHILD

WITH 2 PLATES

Leila Jackson

From the John McCormick Institute for Infectious Diseases, Chicago

The discovery of a protozoon invasion of the kidneys of a child who died suddenly in a convulsion while seemingly not in a serious condition seems worthy of description.

A colored boy, 15 months old, entered the Durand Hospital on the evening of Sept. 1, 1921. He had a history of fever with swelling of the gums about the lower bicuspid teeth and accompanied by a convulsion on August 25, which lasted 15 minutes. He had never had a convulsion previous to this time. He seemed better for the next day, but on September 1 was worse again, and a physician was called who said something was wrong with the tonsils. The temperature was normal on admittance, and he did not appear especially sick but was drowsy. A throat culture was taken which later was reported positive for diphtheria bacilli. The following day was uneventful, the patient receiving the usual treatment for diphtheria. At 11 o'clock that evening he was sleeping well, and the pulse was reported good, but 20 minutes later he wakened while the temperature was being taken, began to cry, had a convulsion and died within a few minutes. No urinalysis had been made as a specimen of urine had not been obtained.

Anatomic diagnosis (Dr. Mulsow): Bronchopneumonia; enlarged mesentric lymphnodes; congestion and fatty changes of the liver; parenchymatous nephritis; edema of the glottis; accessory spleen.

Cultures of the heart blood and pericardical fluid on blood-agar plates and Loeffler's blood serum were sterile; cultures from the lung on the same mediums grew hemolytic streptococci.

The chief changes found in microscopic sections of the tissues are a mild edema of the lungs, small regions of focal necrosis in the spleen and some of the lymph nodes, and a parenchymatous nephritis. Whether the lesions in the spleen and lymph glands bear any relation to those in the kidney I am unable to state. They seemed to have an entirely different character, resembling the necroses found in diphtheria, and no forms resembling those found in the kidneys are seen. The changes in the kidneys are limited almost entirely to the epithelium of the

Received for publication Feb. 13, 1922.

tubules, being most marked in the tubules of the cortex. Only occasionally organismal forms are found in the glomeruli, but there are no observable alterations in them. In some of the secreting tubules the epithelial cells are almost totally destroyed or displaced by the round eosin-stained bodies (hematoxylin and eosin preparations) which first arrested attention. As in the case of a parasitic invasion of the salivary glands,[1] the tissue reaction is mild. There is little infiltration with leukocytes; a moderate number of plasma cells are present in places; the cells of the tubules seem to be partially or completely absorbed rather than destroyed by the action of the organism, and for this reason a casual glance at the section does not reveal the real extent of the damage.

In a well differentiated hematoxylin and eosin preparation the cytoplasm of the organism stains a deeper pink and is more granular than that of the kidney cells, and they are easily distinguished even with a rather low power lens. Stained with polychrome methylene blue without eosin the parasite stains a light robin's egg blue which readily distinguishes it from the deeper purplish blue of the kidney cells. With the Giemsa stain the organism takes a salmon pink color quite different from the bluish pink of the kidney cells and the distinctly yellowish red blood cells.

The forms assumed by the parasite are varied. Certain forms which have been interpreted as representing the schizogonic or vegetative form of the parasite are present chiefly in the outer portion of the cortex. The cells of some of the convuluted tubules are entirely displaced by small, round rather homogeneous bodies, 2-6 mikrons in diameter, nothing remaining except the cell walls (Fig. 30). Different stages in the development of the bodies are present in a tubule or even in a single cell. There are the small round bodies just mentioned, which are of fairly uniform size in the same group but differ considerably in size in the various groups or cells and are apparently simply confined by the epithelial cell membrane, while in other cells there are one or more bodies varying in size 10-18 mikrons in diameter, which contain small round bodies similar to those found free in the cells but in various stages of development. Frequently the large bodies appear to be without nuclei but nuclear fragments are frequent or a dimly outlined nucleus seeming to indicate that a nucleus is probably always present but is to a greater or less extent used up in the development of the small bodies. When the development of the large body or

[1] München. med. Wchnschr., 1904, 43, p. 1905.

schizont is complete, the limiting membrane disappears, and the small bodies become free in the kidney cell where they continue their growth. There is a considerable variation in the depth of stain taken by these bodies, some of them staining decidedly purplish while the majority are pink. With some stains they appear quite homogeneous but with others they are granular, especially about the periphery; even with the same stain there may be some difference in this respect. As before intimated, these smaller forms are regarded as merozoites since it seems that through their development a continuous reinfection of the host is brought about.

Another form which is quite numerous and more widely distributed than the former is a nucleated body which may be round, oval or quite irregular in shape, with a coarsely granular cytoplasm and a relatively small, deeply stained nucleus either eccentrically or centrally placed. These forms vary from 2 to 15 or 18 mikrons in diameter. The small nucleated forms are not very numerous (Figs. 1 and 2). Some have proportionately large nuclei with little cytoplasm while others have small deeply stained nuclei and much cytoplasm with few granules. These are usually found imbedded in the epithelial cells of the tubules but may be free in the lumen or in the tissues outside the tubules. From these forms there are all gradatious in size to bodies 15-20 mikrons in diameter, those about 12-15 in diameter being most numerous. These larger forms are also present both in the epithelial cells and in the lumen of the tubule and quite as often in the latter as in the former. They are sometimes found partly inside and partly outside of the epithelium and sometimes the main part of the parasite is still outside the epithelium while a finger-like process is apparently forcing its way into the cell. Such appearances seem to warrant the assumption that the organism possessed a certain amount of ameboid motion. Besides the difference in size there is considerable variation in appearance. They are often quite irregular in shape often with quite definite processes or pseudopods and frequently contain one or several round, definitely outlined bodies which in appearance and staining reaction resemble the merozoites described, but they are not present in such large numbers. Occasionally there appears to be one or more vacuoles, and in some of the larger forms there is present in the cytoplasm a circular, more lightly pink stained, granular, nonnucleacted body surrounded by a wide unstained halo.

The nucleus apparently undergoes many changes. Sometimes a small round mass of chromatin is seen budding off from the nucleus, and occasionally this small portion of nuclear material may be seen entirely outside the mother cell but still attached to the nucleus by a thin strand of nuclear material. Rarely one sees a nucleus with 3 or 4 processes budding off and in various stages of separation (Fig. 8). There is generally a massing of the chromatin at various points in a nucleus concerned in this process. Little cytoplasm seems to be carried away with the buds. The small nucleated bodies so produced may be one source of the small nucleated bodies I have mentioned. There is also the somewhat larger nucleus usually with chromatin massed at the periphery which is seen in various stages of simple division (Figs. 5, 6 and 7). In some cases the nucleus is simply elongated and becoming slightly constricted at the middle portion without change in the contour of the cell; in others the cytoplasm is also being constricted, and in the final stage the two nucleated portions are seen connected by a thin threadlike strand of chromatin surrounded by a narrow margin of cytoplasm, making it apparent that the bodies reproduce by simple division.

Besides the nuclei just mentioned, there are those with no other apparent change than a rather symmetrical massing of the chromatin about the margin of the nucleus. There are often 4 masses of about equal size; sometimes there is also a central mass connected by narrow chromatin bands with the peripheral masses giving the appearance of a Greek cross; or the nucleus may be oval with a larger mass at either end and two smaller ones between them on either side; or there may be 8 masses of nearly equal size with a more or less symmetrical arrangement. One not infrequently sees two nuclei of this type apparently within the same body or two bodies of similar appearance lying in contact within a cystlike cavity in a kidney cell.

Nuclei apparently in the various stages of mitosis are numerous. They stain deeply and are quite irregular in shape. Among these are nuclei showing a more or less perfect spindle formation. There is elongation of the nucleus with heavily staining polar caps, the intervening portion staining more lightly and seemingly arranged in strands connecting the deeper stained terminal portions. In a number of instances organisms have been seen in the same stage of division described and illustrated by Janicki as occurring in Paramoeba chaetogathi [2] (Fig. 10).

Microgametes have not been identified in these sections beyond a reasonable doubt. Forms have been seen which resemble somewhat

[2] Handbuch der path. Mikroorganismen, 1913, 7, p. 59.

microgametocytes, but in no case have forms been seen with a structure sufficiently definite to be convincing. It seems, therefore, that we are concerned here with reproduction by antogamy rather than by anisogamy.

Encysted forms are fairly numerous (figs. 17-24). An apparently early form consists of a large granular body which contains a lightly stained but clearly outlined eccentrically placed cystlike body. It is separated from the rest of the body by a thick wall inside of which is a clear unstained space, and occupying the central part is an irregularly shaped not very deeply stained mass. The cytoplasm of these cells usually contain none of the small round bodies. Other medium sized forms 8-10 mikrons in diameter contain a lightly stained, round or oval cystlike body within which are 2 to 8 or 12 small round deeply stained bodies usually surrounded by a halo, which vary somewhat in size. The apparently fully developed cyst is oval and contains about 12 of the small bodies and is sometimes seen, freed from the granular portion, in the lumen of the tubule. Occasionally one sees these small bodies apparently freed from the cyst and surrounded by granular material, probably the remnants of the mother cell. If they become free in the kidney, as it seems likely they do, they may easily be one source of the small nucleated bodies before mentioned which have been looked on as gametes.

In some of the large nucleated forms there is a fragmentation of the nucleus and a scattering of the nuclear material of the merozoits, although in some of the bodies which apparently give rise to merozoits no trace of a nucleus is found.

It is interesting to speculate as to the part played by the kidney infection in the fatal issue in this case. Both from the clinical and pathologic points of view the diphtheritic infection does not seem to have been of sufficient severity to cause the sudden death, whereas the parenchymatous nephritis was marked enough to be observable in the gross specimen, and histologically the changes in the epithelium of many of the secreting tubules are striking, seemingly making symptoms inevitable. However, in view of our scanty knowledge of infection of this kind, it would be unwise to draw any definite conclusion.

Three reports of the presence of somewhat similar protozoon-like bodies in the kidneys have been found in the literature. In 1904, Jesionek and Kiolemenoglou [1] report finding large protozoon-like cells in the kidneys, liver and lungs of an 8 months syphilitic fetus. These cells were 20-30 mikrons in diameter with large nuclei and granular cytoplasm. In the kidneys they usually occurred in groups and sometimes in tubular formation with surrounding connecting tissue forming a kind of capsule. These cells showed no genetic relationship to the body cells and are therefore not to be regarded as modifications of them. R. Hertwig also examined the specimens and expressed the opinion that these bodies were protozoa probably to be classified among gregarines.

Later in the same year, encouraged by this report, Ribbert [3] reports 3 cases in which similar bodies were found. In 2 cases these were in the parotid glands of 2 young children neither of whom were syphilitic, and in the third case in the lumen of the tubules in the kidneys of a new-born syphilitic child. The tubules containing these cells were dilated and the epithelium considerably changed. The bodies were not seen outside the tubules in the connective tissue or in the glomeruli or collecting tubules. They had large homogeneous nuclei with nucleoli and between the nucleus and protoplasm was a clear zone as though the nuclear material had contracted and separated itself from the nuclear membrane. The author thinks that the location of the bodies in the lumen of the tubules speaks against their being body cells and that their presence in injured tubules suggests some connection with the injury. He cites Ehlers and Rhumbler as not venturing to decide what the bodies were, being of the opinion that their morphology spoke neither for nor against their being protozoa and suggesting that they might belong among ameba or sporozoa on account of the character of the nucleus and their location.

Smith and Weidman [4] found peculiar cells in the kidneys, liver and lungs of an apparently full term dead fetus in which there was no maceration and the tissues were in a good state of preservation. The mother's history was negative both prior to and after the birth of the fetus. In the kidneys there were minute foci of leukocytes in the interpyramidal cortex, chiefly of mononuclear cells with a few polymorphonuclears. Large prominently nucleated cells occurred in dilated tubules within these foci. These cells were coarsely granular, round or oblong, pyriform or irregular in shape and about 38x25 mikrons in their diameters and possessed short thick pseudopods. The nuclei were relatively large, ⅓-½ the diameter of the cell and without evidence of nuclear division. Some forms were apparently without nuclei and encysted forms were present. The authors believed the parasite was an ameba but did not classify it among known forms, and the name Entamoeba mortinatalium was suggested.

[3] Centralbl. f. allgem. Path., 1904, 15, p. 45.
[4] Univ. Penn. Med. Bull., 1910-11, 23, p. 285.

The bodies found in these cases, while agreeing in some respects with the ones described by me, are somewhat larger, vary less in size, and present much fewer variations in form. It seems probable, however, that in all of these cases we are dealing with organisms of similar nature. In a careful examination of the literature on protozoa in the kidneys, in an effort to classify the organism, I have been impressed with its resemblance to ameba. Many of the forms observed make it evident that they move about by means of pseudopods and exhibit a great variety of form. Multiplication of the organism is brought about by simple division, schizogony and sporulation. Certain appearances also suggest that the parasite reproduces by autogamy. All of which points to at least a close relationship with ameba. A point of interest in these cases would seem to be that we are dealing with a condition which may have been frequently overlooked. The character of the organism is such that at a casual glance one might easily mistake them for body cells, especially if there has not been careful differential staining, as the leukocytic reaction is not very marked, as some of the nuclei resemble those of plasma cells and as the process is more one of absorption and replacement of the epithelium than necrosis of it.

SUMMARY

An ameba-like organism, the apparent cause of an acute parenchymatous nephritis, was found in the kidneys of a child, 15 months old, who died suddenly in a convulsion. Neither the gross nor histologic examination of the tissues revealed any other apparently sufficient cause of death.

Three reports are found in the literature of the occurrence of somewhat similar organisms in the kidneys, twice in syphilitic fetuses and once in a stillborn, nonsyphilitic child.

The character of the organism and the nature of the reaction in the tissues are such that the condition might easily be overlooked.

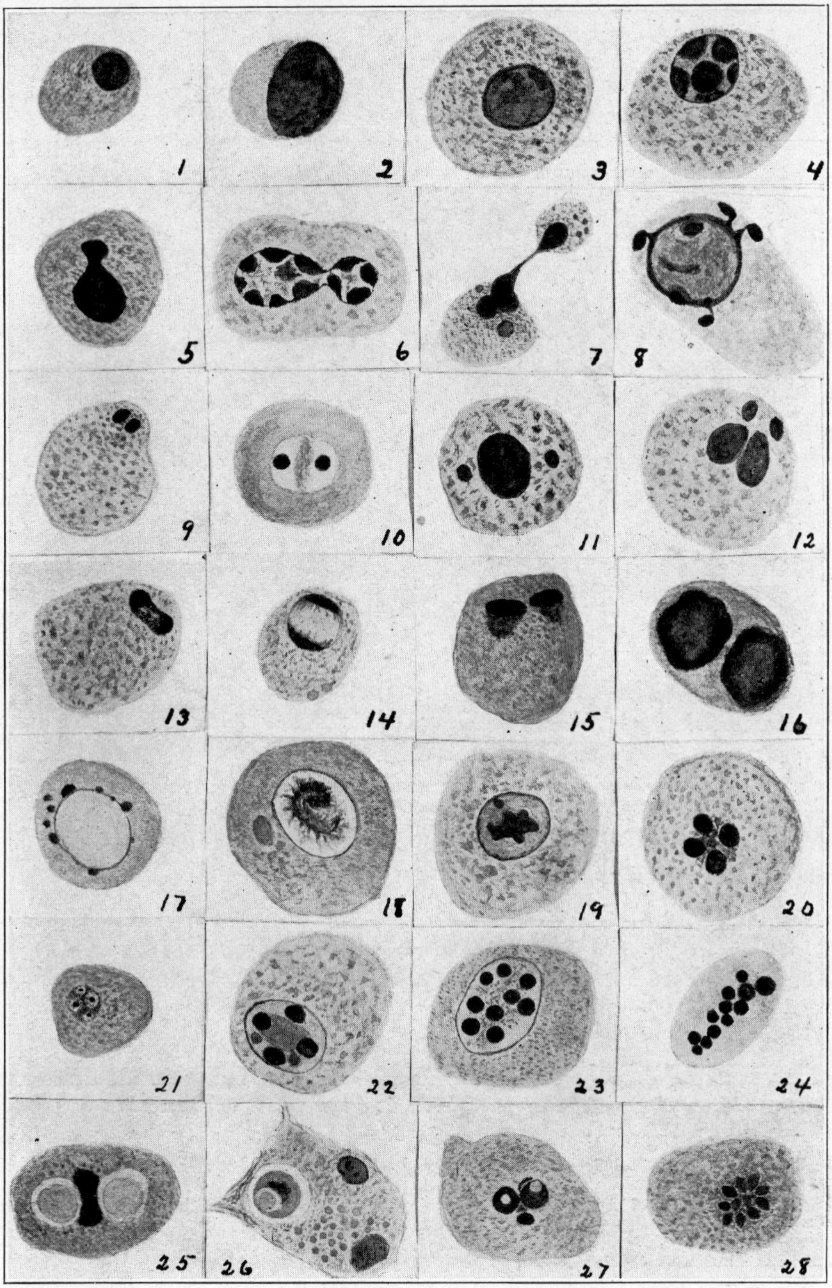

PLATE 1

Figs. 1-4.—Small and large stable forms of parasites.
Figs. 5-7.—Stages of simple binary fission.
Figs. 9-16.—Various forms of mitotic nuclei.
Figs. 17-24.—Encysted forms.
Figs. 25-28.—Unclassified forms.

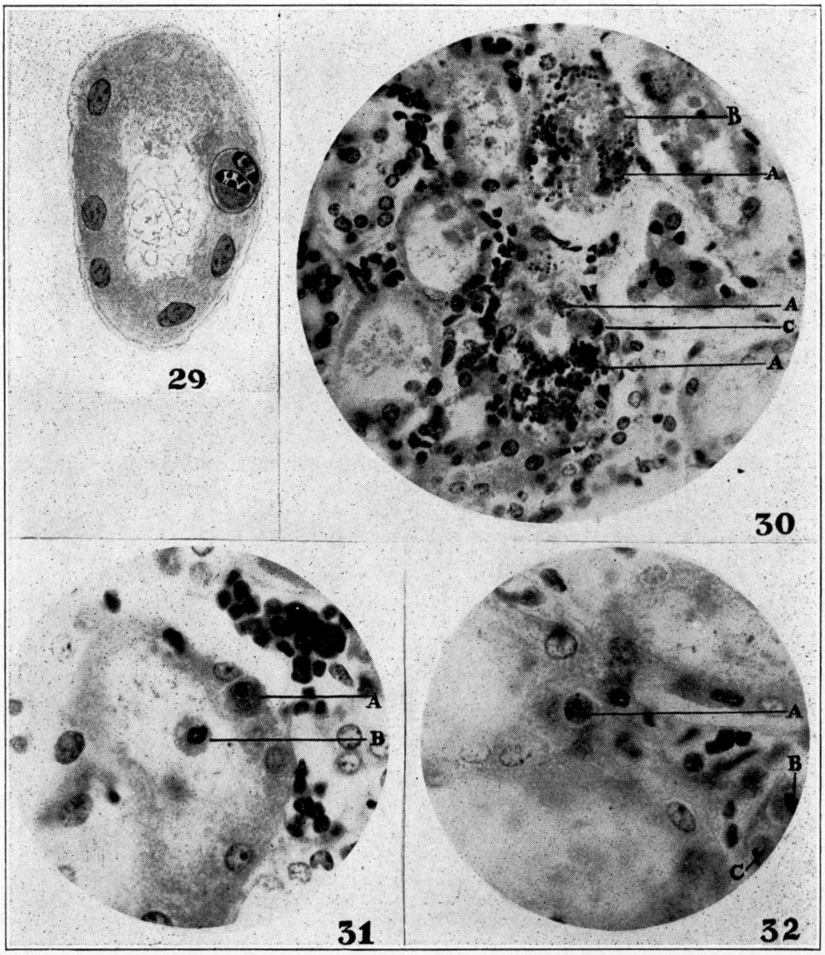

PLATE 2

Fig. 29.—Kidney tubule with a cystlike cavity containing two parasites of similar appearance.

Fig. 30.—Portion of the cortex showing tubular epithelium filled with schizogonic forms; *A*, merozoites; *B*, small nucleated form; *C*, large form; × 425.

Fig. 31.—Tubule containing two parasites; *A*, parasite within an epithelial cell; *B*, parasite in the lumen of tubule; × 780.

Fig. 22.—*A*, parasite in a tubular cell with nuclear material arranged in four round masses as illustrated in Fig. 20; × 780; *B*, parasite with large oval nucleus; *C*, parasite with small round nucleus.

BACTERIOPHAGE PHENOMENA WITH STAPHYLOCOCCUS AUREUS

Bessie R. Callow

From the Department of Bacteriology, College of Physicians and Surgeons, Columbia University, New York

A few months ago I began the study of staphylococcus "bacteriophage" processes, following at first the method by which Twort[1] observed these phenomena in 1914. After several weeks' work with unripened or "green" vaccinia virus from calves, a "lytic" strain was isolated, and most of the observations previously made by Twort and, in part, confirmed by Gratia,[2] were repeated. Meanwhile, the work of most of the observers, who have studied the d'Herelle phenomenon, and especially that carried on in this laboratory by Miss Kuttner[3] on lytic processes in gram-negative bacilli of the typhoid-colon group, seemed to indicate that the most important factor in the initiation of bacteriophage activity was contact with tissues in a state of disintegration, perhaps with tissue enzymes. For this reason, it seemed worth while to attempt the direct isolation of a lytic principle for staphylococcus from boils and other staphylococcus infections.

D'Herelle[4] himself recently reported a staphylococcus bacteriophage from a finger infection of 4 days' duration. Eight drops of the pus were put into 20 c c broth, incubated 24 hours, and filtered. The filtrate, after 5 generations, was active on albus, but not on aureus, both staphylococci having been obtained from the pus.

A total of 14 acute Staphylococcus aureus infections have been examined up to the present time. From 6 of these a bacteriophage specific for one or more strains of staphylococcus was isolated.

The following general technic was found most successful:

Sterile swabs containing pus from the boils were streaked directly on plain and blood-agar plates. Growths were examined on the next day and the individual colonies minutely searched for irregularities suggesting lytic changes.

In two cases to be noted in detail later, typical irregular colonies were found in the streaks made directly from the lesions in this way. Normal colonies were always fished to agar slants for the stock collection.

Received for publication Feb. 23, 1922.

[1] Lancet, Dec. 4, 1915, pp. 1241-1243.

[2] Proc. Soc. Exper. Biol. and Med., 1921, 18, p. 217.

[3] Ibid., p. 222.

[4] Le Bacteriophage, Monographies de L'Institut Pasteur, 1921.

Except in the two cases mentioned, direct streaks from the boils did not yield irregular colonies, and the lytic material was obtained only after the following manipulations. Swabs containing the pus were placed each in 10 c c of extract broth having a reaction of P_H 8, and then were incubated at 37 C. for about 4 hours. Previous experiments with vaccinia bacteriophage showed that longer incubations of the original material obscured the results. Recent observations render it questionable whether incubation is necessary; extraction by shaking and preservation in the icebox until use seems to be entirely satisfactory (see cases 13 and 15).

After incubation, the tubes were placed in the icebox over night or longer, as convenient, and before use were centrifuged and filtered through a Berkefeld candle. The filtrates so obtained were tested for "lytic" properties as described later.

Eighteen-hour broth cultures of 6 or more stock Staphylococcus aureus strains all recently isolated from boils were used. Each filtrate was tested against the autogenous strain, that is, against a strain derived from a normal colony of the same boil. In routine examination of the filtrates inhibition tests were found satisfactory; 0.1 c c of culture was added to each of 2 tubes containing 2 c c extract broth, P_H 8. Tube 1 was set aside as a control. To tube 2 was added 0.5 c c of the suspected lytic filtrate. With several strains of staphylococcus, a series of tubes with their controls were set up for the experiment. They were then incubated for two hours at 37 C.

During the short incubation period the tubes containing the filtrate were from time to time compared with the controls containing culture without filtrate for evidence of inhibition of growth. To prevent heavy growths, the tubes were removed from the incubator after 2 hours and left at room temperature over night and again observed at 18 hours.

Streaks of tubes and controls were made to plain agar plates at 2-hour and 18-hour intervals. Lytic action was recognized by characteristic "moth eaten" areas in the streaks, by irregular colonies with edges showing evidence of lytic changes, and by colonies with mottled surfaces. Whenever the action was marked, innumerable transparent or glassy colonies totally lacking in pigment were present, and there were few if any normal colonies. Occasional streaks showed no growth.

Two-hour streaks were generally more reliable than the 18-hour ones. This may be due to the fact that the normal resistant organisms predominate and overgrow the filtrates in cases in which small amounts of the lytic principle are present. Complete inhibition of growth or subsequent clearing after growth does not mean sterility. These tubes will, on standing, again become clouded. This is due to the fact, now well known, that a culture is made up of 2 types of organisms, a sensitive and a resistant type. The sensitive ones are destroyed by the bacteriophage, the resistant survive and multiply slowly.

In the absence of any evidence of lytic action in the first generation, the experiment was carried through a second or a third generation, and so forth. Tubes containing the original filtrate and the control tubes after 18 hours were centrifuged one hour at high speed. Five tenths c c of each supernatant fluid was pipetted into tubes of broth containing 0.1 c c of corresponding 18-hour broth cultures of staphylococci, and the preceding routine examination was made. In one case marked "lytic" action did not take place until the fourth or fifth generation. The low concentration of the "bacteriophage" in the original filtrate was probably the reason for this.

The following cases of acute staphylococcus infections were examined, and a bacteriophage was obtained from each patient. The method of procedure in every instance followed exactly the routine technic which has been described in the foregoing. Successive steps in that procedure are indicated briefly with each experiment, and the results of each are summarized.

Case 1. No. F 3104.—A man, aged 39, had a carbuncle on the back of his neck for about 5 days. This was incised and drained under local anesthesia. There was very little pus on the swab.

Direct streaks of the pus onto agar plates showed a pure growth of Staphylococcus aureus, but no colonies suggested lytic changes. The swab containing the pus was placed in 10 c c of broth P_H 8.0, and incubated for 3 days at 37 C. After preservation in the icebox over night the culture was filtered through a Berkefeld candle, and the filtrate so obtained was tested against 6 strains of Staphylococcus aureus for the presence of lytic material. The autogenous strain was lost.

The filtrate was active only against the laboratory stock strain of staphylococcus. A few colonies suggesting lytic action were obtained in the streaks made from the tube of the third generation. No inhibition of growth was noted. In the fifth generation a majority of the colonies showed irregularities. Partial but not complete inhibition of growth was evident. The experiment was continued in series through nine generations, but no further increase of lytic material was observed. The streaks still showed innumerable irregular colonies and many transparent ones, but complete inhibition of growth or subsequent clearing after growth did not take place.

Case 2. No. F 2643.—A boy, aged 4, had a submaxillary abscess for 2 weeks with swelling and pain, and accompanied by a few eruptions on the face. It was incised and drained under ether anesthesia. There was about 0.5 c c of heavy pus.

The pus was streaked directly on to agar plates. Growths showed a pure culture of staphylococcus. The examination of individual colonies for evidence of lytic changes proved negative.

Ten c c of broth, P_H 8.0, containing the pus were incubated for 4 hours at 37 C. It was then preserved in the icebox for 3 days and filtered. The filtrate was tested against 6 strains of Staphylococcus aureus. The autogenous strain was lost.

The experiment demonstrated that the lytic material was active against only 2 of the 6 strains used, Nos. 1 and 4. A small amount of lytic action was apparent in the first generation. This was greatly increased in the second generation with both strains. However, total inhibition of growth or subsequent clearing after growth was never obtained even in the ninth generation.

Case 3. No. F 4745.—A boy, aged 17, had a boil on his neck for 2 or 3 days. It was incised, and there was a moderate amount of pus.

A pure culture of Staphylococcus aureus was obtained from the pus. No colonies, however, suggested lytic changes. The swab containing the pus was placed in 10 c c of broth, P_H 8.0, and incubated for 4 hours at 37 C., preserved in the icebox for 3 days, and filtered.

The filtrate so obtained was tested against 7 strains of Staphylococcus aureus, including the autogenous strain from the same boil. Of these only 2 strains, strain 2 and the laboratory stock strain, were effected. Excellent lysis of both was obtained in the first generation.

As a further check on the autogenous strain, 4 other normal colonies from the direct streaks were fished to broth and the filtrate tested against each one of them. These experiments were carried on in series through 5 generations, but no lysis was observed in any instance.

Case 4. No. 13.—A child, aged 8, had submaxillary abscesses, left and right, following an injury to the tongue; death in about 10 days; 3 c c of pus aspirated.

Direct streaks of the pus onto agar plates showed pure Staphylococcus aureus. There was a marked indication of lytic action throughout the streaks. The individual colonies were round but mottled in appearance. On restreaking these irregularities were duplicated. The heavy streaks contained a few clear areas and some colonies had uneven edges showing evidence of lytic changes.

Twenty-five hundredths c c pus in 10 c c of broth, P_H 8.0, was incubated 4 hours at 37 C., placed in the icebox for 4 days and filtered. Streaks made of the broth culture at the 2-hour and the 4-hour intervals showed typical irregular colonies and innumerable transparent ones. The filtrate was tested against 9 strains of Staphylococcus aureus, including the autogenous strain.

It was demonstrated that the filtrate was specific for the autogenous strain and 3 others, namely, 1, 4 and 11. Complete lysis, that is to say, a majority of irregular and transparent colonies in the streaks and a total clearing of the growths in the tubes after a few hours, was observed with each strain in the second generation. The autogenous strain seemed to be most susceptible.

In this experiment a comparison of the results obtained in 3 generations was made, as shown in table 1. It is interesting to note in the first generation experiments that there was no evidence of lytic action in streaks or tubes. The second generation showed complete lysis of the 4 strains, as mentioned in the foregoing. This was considerably diminished in the third generation.

A parallel experiment was also carried out in which the 4-hour incubation period used in the preparation of the filtrate was eliminated. Instead, 0.25 c c of the pus was put into 10 c c of broth, P_H 8, and was shaken vigorously by hand for about 15 minutes, preserved in the icebox over night, and filtered. The filtrate so obtained was tested against autogenous strain 13. Extensive lytic action in the streaks and almost complete inhibition of growth was shown in the first generation.

TABLE 1

COMPARISON OF LYSIS IN THREE GENERATIONS

Strains of Staphylococcus aureus	1st Generation				2d Generation				3d Generation			
	Streaks		Tubes		Streaks		Tubes		Streaks		Tubes	
	2 Hrs.	18 Hrs.	2 Hrs.	18 Hrs.	2 Hrs.	18 Hrs.	2 Hrs.	18 Hrs.	2 Hrs.	18 Hrs.	2 Hrs.	18 Hrs.
Laboratory	—	..	H	H	—	—	H	H	—	—	H	H
Clinic 1	—	..	H	H	+	++++	H	Clear	+	—	H	Mod.
Clinic 2	—	..	H	H	—	—	H	H	—	—	H	H
Clinic 3	—	..	H	H	—	—	H	H	—	—	H	H
Clinic 4	—	..	H	H	+++	++++	V.F.	Clear	+	±	H	Mod.
Clinic 5	—	..	H	H	—	—	H	H	—	—	H	H
Clinic 10	—	..	H	H	—	—	H	H	—	—	H	H
Clinic 11	—?	..	H	H	++	++++	F.	Clear	+	—	H	Mod.
Autogenous 13	—?	..	H	H	++++	++++	Clear	Clear	++	±	H	Mod.

— = all normal colonies; + = an indication of lytic action; ++++ = many irregular colonies, very few normal ones; H = turbidity same as control; F. = faint turbidity as compared with control; V.F. = very faint turbidity; Mod. = moderate turbidity. The control protocols are not given. Streaks were always made at 2-hour and 18-hour intervals.

CASE 5. No. 14.—A woman, aged 26, had a carbuncle on the lower lip, accompanied by multiple abscesses on the face, staphylococcus septicemia. The lip infection had suffered a run down condition due to chronic general eczema. The patient had suffered with eczema since childhood with a series of boils each winter. She recovered.

Direct streaks of the swabs onto plain and blood agar plates gave a heavy hemolytic Staphylococcus aureus growth. The plates also showed several definite transparent areas in the streaks which suggested lytic action. These areas were fished from the center, and the material was streaked on agar plates. The growth showed innumerable irregular and transparent colonies. This proved for the second time that lytic material could be demonstrated in the streaks made directly from the lesion.

A filtrate was made in the usual way by incubating the swab containing the pus in 10 c c of broth, P_H 8.0, for 4 hours and filtering. Streaks from the broth culture again showed irregularities due to the action of a lytic principle.

The filtrate was tested against 11 strains of staphylococcus. Of these only 3 were susceptible to the action of the lytic material, namely, the autogenous strain Nos. 14, 1 and 4. This action was very definite in the first generation and was only slightly increased in the second generation. The autogenous strain proved most susceptible.

A blood culture was taken on the same day. This showed on incubation a heavy growth of Staphylococcus aureus. A transplant was made from this to broth. After standing for two days at room temperature a partial clearing of the growth was noticed. Streaks were made immediately and showed colonies with typical irregularities. This proved that lytic material specific for that strain of staphylococcus was also present in the blood.

Fresh samples of blood and pus from the same patient were taken 5 days later. It was impossible to demonstrate again a lytic principle in either sample. Direct streaks showed regular normal colonies, and inhibition tests with filtrates carried through 2 generations were entirely negative.

A third blood culture taken 5 days later was sterile. The patient made a rapid recovery.

CASE 6. No. 15.—An infant, 10 days old, had cellulitis of the back of the neck, cerebral hemorrhage, cord infection and septicemia with secondary localization in the neck. Pus was taken 4 days after the swelling was first noticed.

Plate cultures made from the pus showed normal Staphylococcus aureus colonies, but no colonies suggested lytic action.

In this experiment 2 filtrates were made and compared. Into each of 2 tubes containing 10 c c of broth, P_H 8.0, 3 c c of pus were added. Tube A was shaken vigorously for 15 minutes, centrifuged and filtered on the same day. Tube B was incubated for 4 hours, preserved in the icebox over night, and filtered. A and B filtrates were then set up in parallel against 11 strains of staphylococcus, including the autogenous strain. Of these, only the laboratory stock strain was susceptible to the action of the lytic material in the 2 filtrates. Filtrate A was more active than B. Streaks from the tube containing filtrate A and culture showed a larger number of irregular and transparent colonies than streaks from the corresponding tube containing filtrate B. Also, filtrate A gave complete clearing after growth, filtrate B only partial clearing.

It is evident from the preceding experiments that a bacteriophage specific for one or more strains of staphylococcus can be isolated from acute staphylococcus infections. This again emphasizes the fact that when a pathogenic organism comes in direct contact with body cells, as is the case in an infection of any kind, a bacteriophage specific for that organism may be produced.

It is important to note that the filtrates which contained the lytic principle were not alike in their action on the several strains of staphylococcus used, that is, each one was active on a different strain or on a different group of strains and showed no action on the others. In other words, the different strains showed great variability to the action of a given lytic agent. Table 2 summarizes these observations.

In this table it is also shown that a staphylococcus bacteriophage isolated from vaccinia and carried through several generations was specific for all the strains with which it came in contact. This proved that a strain which was resistant to the lytic material in the filtrates was not necessarily immune to all bacteriophage activity.

It was also difficult to increase the action of the bacteriophage isolated from the boils beyond the second or third generation. In successive generations it either remained constant or diminished in strength. Also, growth was seldom completely inhibited in the presence of the lytic agent nor were the cultures after growth completely cleared except in one or two instances. Experiments with the vaccinia bacteriophage, on the other hand, showed a marked increase through the fourth generation, at least, and did not deteriorate. A dilution

TABLE 2

REACTION OF VARIOUS STRAINS TO LYTIC AGENTS

Staphylococcus Strains	Filtrates						Vaccinia* Bacteriophage	SPA Controls
	F 3104	F 2643	F 4745	No. 13	No. 14	No. 15		
Laboratory	+	..	+	..	..	+	+	—
Clinic 1	..	+	..	+	+	..	+	—
Clinic 2	..	..	+	..	..	..	+	—
Clinic 3	..	..	..	..	..	..	+	—
Clinic 4	..	+	..	+	+	..	+	—
Clinic 5	..	..	..	..	..	..	+	—
Clinic 10 (Autogenous of F 4745)	..	..	—	..	..	..	+	—
Clinic 11	..	..	..	+	..	..	+	—
Clinic 12	..	..	..	..	..	..	+	—
Clinic 13 (Autogenous of 13)	..	..	..	+	..	..	+	—
Clinic 14 (Autogenous of 14)	..	..	..	..	+	..	+	—
Clinic 15 (Autogenous of 15)	..	..	..	..	..	—	+	—

+ = typical lytic action present; — = no lytic action present.

* This lytic extract was originally derived from untreated calf vaccinia and used against the laboratory stock staphylococcus strain through several generations.

of one to one-million still caused inhibition of growth and complete lysis after growth.

Only two of the filtrates containing the lytic agent showed any action on the autogenous strain, that is, on the strain of staphylococcus derived from a normal colony of the same lesion. Material from these cases was probably taken before all the organisms susceptible to the bacteriophage had been destroyed. The other cases in which the action was negative probably represented a stage in which only the resistant organisms remained. Samples taken earlier in the course of the infection would no doubt have given positive results.

It has been impossible with so few experiments to judge during what period of an infection a bacteriophage appears, or how long it persists. Case 14, in which lytic material was demonstrated in both blood and pus at one time and not at all a few days later, seems to indicate that the presence of a bacteriophage in an infected lesion may last for a limited period only, perhaps only until the susceptible organisms have all been destroyed.[4]

SUMMARY

The presence of a bacteriophage principle transmissible in series against Staphylococcus aureus has been demonstrated in the pus of a series of sixteen staphylococcus infections. In two of these the lytic principle was active against the autogenous strain as well as against other staphylococcus strains. In six others it proved lytic for one or more heterologous strains, but not for the homologous strain, in spite of repeated tests.

[4] Two cases which have been examined since this article was written showed the presence of a bacteriophage. The first was a case of empyema with a positive blood culture following an attack of influenza. A hemolytic Staphylococcus aureus was obtained, and a bacteriophage was isolated from both fluid and blood. It was not, however, specific for the autogenous strain. The patient did not recover.

The second case was a finger infection of 2 or 3 days' duration, from which a bacteriophage was obtained in the second generation. No lytic action on the autogenous strain was noted, even in the fourth generation.

HYDROGEN-ION STUDIES

III. HYDROGEN-ION CHANGES IN THE AGGLUTINATION OF BACTERIA BY IMMUNE SERUM *

Edwin F. Hirsch

From the Pathological Laboratory of St. Luke's Hospital, Chicago

The agglutination of a suspension of bacteria by homologous immune serum in the presence of a salt is one of the best known of the immune reactions. A highly potent immune serum in proper dilutions agglutinates the suspended bacteria into masses which collect at the bottom and sides of the test tube, and the liquid in which the bacteria are suspended becomes clear. Until nonmotile bacteria were observed to agglutinate with immune serum, agglutination was thought to result from some change of the flagella. Then some alteration of the ectoplasm by the immune serum whereby the bacteria became adhesive was considered the cause of agglutination. That bacteria are purely passive however, was learned by observing agglutination with bacteria killed by heat or by various chemicals.

Bordet [1] made the important observation that a salt such as sodium chlorid is necessary for the agglutination of bacteria by immune serum. He also observed that the agglutinins combined with the bacteria in the absence of salt and that the compound so formed was precipitated by the addition of small quantities of salt.

Bechhold [2] and others have shown that bacteria in salt solution carry a negative electrical charge. After having been acted on by agglutinin, they precipitate between the electrodes. In all respects, Wells [3] says, the behavior of bacteria and agglutinins resembles the behavior of colloidal suspensions which form an electrically amphoteric colloidal suspension so that the ions of the electrolytes, or the electrical currents by discharging them unequally, cause precipitation. According to Stieglitz,[4]

Received for publication Feb. 23, 1922.

* Aided by the Winfield Peck Memorial Fund.

[1] Ann. de l'Inst. Pasteur, 1899, 13, p. 225.

[2] Ztschr. f. physik. Chem., 1904, 48, p. 385. Colloids in Biology and Medicine, Trans. by J. G. M. Bullowa, 1919.

[3] Chemical Pathology, 1920.

[4] Qualitative Chemical Analysis I, 1913.

colloids which in a solution carry a negative electrical charge are readily precipitated by the action of positive ions, positively charged colloids by the action of negative ions (Hardy's rule). The precipitated colloid carries with it a part of the precipitating ion (absorption), and the weights of the ions carried down by a given quantity of a given colloid are proportional to the equivalent weights of the ions. The precipitation thus appears to be intimately associated with the neutralization of the charge on the colloid. In accordance with this conclusion, it has been found that a colloid may be precipitated by a colloid carrying an opposite electrical charge.

Colloidal protein solutions now are generally considered to be solutions of amphoteric electrolytes, and the colloidal particles carry a negative electrical charge in an alkaline medium and a positive charge in an acid medium. At a hydrogen-ion concentration specific for the protein there exists no difference in the electrical potential between the particles and the medium, so that the particles appear to be without an electrical charge. This is known as the iso-electric point. Loeb [5] has demonstrated that this marks the turning point of the chemical change which determines the nature of ionization, and the ionization determines the electrical charge. When ionized as an acid and combined with a cation on the alkaline side of the iso-electric point, the protein particle behaves as an anion and carries a negative electrical charge; when ionized as a base and combined with an anion at reactions more acid than the iso-electric point, the protein carries a positive charge.

Coulter [6] determined P_H 4.6 as the iso-electric point for red blood cells (sheep). At hydrogen-ion concentrations less than P_H 4.6, the charge carried by the red blood cells is negative and increases in amount with the alkalinity; at concentrations greater than P_H 4.6, the electrical charge is positive and increases with the acidity. He observed further, that the chlorine ion in the presence of sodium chloride, combines with both normal and sensitized cells in much larger amounts on the acid side of P_H 4.7 than on the alkaline side. Adding sodium hydroxide actually liberates chlorine from the cells between the reactions of P_H 5.7 and P_H 6.2. Similar observations have been made by Loeb,[5] who found that gelatin on the alkaline side of its iso-electric point combines only with a cation, and on the acid side only with an anion. These observations suggest that similar ionization changes occur with bacterial pro-

[5] Jour. Gen. Physiol., 1919, 1, pp. 39, 237, 363, 483, 559.
[6] Ibid., 1920, 3, p. 309.

teins, and that in the presence of an electrolyte such as sodium chloride, a salt of the bacterial protein and the cation of the electrolyte is formed on the alkaline side of its iso-electric point.

In another study Coulter [7] observed the equilibrium between hemolytic sensitizer and red blood cells in relation to the hydrogen-ion concentration. He says that the amphoteric electrolytes with which the immune bodies must be classed on the basis of their behavior in the electrical field owe their electrical charge to ionization, and the combination of sensitizer and cells is related intimately with the ionization of the immune body. In a salt-free medium, he finds the proportion of the total amount of hemolytic sensitizer present and combined with the homologous cells is almost 100% at P_H 5.3. On the alkaline side of this reaction, the proportion diminishes with increasing alkalinity to about 5% at P_H 10. On the acid side, the same decrease occurs, but somewhat less rapidly. The presence of sodium chloride greatly increases the proportion of sensitizer combined with cells at all reactions except those about P_H 5.3. At this point the combination of sensitizer with cells is independent of the electrolyte.

Loeb [8] regards the difference in the hydrogen-ion concentration between the micellae of protein and the surrounding solution as the only cause of the electrical charges of the micellae of protein or of their models. The electrical charges of powdered gelatin suspended in an aqueous solution are determined by the fact that acid is forced into the water solution when the particles consist of gelatin chloride, and that alkali is forced into the water when they consist of sodium gelatinate. The P_H inside minus the P_H outside the particles is positive as long as the P_H of the gelatin is on the acid side of its iso-electric point, while it is negative when the gelatin is on the alkaline side of its iso-electric point. Addition of salt to solutions containing powdered gelatin chloride diminishes the potential difference between the particles and the surrounding liquid, and this is due to a diminution of the value of P_H inside minus P_H outside.

Since many chemical reactions are accompanied by changes in the hydrogen-ion concentration of the medium in which they occur, and as such changes are significant in understanding these chemical reactions, it seems possible that a study of the hydrogen-ion concentration of the medium in which agglutination of bacteria by immune serum

[7] Ibid., 1920, 3, p. 513.
[8] Ibid., 1922, 4, p. 351.

takes place may add new facts which will aid in understanding better the nature of this and similar reactions.

The immune serums were prepared in rabbits. The bacterial suspensions were made with normal salt solution, and the growth of bacteria obtained from 24-hour plain agar slant cultures. Such suspensions were diluted to a medium density and then heated to 56 C. for half an hour to kill the bacteria. To 1 c c quantities of serum diluted with normal salt solution beginning with 1:25 and continuing to 1:6,400 were added 1 c c quantities of the suspension. This system of preparing the dilutions was followed throughout. The mixtures were incubated with their controls (similar dilutions of nonimmune serum) at 37 C. overnight, and the hydrogen-ion concentration of each was determined the next morning. These estimations were made at a constant temperature (25 C.) by the gas-chain method.

The chart illustrates graphically the results of such an experiment and its control with normal serum.

Results which in graphs make curves of similar contour have been obtained with suspensions of typhoid bacilli, colon bacilli, dysentery bacilli, and paratyphoid bacilli, and their homologous immune serums.

COMMENT

The interpretation of the changes in the reaction of the medium in which agglutination occurs involves consideration of certain ionization principles. When sodium chloride is added to water, ionization occurs as follows:

$$\begin{array}{ccc} NaCl & Na^{+} & Cl^{-} \\ HOH & OH^{-} & H^{+} \\ & \downarrow\uparrow & \downarrow\uparrow \\ & NaOH & HCl \end{array}$$

Since the dissociation constants of sodium hydroxide and hydrogen chloride are so nearly equal, such a solution contains an equal concentration of hydrogen and hydroxyl ions and reacts neutral. The addition of bacteria (living or killed) renders the reaction alkaline, as for example the medium changes from P_H 7 to P_H 8.25, a change not due to substances dissolved from the plain agar on which the bacteria were cultivated. The bacteria themselves carry negative electrical charges. Similar changes in reaction are observed when the salt of a strong base and a weak acid is ionized in water. This behavior of bacteria in salt solution suggests that the bacterial protein combines with the Na ion to form a salt, or that this salt already exists when the bacteria are added, and that it then dissociates. The latter seems quite likely because practically all mediums contain salt.

Bacteria in salt solution must be considered to be in two phases, a dissolved portion [9] and an undissolved portion. The latter is concerned especially with the physical changes of agglutination. The dissolved portion ionizing as the salt of a strong base and a weak acid probably causes the alkaline reaction. Letting NaBa represent the dissolved protein salt, its ionization would occur as follows:

Na Ba	Na^+	Ba^-
H OH	OH^-	H^+
	↓↑	↓↑
	NaOH	HBa

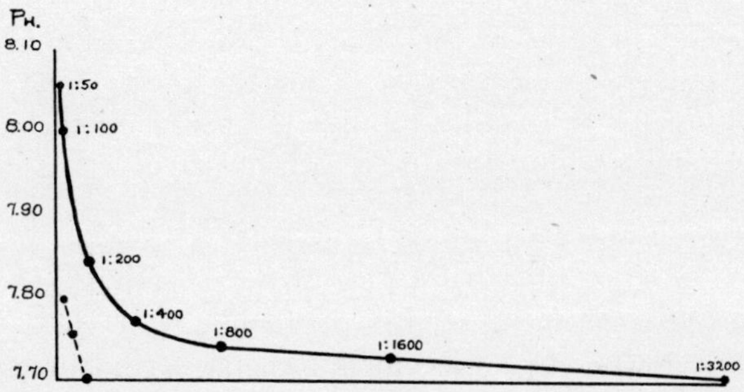

Chart 1.—Graphs representing the reaction of dilutions of serum and colon bacillus suspension; the solid line represents those with immune serum, the interrupted line those with nonimmune serum. Agglutination was complete in dilutions of 1:50 and 1:100 and decreased to slight in dilution of 1:3,200. No agglutination with control serum.

The dissociation of sodium hydroxide is so nearly complete that very little sodium hydroxide exists as such in the liquid. The dissociation of many weak organic acids, however, is much less, and in a medium in which it is establishing its equilibrium, hydrogen-ions are used up, more water ionizes to satisfy its dissociation constant, and the formation of undissociated weak acid continues until its dissociation constant and the dissociation constant of water are satisfied. The hydrogen ion is therefore used up to a much greater degree than is the hydroxide ion. The latter accumulates and the solution becomes alkaline.

[9] See discussion of soluble bacterial substances by Martin Ficker, Kolle and Wassermann, Handbuch der path. Mikroorganismen, 1913, 2.

The mixtures of bacteria and homologous immune serum in the agglutination experiments mentioned are as follows:

Bacterial suspension.	1.0 c c	1.0 c c	1.0 c c
Salt solution.........	0.96 c c	0.98 c c	0.99 c c, etc.
Immune serum	0.04 c c	0.02 c c	0.01 c c

As the amount of immune serum decreases in each tube, the extreme limit of reaction on one end of the series of dilutions (greatest) is that of the bacterial suspension diluted with an equal volume of salt solution, and at the other end of the series it is this reaction modified by the substitution of 1/50th volume salt solution by immune serum. Similar relations exist for mixtures of nonimmune serum and bacterial suspension.

The curve representing the hydrogen-ion concentration of the dilutions of the homologous immune serum and bacterial suspension demonstrates an increase in the alkalinity of the medium where this occurs, while that representing those for the nonimmune serum is a straight line, in all respects like a graph of hydrogen-ion concentrations obtained by similar dilutions of two chemically inert solutions with different reactions.

The negative electrical charges carried by bacteria probably are acquired in much the same way as are similar electrical charges by the colloidal particles of a metal such as platinum. Such colloidal particles react with water whereby an incomplete chemical combination with the liquid occurs. $_nPt.^+ H.OH = (Pt_n H^+)^+ OH^-$. This platinum-hydrogen aggregate dissociates slightly and gives rise to a negative charge on the metal.[10]

Bordet's [1] observation that the presence of a salt is necessary for agglutination may be taken to mean that in distilled water the bacterial protein is not ionized to an appreciable extent. In order to react with immune serum and agglutinate, ionization is necessary and occurs when the bacterial protein is combined with a base to form a salt. The distribution of electrical charges is represented then by $Na^+ Ba^-$.

The agglutination of bacteria is associated with the neutralization of their electrical charges by the immune substance. It is fair to believe that the immune body carries a positive electrical charge, that it possesses basic properties, and that it ionizes according to the formula $\frac{\text{Immune substance x OH}}{\text{Immune substance OH}^-} = K_{\text{I. S.}}$ The dissociation constant $K_{\text{I.S.}}$ is satisfied in the serum, so that adding serum to the salt solution-

[10] Burton, E. F.: The Physical Properties of Colloidal solutions, 1916.

bacterial suspension mixture alters the reaction only in so far as its dissociated products are able. The neutralization of the negative charge of the bacteria by the immune body liberates the cation of the bacteria (Na) and the anion of the immune body (OH). The dissociation constant of the sodium hydroxide resulting from this interaction is probably so much greater than the dissociation constant of the immune substance that more hydroxyl ions are contained in the liquid after agglutination than before, and the medium becomes more alkaline.

The contour of the graph representing this reaction strikingly resembles others representing titration and dissociation curves.[11]

The intravenous injection of a suspension of bacteria [12] has been found to lower temporarily the alkaline reserve of the blood. Within 24 hours, when recovery is prompt, the alkaline reserve of the blood returns to normal, sometimes after having reached a higher than normal value. These changes have been regarded as significant in the establishing of immunity. Since bacteria in their chemical activity resemble the salts of weak acids, the lowering of the alkaline reserve of the blood by their presence is not difficult to correlate. Nor is it unlikely that the immune substance of an acid salt is basic in reaction. In regarding the balanced P_H of the blood, it is necessary to consider the inorganic substances, carbonates (notably) and the phosphates, which fluctuate rapidly and easily to maintain the P_H equilibrium, and another group (proteins), the basic immune substances, which appear in defense against infections, and which alter by their dissociation products the reaction of the blood. The latter changes probably are very small and are readily compensated by the inorganic substances first mentioned.

SUMMARY

Bacteria suspended in normal salt solution behave chemically and electrically like the anion of the salt of a strong base and a weak acid.

When bacteria are agglutinated by homologous immune serum, the medium in which this reaction occurs increases in alkalinity.

This change in reaction is regarded to result from differences in the dissociation constants of the reacting substances and their products.

[11] Clark, W. Mansfield: The Determination of Hydrogen Ion, 1920.

[12] Hirsch, E. F.: Jour. Am. Med. Assn., 1920, 75, p. 1204; Jour. Infect. Dis., 1921, 28, p. 275.

HYDROGEN-ION STUDIES

IV. CHANGES IN REACTION ACCOMPANYING THE PRECIPITATION OF COLLOIDAL GOLD BY SPINAL FLUID (LANGE TEST) *

From the Pathological Laboratory of St. Luke's Hospital, Chicago

EDWIN F. HIRSCH

The colloidal gold test with spinal fluid, commonly known as the Lange test, is an important aid in the diagnosis of cerebrospinal syphilis. The results of the test are expressed in color changes from the pink-red of the prepared colloidal gold suspension, and these in turn are plotted in graphs, or are designated by numbers (chart 1). The color of the colloidal gold suspension is dependent on the dispersion of the finely divided gold particles, and changes from the pink-red color are accompanied by an increase in the size of the aggregates.

Faraday[1] observed these color changes in his gold solutions on the addition of a salt, and correctly regarded the changes as due to an increase in the size of the gold particles. Jevons[2] (1868), studying the Brownian movement of particles in suspension, observed that this movement ran parallel with the stability of the suspension, and that the addition of acids, alkalis, or salts, regardless of their chemical composition caused the cessation of the movement and coagulated the suspensions. These results suggested to Jevons that the particles were electrically charged, and that the coagulating action of the electrolytes is due to the neutralizaion of an electrical charge carried by the particles of gold. Billitzer,[3] experimenting with the electrical migration of colloidal particles of gold and other metals, found that this gradually decreases and finally changes its direction on the addition of electrolytes, demonstrating that even the sign of the charge on the colloidal particle may be changed by adding enough oppositely charged electrolyte ions.

Particles of gold in colloidal suspension carry a negative electrical charge, and ions, metallic or colloidal, precipitating them are positively charged. Burton[2] studied the mobility of colloidal gold particles after the addition of varying amounts of 0.001 N aluminum sulphate (Al^{+}), and the results obtained indicate clearly the presence of an iso-electric point for the gold suspensions, and that the gold particle passes through a state of maximum instability at the time its electrical charge is changing from negative to positive. After passing through the iso-electric point, an increase in the quantity of electrolyte added increases the stability of the suspension. When the smallest traces of aluminum sulphate are added to the colloidal gold, all of the aluminum ions go to decrease the charge on the gold particles, and when aluminum is added in quantities just

Received for publication March 17, 1922.

* Aided by the Winfield Peck Memorial Fund.

1 Philosophical Mag., 1857, 4, pp. 401 and 512.

2 See Burton, E. F.: The Physical Properties of Colloidal Solutions, 1916, p. 145.

3 Ann. d. Physik, 1903, 11, p. 902.

sufficient to neutralize that charge, coagulation of the particles is most rapid. If the electrolyte is added at once in excess, the particles absorb the metallic ion, and the charge is changed from a large negative to a large positive, the positive charge inducing the same stabilizing effects as the negative, and so maintaining the colloidal particle in a state of fine subdivision. Hardy[4] suggests that the coagulation of a colloidal suspension by electrolytes takes place because the electrical charges of the particles are neutralized by the absorption of oppositely charged ions of the electrolyte solution, and at the iso-electric point where the charge becomes zero, the colloidal coagulates. Burton,[2] summarizing the work on the ultramicroscopic observations of electrolytic coagulation of colloids, says that electrolyte coagulation progresses by the condensation of small particles on those of larger size, and not by the coalescence of particles of equal size. The larger ultramikrons act as condensation nuclei for the smaller particles. The color changes of the gold solution follow parallel with the ultramicroscopic changes in that the size of the particles increases and their number

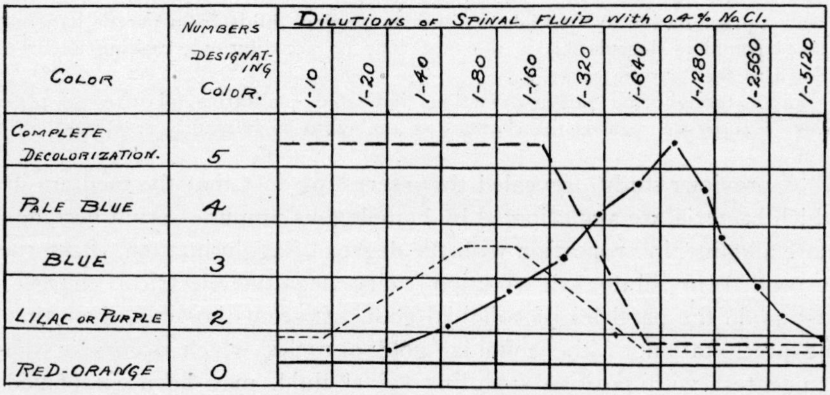

Chart 1.—Typical curves with the Lange test. The continuous line indicates a normal spinal fluid; the long dashes, a paretic spinal fluid; the short dashes, a syphilitic spinal fluid; and the dot and dash line, precipitation in higher dilutions.

decreases as more and more of the electrolyte is added. Gold solutions, as observed by Faraday,[1] Zsigmondy[5] and others, pass through a series of color changes on the addition of coagulating agents. These are red, purple-red, red-violet, blue-violet and deep blue. The suspension becomes turbid, and finally the gold separates in the form of powder or flakes.

Certain organic colloids when added in small quantities to a metal solution prevent the coagulation of the suspended particles by electrolytes. Zsigmondy[6] found this protection specific for each protein examined, and he expressed this relation in terms of milligrams of protein capable of protecting 5 cc of his colloidal gold solution against precipitation by 0.5 cc of a 10% sodium chlorid solution. Lange,[7] with the possibility of clinical application in mind, after having failed with blood serum, attempted its application in a quantitative study of the

[4] Jour. Physiol., 1905-6, 33, p. 251.
[5] Zur Erkenntniss der Kolloide, 1905.
[6] Ztschr. f. Anal. Chem., 1901, 40, p. 697.
[7] Ztschr. f. Chemotherapie, O., 1912-13, 1, p. 44.

proteins of the cerebrospinal fluid. His first attempts were unsuccessful because in using distilled water to make the spinal fluid dilutions, certain proteins, particularly the globulins, were thrown out of solution. However, with a weak salt solution (0.4% sodium chlorid) the spinal fluid proteins did not precipitate, and the salt concentration was too low to agglutinate the gold particles. With this procedure, Lange obtained results which were as interesting as they were startling to him. He found that normal spinal fluid diluted with 0.4% sodium chlorid solution caused no color change with the colloidal gold, while abnormal fluids, which reasonably could be expected to protect against precipitation because of their protein content, caused partial or complete precipitation of the gold particles with resultant color changes. These, plotted in curves according to dilutions, seem to be almost specific for certain diseases, particularly syphilis. Fluids from patients with tabes or cerebrospinal syphilis reacted within a range of dilutions regularly enough to suggest the term "syphilitic curve," while fluids from certain types of meningitis reacted in such a way as to make curves characterized by the term "Verschiebung nach Oben" or reactions with the greatest precipitation in the highest dilutions. Spinal fluids from paretic patients caused complete flocculation in the first four or six dilutions, making a curve known as the "paretic curve."

Lange thought the various reactions indicated qualitative mixtures of proteins. Zalozieki [8] regards the changes as analogous to immunity reactions.

A previous study [9] revealed the interesting fact that the medium in which bacteria are agglutinated by homologous immune serum becomes more alkaline, in proportion with the degree of agglutination. Bacteria suspended in dilute salt solution carry negative electrical charges, just as do the particles of colloidal gold. It seems possible, then, that the precipitation of the colloidal gold particles which occurs in the Lange test with positive syphilitic spinal fluid, may be accompanied by changes in the reaction of the medium similar to the changes occurring with the agglutination of a suspension of bacteria by homologous immune serum. The gold solution was prepared chemically [10] and its reaction adjusted to approximate neutrality. The spinal fluid dilutions and mixtures with the gold solution were made in clean glass tubes as follows:

Gold Solution	5 c c	5 c c	5 c c
0.4% NaCl	0.9 c c	0.95 c c	0.975, etc.
Spinal fluid	0.1 c c	0.05 c c	0.025

These tubes stood at room temperature over night, and their reactions were determined the next morning at constant temperature (25C.) by the gaschain method. Chart 2 illustrates graphically the results

[8] Deutsch. Ztschr. f. Nervenh., 1913, 47, p. 783.
[9] Jour. Infect. Dis., 1922, 30, p. 651.
[10] Bull. Johns Hopkins Hosp., 1915, 26, p. 391.

of such an experiment with a spinal fluid giving a modified paretic curve. The Wassermann reaction was 100% positive with the acetone-insoluble and cholesterinized antigens. With it is plotted a normal negative control. In the table are included the results obtained with other spinal fluids.

All of these results demonstrate that the agglutination of the gold particles as manifested by color changes, turbidity or complete precipitation is accompanied by a parallel increase in the alkalinity of the medium.

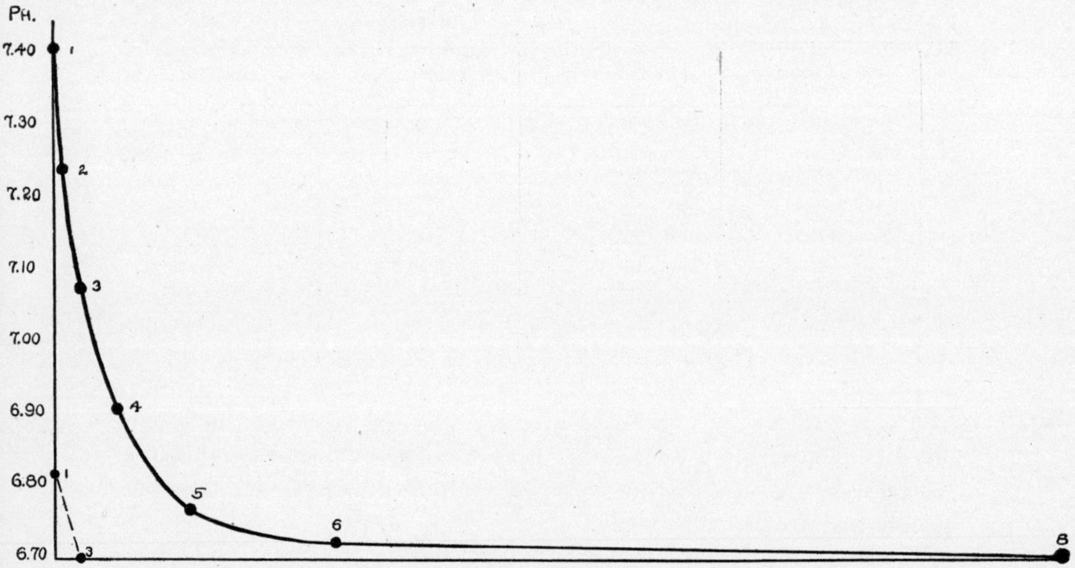

Chart 2.—Curve showing the reactions in dilutions of spinal fluid and colloidal gold giving a modified paretic curve. Complete precipitation of the colloidal gold in the first two tubes; no color change after the seventh tube.

COMMENT

The negative electrical charges of the colloidal particles of a metal such as gold are thought to arise from an incomplete chemical combination with water as follows: $Au + H.OH = (Au_n.H^+) + OH^-$. The gold-hydrogen aggregate dissociates slightly and gives rise to a negative electrical charge on the metal. In the presence of a small amount of sodium chloride, it is possible that the dissociated Na-ions carry the positive charges in equilibrium with the negative electrical charges of the colloidal gold. The addition of syphilitic spinal fluid precipitates the gold particles like aluminum sulphate. The reacting ion (Al) carries a positive electrical charge, and it is reasonable to conclude that the ions in the spinal fluid reacting with the gold also carry a positive electrical charge. Linder and Picton [11] classified colloids into anionic and cationic according to the migration of the particles to the positive or negative electrode. They observed also that under certain conditions a colloid bearing a charge of one sign is precipitated by the addition of a colloid of an opposite sign, and that both colloids are

TABLE 1

RESULTS OF THE PRECIPITATION OF A SPINAL FLUID MANIFESTING A STABILIZING EFFECT

	Precipitation in Higher Dilutions		Paretic Curve		Syphilitic Curve		Normal	
	Color Change	PH	Color Change	PH	Color Change	PH.	Color Change	PH
1	Pink, some precipitate	7.61	Complete precipitate	7.49	Rose	6.92	0	6.82
2	Pink, some precipitate	7.38	Complete precipitate	7.46	Rose	6.84	0	6.82
3	Complete precipitate	7.12	Complete precipitate	7.22	Purple	6.83	0	6.71
4	Blue	6.96	Complete precipitate	7.18	Blue	6.82	0	6.70
5	Lilac	6.93	Complete precipitate	6.95	Purple	6.80	0	
6	Purple	6.87	Blue	6.74	Red blue	6.75	0	
7	0		Purple		0	6.70	0	
8	0	6.84	0		0	6.70	0	
9	0		0		0	6.70	0	
10	0	6.70	0	6.70	0	6.70	0	6.70

carried down in the precipitate. Biltz [12] suggests that the following rules govern the precipitating and precipitated colloids, mixed together quickly and treated uniformly.

> If to a given colloid one of opposite sign is added in small proportion there is no precipitating action. As the quantity of the second increases, the coagulative action follows parallel until a proportion is reached which causes immediate coagulation. As this amount is still further increased, coagulation ceases, that is, there is an optimum precipitation for certain proportions, and if these favorable proportions are exceeded on either side, no precipitation occurs.

It seems, then, that the precipitation of the colloidal gold particles is dependent on the presence of positively charged ions in the spinal fluid, probably protein substances. The neutralization of the negative charges of the ionized gold-sodium aggregate by the positive charges of the substances contained in the spinal fluid liberates the base sodium, which in water dissociates to satisfy its own constant. The

[11] Jour. Chem. Soc., 1892, 61, p. 148; 1895, 67, p. 63; 1897, 71, p. 568; 1905, 87, p. 1906.

[12] Berichte d. Deutsch. chem. Gesellschaft., 1904, 37, p. 1095.

protein substance dissociated in water may be represented by the formula $\frac{(\text{protein}) \times (\text{OH})}{(\text{protein OH})} = K$. The dissociation constant of the sodium hydroxide is probably so much greater than that of the protein substance that when it (K_{Na}) is satisfied, the medium contains a much greater number of dissociated hydroxyl ions, and consequently is more alkaline in reaction. The amount of base liberated depends on the degree of gold precipitation.

In accordance with the observations that an excess of an oppositely charged colloid stabilizes the gold solution are those results with spinal fluids which form curves with precipitation in the higher dilutions. In the table are given the results of a spinal fluid manifesting this stabilizing effect in the first two dilutions. The alkalinity is greater than that of any others in similar dilutions. This curve in the Lange test results when a large negative charge on the gold particles is suddenly replaced by a large positive, the solution being stabilized in the lower dilutions, but precipitated in the higher dilutions.

The color in the first two dilutions of the syphlitic curve is said to be unchanged. Careful comparison, however, demonstrates that it is rose-red and that the medium often is slightly turbid. The reaction curve of fluids in such a series of tubes conforms in outline if not in length with the paretic and other curves.

CONCLUSIONS

The agglutination of colloidal gold particles by spinal fluid (Lange test) is accompanied by an increase in the alkalinity of the medium in which this reaction occurs.

This change in reaction is similar to that observed on the agglutination of bacteria by homologous immune serum.

HYDROGEN-ION STUDIES

V. CHANGES IN THE REACTION OF THE BLOOD IN EXPERIMENTAL INFECTIONS *

Edwin F. Hirsch

and

J. Lisle Williams

From the Pathological Laboratory of St. Luke's Hospital, Chicago, Ill.

Although there are many statements to the effect that acidosis accompanies acute infections, there seems to be in the literature only the work of Dragstedt [1] on the reaction of the blood in experimental infections, measured by the Levy, Rowntree, and Marriott colorimetric method, and the studies by Means [2] and his associates on the acid-base balance of the blood in pneumonia in which the reaction of the blood was determined by constructing carbon dioxid diagrams according to Haggard and Henderson. These reports all mention changes in the reaction of the blood; namely, a decrease in its alkalinity. The gas-chain method for determining the H-ion concentration of the blood, when properly carried out, probably detects minute changes in reaction more precisely than either of the methods mentioned, or others whereby the P_H is determined directly or indirectly. Since the entire range of reaction of the blood compatible with life lies between P_H 7 and P_H 7.8,[3] minute changes are significant. Other studies [4] have demonstrated that the alkali reserve of the blood in rabbits is lowered in experimental infections. This is a similar study in which the reaction of the blood has been determined directly according to the gas-chain method.

The bacteria were grown on plain agar, and fractional amounts of an 18-hour growth, suspended in sterile 0.9% sodium chlorid solution (not more than 2 c c volume), were injected intravenously into rabbits. The blood in 10 c c quantities was drawn aseptically without anesthesia from the heart into a defibrinating tube, all of the air being displaced. After defibrination by shaking, the blood was introduced directly into

Received for publication March 25, 1922.

* Aided by the Winfield Peck Memorial Fund.

[1] Jour. Infect. Dis., 1920, 27, p. 452.

[2] Jour. Exper. Med., 1921, 33, p. 201; Jour. Biol. Chem., 1922, 50, p. 413.

[3] Jour. Biol. Chem., 1921, 48, p. 154.

[4] Hirsch, E. F.: Jour. Am. Med. Assn., 1920, 75, p. 204; Jour. Infect. Dis., 1921, 28, p. 275.

a McClendon electrode vessel without loss of carbon dioxid or the introduction of air. All of the readings were made at a constant temperature of 25 C. The carbon dioxid binding power of the blood was estimated according to the method of Van Slyke and Cullen.[5] Each rabbit was bled immediately before receiving the injection of bacteria, and once again 2 to 4 hours after, as a rule, but sometimes again during the next day.

TABLE 1

RESULTS OF EXPERIMENTS

Organisms	Before Injection		After Injection		Result
	P_H	CO_2	P_H	CO_2	
B. typhosus..................	7.46	64.31	7.22	49.26	Recovered
B. typhosus..................	7.50	41.44	6.74	17.76	Died
B. dysenteriae (Flexner).....	7.42	53.61	7.46	49.26	Recovered
B. dysenteriae (Flexner).....	7.42	64.14	7.22	26.39	Died
B. paratyphosus A..........	7.50	43.85	7.34	48.24	Died after 3 days
B. paratyphosus B..........	7.58	60.32	7.41	43.99	Died
			7.49	37.28	
B. enteritidis................	7.55	47.57	6.87	26.21	Died
B. mucosus..................	7.49	59.55	7.32	37.34	Died
10 c c 0.9% NaCl solution....	7.52	65.25	7.44	62.37	No unusual symptoms

The results of these experiments are collected in the table, and they show that the intravenous injection of a suspension of pathogenic bacteria is followed not only by a depression of the alkaline reserve of the blood, but also by a diminution of its alkalinity. The blood of rabbits subjected only to the manipulation incident to bleeding from the heart and the intravenous injection of 10 c c of a 0.9% sodium chlorid solution changed slightly in reaction and in alkaline reserve, but not so much as that of rabbits injected with the bactera. Those rabbits whose blood reaction and alkaline reserve were changed moderately recovered, those with marked changes died, and in some death occurred at a time when further determinations could not be made. Probably, therefore, some of the values obtained after the injection of the bacteria are much higher than those which actually existed at death.

SUMMARY

The intravenous injection of pathogenic bacteria into rabbits diminishes the alkalinity of the blood as well as the alkaline reserve.

The hydrogen-ion concentration of the blood may become so great that the reaction becomes slightly acid.

[5] Jour. Biol Chem, 1917, 30, p. 289.

HYDROGEN-ION STUDIES

VI. HYDROGEN-ION CHANGES ON PRECIPITATION OF HUMAN SERUM BY IMMUNE SERUM *

Edwin F. Hirsch

From the Pathological Laboratory of St. Luke's Hospital, Chicago

Proteins are regarded, generally, as amphoteric electrolytes, that is, substances which are able to unite with acid as well as alkali.[1] The hydrogen-ion concentration of the surrounding solution determines whether they unite with the one or the other. When the hydrogen-ion concentration of the solution exceeds a critical point which is known as the iso-electric point of the protein, the protein combines with acid to form a salt which, dissociating, gives rise to a protein cation carrying a positive electrical charge and an acid anion with a negative electrical charge. When the hydrogen-ion concentration of the solution is on the alkaline side of the iso-electric point of the protein, the protein combines with metals to form a salt such as sodium proteinate which dissociates into negatively charged protein ions, and positively charged ions of the metal.

That precipitation of a colloid bearing an electrical charge of one sign is accomplished by the addition of a colloid bearing an opposite charge, and that both colloids are carried down in the precipitate, is generally recognized. The precipitin reaction on mixing an antigen in solution with its homologous immune serum probably belongs to the same group of reactions. Biltz [2] suggests the following rules regarding the precipitation of one colloid by another when mixed together quickly and uniformly:

> If to a given colloidal solution, one of the opposite sign is added in small proportion, there is no precipitation. As the quality of the second increases the coagulative action follows parallel until a proportion is reached which causes immediate coagulation. As the amount is still further increased, coagulation ceases; that is, there is an optimum precipitation for certain proportions, and when these favorable proportions are exceeded on either side, no precipitation occurs.

Changes in the hydrogen-ion concentration of a medium frequently occur with the chemical interaction of the substances contained, and

Received for publication, March 25, 1922.

* Aided by the Winfield Peck Memorial Fund.

[1] Loeb, Jacques: Jour. Gen. Physiol., 1918-19, 1, pp. 39, 237, 363, 483, 559.

[2] Berichte d. Deutsch. Chem. Gesellschaft, 1904, 37, p. 1095.

these changes in reaction are important in understanding the nature of the chemical change. Previous studies [3] of the hydrogen-ion changes on agglutination of bacteria by homologous immune serum, and of the changes in reaction on the precipitation of a colloidal gold solution by spinal fluid (Lange test) demonstrated that these chemical reactions are accompanied by an increase of the hydroxyl-ion (alkalinity) content of the medium. Since both the bacteria in a suspension in salt solution and the colloidal gold particles of the gold solution carry negative electrical charges, it is likely that their agglutination or precipitation are similar chemical reactions, that the changes are governed by well-known laws obtaining in the precipitation of a colloid bearing an electrical charge of one sign by the addition of a colloid with an opposite electrical charge, and that the precipitate contains both the precipitating and the precipitated colloids. The precipitin reaction is analogous, at least to a certain extent, with these reactions, and therefore experiments were made to determine whether similar changes occur in the hydrogen-ion concentration of the medium.

Human serum and homologous immune rabbit serum were used in these experiments, the amounts in c c being as follows:

				Control
Immune rabbit serum	0.1	0.1	0.1	0.1
Human serum	0.1	0.05	0.025 etc.	0
NaCl, 0.9%	1.8	1.85	1.875	1.9
Normal rabbit serum	0.1	0.1	0.1	0.1
Human serum	0.1	0.05	0.025 etc.	0
NaCl, 0.9%	1.8	1.85	1.875	1.9

The dilutions were made in clean, sterile, glass test tubes with precautions against bacterial contamination, and then kept at icebox temperature over night, the reactions of the tubes being determined after about 18 hours, according to the gas-chain method, at a constant temperature (25 C.).

Table 1 gives the results of one experiment which are like those obtained in others. The experiments demonstrate that there is an increase of the hydroxyl-ion content of the medium with the precipitation of human serum by homologous immune rabbit serum. The changes in reaction are similar to those on agglutination of bacteria by homologous immune serum, and on precipitation of colloidal gold solution by spinal fluid (Lange test). When plotted they form curves like those in the other studies.[3] The reactions of the control series fall in a straight line like a graph of hydrogen-ion concentrations obtained by similar dilutions of two chemically inert solutions with different reactions. The inhibition of precipitation in the first antigen-

[3] Jour. Infect. Dis., 1922, 30, pp. 259, 263.

antibody dilution corresponds with observations already well known and probably results from an excess of antigen in the mixture.

TABLE 1
RESULTS OF EXPERIMENT

Dilution of Human Serum	Immune Rabbit Serum		Normal Rabbit Serum	
	P_H	Precipitation	P_H	Precipitation
1:20	8.08	Turbid only	7.90	0
1:40	7.98	+++	7.84	0
1:80	7.93	+++	7.74	0
1:160	7.85	++	7.74	0
1:320	7.82	++	—	—
1:640	7.80	++	—	—
1:1280	7.76	+	—	—
Control	7.74	0	7.74	0
Salt solution				

Each tube contains 1/20th volume rabbit serum.

COMMENT

Since the results obtained with the precipitation test are like those obtained with the agglutination of bacteria, it is fair to regard the two phenomena as chemically similar. The presence of an inorganic salt such as sodium chloride is as essential for precipitation in the precipitin test as it is for the agglutination of bacteria by homologous immune serum. Bacteria in sodium chloride solution carry negative electrical charges; that is, they are ionized as the acid anion of a salt. When they are added to a sodium chloride solution, the reaction of the medium becomes more alkaline, a change similar to that observed when a salt of a strong base and a weak acid is added to water. This alkalinity results because of dissociation changes of the salt and water in establishing their equilibrium and in satisfying their dissociation constants. The protein substance or substances in human serum concerned with the precipitin reaction may be represented as dissociating in salt solution according to the formula:

$$\begin{array}{lll} \text{Na proteinate} & Na^{+} & \text{Proteinate}^{-} \\ \text{HOH} & OH^{-} & H^{+} \\ & \downarrow\uparrow & \downarrow\uparrow \\ & \text{NaOH} & \text{Hproteinate} \end{array}$$

$$\frac{H \times \text{proteinate}}{H \quad \text{proteinate}} = K$$

and the immune substance in the homologous serum according to the formula:

$$\begin{array}{lll} \text{Immune substance Cl} & \text{Immune}^{+}\ \text{substance} & Cl^{-} \\ \text{HOH} & OH^{-} & H^{+} \\ & \downarrow\uparrow & \downarrow\uparrow \\ & \text{Immune substance OH} & \text{HCl} \end{array}$$

$$\frac{\text{Immune substance} \times OH}{\text{Immune substance} \quad OH} = K$$

The mutual precipitation of colloids bearing opposite electrical charges is generally known, and the laws governing this chemical action probably apply equally well in the precipitin reaction.

The increase of hydroxyl ions on the precipitation of human serum by homologous immune serum probably results from a liberation of the base (Na) whose dissociation constant is greater than that of the immune substance.

SUMMARY

The precipitation of human serum by homologous immune serum is accompanied by an increase in the alkalinity of the medium similar to that observed on the agglutination of bacteria by immune serum and on the precipitation of colloidal gold by spinal fluid (Lange test).

THE PRODUCTION OF LUNG HEMORRHAGES AND ASSOCIATED PHENOMENA IN RABBITS AND GUINEA-PIGS

Sara Elizabeth Branham

From the Department of Hygiene and Bacteriology of the University of Chicago

During the influenza epidemic in the winter of 1920 an attempt was made to cultivate a filtrable organism from material from several patients with influenza.[1] The number of cases available was too small to have much significance, but the negative results obtained made it seem desirable to employ other methods of attack in addition to the attempts at direct cultivation. By this time the epidemic had passed and no fresh influenza material was available for direct inoculation of animals. It seemed, however, of importance to begin this work with normal animals and noninfluenzal material, for the data thus collected would serve to control later work, should another wave of influenza come, and would prove a valuable basis for further experiment.

Both rabbits and guinea-pigs were used, the larger number of rabbits being due to the fact that they were much more conveniently handled. Following the line of experiment initiated by others working in this field,[2,3] the effect of the inoculations on the total leukocyte count was noted in the first series of animals, since leukopenia is considered one of the outstanding features in influenza in man. These leukocyte counts were accompanied by records of weight and temperature.

The materials used for inoculation were sterile physiologic salt solution and nasal washings both from normal persons and persons with colds. With three of the last named, the material was collected within the first 24 hours after the onset, but in one case the cold was 4 days old. These nasal washings were obtained by washing out the nose with about 50 c c of warm sterile physiologic salt solution, collecting this material in a sterile glass-stoppered bottle containing beads. The nasopharynx was also swabbed and the swab shaken with the saline nasal washings. After being thoroughly shaken, the mixture was passed

Received for publication Feb. 1, 1922.

1 Branham and Hall: J. Infect. Dis., 1921, 28, p. 143.

2 Olitsky and Gates: Jour. Am. Med. Assn., 1920, 74, 74, p. 1497; 1921, 76, 640; J. Exper. Med., 1921, 33, pp. 125, 361, 373, 713; 34, p. 1; 1922, 35, p. 1.

3 Loewe and Zeman: J. Am. Med. Assn., 1921, 76, p. 986.

through a tested Mandler filter. Five c c of the filtrate was inoculated into about 20 c c of a 1% dextrose broth to determine its freedom from ordinary bacteria. The constricted tube with marble seal designed by Hall [4] was used for this, and the broth was boiled just before use

EXAMPLE OF A RABBIT SHOWING A LEUKOCYTOSIS. OBSERVATIONS MADE 11 TO 12 A. M.

Rabbit 30	Temperature, F.	Weight, Kg.	Leukocytes
July 25	104.0	1.724	8 000
July 26	104.2	1.740	7,000
July 27 (3 p. m. inoculation 4 c c salt solution)	104.6	1.719	8,800
July 28	104.0	1.695	12,000
July 29	103.8	1.708	15,000

Killed by a blow, July 29. Extensive bright red hemorrhages involved all lobes, even the collapsed ones. Greater part of lungs uncollapsed. Cultures from lung in dextrose broth were sterile.

EXAMPLE OF A RABBIT SHOWING A LEUKOPENIA. OBSERVATIONS MADE 2 TO 3 P. M.

Rabbit 22	Temperature, F.	Weight, Kg.	Leukocytes
July 11	103.0	2,920	12,000
July 12	103.2	2,951	13,000
July 13	103.3	2.955	11,800
July 14	103.4	2.939	12,100
July 15 (11 a. m. inoculation 3 c c salt solution)	103.0	2.986	12,200
July 16	103.1	.....	8,000

Killed by a blow, July 16. Lungs not collapsed and with abundant and extensive hemorrhages, varying in size from pinhead dots to areas several square centimeters in size. Cultures in dextrose broth yielded a tiny gram negative, bipolar organism.

EXAMPLE OF A RABBIT WITH A VERY SLIGHT, BUT DEFINITE, LEUKOPENIA. OBSERVATIONS MADE 11 TO 12 A. M.

Rabbit 39	Temperature, F.	Weight, Kg.	Leukocytes
August 8	103.4	1.765	7,060
August 9	103.0	1.819	6,400
August 10 (3 p. m. inoculation 3 c c salt solution)	103.3	1.850	6,400
August 11	103.3	1.807	5,220
August 12	103.3	1.911	7,000

Killed with ether, Aug. 12. Lungs well collapsed and normal in appearance. Cultures in dextrose broth were sterile.

to expel the dissolved oxygen, so that both aerobic and anaerobic conditions could be obtained.

Each animal was under observation for at least 3 days, and often longer, before inoculation. Daily records of weight, temperature, and

[4] Univ. Calif. Pub. in Path., 1915, 2, p. 147.

total white blood count were kept, these observations being made at the same hour every day for each animal, so that the conditions might be as uniform as possible. In order to avoid any irregularity in leukocyte count which might result from differences in vasodilation, each animal's ear was flushed with water at 45 C. for about 2 minutes, after the method of Clark.[5] Two blood dilutions were then made and duplicate counts thus obtained.

Inoculations were made directly into the trachea with an ordinary Luer syringe and hypodermic needle, and were made under ether anesthesia. The amount of material used depended on the size of the animal, about 1 c c being given to a small guinea-pig, and 3, 4, and even 5 c c to rabbits.

TABLE 1

CHANGES IN LEUKOCYTE COUNT ASSOCIATED WITH INTRATRACHEAL INOCULATIONS WITH DIFFERENT MATERIALS

Inoculum	Leukopenia	Leukocytosis	Unchanged	Total
Salt solution	10	4	3	17
Washings from persons with colds	3	3	3	9
Washings from normal persons	2	1	1	4
Lung emulsion	—	1	1	2
	15	9	8	32

As a rule, these inoculations seemed to have no effect on either temperature or weight. With 4 rabbits there was a slight rise in temperature accompanying leukopenia after inoculation, 2 of these with filtrates from colds, and 2 with sterile salt solution. Changes equally great occurred often with no apparent cause, though as a rule the temperature curves were much more uniform than one would expect in rabbits.

A marked change in white blood count following inoculation was shown by 24 of the 32 animals in this series, 15 having leukopenia and 9 leukocytosis. Eight seemed unaffected. The changes were more marked in some cases than in others. Just how much change in the white count was considered a leukopenia or leukocytosis may be seen in the protocols of several of the animals as given. Generally speaking, the differences shown here were not so great as those observed by several workers in similar experiments with influenza material [2,3], but they were clear cut and definite. Sometimes this change was evident in 6 or 8 hours; more generally it did not appear until the next day. By the third day the count had usually returned to its normal level.

[5] Am. J. Hyg., 1921, 1, p. 39.

Three of the 15 animals showing leukopenia had been inoculated with the sterile filtered nasal washings from colds, 2 with similar washings from normal people, and 10 with sterile physiologic salt solution. Of the 9 showing leukocytosis, 3 were inoculated with nasal washings from colds, 1 from a normal person, 1 from the lung filtrate, and 3 with salt solution. It can be seen from table 1 that while no definite blood change was associated regularly with any one inoculum, the outstanding feature here was the common occurence of leukopenia after inoculations with salt solution.

Three of the leukopenias were accompanied by an acute conjunctivitis from which no bacteria could be isolated on blood agar. Two of these occurred in animals inoculated with salt solution, and the third in one which had received a filtrate from a cold.

Sixteen of this series of 32 inoculated animals were killed, 3 with ether and 13 by a sharp blow on the back of the neck, which dislocated the cervical vertebrae, causing death quickly and bloodlessly. In only one case was the skull injured. Some of these animals were killed as soon as a change in blood count was noted, this period varying from 18 hours to 2 days, but some of them had shown no such change. With others a delay of 3 or 4 days gave time for the total white count to return to normal.

The lungs of the etherized animals seemed well collapsed and were of a normal pinkish color. Of the 13 animals killed by a blow on the neck, 8 showed an interesting lung picture. The most outstanding features were: 1. The lungs did not usually collapse, but remained quite large in volume. Sometimes one lung would be well collapsed and the other voluminous; at other times only one lobe or part of a lobe would show this emphysema. 2. The lungs were more or less mottled by bright red areas of hemorrhage, sometimes diffuse and sometimes patchy, varying in size from that of a pinhead to several square centimeters, and sometimes entirely involving a lobe. These were not superficial, but extended into the deeper portions of the lung. The bright red color gave the impression that these hemorrhages were very fresh. As a rule, they occurred on those lobes which were emphysematous, but several times they were on those that were fairly well collapsed. Occasionally darker and more purplish hemorrhages accompanied the brighter ones. There was no consolidation nor congestion anywhere.

Sections for microscopic study showed marked emphysema and varying degrees of hemorrhage, sometimes patchy and sometimes diffuse, in the interstitial tissue and into the alveoli. In some only about 5% of the alveoli contained blood; in others 50 to 70%. Some showed more leukocytes than others, but in none was there an excess over normal limits. Desquamated cells from the alveolar walls were present in all to a varying degree. There was no evidence of any pneumonic consolidation.

TABLE 2

THE ASSOCIATION OF HEMORRHAGIC LESIONS WITH OTHER SYMPTOMS IN INOCULATED ANIMALS

Animal	Hemorrhagic Lesions	Temperature Rise	Leukopenia	Leukocytosis	Conjunctivitis	Inoculum	Method of Killing
GP 1	−	−	−	+	−	Salt solution	
GP 2	−	−	+	−	−	Salt solution	
R 1	−	+	+	−	+	Salt solution	
R 2	−	−	+	−	+	Salt solution	
R 3	−	−	−	+	−	Cold 1	Head down
R 4	−	−	−	−	−	Cold 1	
R 5	−	−	−	+	−	Lung	Head down
R 6	−	−	−	−	−	Lung	
R 7	−	−	+	−	−	Normal	
R 8	+	+	+	−	−	Normal	Head down
R 9	−	−	−	+	−	Cold 2	Head down
R 10	−	−	+	−	−	Cold 2	
R 11	−	−	+*	+*	+	Cold 2	Head down
R 15	−	−	+	−	−	Salt solution	
R 16	−	−	+	−	−	Salt solution	
R 17	−	−	−	−	−	Salt solution	
R 18	−	−	−	−	−	Normal	
R 19	−	−	−	−	−	Normal	
R 21	−	−	−	+	−	Salt solution	
R 22	+	−	+	−	−	Salt solution	Head up
R 23	+	−	−	+	−	Salt solution	Head up
R 24	+	−	−	−	−	Salt solution	Head up
R 25	+	−	+	−	−	Cold 4	Head up
R 26	+	−	−	−	−	Cold 4	Head up
R 27	−	−	−	−	−	Cold 4	Ether
R 28	−	−	−	+	−	Cold 3	
R 29	−	−	+	−	−	Salt solution	
R 30	+	−	−	+	−	Salt solution	Head up
R 31	+	−	+	−	−	Salt solution	Head up
R 32	−	−	+	−	−	Salt solution	
R 37	−	−	−	−	−	Salt solution	Ether
R 39	−	−	+	−	−	Salt solution	Ether

* This rabbit showed a leukocytosis a few hours after inoculation, but after 24 hours a decided leukopenia.

This emphysema and hemorrhage occurred sometimes in conjunction with the changes in leukocyte count and the conjunctivitis described in the foregoing, and sometimes without them. Four of the 8 animals with the lung lesions also showed leukopenia, and two leukocytosis. In one a decided rise in temperature accompanied leukopenia and hemorrhagic lesions. Three leukopenias were accompanied by conjunctivitis, but in no case were all 4 phenomena observed together (table 2).

It is interesting to note here that of 7 rabbits which were held by the ears with the head up when they were struck on the back of the neck, every one showed the emphysema and hemorrhagic lesions, while of 6 held by the feet with the head down, only one showed them.

The 8 rabbits with these lesions had been inoculated with the following material: 5 with sterile salt solution, 2 with filtrates from colds, and 1 with a filtrate from a normal person. The 5 without hemorrhage had been given: 3, filtrates from colds; 1, salt solution; and 1, a filtered emulsion of a pair of hemorrhagic lungs. The nature of the inoculum was evidently not the controlling factor in their production here (table 3).

TABLE 3

THE OCCURRENCE OF HEMORRHAGIC LESIONS IN RELATION TO THE NATURE OF THE INOCULUM

	Salt Solution	Normal Filtrate	Cold Filtrate	Lung Emulsion	Total
Lesions	5	1	2	—	8
No lesions	1	—	3	1	5

In order to determine a possible relationship between these lesions and the intratracheal inoculation in itself, 4 rabbits which had been under the usual observation for several days were killed, without previous inoculation, by a blow on the back of the neck. All showed emphysema and hemorrhagic areas as striking and extensive as any of those found in the inoculated animals. There seemed to be no relation between the inoculations and the lesions.

The idea that these lesions might have some connection with the method of killing the animals had been suggested before.[6] Four new rabbits were kept under the usual observation for a week. After 3 days 2 were given intratracheal inoculations of salt solution and 2 were allowed to remain uninoculated. On the sixth day all were anesthetized and the chest cavities opened while the animals were still alive. None of these showed hemorrhage. The lungs were well collapsed and of a uniform pinkish gray color.

Subsequently a number of other animals were killed in different ways. Most of these were healthy young rabbits and guinea-pigs just from the breeding farms, which had never been used in any previous experiment. None of those killed by ether showed either emphysema or hemorrhages, but the lungs were well collapsed and of normal color. On the contrary, of the rabbits killed by a blow on the neck,

[6] Maitland, Cowan, and Detweiler: Brit. J. Exper. Path., 1920, 1, p. 263; 1921, 2, p. 8.

87% of those that were held with the head up when struck showed extensive hemorrhage and emphysema, and 14% of those held with the head down. This greater frequency of lesions in rabbits held with the head up might possibly be due to the fact that a sharper blow is usually required to kill an animal in that position. Also 66% of the guinea-pigs, all held head downward, showed these lesions.

In all 46 animals were killed. The occurrence of the lesions in connection with the method of killing the animals is shown in table 4, the presence of hemorrhage and emphysema being considered positive and their absence negative. Although the lesions were found in 66% of guinea-pigs, held with head down, no conclusion should be drawn concerning the relative frequency of this phenomenon in guinea-pigs as compared with rabbits, since the number of these animals used was small.

TABLE 4

The Occurrence of Lung Lesions in Connection with the Mode of Death

	Head Up				Head Down				Ether			
	Total	+	—	%+	Total	+	—	%+	Total	+	—	%+
Rabbits	23	20	3	87	8	1	7	14	8	0	8	0
Guinea-pigs	—	—	—	—	6	4	2	66	1	0	1	0
Both	23	20	3	87	14	5	9	36	9	0	9	0

The microscopic appearance of these lesions in inoculated animals has already been described. Sections from the lungs of uninoculated animals showing emphysema and hemorrhage were the same, save that there was even less edema. It is questionable whether any of these were true edema in the sense of being part of an inflammatory process, or merely serum escaping from the vessels, as did the blood. Sections from the negative animals, both those killed with ether and otherwise, were atelectatic, free from hemorrhage, and appeared normal. The lungs from 24 animals were studied microscopically, 19 rabbits and 5 guinea-pigs.

No hemorrhage was observed in any of the organs other than the lungs. The circumstances under which this pathologic picture was found seemed to indicate that it was an agonal phenomenon. This conclusion has been similarly reached by Foord [7] and by Maitland, Cowan, and Detweiler [6] in their recent experiments.

[7] J. Infect. Dis., 1918, 23, p. 159.

Since it was possible that the relation between these lesions and the mode of death might have been more apparent than real, an attempt was made to observe the effects of first ether and then a blow on the same animal. This was tried with four rabbits. Each animal was anesthetized and a cannula put into the trachea so that artificial respiration could be applied. The chest cavity was opened and the lungs examined in situ. While artificial respiration was continued the animal was held up by the ears and given a sharp blow on the back of the neck. Then the lungs were removed and reexamined. The results were not conclusive. In each of the rabbits the lungs after the ether

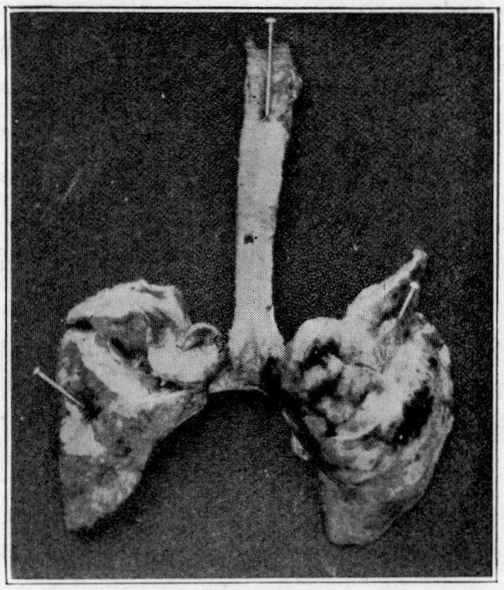

Fig. 1.—Lungs of a normal rabbit killed by a blow on the neck, showing marked hemorrhagic areas and emphysema.

only appeared normal and quite free from hemorrhage. After the blow and the removal of the lungs from the body there were a few small bright red pinhead sized hemorrhages scattered here and there. These were so few and far between that they might have been overlooked when the lungs were examined in situ. The fourth animal showed these more strikingly than any of the others, so it is possible that with a larger number of animals and the acquisition of more skill in handling them, more satisfactory results would be obtained.

Hemorrhages apparently like those described in the foregoing have been reported by a number of other workers [2,3,6,7,8] sometimes in

[8] Gibson, Bowman, and Connor: Brit. M. J., 1918, 2, p. 645; 1919, 1, p. 331. Bradford, Bashford and Wilson: Brit. M. J., 1919, 1, p. 599; 1919, 1, p. 602; Jour. Am. Med. Assn., 1919, 73, p. 67. Hall: Arch. Int. Med., 1920, 26, p. 612. Aufrecht: Deutsch. Arch. f. klin. Med., 1915, 117, p. 602. Flexner and Noguchi: J. Exper. Med., 1913, 18, p. 461.

animals killed in others ways. Foord[7] found them abundantly in rabbits killed with KCN, and to a much less extent in those killed with chloral.

Both emphysema and hemorrhages have been found to occur in anaphylaxis. There was no possible anaphylaxis here. The variety of sources from which these animals came, and their healthy appearance, made it seem unlikely that they were the victims of a peculiar epidemic.

Cultures were made from the lungs of 31 animals, 20 showing hemorrhages and emphysema, and 11 appearing normal. Two mediums were employed, a plain 1% dextrose broth in a constricted tube with a marble seal, and ascitic fluid with sterile rabbit kidney. At first the ascitic fluid medium was prepared in long straight culture tubes as prepared by Noguchi, but the difficulty of obtaining strict anaerobiosis in these with the air-filled floating bits of lung tissue resulted in the adoption of the mechanically sealed constricted tube for this also. These tubes of ascitic fluid containing large pieces of rabbit kidney were incubated for several days before use. Before being inoculated, the tubes of dextrose broth were boiled to drive out the dissolved oxygen. As thus prepared, these mediums gave opportunity for both aerobic and anaerobic growth. Sufficient blood was introduced, both in the kidney tissue and in the piece of lung to give a favorable condition for growth for any hemoglobinophilic organisms which might have been present. The piece of lung used for inoculation was chosen from one of the hemorrhagic areas, if such were present, was snipped off aseptically into the culture tube, and introduced below the marble seal.

Cultures from 12 of these animals remaining sterile after a number of days. Nineteen showed bacterial growth, usually after 48 or 72 hours' incubation. The most common organisms, found in 12 cases, were extremely tiny gram-negative rods, sometimes bipolar, with a strong preference for aerobic conditions, though they could grow anaerobically. An intensive study of these strains was not undertaken at this time. Similar organisms have been frequently described in connection with experimental work on the respiratory flora of guinea-pigs and rabbits, as well as in some other animals.[9] Cultures from 5 animals gave gram-positive diplococci, and 4 staphylococci. In 2 cases a tiny gram-

[9] Smith: J. Comp. Med. & Surg., 1887, 8, p. 24; J. Med. Res., 1913-14, 29, p. 291. McGowan: J. Path. & Bact., 1911, 15, p. 372. Davis: J. Infect. Dis., 1913, 19, p. 42. Hoskins, J.: Am. Vet. Med. Assn., 1920, 57, p. 317. Ferry and Hoskins: J. Lab. & Clin. Med., 1920, 5, p. 311. Hoskins and Stout: Ibid., 1920, 5, p. 307. DeKruif: J. Exper. Med., 1921, 33, p. 773. Saelhof: J. Infect. Dis., 1921, 28, p. 374.

positive diplococcus grew only at first under anaerobic conditions, but after several generations it finally grew aerobically.

These organisms were found as often in lungs of normal appearance as in those with hemorrhage. Usually they were in pure culture, but in two cases the tiny bacilli occurred in connection with some other organism. The occurrence of these bacteria in the hemorrhagic and nonhemorrhagic lungs is shown in table 5.

TABLE 5

THE OCCURRENCE OF BACTERIA IN HEMORRHAGIC AND NONHEMORRHAGIC LUNGS

	Hemorrhagic		Nonhemorrhagic		Total
	Guinea-Pigs	Rabbits	Guinea-Pigs	Rabbits	
Gram-negative rods..........	—	7	—	5	12
Staphylococcus..............	—	2	—	2	4
Gram-positive diplococci.....	1	2	—	2	5
Sterile......................	2	3	2	5	12

SUMMARY

Of the 70 animals included in this study, 32 received intratracheal inoculations, chiefly with salt solution and filtered saline nasal washings; 75% of these showed a marked change in the total white blood count within 6 to 48 hours after inoculation. Leukopenia occurred almost twice as often as leukocytosis. Three times the leukopenia in inoculated animals was accompanied by an acute conjunctivitis.

Sixteen of the 32 animals were killed, and the lungs of 8, or 50%, showed striking hemorrhagic areas and a marked emphysema. Four of these were animals which had shown leukopenia, 1 a leukocytosis, and 3 no blood change at all.

In all, 50 of the 70 animals of this series have been killed. The emphysema and hemorrhages were found to a marked degree in 50%. These lesions occurred with equal frequency in normal uninoculated animals and in those injected intratracheally. They were not found in any killed with ether.

These hemorrhages have not been found constantly in animals killed by a blow on the back of the neck. They have been reported in some killed in other ways. But finding them in 67% of all animals killed by a blow, and in 87% of those which were held head up when the blow was given, seemed to indicate that the mode of death had something to do with their occurrence.

There seemed to be no evidence that the association of these lung lesions with changes in the leukocyte count and conjunctivitis was anything more than accidental.

No explanation of the occurrence of these lesions is here offered. The fact that hemorrhages and other associated phenomena are produced with considerable frequency in apparently normal rabbits and guinea-pigs killed in certain ways should be borne in mind when using these animals for experimental purposes.

CORRECTION

In the paper by Bie and Schwensen, which appeared in the issue of March, 1922, on page 311, the tracing labeled Chart 5, Case 2, was inserted through error. The correct tracing for the legend does not appear with the article.

GENERAL INDEX

A

PAGE
Actinomyces - - - - - - - - - - - - - - - - 99
Agglutination, changes in hydrogen-ion concentration in - - - - 651
ALBERT, HENRY. See ERICKSON, MARY J. - - - - - - - - - 268
Ameba-like organism in kidneys of child - - - - - - - - - 636
Anaerobic bacteria - - - - - - - - - - - 1, 18, 33, 445
Anaerobes, sporulating - - - - - - - - - - - - - 445
Anaphylatoxin - - - - - - - - - - - - - - 107
Anaphylaxis - - - - - - - - - - 50, 107, 259, 333, 418
Anaphylaxis, by eye tissues - - - - - - - - - - - - - 418
Anaphylaxis, effect of roentgen ray and mustard gas on, in guinea-pigs 50
Anaphylaxis, serum, specificity of desensitized state in - - - - - 333
Antibody production after intratracheal injection of antigen - - - 347
ARMANGUÉ, MANUEL, AND GONZALES, PEDRO. Studies on the formol and Wassermann reactions - - - - - - - - - - - - - 443
AYERS, S. HENRY, AND RUPP, PHILIP. Differentiation of hemolytic streptococci from human and bovine sources by the hydrolysis of sodium hippurate - - - - - - - - - - - - - 388

B

B. aerofoetidus, metabolism of - - - - - - - - - - - 190
B. alkalescens, nitrogenous metabolism of - - - - - - - - 248
B. bifermentans, metabolism of - - - - - - - - - - - 182
B. botulinus, metabolism of - - - - - - - - - - - - 177
B. botulinus, pathogenicity of - - - - - - - - - - - 118
B. coli, nitrogenous metabolism of - - - - - - - - - - 239
B. diphtheriae, effect of peptone on toxigenic property of - - - 536
B. dysenteriae (Shiga) metabolism of - - - - - - - - - 226
B. fallax, metabolism of - - - - - - - - - - - - 163
B. histolyticus, metabolism of - - - - - - - - - - - 199
B. lactimorbi in throats of cats - - - - - - - - - - 505
B. oedematiens, metabolism of - - - - - - - - - - - 185
B. paratyphosus, metabolism of - - - - - - - - - - - 233
B. paratyphosus B., epizootic of guinea-pigs due to - - - - - 516
B. paratyphosus B, metabolism of - - - - - - - - - - 236
B. proteus, nitrogenous metabolism of - - - - - - - - - 251
B. pseudotetani, metabolism of - - - - - - - - - - - 175
B. putrificus, metabolism of - - - - - - - - - - - - 204
B. sporogenes, metabolism of - - - - - - - - - - - 193
B. tertius, metabolism of - - - - - - - - - - - - 167
B. tetani (genus Nicolaierillus) - - - - - - - - - - 13, 33
B. tetani, metabolism of - - - - - - - - - - - - 170
B. tuberculosis, ammonia production by - - - - - - - - 357
B. tuberculosis, cultivation of - - - - - - - - - - - 58
B. typhosus, metabolism of - - - - - - - - - - - - 229
B. typhosus, production of CO_2 by - - - - - - - - - 320
B. welchii, metabolism of - - - - - - - - - - - - 141
Bacteria, metabolism of 141, 155, 163, 167, 170, 175, 177, 182, 185, 190, 193, 199, 204, 211, 225, 226, 229, 233, 236, 239, 245, 248, 251

PAGE
Bacteria, nitrogenous metabolism of - - - - - - - - - - - 211
Bacterial cells, conductivity of - - - - - - - - - - - - - 550
Bacteriophage phenomena with staphylococcus aureus - - - - - 643
BEACH, B. A., AND HASTINGS, E. G. Johne's disease and its detection - - 68
BELL, HOWARD H. Infection of the meninges and lungs by a species of actinomyces - - - - - - - - - - - - - - - - - 99
BIE, V., AND SCHWENSEN, CARL. The effect of digitalis in two cases of arrhythmia in diphtheria - - - - - - - - - - - - 308
BLACK, LOUISA T. See CORPER, H. J. - - - - - - - - - - 50
BLANCHARD, MARGUERITE E. See BOSWORTH, ALFRED W. - - - - - 357
Blood, changes in reaction of, in infections - - - - - - - - 664
Blood, reaction of, in anaphylactic shock - - - - - - - - - 259
BLY, ROBERT S. See KENDALL, ARTHUR ISAAC - - - - - - - - 239
BOSWORTH, ALFRED W.; ELKINS, MARION G., AND BLANCHARD, MARGUERITE E. A study of ammonia production by a certain strain of avirulent human tubercle bacillus - - - - - - - - - - - - - - - - 357
BRANHAM, SARA ELIZABETH. The production of lung hemorrhages and associated phenomena in rabbits and guinea-pigs - - - - - 670
BURKY, EARL. See FISK, ETTA - - - - - - - - - - - - - 128

C

CALLENDER, G. R., AND COUPAL, J. F. An unusual case of nocardiosis - 601
CALLOW, BESSIE R. Bacteriophage phenomena with staphylococcus aureus 643
CHETHAM, HAROLD C. See KENDALL, ARTHUR ISAAC - - - - - 251
Clostridium botulinum - - - - - - - - - - - - - - - 118
COHEN, CECILE. See HODGE, W. RAY - - - - - - - - - - 400
Complement fixation - - - - - - - - - - - - - - - 313
CORPER, H. J.; BLACK, LOUISA T., AND MOORE, MARY. The effect of the Roentgen ray and mustard gas (dichlorethylsulphid) on active anaphylaxis in the guinea-pig - - - - - - - - - - - - 50
COUPAL, J. F. See CALLENDER, G. R. - - - - - - - - - - 601
Cresol and phenol in biologic products - - - - - - - - - 379

D

D'AUNOY, RIGNEY. Antibody production after intratracheal injection of antigen - - - - - - - - - - - - - - - - - - 347
DAY, ALEXANDER ALFRED. See KENDALL, ARTHUR ISAAC - - - - 141, 248
DEWITT, LYDIA M. The inhibitory action of certain organic mercury compounds on the growth of human tubercle bacilli. Studies on the biochemistry and chemotherapy of tuberculosis. XXII - - - - - 363
Dichlorethylsulphid (mustard gas), effect of, on anaphylaxis in guinea-pigs 50
Digitalis, effect of, in arrhythmia in diphtheria - - - - - - 308
Diphtheria, heart rhythm in - - - - - - - - - - - - 279, 308
Dysentery, entamoeba histolytica in testis and epididymis in chronic - 559

E

ECKER, ENRIQUE E. See KARSNER, HOWARD T. - - - - - - - - 333
ELKINS, MARION G. See BOSWORTH, ALFRED W. - - - - - - - 357
Entamoeba histolytica in testis and epididymis in chronic dysentery - 559
ERICKSON, MARY J., AND ALBERT, HENRY. Cultivation of the gonococcus 268
EVANS, ALICE C. A buffered physiologic salt solution - - - - - 95

F

PAGE
FISK, ETTA, AND BURKY, EARL L. Study on the classification of streptococci 128
Formal reaction - - - - - - - - - - - - - - - 443

G

Gastric juice, bacteria in - - - - - - - - - - - - - 613
GERMAN, W. M. Anaphylatoxin and anaphylaxis. XII. Studies on the chemistry of the blood - - - - - - - - - - - - - 107
Gonococcus, cultivation of - - - - - - - - - - - - - 268
Gonorrheal discharges, determination of infectivity of, by precipitin reaction 623
GONZALES, PEDRO. See ARMANGUÉ, MANUEL - - - - - - - - - 443
GOODMAN, E. LOUIS, AND MOORE, MARY. Cultivation of tubercle bacilli - 58
GORDON, JOHN E. See SHARP, WILLIAM B. - - - - - - - - 372
GREEN, R. G., AND LARSON, W. P. Conductivity of bacterial cells - - 550
GRUND, M. Susceptibility of rabbits to the virus of measles. Inoculations with nasopharyngeal material - - - - - - - - - - 86

H

HALL, IVAN C. Differentiation and identification of the sporulating anaerobes - - - - - - - - - - - - - - - 445
HAMILTON, CLIFF S. See KENDALL, ARTHUR ISAAC - - - - - - 251
HANER, REBA CORDELIA. See KENDALL, ARTHUR ISAAC - - - 225, 245
HASTINGS, E. G. See BEACH, B. A. - - - - - - - - - - 68
HAYASHI, N., AND KIBATA, T. Spirochetal organisms in the tissues in acute yellow atrophy of the liver - - - - - - - - - - 64
Heart rhythm in diphtheria - - - - - - - - - - - - 279
HEINEMAN, P. G., AND HIXSON, CHARLES R. Observations on the preparation of toxin-antitoxin mixture - - - - - - - - - - 508
HELLER, HILDA HEMPL. Mutations in the genus Nicolaierillus (B. Tetani) Studies on pathogenic anaerobes, VIII - - - - - - - - 33
HELLER, HILDA HEMPL. Notes on the genus Nicolaierillus (B. Tetani). Studies on pathogenic anaerobes, VII - - - - - - - - - 18
HELLER, HILDA HEMPL. The study of colony formation in deep agar. Studies on pathogenic anaerobes, VI - - - - - - - - - 1
HERROLD, RUSSELL D. A study of streptococci from post-gonorrheal prostatitis by a quantitative method of agglutination and absorption - 80
HIRSCH, EDWIN F., AND WILLIAMS, J. LISLE. Hydrogen-ion studies. I. changes in the reaction of the blood during anaphylactic shock - 259
HIRSCH, EDWIN F., AND PETERS, EBBA C. Hydrogen-ion studies. II. Changes in the reaction of serum with the thermal destruction of complement - - - - - - - - - - - - - - - 263
HIRSCH, EDWIN F. Hydrogen-ion studies. III. Hydrogen-ion changes in the agglutination of bacteria by immune serum - - - - - 651
HIRSCH, EDWIN F. Hydrogen-ion studies. IV. Changes in reaction accompanying the precipitation of colloidal gold by spinal fluid (Lange test) 658
HIRSCH, EDWIN F., AND WILLIAMS, J. LISLE. Hydrogen-ion studies. V. Changes in the reaction of the blood in experimental infections - 664
HIRSCH, EDWIN F. Hydrogen-ion studies. VI. Hydrogen-ion changes on precipitation of human serum by immune serum - - - - - 666
HIXSON, CHARLES R. See HEINEMAN, P. G. - - - - - - - 508
HODGE, W. RAY, AND COHEN, CECILE. Streptococci in chronic respiratory infections - - - - - - - - - - - - - - - 400

PAGE

HOWELL, KATHARINE M. A study of two distinct strains of streptococcus isolated from the same heart-valve lesion - - - - - - - 299
HOWELL, KATHARINE M., AND SCHULTZ, OSCAR T. An epizootic among guinea-pigs due to a paratyphoid B bacillus - - - - - - 516
HUDSON, N. PAUL. Inoculation of white mice with Pfeiffer's bacillus. Influenza studies. IX - - - - - - - - - - - - - 433
Hydrogen-ion changes in agglutination - - - - - - - - - 651
Hydrogen-ion changes in anaphylactic shock - - - - - - - 259
Hydrogen-ion changes in Lange test - - - - - - - - - - 658
Hydrogen-ion changes in specific precipitation - - - - - - - 666
Hydrogen-ion changes in infections - - - - - - - - - - 664
Hydrogen-ion changes of serum on destruction of complement - - 263

I

Influenza - - - - -- - - - - - - - 372, 433

J

JACKSON, LEILA. An ameba-like organism in the kidneys of a child - 636
Johne's disease - - - - - - - - - - - - - - - 68

K

KAHN, R. L., AND WHITE, ETHEL D. Studies on complement fixation. V. The hemolytic versus fixability powers of complement - - - - 313
KARSNER, HOWARD T., AND ECKER, ENRIQUE E. The specificity of the desensitized state in serum anaphylaxis - - - - - - - - 333
KELLEY, MARGARET F. The precipitin reaction in the determination of the infectivity of gonorrheal discharges - - - - - - - - 623
KENDALL, ARTHUR ISAAC; DAY, ALEXANDER ALFRED, AND WALKER, ARTHUR WILLIAM. Studies in bacterial metabolism, XLIV-LVI - - - - 141
B. welchii - - - - -- - - - - - - - 141
Vibrion septique - - - - - - - - - - - - 155
B. fallax - - - - - - - - - - - - - - 163
B. tertius - - - - - - - - - - - - - - 167
B. tetani - - - - - - - - - - - - - - 170
B. pseudotetani - - - - - - - - - - - - - 175
B. botulinus - - - - - - - - - - - - - 177
B. bifermentans - - - - - - - - - - - - 182
B. oedematiens - - - - - - - - - - - - - 185
B. aerofoetidus - - - - - - - - - - - - - 190
B. sporogenes - - - - - - - - - - - - - 193
B. histolyticus - - - - - - - - - - - - - 199
B. putrificus - - - - - - - - - - - - - 204
KENDALL, ARTHUR ISAAC. The significance and quantitative measurement of the nitrogenous metabolism of bacteria. Studies in bacterial metabolism, LVII - - - - - - - - - - - - - 211
KENDALL, ARTHUR ISAAC, AND HANER, REBA CORDELIA. Studies in bacterial metabolism, LVIII-LXI - - - - - - - - - - - 225
B. dysenteriae (Shiga) - - - - - - - - - - 226
B. typhosus - - - - - - - - - - - - - 229
B. paratyphosus alpha - - - - - - - - - - 233
B. paratyphosus beta - - - - - - - - - - 236

PAGE

KENDALL, ARTHUR ISAAC, AND BLY, ROBERT S. The nitrogenous metabolism of Bacillus coli. Studies in bacterial metabolism, LXII - - - - 239
KENDALL, ARTHUR ISAAC; HANER, REBA CORDELIA, AND BLY, ROBERT S. The nitrogenous metabolism of the Schmitz bacillus. Studies in bacterial metabolism, LXIII - - - - - - - - - - - - - 245
KENDALL, ARTHUR ISAAC, AND DAY, ALEXANDER ALFRED. The nitrogenous metabolism of Bacillus alkalescens. Studies in bacterial metabolism, LXIV - - - - - - - - - - - - - - - - 248
KENDALL, ARTHUR ISAAC; CHEETHAM, HAROLD C., AND HAMILTON, CLIFF S. The nitrogenous metabolism of Bacillus proteus. Studies in bacterial metabolism, LXV - - - - - - - - - - - - - - 251
KIBATA, T. See HAYASHI, T. - - - - - - - - - - - - - 64
Kidney, amebae in - - - - - - - - - - - - - - - 636
Kidneys, excretion of spirochaeta pallida through - - - - - - 569
KODOMA, RYUZO. Anaphylaxis produced by eye tissues. Primary toxicity of eye tissues—organ specificity and group reactions of eye tissues—anaphylactic theory of sympathetic ophthalmia - - - - - - 418
KOPELHOFF, NICHOLAS. Bacteriologic studies of gastric fractions obtained by the Rehfuss method - - - - - - - - - - - - 613

L

Lange test, changes in reaction in precipitation of colloidal gold by spinal fluid - - - - - - - - - - - - - - - - - 658
LARSON, W. P. See GREEN, R. G. - - - - - - - - - - - 550
Leukocytes, action of neo-arsphenamin and neo-salvarsan, on phagocytic activity of - - - - - - - - - - - - - - - - 545
Leukocytes, effect of pneumococcus on - - - - - - - - - 323
Liver, acute yellow atrophy of, spirochetal organism in - - - - - 64
Lung hemorrhages in rabbits and guinea-pigs - - - - - - - 670
Lungs, infection of, by actinomyces - - - - - - - - - - 99

M

MASUCCI, PETER. Phenol and cresol as preservatives in biologic products - 379
Measles, susceptibility of rabbits to virus of - - - - - - - - 86
Meninges, infection of, by actinomyces - - - - - - - - - 99
Meningo-encephalitis, spontaneous chronic, of rabbits - - - - - 91
Metabolism, bacterial 141, 155, 163, 167, 170, 175, 177, 182, 185, 190, 193, 199, 204, 211, 225, 226, 229, 233, 236, 239, 245, 248, 251
MOORE, MARY. See CORPER, H. J. - - - - - - - - - - - 50
MOORE, MARY. See GOODMAN, E. LOUIS - - - - - - - - - 58
Mustard gas, effect of, on anaphylaxis in guinea-pigs - - - - - 50

N

Neo-arsphenamin, action of, on phagocytic activity of leukocytes - - 545
Neo-salvarsan, action of, on phagocytic activity of leukocytes - - - 545
NICHOLS, HENRY J., AND WOOD, CYRUS B. The production of CO_2 by the typhoid bacillus and the mechanism of the Russell double sugar tube. II. Fermentation or respiration. Phenol red as an indicator - - 320
Nicolaierillus (B. Tetani) - - - - - - - - - - - - - 18
Nicolaierillus, genus (B. Tetani), mutations in - - - - - - - 33
Nocardiosis - - - - - - - - - - - - - - - - - - 601
NORTON, JOHN F. See SHARP, WILLIAM B. - - - - - - - - 372

O

PAGE
OLIVER, JEAN. Spontaneous chronic meningo-encephalitis of rabbits - 91
ORR, PAUL F. The pathogenicity of Bacillus botulinus - - - - - 118

P

PERKINS, ROGER G., AND SHEN, JAMES K. Presence of B. lactimorbi in the throats of cats - - - - - - - - - - - - 505
PETERS, EBBA C. See HIRSCH, EDWIN F. - - - - - - - - 263
Pfeiffer's bacillus, inoculation of white mice with - - - - - - 433
Phenol and cresol in biologic products - - - - - - - - 379
Pneumococcus type I, effects of, on leukocytes and hemopoietic organs - 323
Precipitation, specific, hydrogen-ion changes in - - - - - - 658
Precipitin reaction and infectivity of gonorrheal discharges - - - 623
Prostatitis, post-gonorrheal, streptococci in - - - - - - - 80

R

Rabbits, spontaneous meningo-encephalitis - - - - - - - - 91
Rehfuss method, bacteriologic studies of gastric fractions obtained by - 613
Roentgen ray, effect of, on anaphylaxis in guinea-pigs - - - - - 50
RUPP, PHILIP. See AYERS, S. HENRY - - - - - - - - - 388
Russell double sugar tube - - - - - - - - - - - - 320

S

Salt solution, buffered - - - - - - - - - - - - - 95
Schmitz bacillus, nitrogenous metabolism of - - - - - - - 245
SCHULTZ, OSCAR T. See HOWELL, KATHARINE M. - - - - - - 516
SCHWENSEN, CARL. The heart rhythm in diphtheria - - - - - - 279
SCHWENSEN, CARL. See BIE, V. - - - - - - - - - - - 308
Serum, reaction of, on thermal destruction of complement - - - 263
SHARP, WILLIAM B.; NORTON, JOHN F., AND GORDON, JOHN E. A sore throat epidemic of unusual type. Influenza studies. VIII - - - 372
SHEN, JAMES K. See PERKINS, ROGER G. - - - - - - - - - 505
Silver-agar method for staining spirochetes - - - - - - - 592
Sore throat - - - - - - - - - - - - - - - 372
Spirochetes, staining of, by silver-agar method - - - - - - 592
Spirochaeta pallida, excretion of, through kidneys - - - - - - 569
Spirochetal organism in acute yellow atrophy of liver - - - - - 64
Staphylococcus aureus, bacteriophage phenomena with - - - - - 643
STARRY, A. C. See WARTHIN, A. S. - - - - - - - - - - 592
Streptococci, classification of - - - - - - - - - 128, 358
Streptococci in post-gonorrheal prostatitis - - - - - - - - 80
Streptococci in respiratory infections - - - - - - - - - 400
Streptococcus, differentiation of hemolytic, by hydrolysis of sodium hippurate - - - - - - - - - - - - - - - 388
Streptococcus, hemolytic, failure of hemolytic action in strain of - - 610
Streptococcus, two strains of, from heart valve - - - - - - 299

T

TONGS, M. S. Effects of pneumococcus type I on leukocytes and hemopoietic organs - - - - - - - - - - - - - - 323
Toxin-antitoxin - - - - - - - - - - - - - - 508

PAGE
Treponema pallidum, excretion through kidney - - - - - - - - 569
Tuberculosis, biochemistry and chemotherapy of - - - - - - 363
TUNNICLIFF, RUTH. The action of neo-arsphenamin and neo-salvarsan on the phagocytic activity of leukocytes - - - - - - - - 545

V

VALENTINE, EUGENIA. A peculiar failure of hemolytic action in a strain of hemolytic streptococcus - - - - - - - - - - 610
Vibrion septique, metabolism of - - - - - - - - - - 155

W

WALKER, ARTHUR WILLIAM. See KENDALL, ARTHUR ISAAC - - - 141
WARTHIN, ALDRED SCOTT. The occurrence of entamoeba histolytica with tissue lesions in the testis and epididymis in chronic dysentery - 559
WARTHIN, ALDRED SCOTT. The excretion of spirochaeta pallida through the kidneys - - - - - - - - - - - - - 569
WARTHIN, A. S., AND STARRY, A. C. The staining of spirochetes in cover-glass smears by the silver-agar method - - - - - - - 592
Wassermann reaction - - - - - - - - - - - - - 443
WHITE, ETHEL D. See KAHN, R. L. - - - - - - - - - - 313
WILCOX, HARRIET LESLIE. The effect of peptone on the toxigenic property of B. diphtheriae No. 8 - - - - - - - - - - - - 536
WILLIAMS, J. LISLE. See HIRSCH, EDWIN F. - - - - - - - 259
WOOD, CYRUS B. See NICHOLS, HENRY J. - - - - - - - - 320